Gynecological and Breast Cytopathology Board Review and Self-Assessment

Walid E. Khalbuss • Marilee Means
Editors

Gynecological and Breast Cytopathology Board Review and Self-Assessment

Springer

Editors
Walid E. Khalbuss, MD, PhD, FIAC
Director of Cytology and Cytopathology
Fellowship Program
University of Pittsburgh Medical Center
Shadyside Hospital
Pittsburgh, Pennsylvania, USA

Marilee Means, PhD, SCT(ASCP)
School of Health Professions
University of Kansas Medical Center
Kansas City, Kansas, USA

ISBN 978-1-4614-7269-8 ISBN 978-1-4614-7270-4 (eBook)
DOI 10.1007/978-1-4614-7270-4
Springer New York Heidelberg Dordrecht London

Library of Congress Control Number: 2013941370

Printed on acid-free paper

Springer is part of Springer Science+Business Media (www.springer.com)

I dedicate this book to my beloved family, my teachers, mentors, and trainees.

Walid E. Khalbuss

I dedicate this book to my parents, my children, and my supportive husband as well as the many great pathologists who have shared both their knowledge and their friendship with me.

Marilee Means

Preface

This book provides a comprehensive in-depth systems-based review of gynecological cytology including cytomorphology, pitfalls, and ancillary testing presented in a high-yield review followed by board-type questions and discussions. It is an excellent review and self-assessment for pathologists, cytopathologists, and cytologists, as well as cytology trainees (e.g., pathology residents, cytopathology fellows, and cytotechnology students). The book includes ten chapters covering technique, cytomorphology, ancillary testing, management, legal, and QA topics. Each chapter contains introductory high-yield review on the subject with tables and key points emphasizing useful criteria and concepts needed to make diagnoses in common and uncommon cases and to avoid diagnostic pitfalls.

- The book contains 64 summary tables, a wealth of full high-quality color photomicrographs of over 784 images, and review questions of 736 text-based and image-based multiple-choice questions (MCQs) that focus on practical diagnostic knowledge that will be useful to cytology trainees seeking basic information and also those with more experience who would like to fine-tune their skills.
- The book also features chapters dedicated to breast FNA, Pap test clinical management, laboratory management, and quality assurance as related to gynecological cytology.

Pittsburgh, PA, USA — Walid E. Khalbuss
Kansas City, KS, USA — Marilee Means

Acknowledgement

We are indebted to Dr. Laura Z. Tabatabai for her meticulous review of this entire book and for sharing her pearls of wisdom with us.

Contents

Contributors

Walid E. Khalbuss, MD, PhD, FIAC Director of Cytology and Cytopathology Fellowship Program, University of Pittsburgh Medical Center Shadyside Hospital, Pittsburgh, PA, USA

Marilee Means, PhD, SCT(ASCP) School of Health Professions, University of Kansas Medical Center, Kansas City, KS, USA

Reda S. Saad, MD, PhD, FRCPC Department of Pathology, Hotel Dieu Grace Hospital, Windsor, ON, Canada

Huaitoa Yang, MD, PhD Department of Pathology, University of Pittsburgh Medical Center, Pittsburgh, PA, USA

Jing Yu, MD, PhD Department of Pathology, University of Pittsburgh Medical Center, Pittsburgh, PA, USA

Chengquan Zhao, MD Department of Pathology, Magee-Womens Hospital, University of Pittsburgh Medical Center, Pittsburgh, PA, USA

Noreen Akhtar, FCPS, MBBS Department of Pathology, Shaukat Khanum Memorial Cancer Hospital and Research Center, Lahore, Punjab, Pakistan

Asif Loya, MD, MBBS Department of Pathology, Shaukat Khanum Memorial Cancer Hospital and Research Centre, Lahore, Punjab, Pakistan

Pamela Michelow, MBBCh, MSc Cytology Unit, Department of Anatomical Pathology, National Health Laboratory Service, University of Witwatersrand, Johannesburg, Gauteng South Africa

The Pap Test: Technique and Reporting 1

Marilee Means and Walid E. Khalbuss

Contents

M. Means, PhD, SCT(ASCP) (✉)
School of Health Professions,
University of Kansas Medical Center,
3901 Rainbow Blvd., Mail Stop 4048,
Kansas City, KS 66160, USA
e-mail: mmeans@kumc.edu

W.E. Khalbuss, MD, PhD, FIAC
Director of Cytology and Cytopathology Fellowship Program,
University of Pittsburgh Medical Center Shadyside Hospital,
5150 Centre Avenue, 2, Suite 201,
Pittsburgh, PA 15232, USA
e-mail: khalbussw2@upmc.edu

1.1 Tables and Summary

Table 1.1 Bethesda 2001 reporting terminology

Reporting terminology	Description
NILM	Negative for intraepithelial lesion or malignancy
ASC-US, ASC-H	Atypical squamous cells of uncertain significance, atypical squamous cells, cannot r/o HSIL
LSIL	Low-grade squamous intraepithelial lesion. Includes slight dysplasia, CIN I, and HPV
HSIL	High-grade squamous intraepithelial lesion. Includes moderate and severe dysplasia, CIS, CIN II, and CIN III. HSIL, cannot r/o invasion
SCCA	Squamous cell carcinoma
Glandular cell abnormalities	This category includes atypical glandular cells (endocervical, endometrial, or not specified); atypical endocervical cells, favor neoplastic; glandular cells, favor neoplastic; endocervical adenocarcinoma in situ; adenocarcinomas of endocervical, endometrial, or extrauterine origin; or adenocarcinomas which are not otherwise specified
Adequacy	All reports must be classified as satisfactory or unsatisfactory If unsatisfactory, a diagnosis cannot be reported. If, however, abnormal cells are identified, a specimen cannot be called unsatisfactory Comments may be made regarding the presence or absence of endocervical component (at least 10 squamous metaplastic and/or endocervical cells) in those patients in which one would expect to find them. If the endocervical component is inadequate, then the report should include this information as a quality indicator, but the slide should be categorized as satisfactory Conventional slides should have at least 8,000–12,000 well-visualized cells, and liquid-based preparations should have at least 5,000 such cells. Less cellularity than this should be classified as unsatisfactory
Other	The specimen type (conventional vs. liquid based), general categorization (optional), organisms, reactive findings, normal-appearing endometrial cells in women over 40, ancillary testing details, indication of automated review, and educational notes and suggestions (optional) are all components of the newest Bethesda System for Reporting Cervical Cytology

W.E. Khalbuss, M. Means (eds.), *Gynecological and Breast Cytopathology Board Review and Self-Assessment*, DOI 10.1007/978-1-4614-7270-4_1, © Springer Science+Business Media New York 2013

Table 1.2a Colposcopic findings and concomitant cytopathology results: part 1

Cytology Dx	Colposcopic findings
Normal	Smooth, pink, glistening cervical surface with a deeper pink near the external os, indicating the squamocolumnar junction. Iodine staining in a normal cervix shows dark purple-black or brown coloration as the normal glycogenated cells react with the iodine
Infection – *Trichomonas*	Inflamed cervix with multiple small hemorrhagic ulcers, greenish discharge, "strawberry cervix"
Infection – *Candida*	Inflamed cervix with thick, white to yellowish discharge on cervix and in vagina
Hyperkeratosis or parakeratosis	Raised, bright white areas of the cervix PRIOR to the application of acetic acid solution. These areas usually reflect a benign protective reaction but may need to be biopsied if neoplasia is suspected
Atrophy	Thin, delicate, easily damaged epithelium. Lack of or partial iodine uptake; fine, branching capillaries
LSIL – dysplasia	Mostly flat lesions with a smooth surface, usually occurring within the squamocolumnar junction. May appear white PRIOR to the application of acetic acid, reflecting a lesion which is beneath a layer of HK or PK. After the application of acetic acid, the degree of whitening may be faint, brief, or slow to develop. Lesions are typically smooth with indistinct borders. May have fine mosaicism or punctuation or may be without endothelial features. Vascular changes are more regular and less abnormal than higher-grade lesions. Less reliable appearance on colposcopy than higher-grade lesions. Lugol's iodine solution results are often speckled without the complete absence of uptake more commonly seen in HSIL lesions. Requires considerable training to differentiate benign from LSIL lesions
LSIL – HPV	Bright white acetowhitening AFTER application of acetic acid solution is typical. Central loops of vascularity are seen within the projections of condyloma. Other abnormal vascularities are seldom seen in HPV lesions and more often seen in HSIL

Note: This information contains a broad overview of some of the most obvious and frequently seen findings in colposcopy. However, expertise in this area can only be obtained by thorough training and extensive study. This summary is not meant to replace the hours of practice under the supervision of a trained colposcopist needed to develop competency in this area.

Table 1.2b Colposcopic findings and concomitant cytopathology results: part 2

Cytology Dx	Colposcopic findings
HSIL	Usually found within the transformation zone and may extend into the endocervical canal. May coexist with LSIL lesions. Abnormal vascular patterns, erosions, and abnormalities of the surface configuration of the cervix are seen. Examination should begin with a green filter to assist in the evaluation of these features. The margins of the lesion, its size, and vascular patterns should be observed AFTER the application of acetic acid solution. Sharp borders, raised edges, peeling areas of epithelium, with more distinct acetowhitening and a dull surface (due to the increase in numbers of nuclei), and a gray or gray-white color are seen. The vascularity is coarse with frequent, pronounced abnormalities in the variability of the width of the capillaries, mosaic patterns, distance between capillaries, and punctuation. Iodine solutions are usually completely negative (appearing bright yellow or pink)
Invasive SCCA	Unevenly dense, thick layers which may contain ulceration, multiquadrant evidence of HSIL disease, highly atypical vessels with punctuation, coarse mosaicism, and irregular, abnormal forms (hairpin, comma shapes). The lesion may extend into the canal and may have a very irregular surface. Leukoplakia may be observed PRIOR to the application of acetic acid, or prominent prompt acetowhitening after the acetic acid is applied may occur

Note: This information contains a broad overview of some of the most obvious and frequently seen findings in colposcopy. However, expertise in this area can only be obtained by thorough training and extensive study. This summary is not meant to replace the hours of practice under the supervision of a trained colposcopist needed to develop competency in this area.

Table 1.3 The technique for collection of gynecologic cytology samples

Patient instructions	
	Avoid scheduling the exam during the menstrual cycle as blood may interfere with the exam
	Avoid intercourse the day prior to the exam
	Avoid the use of douches, vaginal medication, or vaginal contraceptives for 2 days prior to the exam
Collection	
	Avoid the use of lubricant other than warm water
	Remove excessive mucus or other discharge gently with a gauze prior to taking the sample
	Ideally the sample should include cells from both the endocervix and the ectocervix to assure that the squamocolumnar area is sampled
	Collect the specimen prior to the application of iodine or acetic acid solution
Conventional smears	
	Rotate the spatula in a full circle with the tip of the spatula at the external os and the curved edge of the spatula in contact with the cervix
	Obtain a sample from the endocervix using an endocervical brush. Some of the outermost bristles should be visible to avoid collecting material from the lower uterine segment. Rotate gently only ¼ turn
	Both samples should be applied to the slide smoothly and gently with the immediate application of a fixative solution. The brush should be rolled to dislodge material collected on all sides of the brush
	A broom device may be used in place of the dual spatula and brush technique. The broom is used by having the central longer plastic tips inserted into the endocervical canal while the shorter, outer tips collect material from the ectocervix. It is rotated three to five times and gently applied to the slide with immediate fixation
Liquid-based cytology	
	In the USA, most cervical cytology is done using a liquid-based collection technique. The specimens are collected as outlined above for the conventional smears
	The SurePath™ method utilizes the plastic broom device, the tip of which is detached and immediately immersed into the sample vial. The entire vial is then labeled and sent to the laboratory with the collection device inside
	The ThinPrep™ method may use either the broom device or the combination of the spatula and cytobrush to collect the sample. The sample is then dislodged from the collection devices by swirling or rinsing into the vial. The vial is then labeled and sent to the laboratory
	Both of these methods have shown increased detection of premalignant lesions when compared to conventional smear techniques
	An advantage to liquid-based methods is the ability to utilize the remaining sample left in the vial for ancillary testing, such as HPV testing, or testing for infectious organisms. Additionally, the more uniform preparations are useful for automated screening devices, as well as somewhat less tiring for cytotechnologists and pathologists to examine

1.2 Text-Based Questions 1–40

Q-1. Since the most likely site for the development of cervical neoplasia is the squamocolumnar junction, the clinician should always attempt to obtain this material which is adequately identified on the Pap sample by the presence of:
(a) Endocervical cells
(b) Squamous metaplastic cells
(c) Neoplastic cells
(d) Superficial squamous cells
(e) At least 10 endocervical and/or metaplastic cells

Q-2. The latest recommendations (2006) from the American Cancer Society for the screening of women using the Pap smear technique suggest that screening begin:
(a) With the onset of menses
(b) Prior to the onset of sexual activity
(c) After the detection of high-risk HPV in women less than 20
(d) No later than age 21 or 3 years after onset of sexual activity

Q-3. The most appropriate stain for routine cervical cancer screening is:
(a) Diff-Quik
(b) H and E
(c) Papanicolaou
(d) p53

Q-4. Excessive amounts of epithelium from the lower uterine segment may be best avoided by:
(a) Making sure to insert the endocervical brush until the lower bristles disappear from view
(b) Using a speculum lubricated with water-soluble lubricant
(c) Rotating the cervical broom device 4 complete rotations
(d) Maintaining visibility of the lower one-third of the endocervical brush device

Q-5. Lubricant may:
(a) Appear in conventional smears as white bubbly background material
(b) Interfere with the proper filtration of ThinPrep preparations
(c) Resemble abnormal cells
(d) Simulate HPV infections

Q-6. After obtaining a cervical sample for preparation by the ThinPrep method, it is most important to:
(a) Smear the material promptly on the slide and immerse in alcohol.
(b) Break off the tip of the collection device and drop it into the vial.
(c) Thoroughly dislodge the material by stirring and compressing the brush against side of the vial.
(d) Allow the smeared material to air dry and then spray with fixative.

Q-7. The SurePath preparation system relies on a _________.
(a) Filtration method
(b) Gravity sedimentation method
(c) Endocervical brush smear
(d) Endocervical broom smear

Q-8. The finding that premalignant and malignant lesions of the cervix occur at increasingly higher ages as the severity of the lesion increases is a part of the epidemiologic evidence that:
(a) Squamous cell carcinoma develops de novo.
(b) Infections from *Trichomonas*, *Candida*, and herpes lead to squamous cell carcinoma.
(c) Sexual activity is a direct cause of cervical cancer.
(d) Premalignant lesions precede and lead to the development of squamous cell carcinoma.

Q-9. In all countries where routine cervical screening has been implemented, it has been found to lead to:
(a) A decrease in the incidence of squamous cell carcinoma of the cervix
(b) A decrease in the incidence of infectious diseases such as *Trichomonas* and herpes
(c) An increase in the diagnosis of reactive and reparative lesions
(d) A decrease in metastatic disease of the cervix

Q-10. All patients who have a diagnosis of ASC-H should first be followed up by immediate:
(a) High-risk HPV testing
(b) Colposcopically directed biopsy
(c) Hysterectomy
(d) Return to the pool of yearly screening

Q-11. After a patient with a Pap diagnosis of ASC-US has received a positive high-risk HPV result, the next immediate follow-up step per 2006 ASCCP guideline is:
(a) Colposcopically directed biopsy
(b) Repeat high-risk HPV test
(c) Endometrial biopsy
(d) FNA of the cervix

Q-12. In patients younger than 20 with previous normal Paps, a diagnosis of ASC-US should immediately be followed by:

(a) A high-risk HPV test
(b) A high-risk and low-risk HPV test
(c) Return to yearly screening
(d) Colposcopically directed biopsy

Q-13. For adolescents (20 and younger), a diagnosis of HGSIL should immediately lead to:
(a) Immediate LEEP
(b) Testing for high-risk HPV
(c) Colposcopy
(d) Return to yearly screening

Q-14. For a patient with a Pap diagnosis of ASC-H, if CIN II–III is not detected on biopsy, the patient may be followed up with:
(a) High-risk HPV testing at 12 months
(b) Return to yearly screening
(c) LEEP
(d) Repeat colposcopy in 6 weeks

Q-15. The Bethesda System (2001) added the following new terminology or categories for inclusion on the report:
(a) Specimen type (conventional or liquid based), ASC-H, and NILM
(b) ASC-US, favor reactive; ASC-US, favor LGSIL; and satisfactory-quality indicators
(c) Moderate dysplasia, carcinoma in situ, CIN II
(d) Ancillary testing, automated review, within normal limits

Q-16. The best location to give appropriate guidance for clinical follow-up in TBS 2001 reporting is:
(a) Other
(b) General categorization
(c) Ancillary testing
(d) Automated review
(e) Educational Notes and Suggestions

Q-17. Numeric criteria proposed for the evaluation of cellularity adequacy in TBS 2001 include which of the following in a liquid-based preparation?
(a) 10 or more endocervical or metaplastic cells
(b) 10 % coverage of the slide
(c) 5,000 cells minimum
(d) 8,000–12,000 cells minimum

Q-18. If a high-grade lesion or cancer is identified on a gynecologic sample, the comment which may be omitted is:
(a) "Endocervical/transformation zone component is not identified."
(b) "HGSIL."
(c) "Squamous cell carcinoma."
(d) "HGSIL with features suspicious for invasion."

Q-19. The best way to determine the adequacy of cellularity in a conventional slide is to:
(a) Compare the 4× field appearance with reference images.
(b) Count the cells.
(c) Count the cells in 100 10× fields.
(d) Use the 10 % slide coverage criterion.

Q-20. The TBS 2001 category of "Other" includes which of the following:
(a) LGSIL
(b) HGSIL
(c) Endometrial cells in a woman ≥40 years of age
(d) ASC-H

Q-21. In TBS 2001, the category of Automated Review should include which of the following?
(a) Brief description of the testing methodology and an understandable result
(b) Notation if review is done with computer-assisted screening, specify the device and the result
(c) Suggestions for clinical follow-up of the patient consistent with professional organizations
(d) Description of the degree of technical interpretability (50–75 % obscured)

Q-22. Which of these findings from a colposcopic examination is considered the most serious?
(a) Mosaic pattern of blood vessels
(b) Dark iodine staining (Schiller's test)
(c) Tissue follows the normal contours of the cervix
(d) Punctuation pattern of blood vessels

Q-23. The coexistence of which of the following is most likely to obscure colposcopic detail?
(a) *Trichomonas*
(b) Lugol's solution
(c) Iodine
(d) Atypical blood vessels

Q-24. Regarding studies of the natural history of CIN 1, 2, and 3 lesions, which of these statements is correct?
(a) Relatively fewer CIN 1 lesions go on to progress to carcinoma in situ or worse than CIN 2 or 3.
(b) Almost all lesions of CIN 1 go on to become carcinoma in situ, if not treated.
(c) CIN 2 is the least likely of these lesions to regress.
(d) CIN 3 almost always becomes invasive without treatment.

Q-25. Currently FDA-approved high-risk HPV tests include:
- (a) Hybrid Capture 1
- (b) Cervista HPV 16/18
- (c) Cervista HPV HR
- (d) PCR detection

Q-26. Per American Cancer Society guidelines (2012), women who have been vaccinated against HPV:
- (a) Are at little risk of developing cervical cancer and may omit Pap testing
- (b) Are protected against HPV even if they have already been infected by the virus
- (c) Need to follow screening recommendations for their age group
- (d) May develop cervical cancer caused by one of the low-risk HPV subtypes

Q-27. The application of a mild vinegar (3–5 % acetic acid) solution to the cervix during colposcopy:
- (a) Shows suspicious areas as a dark brown color
- (b) Shows suspicious areas as intensely white in color
- (c) Shows suspicious areas as iodine negative (yellow in color)
- (d) Removes any reactive or inflammatory material that might confound the examination

Q-28. During colposcopy, the endocervical canal can be sampled for an ECC by using a Kevorkian curette or:
- (a) An Ayre spatula
- (b) A cytobrush
- (c) Forceps
- (d) A Q-tip

Q-29. The reporting of specimen adequacy for excessive obscuring inflammation should be interpreted as "unsatisfactory" if:
- (a) 10–25 % of the cells are obscured.
- (b) 25–50 % of the cells are obscured.
- (c) 50–75 % of the cells are obscured.
- (d) More than 75 % of the cells are obscured.
- (e) More than 90 % of the cells are obscured.

Q-30. If a conventional Pap smear is received broken into many pieces, the suggested wording from the 2006 Bethesda System is which of the following?
- (a) Unsatisfactory: Specimen was processed and examined but breakage of the slide interfered with the interpretation.
- (b) Unsatisfactory: Specimen rejected (not processed) because the slide was broken.
- (c) Unsatisfactory: Specimen was processed and examined but cannot be interpreted.
- (d) Satisfactory: Quality indicator – broken slide.

Q-31. A special population of women who should follow an increased screening frequency is made up of patients who:
- (a) Are older than age 65 and have had a hysterectomy for noncancerous conditions
- (b) Are HIV positive, transplant patients, or on chemotherapy
- (c) Are younger than age 21 and who have had HPV vaccination
- (d) Are between ages 21 and 29

Q-32. To provide the optimum gynecologic sample, patients should be advised to:
- (a) Refrain from douching or use of spermicides within 48 h of exam.
- (b) Cancel the Pap test in the case of noncyclic bleeding.
- (c) Restrict intake of fluids for 10 h prior to the exam.
- (d) Fast for 8 h prior to the exam.

Q-33. Indications for colposcopic examination do NOT include which of the following?
- (a) ASC-US
- (b) LGSIL
- (c) ASC-H
- (d) ASC-US with + HR HPV test

Q-34. In order to determine adequate cellularity on a liquid-based preparation, the usual procedure is to:
- (a) Count the cells on the slide.
- (b) Count the cells in 10 40× fields to determine mean number of cells per field.
- (c) Compare the overall cellularity with reference images.
- (d) Use a digitalized image analysis device to determine cellularity.

Q-35. In the latest (2006) revision of the Bethesda System terminology, radiation effect would be reported as:
- (a) NILM, reactive cellular changes associated with radiation
- (b) ASC-US, changes consistent with radiation therapy
- (c) LGSIL, consistent with radiation therapy
- (d) LGSIL

Q-36. Advantages of utilizing liquid-based preparation methods include:

(a) The ability to test the remaining material in the vial for HR HPV
(b) The ability to place more cells on the slide than conventional slides and so increase accuracy
(c) The elimination of organisms which might obscure the slide
(d) The reduction of HGSIL cases

Q-37. Which of these stains is most frequently used on cell block material from liquid-based gynecologic preps?
(a) Oil red O
(b) Methyl green pyronin
(c) Mucin
(d) p16

Q-38. If HPV subtyping (16/18) is done for a woman (above 30) who is HPV HR positive but cytology negative, the ASCCP recommendations suggests:
(a) Repeating both cytology and the HR HPV test at 12 months if 16/18 test is positive
(b) Returning to annual screening if 16/18 test is positive
(c) Performing colposcopy if the 16/18 result is positive
(d) Returning to screening every 3 years if 16/18 test is positive

Q-39. The reporting of a slide with significant inflammation should be "Satisfactory for evaluation; Quality indicator – Partially obscuring inflammation" if the percentage of obscured cells is:
(a) 5–25 %
(b) 25–50 %
(c) 50–75 %
(d) >75 %

Q-40. If a specimen is unsatisfactory, which of the following would be the best wording for the report?
(a) "Unsatisfactory for evaluation"
(b) " Unsatisfactory for evaluation…(specify reason)"
(c) "Unsatisfactory for evaluation. Specimen rejected/ not processed"
(d) "Unsatisfactory for evaluation. Specimen processed and examined, but unsatisfactory for evaluation because of…(specify reason)"

1.3 Image-Based Questions 41–70

Fig. 1.41

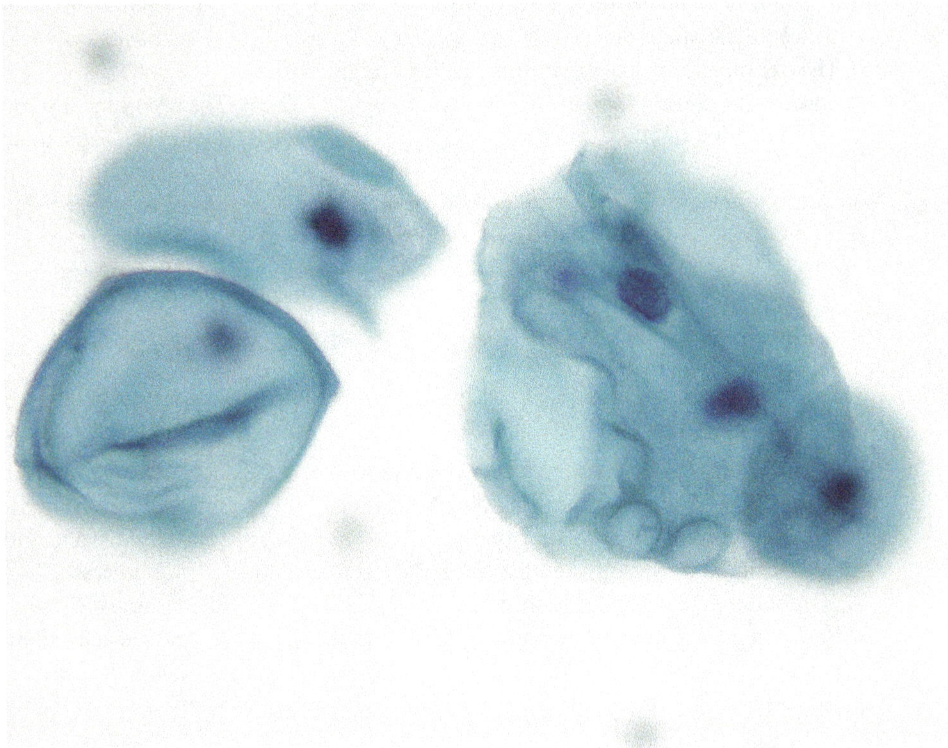

Q-41. (SurePath, high magnification) Many cells with cytomegaly, increased nuclear and cytoplasmic size, and cytoplasmic vacuoles such as this were seen in the gynecologic sample from a 62-year-old female who had been treated for squamous cell carcinoma of the cervix 8 years ago. The appropriate terminology for this lesion according to the Bethesda System 2006 is:

(a) LGSIL encompassing HPV/mild dysplasia/CIN I
(b) Reactive cellular changes associated with radiation
(c) Post-radiation dysplasia
(d) Squamous cell carcinoma
(e) Repair

Fig. 1.42

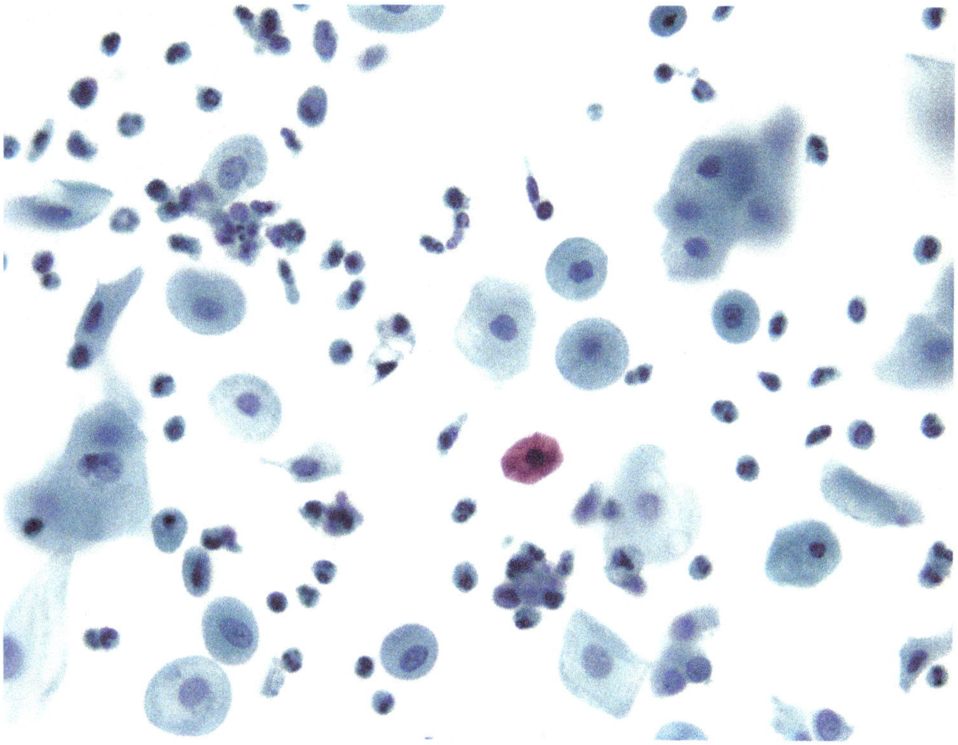

Q-42. (SurePath, low magnification) A 73-year-old woman with no previous abnormal history has a gynecologic sample submitted with many cells similar to those in the image. According to the 2006 Bethesda System, the best diagnosis for this case would be:

(a) Negative for intraepithelial lesion or malignancy. Atrophy.
(b) Negative for intraepithelial lesion or malignancy. Reactive changes consistent with repair.
(c) Negative for intraepithelial lesion or malignancy. Parakeratosis.
(d) Negative for intraepithelial lesion or malignancy. Hyperkeratosis.

Fig. 1.43

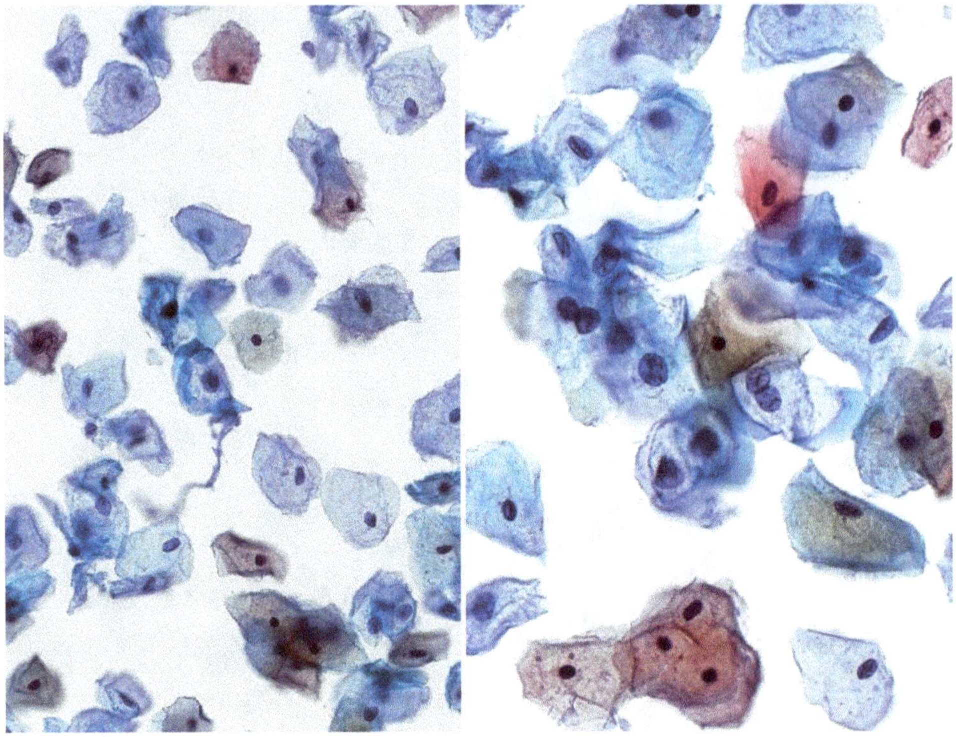

Q-43. (ThinPrep; left, low magnification; right, high magnification) If a number of cells such as these were seen in the gynecologic sample from a 36-year-old woman, the most appropriate diagnosis for this case according to the Bethesda System 2006 would be "Epithelial cell abnormality" and:

(a) Cellular changes of HPV
(b) Mild dysplasia
(c) CIN I
(d) Slight dysplasia
(e) LSIL

Fig. 1.44

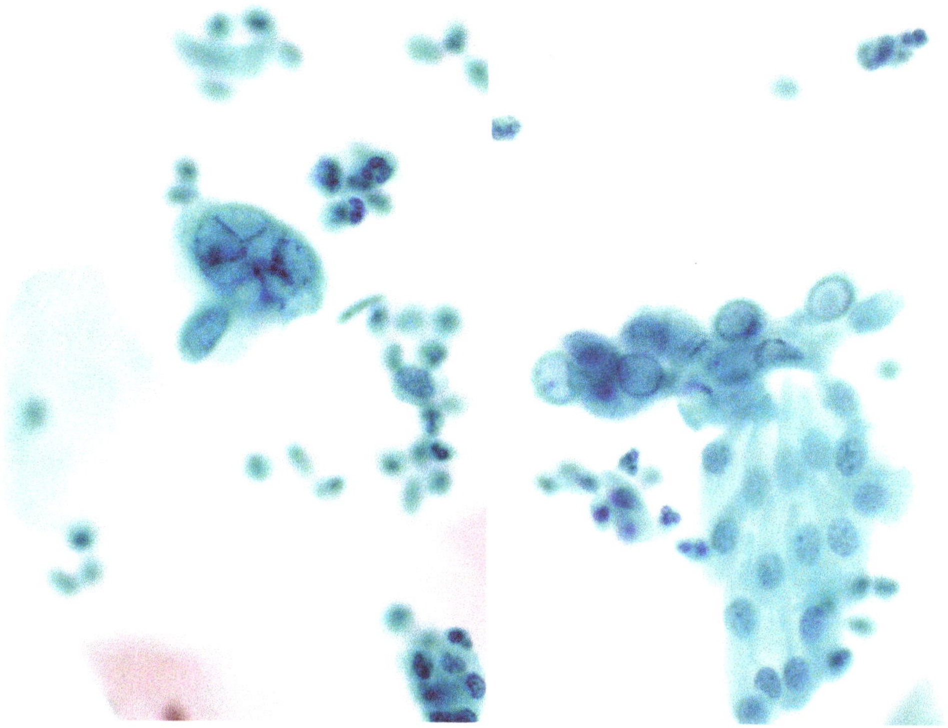

Q-44. (SurePath, high magnification) Cells such as these were found in the gynecologic sample of a 45-year-old woman. The most appropriate interpretation according to the Bethesda System 2006 is:

(a) Herpes
(b) Herpes simplex
(c) CMV
(d) Cellular changes consistent with herpes
(e) Cellular changes consistent with herpes simplex virus

Fig. 1.45

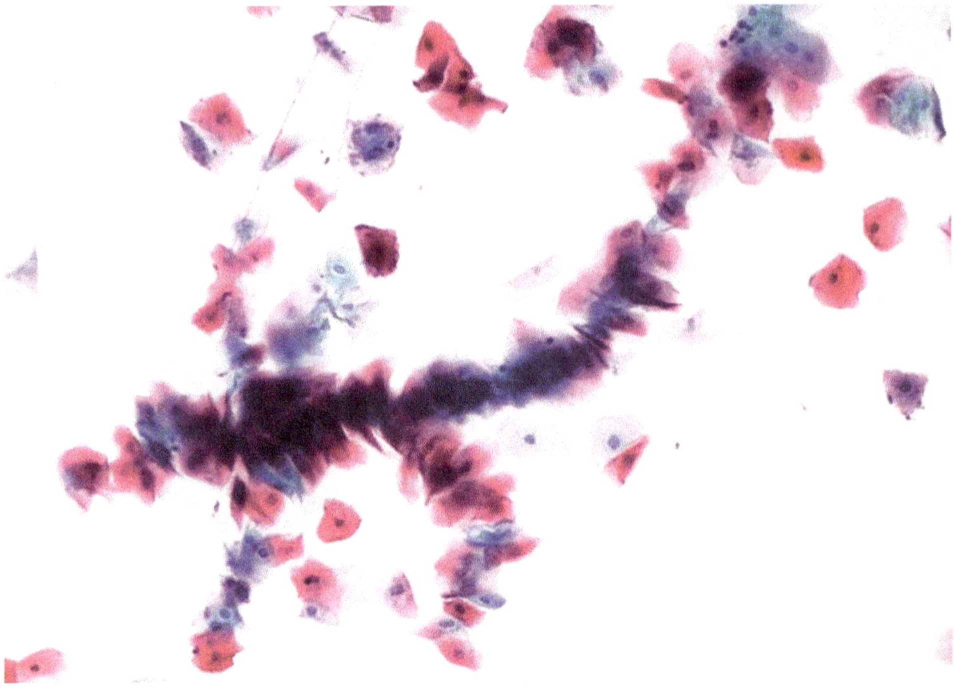

Q-45. (ThinPrep, low magnification) The most appropriate interpretation of this case according to the Bethesda System 2006 is:

(a) String of pearls
(b) *Candida albicans*
(c) *Candida glabrata*
(d) Fungal organisms morphologically consistent with *Candida* species
(e) *Torulopsis*

Fig. 1.46

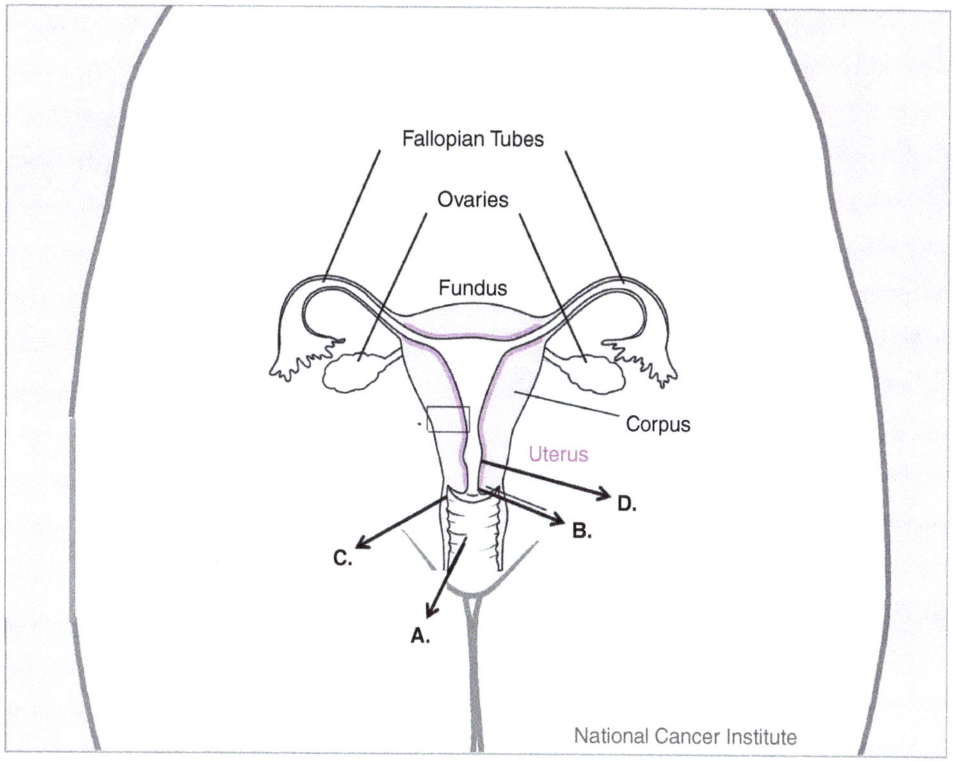

Q-46. In this diagram of the female genital tract, the most likely location to obtain a sample of the transformation zone is:
(a) Location A
(b) Location B
(c) Location C
(d) Location D

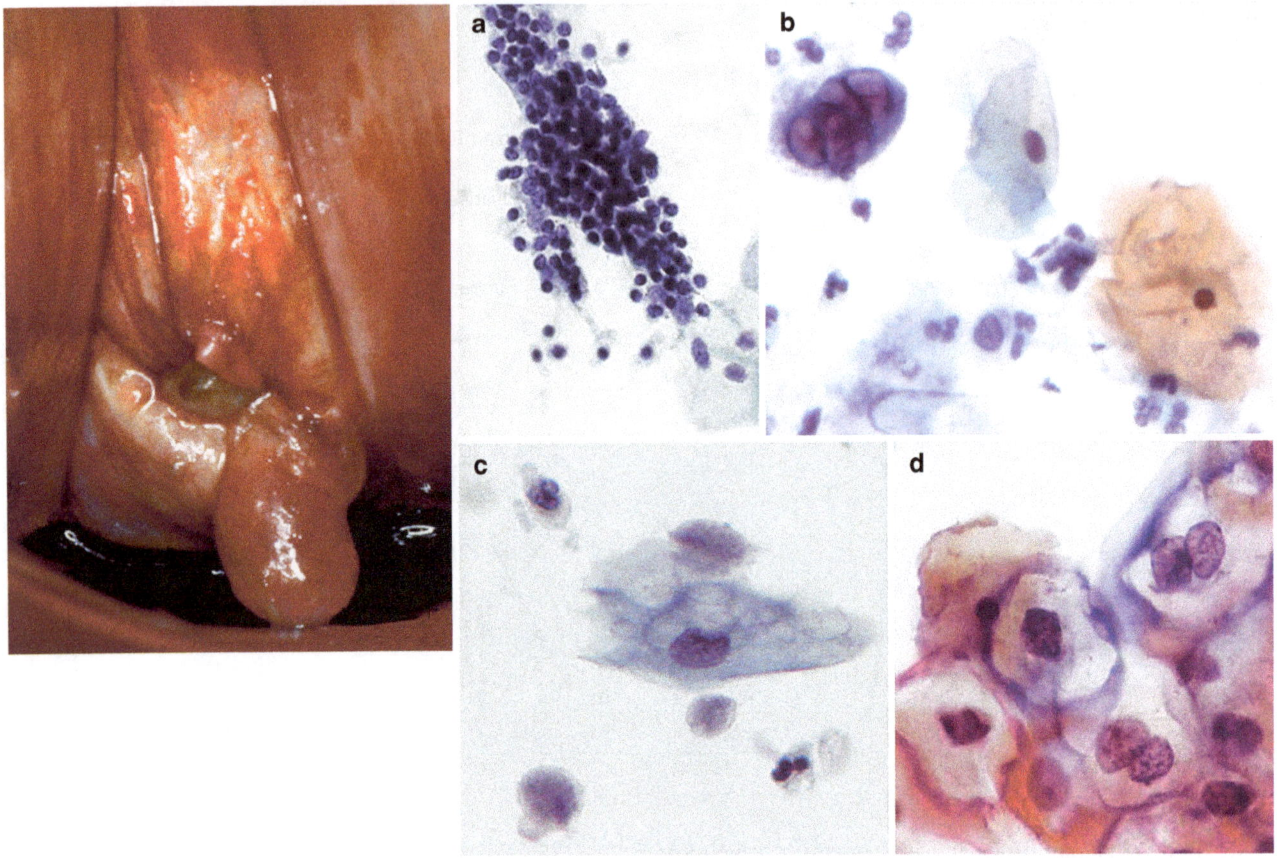

Fig. 1.47 Permission to utilize the colposcopic image, Colposcopy Principles and Practice: An Integrated Textbook and Atlas, Apgar et al. 2nd (ed), 2008. Elsevier

Q-47. This appearance of the cervix under colposcopy is typical for which of the cytologic images displayed?
 (a) Image A
 (b) Image B
 (c) Image C
 (d) Image D

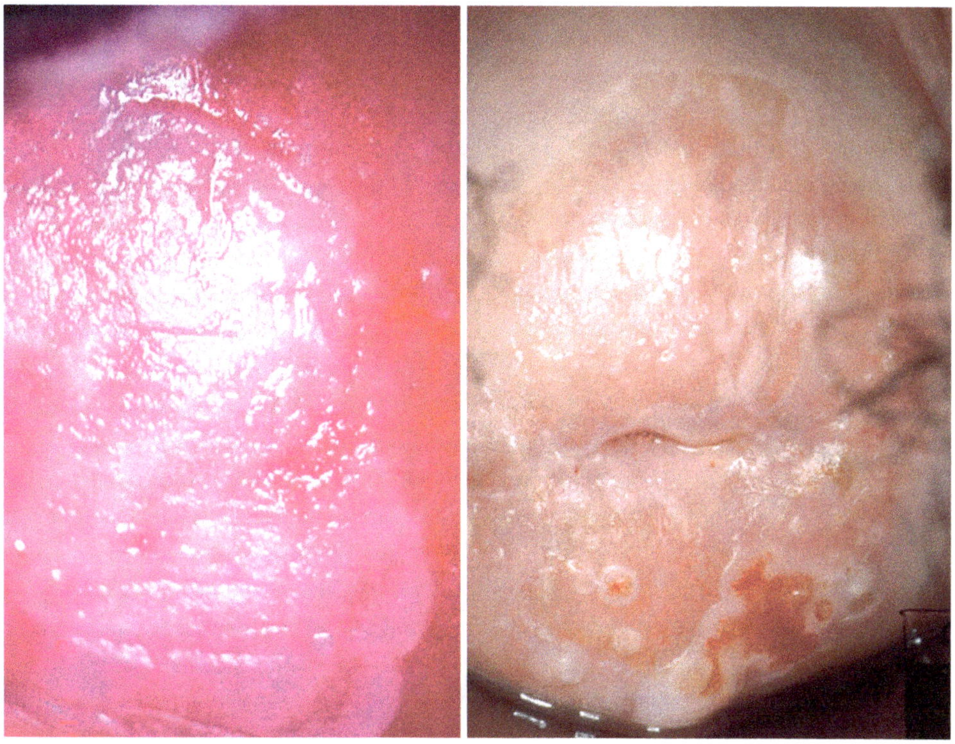

Fig. 1.48 Permission to utilize the colposcopic image, Colposcopy Principles and Practice: An Integrated Textbook and Atlas, Apgar et al. 2nd (ed), 2008. Elsevier

Q-48. This appearance of the cervix under colposcopy PRIOR to the application of acetic acid solution may be caused by a number of conditions. Of the following, which is the most likely to cause this appearance?
(a) *Trichomonas*
(b) *Candida* infection
(c) Follicular cervicitis
(d) Hyperkeratosis

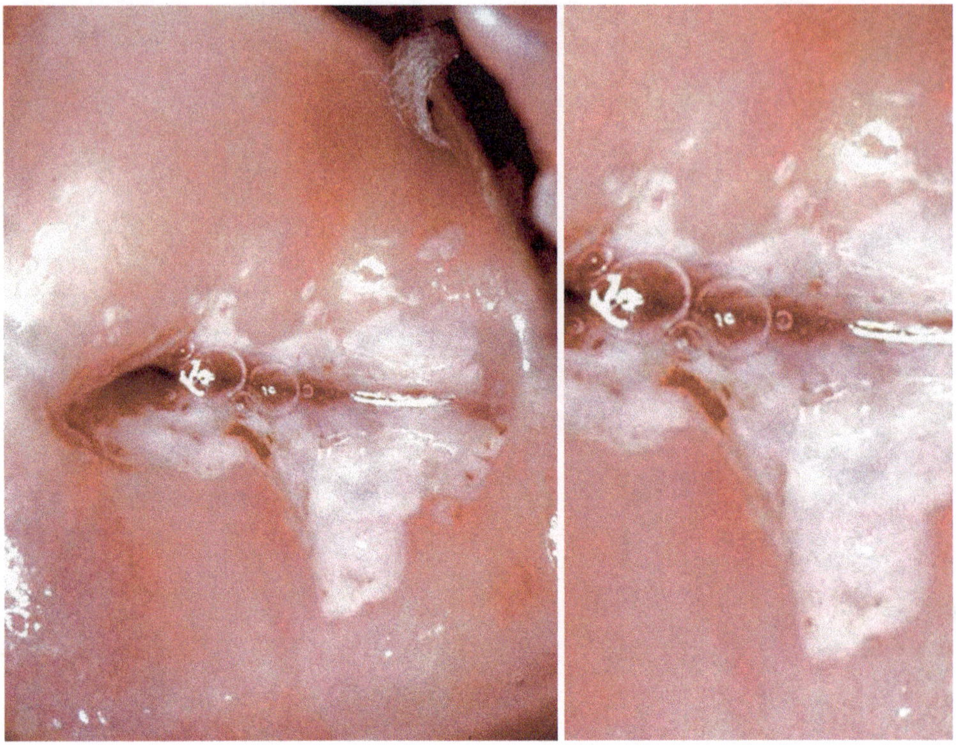

Fig. 1.49 Permission to utilize the colposcopic image, Colposcopy Principles and Practice: An Integrated Textbook and Atlas, Apgar et al. 2nd (ed), 2008. Elsevier

Q-49. This appearance of a cervix during colposcopy AFTER the application of an acetic acid solution shows the bright white, dense, and sharply demarcated edges of an area that is most likely:

(a) HSIL
(b) Atrophy
(c) Normal epithelium
(d) Cervicitis

Fig. 1.50

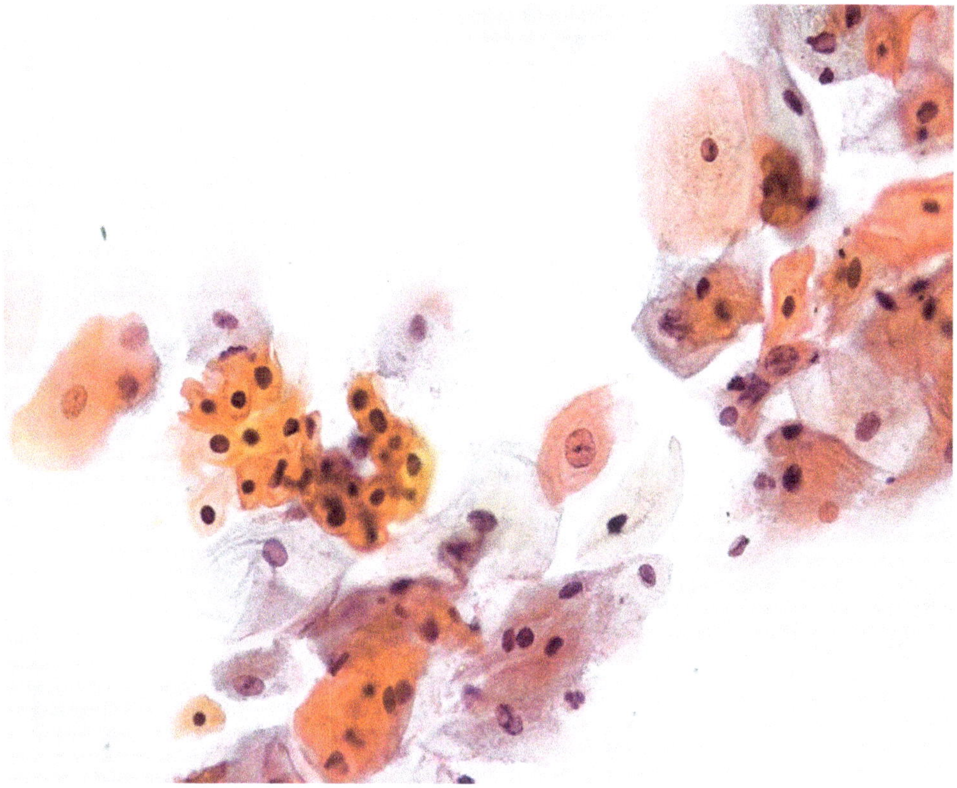

Q-50. Under colposcopy, a cervix which has a layer of cells such as these often will display white plaques PRIOR to the application of acetic acid solution. The best interpretation of these small orange cells is:
(a) HSIL
(b) Squamous metaplasia
(c) Endocervical cells
(d) Parakeratosis

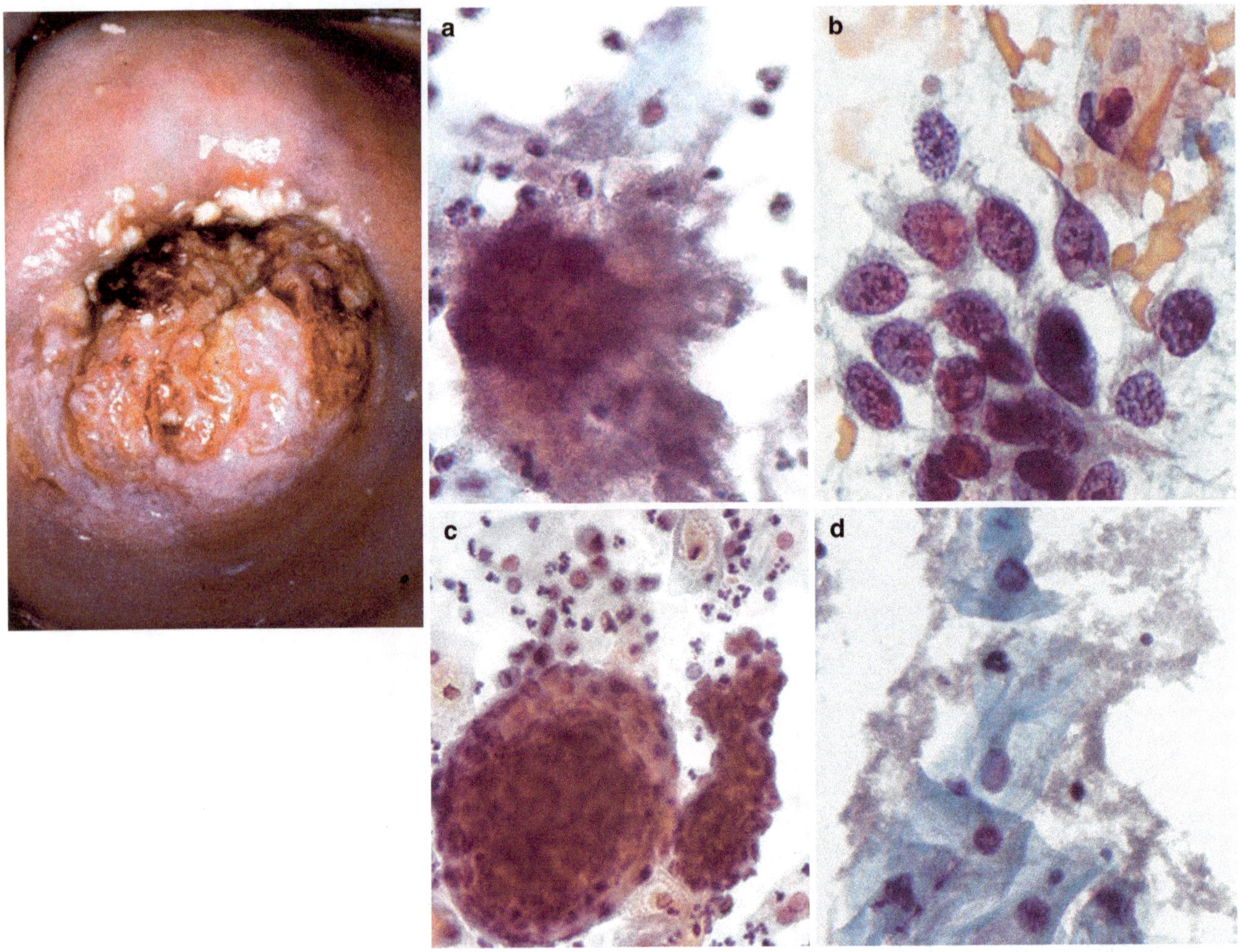

Fig. 1.51 Permission to utilize the colposcopic image, Colposcopy Principles and Practice: An Integrated Textbook and Atlas, Apgar et al. 2nd (ed), 2008. Elsevier

Q-51. Which of the cytologic images displayed is most consistent with this view of the cervix under colposcopy PRIOR to application of acetic acid solution?

(a) Image A
(b) Image B
(c) Image C
(d) Image D

Fig. 1.52

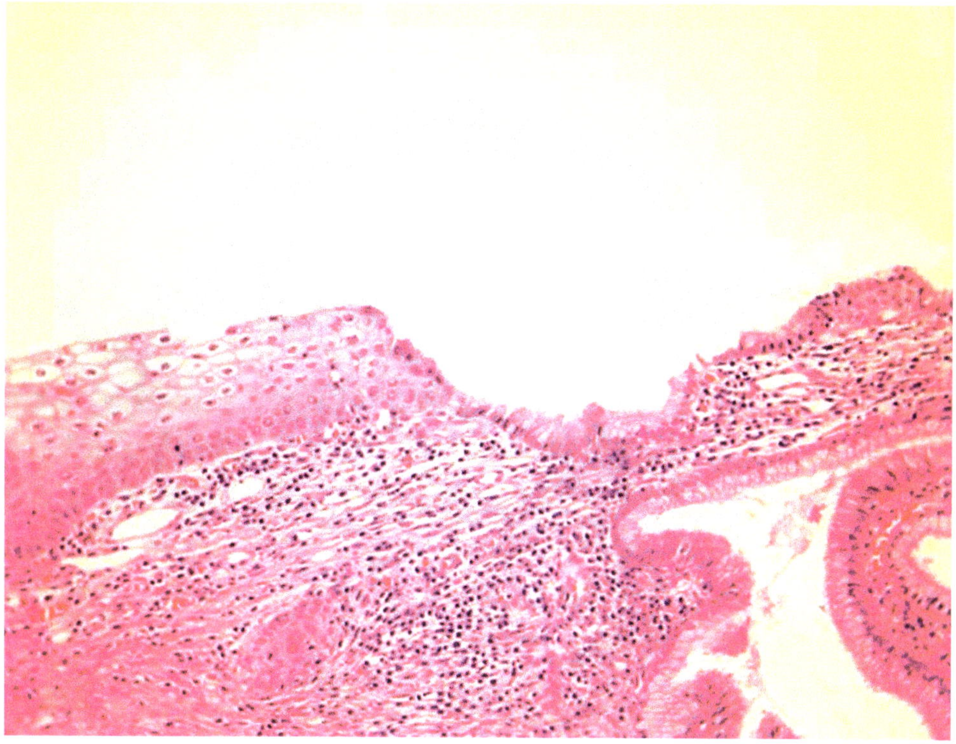

Q-52. It is important for the clinician to obtain material from this area of the cervix because:
(a) This image shows dysplasia.
(b) This image shows invasive squamous cell carcinoma.
(c) This image displays the most frequent site of lesions found on the cervix.
(d) This image shows adenocarcinoma in situ.

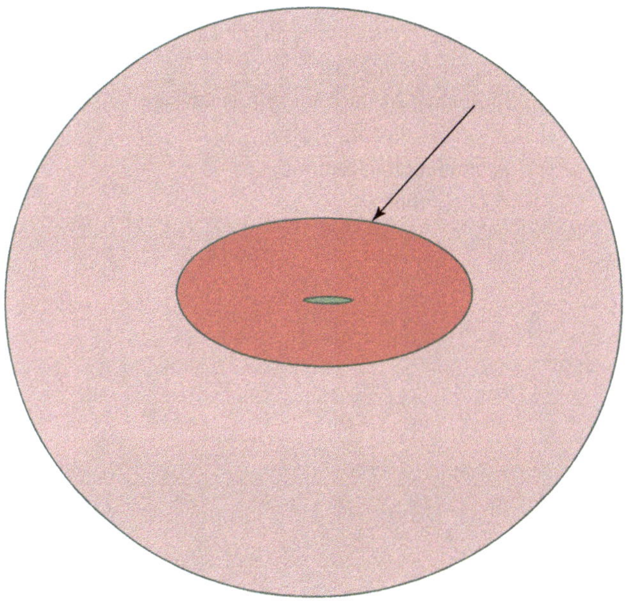

Fig. 1.53

Q-53. In order for a colposcopy to be considered "satisfactory," it is very important that:
(a) The squamous mucosa, at arrow, is seen in its entirety.
(b) The columnar mucosa, at arrow, is seen in its entirety.
(c) The vaginal epithelium, at arrow, is seen in its entirety.
(d) The transformation zone, at arrow, is seen in its entirety.

Fig. 1.54

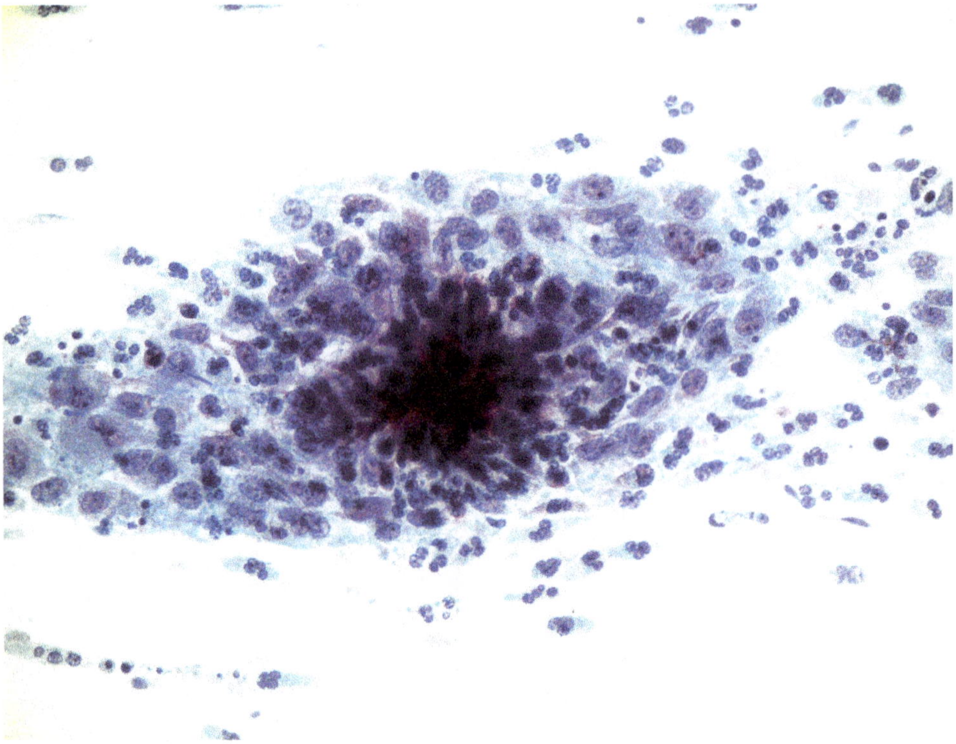

Q-54. This finding on the gynecologic sample of a 25-year-old pregnant female is:
(a) Indicative of impending miscarriage
(b) A syncytiotrophoblast
(c) A small cell carcinoma
(d) A cocklebur

Fig. 1.55

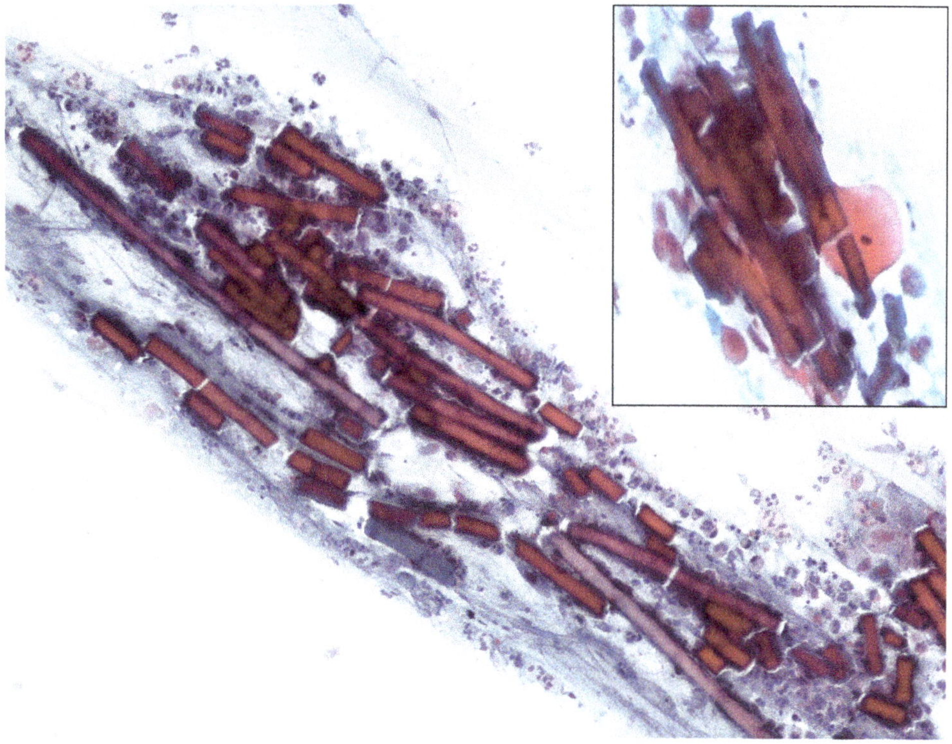

Q-55. These rectangular structures were found in the gynecologic sample of a woman evaluated during a 4 week postpartum examination. The most likely explanation for these structures is:
- (a) *Candida*
- (b) *Actinomyces*
- (c) Muscle fibers
- (d) Suture contaminants

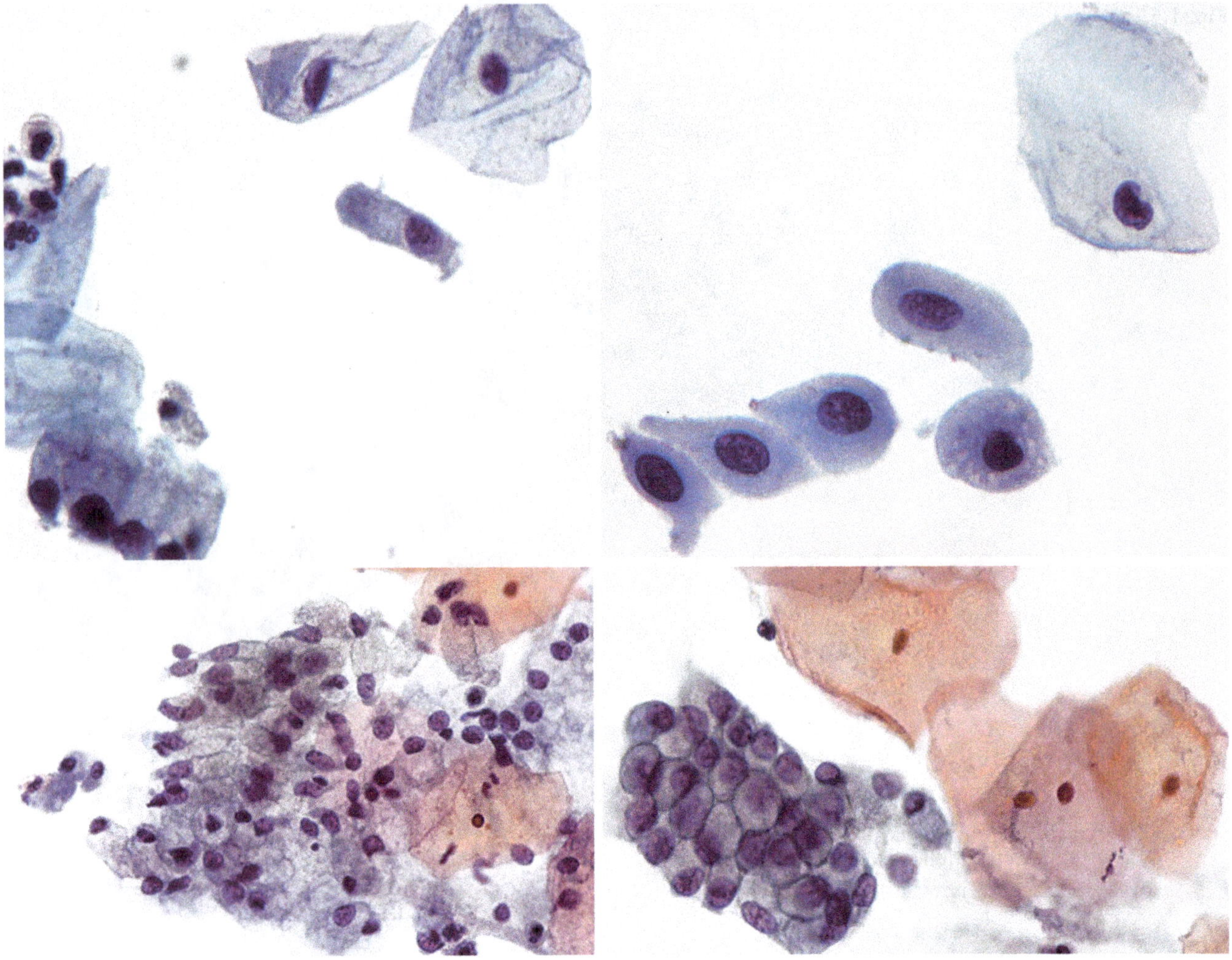

Fig. 1.56

Q-56. In this composite image are elements which need to be identified in order to verify that the transformation zone has been sampled. Which of the following best describes the criteria for identification of the T-zone?

(a) Squamous cells must be present in the appropriate numbers according to the specimen preparation method.

(b) Endocervical cells must be present singly, in picket fence arrangements, or in a honeycomb arrangement.

(c) Squamous metaplastic cells must be present in groups of 5 or more.

(d) 10 endocervical and/or 10 metaplastic cells must be present in any configuration.

Fig. 1.57

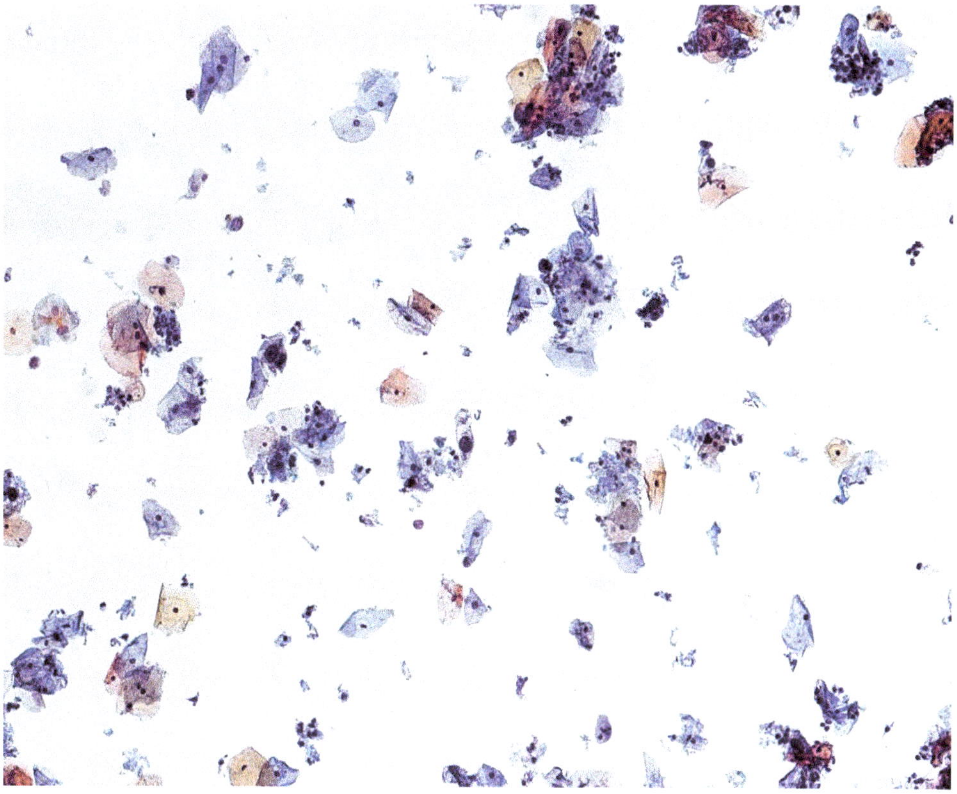

Q-57. This ThinPrep slide (low magnification) was examined, and several areas were found to have "holes" that did not have cellular material. When the slide was examined for adequate cellularity using the method described in *The Bethesda System for Reporting Cervical Cytology, 2nd edition, 2004*, there was a mean of 40 cells per 10× magnification. What is the most appropriate evaluation of this specimen?

(a) Unsatisfactory due to scant squamous cellularity.
(b) Satisfactory for evaluation. NILM.
(c) Unsatisfactory due to "holes" found in the cellular preparation.
(d) Satisfactory for evaluation. Epithelial cell abnormality. LSIL. A more serious lesion cannot be ruled out.

Fig. 1.58

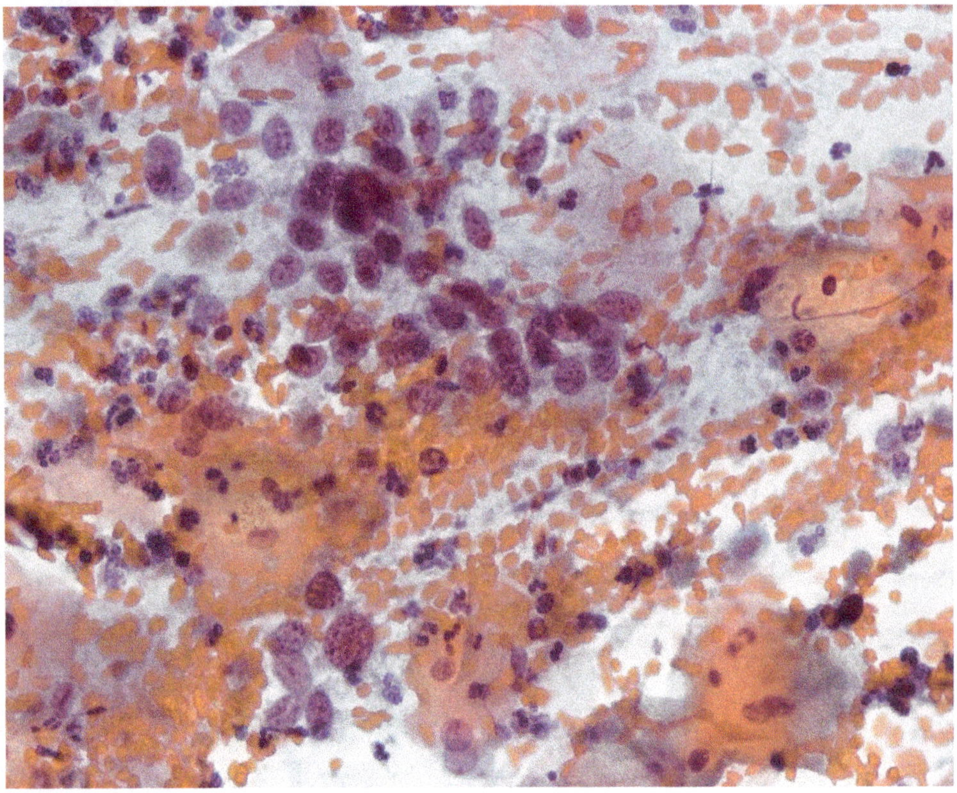

Q-58. In other places on this conventional slide, the blood was found to obscure more than 75 % of the cells. The most appropriate diagnosis for this slide would be:

(a) Unsatisfactory due to blood obscuring more than 75 % of the cells.
(b) Unsatisfactory. Quality Indicator: Blood obscuring from 50 to 75 % of the cells. NILM.
(c) Unsatisfactory due to scant squamous cellularity.
(d) Satisfactory. Quality indicator: Blood obscuring from 50 to 75 % of the cells. HSIL.
(e) Satisfactory. Quality indicator: Blood obscuring from 50 to 75 % of the cells. NILM.

Fig. 1.59

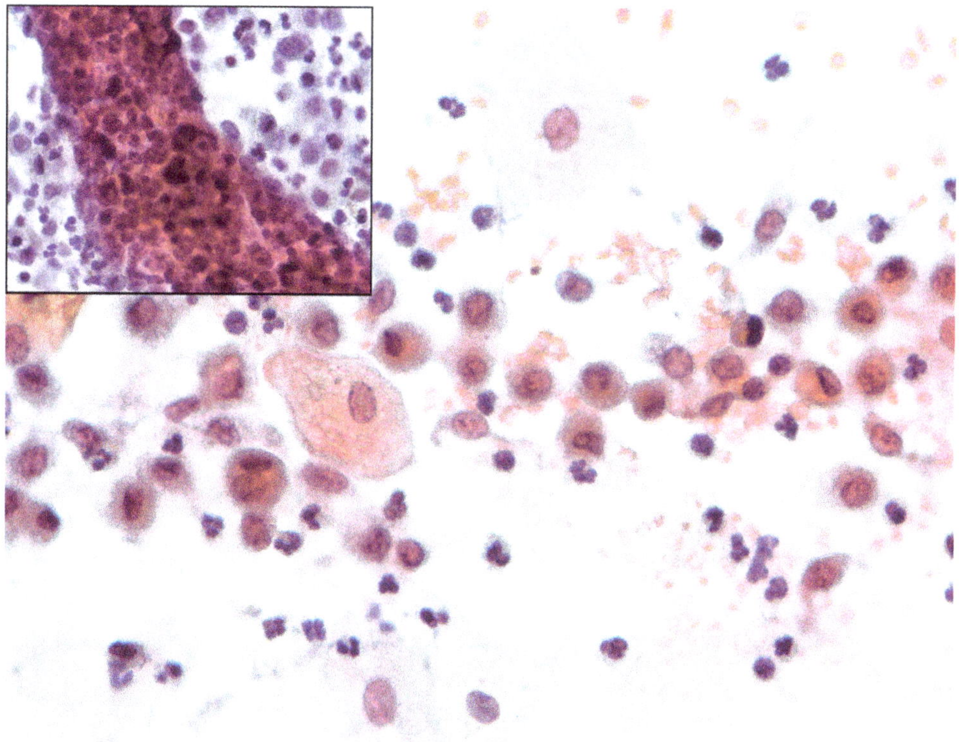

Q-59. This conventional slide was prepared from the gynecologic sample of a 42-year-old woman. Several groups of cells such as these were found on the slide. The best diagnosis for this slide according to the Bethesda System is which of the following?

(a) Satisfactory for evaluation. NILM
(b) Satisfactory for evaluation. Endometrial cells present. NILM
(c) Satisfactory for evaluation. Other: Endometrial cells in a woman over 40
(d) Unsatisfactory for evaluation. Other: Endometrial cells in a woman over 40

Fig. 1.60

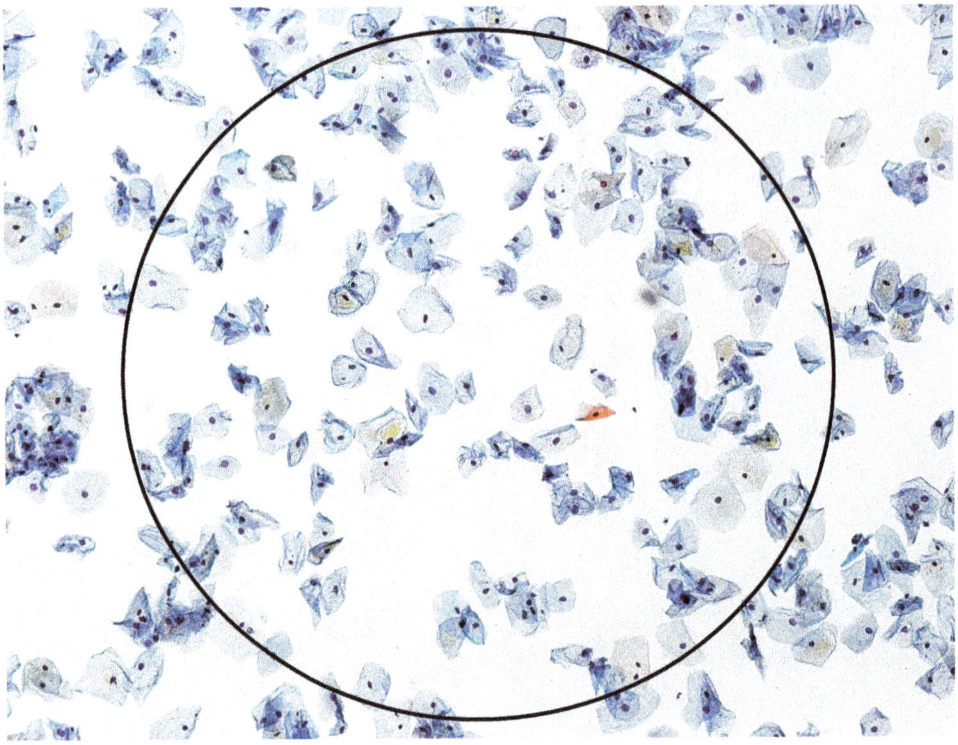

Q-60. This patient is a 38-year-old with a history of hysterectomy but no previous neoplasia. Assuming the entire ThinPrep slide appeared similar to this field and that the circle delineates an area equivalent to a 10× magnification using a FN20 eyepiece, the appropriate reporting terminology according to the Bethesda System is which of the following?

(a) Satisfactory for evaluation. NILM.
(b) Unsatisfactory for evaluation.
(c) Satisfactory for evaluation due to lack of endocervical and/or squamous metaplastic cells.
(d) Unsatisfactory for evaluation due to scant squamous cellularity.

Fig. 1.61

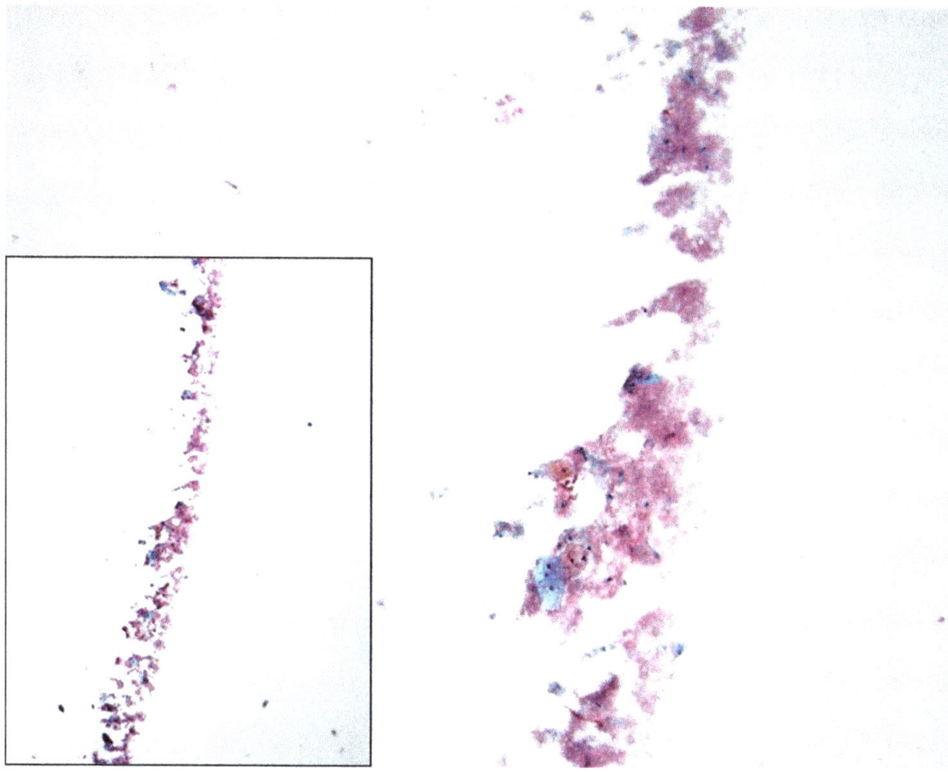

Q-61. This image is from a slide processed by the ThinPrep liquid-based method (left inset, 4x; right, 10x). How could this specimen, which microscopically had very few cells in the central area and would have to be called unsatisfactory, be improved?

(a) Centrifuge prior to processing.
(b) Treat with a 1:4 solution of 3 % glacial acetic acid and CytoLyt, centrifuge, decant, and rerun.
(c) Increase staining time in hematoxylin.
(d) Add equal amount of normal saline, centrifuge, decant, rerun.

Fig. 1.62

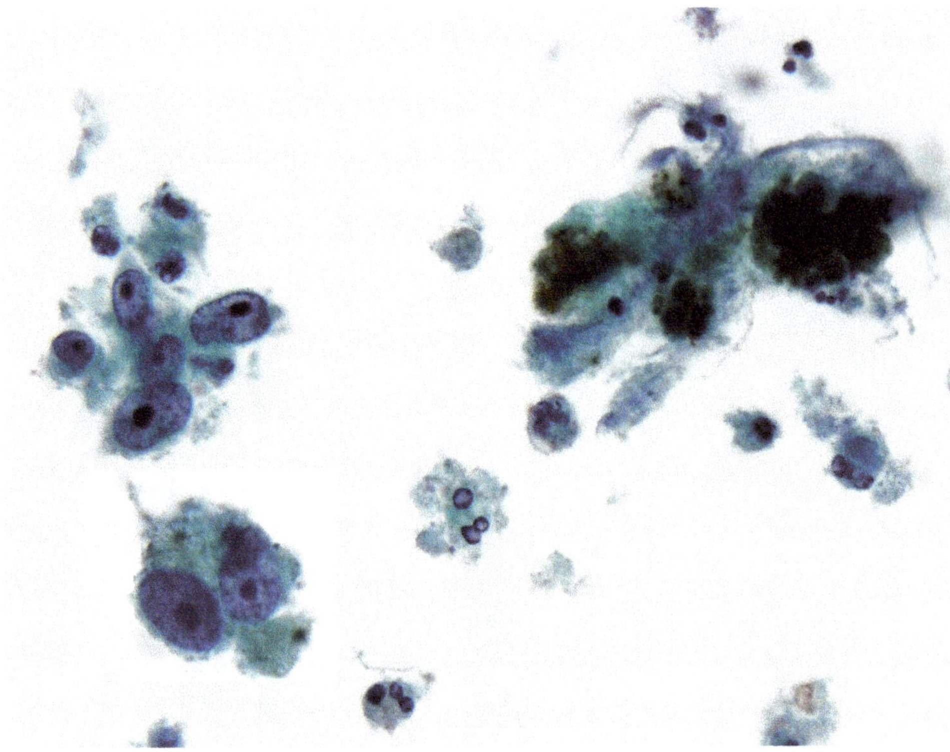

Q-62. This ThinPrep specimen is from an 87-year-old female (left, 40×; inset 40×). Many cells such as these are seen on the slide, along with brownish pigment, both within and outside of the cells. The best stain to utilize in the diagnosis of this case would be:

(a) Mucicarmine
(b) Hale's colloidal iron
(c) HMB-45
(d) pCEA
(e) CD117

Fig. 1.63

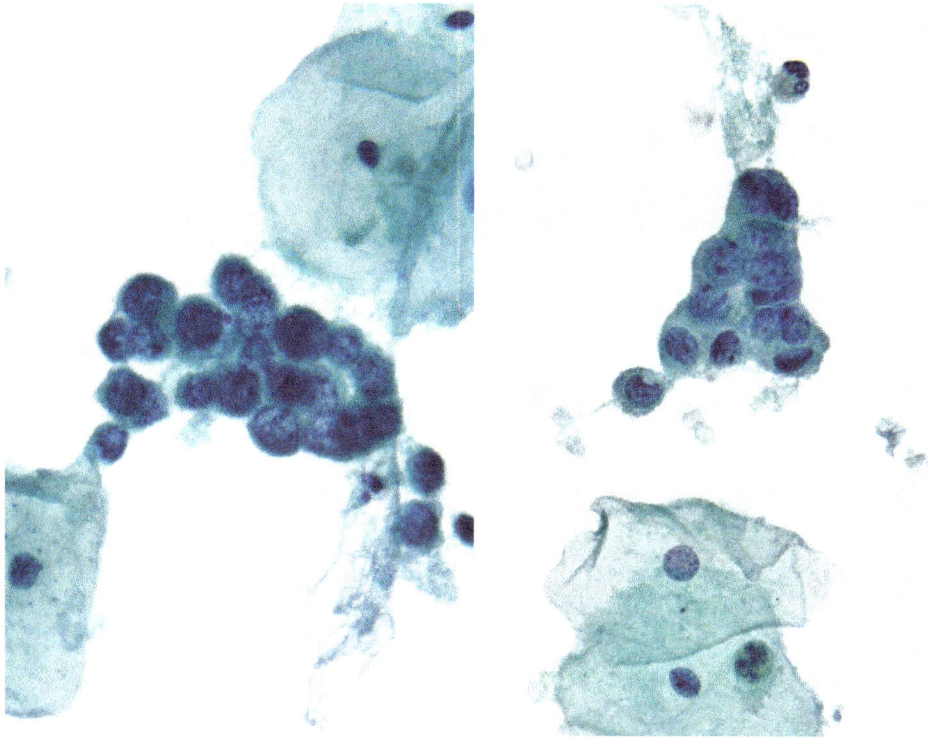

Q-63. This 65-year-old patient had a gynecologic sample with cells such as these (left and right, 40×). The background is clean and these cell clusters are relatively few in number. If endometrial curettage and endocervical biopsy are negative, which of the following might be the most likely source of these cells?

(a) Lobular carcinoma of the breast
(b) Colonic adenocarcinoma
(c) Squamous cell carcinoma of the lung
(d) Serous cystadenocarcinoma of the ovary

Fig. 1.64

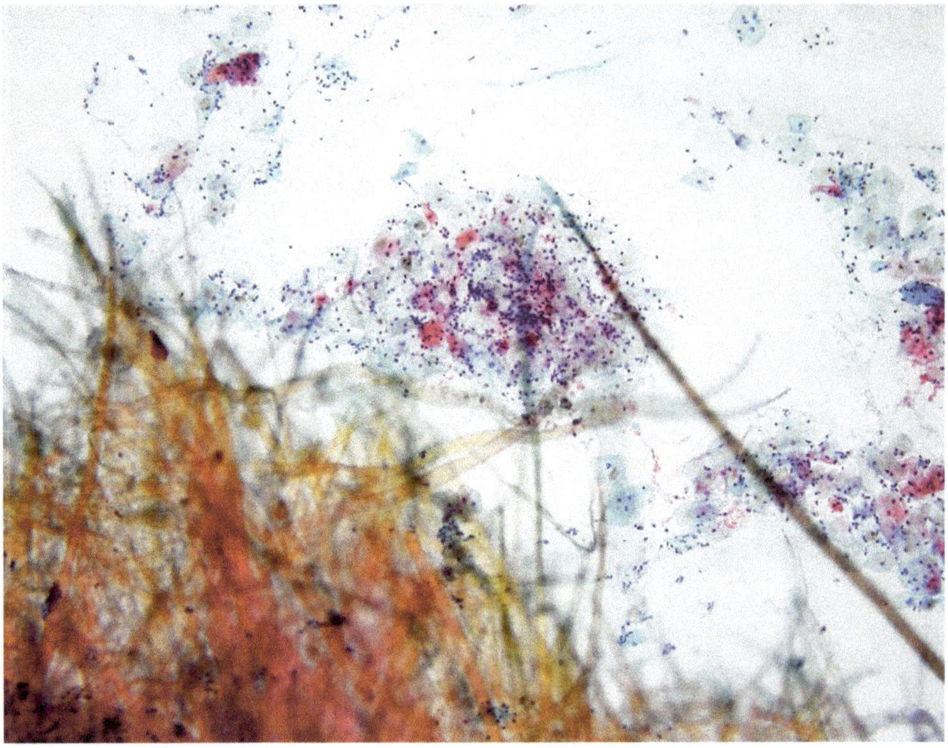

Q-64. This conventional slide is from a 20-year-old female, day 12 (low magnification). A large cluster of these elongated structures are seen on the slide. The most likely interpretation of this image is:

(a) *Candida*
(b) Mucormycosis
(c) Bristles from a cytobrush
(d) Cotton fibers
(e) Mucous strands

Fig. 1.65

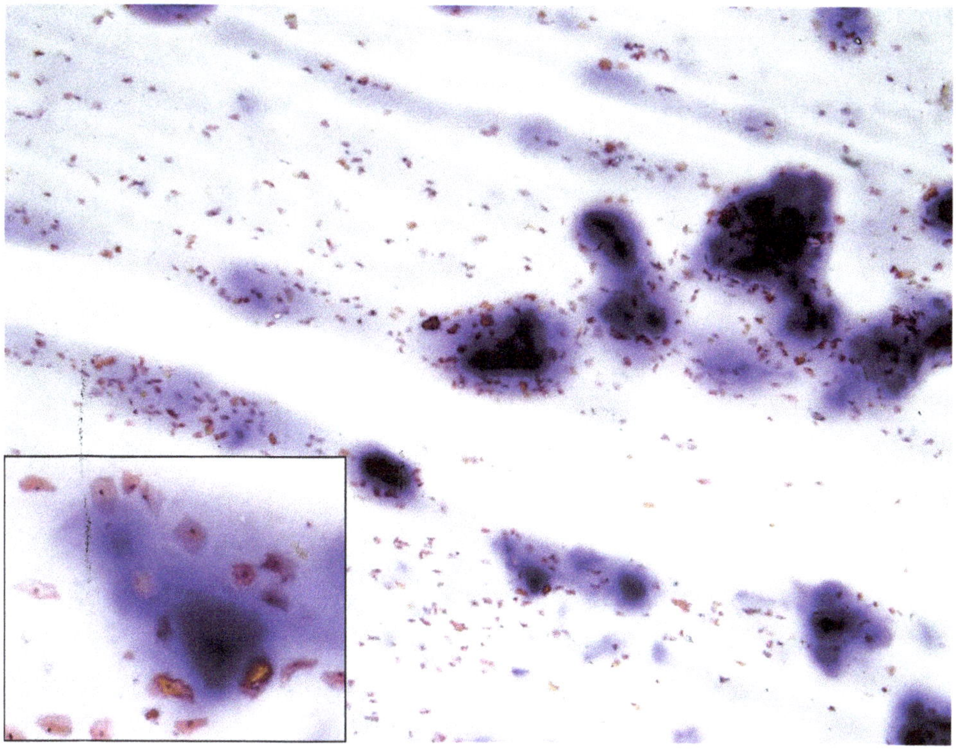

Q-65. This image is from a conventional smear from a 23-year-old woman. The slide contains many areas of lavender material as seen here (main image, 4×; inset, 10×). The most likely explanation of this material is:
(a) Lysed blood
(b) Mucinous discharge
(c) *Actinomyces*
(d) Lubricant artifact
(e) Rectovaginal fistula

Fig. 1.66

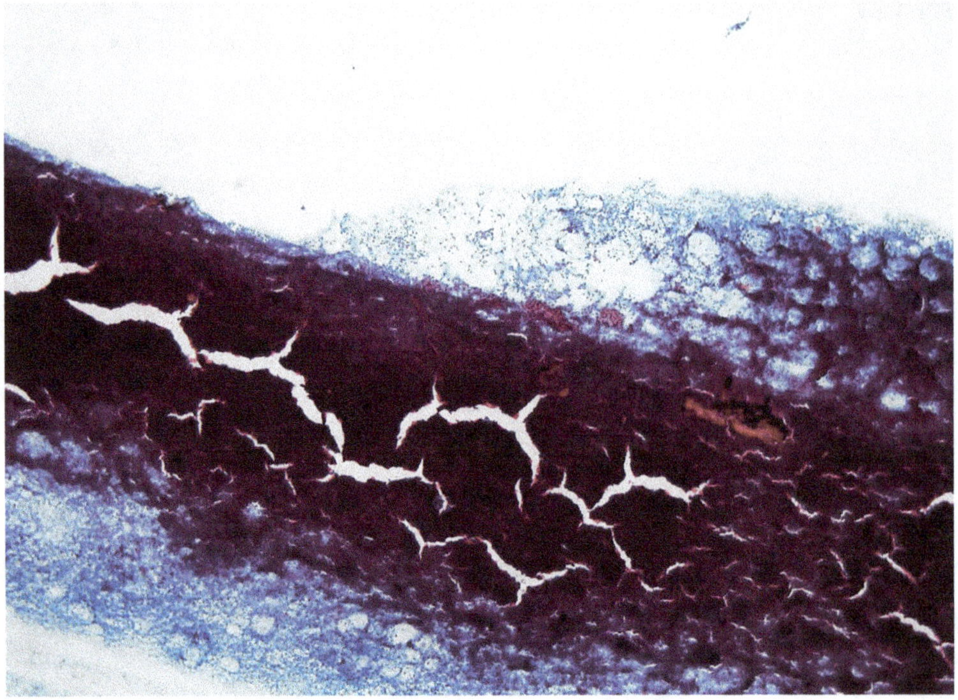

Q-66. This conventional slide is from a 57-year-old female (4x). If the entire slide showed this appearance, with large numbers of neutrophils, the most appropriate diagnosis would be:

(a) Satisfactory, NILM, inflammation.
(b) Satisfactory, quality indicator: 25–50 % of the cells are obscured by blood.
(c) Unsatisfactory, scant cellularity.
(d) Unsatisfactory, over 75 % of the cells are obscured by inflammation.

Fig. 1.67

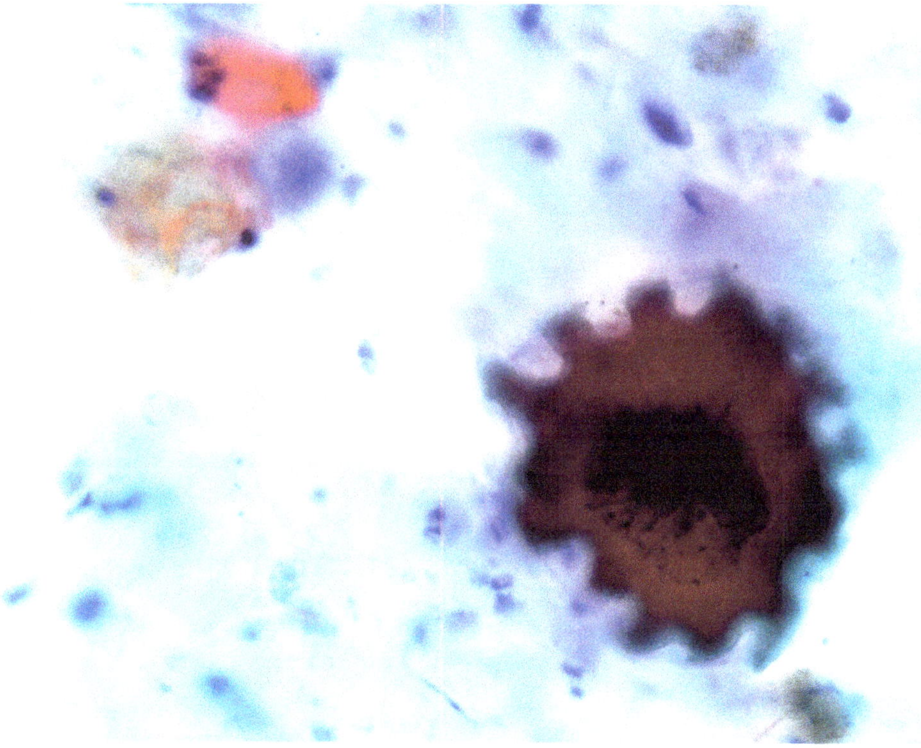

Q-67. This conventional slide is from an 18-year-old female. The orange-staining structure seen is most likely:

(a) Pollen
(b) Ova of a parasite
(c) Part of a plant
(d) A fungus

Fig. 1.68

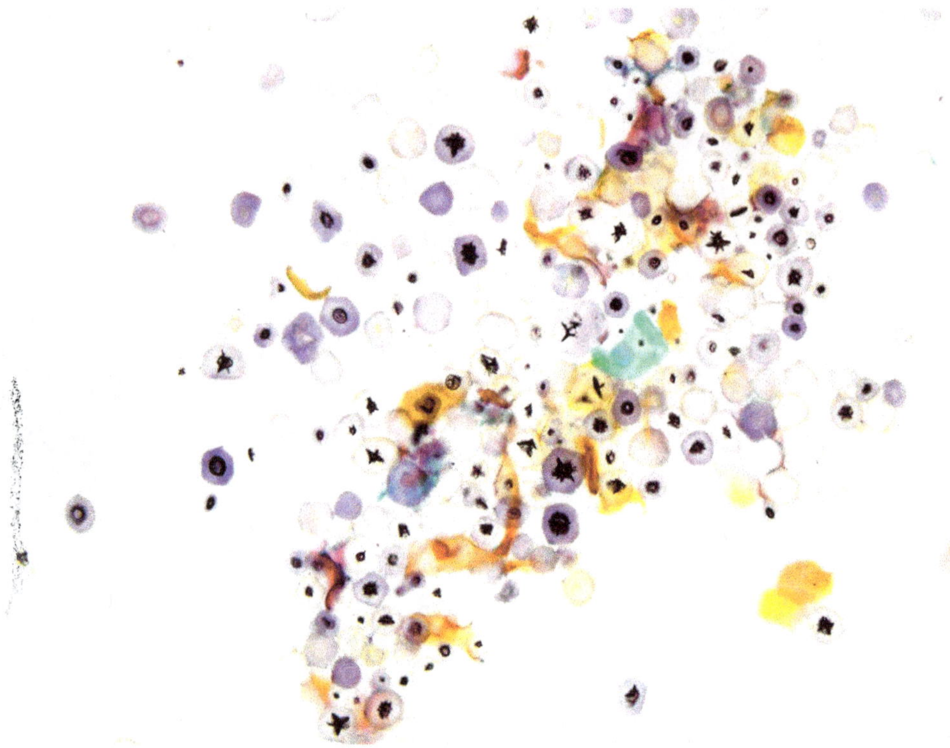

Q-68. This conventional slide is from a 60-year-old female. The pale to lavender rounded structures, some of which have a grayish star-shaped central area, are most likely:

(a) *Blastomyces dermatitidis*
(b) Cryptococcus neoformans
(c) *Coccidioides immitis*
(d) Glove powder
(e) Psammoma bodies

Fig. 1.69

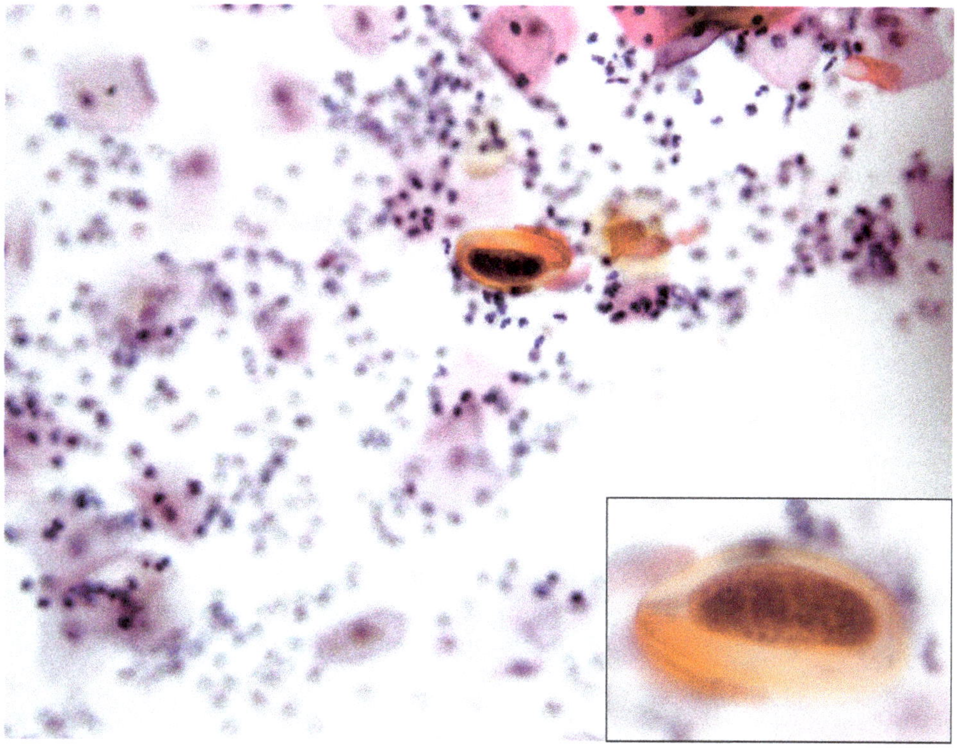

Q-69. These images are from the conventional slide of a 40-year-old woman (main image, 40×; inset, 100×). The oval structure seen is most consistent with an interpretation of:

(a) Keratinizing squamous metaplasia
(b) Pollen
(c) *Enterobius vermicularis* ova
(d) Plant cell

Fig. 1.70

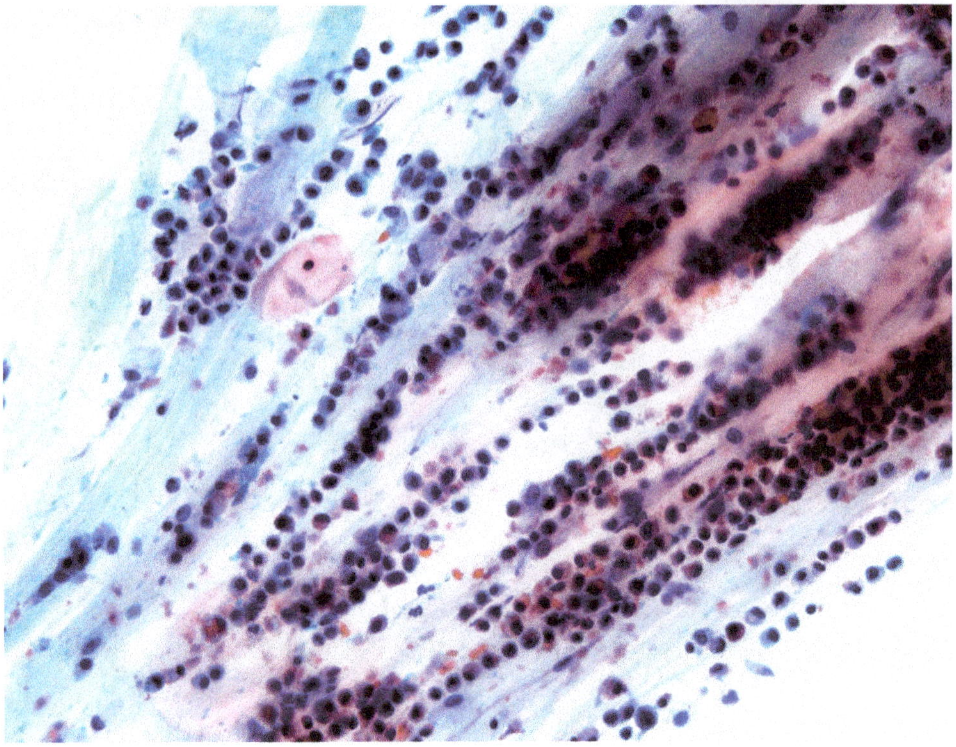

Q-70. This conventional slide (high magnification) is from a 23-year-old patient with a history of oral contraception use. The cells seen in this image appeared in streams and clusters within areas of endocervical mucous. The most likely interpretation is:
(a) Parakeratosis
(b) Hyperkeratosis
(c) Pseudoparakeratosis (microglandular hyperplasia)
(d) Dyskeratosis
(e) Squamous metaplasia

1.4 Answers and Discussion of Text-Based Questions 1–40

A-1. (e) **At least 10 endocervical and/or metaplastic cells**

The Bethesda System indicates that at least 10 cells from the endocervical canal (columnar and/or metaplastic cells) must be found in order to indicate that the squamocolumnar junction has been sampled. In cases in which this is not found, the phrase "Satisfactory for evaluation: endocervical/transformation zone component absent/insufficient" is used to convey this information. In patients who have had a hysterectomy, or in whom cancer or a high-grade lesion is found, this comment may be omitted.

A-2. (d) **No later than age 21 or 3 years after the onset of sexual activity**

The most recent (2012) recommendations from the American Cancer Society state that screening should begin at age 21 or 3 years after onset of sexual activity. Co-testing for HPV, however, should not be performed on the 21–29 age group since there are so many transient HPV infections in this age group which may lead to overtreatment. HPV testing may be performed, however, if the Pap results are abnormal.

A-3. (c) **Papanicolaou**

Per laboratory guidelines in the CAP Cytopathology Checklist, Papanicolaou stain is the most appropriate stain for routine cervical cancer screening.

A-4. (d) **Maintaining visibility of the lower one-third of the endocervical brush device**

By maintaining visibility of the lower one-third of the endocervical brush, the clinical staff is prevented from inadvertently sampling the lower uterine segment, which may be the cause of hyperchromatic crowded groups on the slide. These groups might be overinterpreted as neoplastic, so avoiding the sampling of this area is encouraged.

A-5. (b) **Interfere with the proper filtration of ThinPrep preparations**

Use of lubricant is not recommended by Hologic corporation nor by published guidelines (NCCLS Document CP15-A, ACOG Practice bulletin, no. 45, Aug. 2003) as it may interfere with a ThinPrep slide by causing the clumping of cells, creating a scanty preparation, or obscuring the cellular material. It is recommended that if lubricant is used for patient comfort, it be used sparingly, avoiding the tip of the speculum. Lubricants containing an ingredient known as "carbomers" or "carbopol polymers" should be avoided. Lubricant may appear in a variety of ways in the sample but usually creates lavender, pink, or purple acellular streams in the background of the slide. There is usually no confusion with abnormal cells or HPV infections, but lubricant may make the slide suboptimal due to scant cellularity.

A-6. (c) **Thoroughly dislodge the material by stirring and compressing the brush against side of the vial**.

Material obtained for preparation by the ThinPrep method is never smeared on a slide, nor is the tip of the collection device dropped into the vial. The material obtained should be thoroughly dislodged by vigorous stirring of the vial with the collection device while pressing the device against the side of the vial. This immediate transfer of the cells to the fixative solution helps to preserve nuclear and cytoplasmic detail, which would sometimes be obscured if air drying occurred prior to fixation of a conventional slide.

A-7. (b) **Gravity sedimentation method**

The SurePath preparation system utilizes a series of steps which help to remove material from the collection device, concentrate the material, wash the cells, and then allow the heavier cellular material to deposit onto the glass slide. The ThinPrep method uses a filtration system. Neither method uses a smear of either the endocervical brush or the broom collection device.

A-8. (d) **Premalignant lesions precede and lead to the development of squamous cell carcinoma**.

Early epidemiologic studies that noted the mean age at detection for premalignant and malignant squamous lesions of the cervix increased in relation to their severity were the basis for concluding that most invasive lesions developed from precursor abnormalities. Now that HPV has been shown to be the cause of virtually all squamous cell carcinomas, as well as the precursor lesions, this age progression is further explained. Almost all squamous cell carcinomas develop from these precursor lesions, and infections from other causes have not been shown to play a role in the development of squamous cancer of the cervix. Although sexual activity is the means by which the HPV virus is spread from one to another, most women who get the HPV infection clear it on their own without treatment. Thus, sexual activity itself is not a direct cause of cervical cancer.

A-9. (a) **A decrease in the incidence of squamous cell carcinoma of the cervix**
Where routine screening has been implemented, the incidence of cervical squamous cell carcinoma has decreased, due to the preventative effect of detecting precursor lesions and treating them before invasive lesions develop. The incidence of infectious diseases such as *Trichomonas* and reactive or reparative lesions do not decrease with the implementation of screening. Screening also does not have an effect on cancers metastatic to the cervix.

A-10. (b) **Colposcopically directed biopsy**
Patients with a diagnosis of ASC-H are at a much higher risk of CIN II or above than patients diagnosed with ASC-US. The current recommendation is for immediate colposcopically directed biopsy. High-risk HPV testing is not recommended as these patients have such a high positivity rate that the test is costly and not useful for triage, unlike patients with a diagnosis of ASC-US. Hysterectomy is overtreatment in the absence of a positive biopsy. However, these patients should not be returned to the pool of yearly screening as many of them will display biopsy results of CIN II or higher immediately after this Pap diagnosis.

A-11. (a) **Colposcopically directed biopsy**
The performance of a colposcopically directed biopsy only in those patients with a high-risk HPV result after a diagnosis of ASC-US means that patients with an ASC-US diagnosis who are HPV negative may return to the normal screening pool. This excludes about two-thirds of these patients from colposcopy at a substantial savings and at little to no risk of missing a significant lesion. There is no reason to perform a repeat HPV test as the results would be the same. An endometrial biopsy is not indicated as the endometrium is not the site in which these abnormal cells would develop. An FNA of the cervix is also not warranted in the absence of a cervical mass.

A-12. (c) **Return to yearly screening**
In this young population of patients, as many as 71 % of them would test positive for high-risk HPV, yet almost all of them would clear this infection on their own without treatment. These transient infections usually do not lead to cervical carcinoma in this young age group, and so these patients may return to yearly screening. Low-risk HPV testing is never justified. A colposcopically directed biopsy is also not justified in this young age group.

A-13. (c) **Colposcopy**
HGSIL patients under 20 should first be examined by colposcopy. Immediate LEEP procedures are never justified in these patients without colposcopic examination and biopsy of the cervix, due to the possibility that future fertility may be adversely affected by the procedure. High-risk HPV testing is not appropriate since the results would be costly and almost always positive. A return to yearly screening is also not appropriate without additional examination of the patient's cervix under colposcopy.

A-14. (a) **High-risk HPV testing at 12 months**
Either high-risk HPV testing at 12 months or repeat cytology at 6 and 12 months is acceptable for follow-up of a patient in this scenario. The return to yearly screening is not ideal as it may miss a rare lesion not found on biopsy. LEEP is too aggressive a procedure without a positive biopsy since it may compromise future fertility. A repeat colposcopy in 6 weeks would be costly and not useful in this scenario.

A-15. (a) **Specimen type (conventional or liquid based), ASC-H, and NILM**
The Bethesda System 2001 added to the report a comment on the specimen type, the "new" category of ASC-H, and the term "NILM," negative for intraepithelial lesion or malignancy. The terminology dividing ASC-US into reactive or favor LGSIL was dropped. Moderate dysplasia, carcinoma in situ, and CIN II were omitted in the previous Bethesda System and replaced by LGSIL and HGSIL. The 2001 version also dropped the terminology of "within normal limits." Thus, the best answer is a.

A-16. (e) **Educational Notes and Suggestions**
Clinical follow-up and guidance can be included in the Educational Notes and Suggestions section of the report. Here the pathologist can include suggestions, such as "Recommend colposcopically directed biopsy if clinically indicated," or other helpful indications for difficult or unusual cases. None of the other areas of the report are suggested for these types of comments.

A-17. (c) **5,000 cells minimum**
The 5,000 cells minimum is the number proposed by the Bethesda System for liquid-based preparations. Eight thousand to twelve thousand cells is the minimum number for conventional slides. 10 % coverage was an older suggested minimum for conventional slides. The number of endocervical and/or metaplastic

cells is a proposed guideline for the indication of the adequacy of sampling of the transformation zone. Samples which do not meet this guideline are not considered inadequate, but a comment indicating the presence or absence of this feature is noted. Also, any sample which contains abnormal cells, no matter what the cellularity, is never considered inadequate but is reported out as abnormal.

A-18. (**a**) **"Endocervical/transformation zone component is not identified.**"
In cases in which there is either a HGSIL or cancer, the comment on the presence or absence of endocervical component may be omitted. Depending on the severity of the lesion, any of the other comments might be appropriate.

A-19. (**a**) **Compare the 4× field appearance with reference images**.
The reference image methodology for conventional slides has been shown to have better reliability than using the earlier 10 % slide coverage criterion. It is impractical to count all of the cells on a conventional slide, and even counting 100 10× fields would not be appropriate since most conventional slides have thin and thick areas, unlike liquid-based preparations.

A-20. (**c**) **Endometrial cells in a woman ≥40 years of age**
The "Other" category in the Bethesda System 2001 is used only for endometrial cells in a woman older than 40. This General Categorization is intermediate between a NILM result and an Epithelial Cell Abnormality result, since some women over the age of forty with normal-appearing endometrial cells may require further follow-up. All of the other reporting interpretations listed are Epithelial Cell Abnormalities.

A-21. (**b**) **Notation if review is done with computer-assisted screening**, **specify the device and the result**
The category of Automated Review should only include a specification of the device used and the result. This is only included for those cases evaluated by automated screening. The remaining choices are for the ancillary testing – a, educational notes; c, or specimen adequacy – d.

A-22. (**a**) **Mosaic pattern of blood vessels**
The mosaic pattern of atypical blood vessels is considered a somewhat more serious pattern than the punctuation pattern of blood vessels. The dark iodine staining is indicative of normal tissue, and tissue following the normal contours of the cervix is considered a normal finding, as opposed to roughened or "humped up" areas of tissue.

A-23. (**a**) ***Trichomonas***
Trichomonas is likely to cause severe inflammation, reactive changes in the cervix, and the appearance of reddened "strawberry cervix" in which small punctate hemorrhages simulate the many seeds of a strawberry. These findings may interfere with an adequate colposcopic evaluation of the cervix. Lugol's solution (iodine) is often applied to the cervix during colposcopy. Atypical blood vessels are actually one of the abnormal findings in colposcopy that the clinician can identify so it will not be an obscuring factor.

A-24. (**a**) **Relatively fewer CIN 1 lesions go on to progress to carcinoma in situ or worse than CIN 2 or 3**.
Fewer CIN 1 lesions progress to CIS or worse compared to CIN 2 or 3 lesions. Most CIN 1 lesions regress even without treatment, and only about 10 % go on to become CIS. CIN 3, although it has the highest rate of persistence of all of these lesions, still has about one-third of the cases which regress. Thus, "a" is the best answer.

A-25. (**c**) **Cervista HPV HR**
Cervista HPV HR is the FDA-approved method to test for the presence of HR HPV subtypes, of those listed. "A" is incorrect as the correct name is "Hybrid Capture 2," "b" is incorrect as this is the name for the test which detects ONLY HPV 16 or 18, and "d" is incorrect.

A-26. (**c**) **Need to follow screening recommendations for their age group**
Even though vaccination with HPV vaccine is promising, long-term recommendations currently are for these women to continue to follow whatever screening recommendations exist for their age group. It is not recommended at this time that these women omit screening altogether. Young girls must receive the vaccine in order to develop immunity prior to sexual activity and exposure to the HPV antigen. If already exposed, the vaccine is not worthwhile. The low-risk subtypes of HPV do not appear to cause cancer, even though some of them may cause ASC-US and LGSIL. However, most of these less serious lesions are also caused by the high-risk viruses, especially 16 and 18.

A-27. **(b) Shows suspicious areas as intensely white in color**
The finding of intensely acetowhite areas on colposcopy is considered an abnormal finding. Dark brown would be the color of normal tissue with the iodine solution. Iodine-negative areas (yellow in color) would be abnormal using Lugol's solution. Although a gentle blotting of the cervix might be done prior to colposcopy if excessive discharge or mucous were present, one should not try to remove excessive material by wiping as this might discard valuable diagnostic material.

A-28. **(b) A cytobrush**
A cytobrush can be used in place of a Kevorkian curette to obtain material for an endocervical sample. Some studies have found a similar sensitivity to the curette with a higher specificity.

A-29. **(d) More than 75 % of the cells are obscured**.
The percentage of cells which should be obscured in order to call the specimen "unsatisfactory" is greater than 75 %. The percentage of cells obscured should be the determining factor, not the surface area of the slide. Nuclear detail and visualization are the determining factors in making this determination, so that even cells which are accompanied by a large number of inflammatory cells are not considered to be "obscured" as long as the nuclear detail, nuclear cytoplasmic ratios, etc., are sufficiently visible to evaluate for cytologic interpretation. Slides which have any abnormality (ASC-US or above) are never interpreted as "unsatisfactory," even in the presence of obscuring factors. In that case, the slide would be interpreted as "Satisfactory for evaluation. Quality indicator: Obscuring inflammation. ASC-US." An additional comment could be made that the interpretation may be limited by the obscuring inflammation.

A-30. **(b) Unsatisfactory: Specimen rejected (not processed) because the slide was broken**.
A slide which is broken into many small pieces cannot be adequately processed and repaired for microscopic review. When slides are rejected due to condition of breakage of the slide which is not reparable or due to an unlabeled sample, the report should reflect this and the reason the specimen was rejected. Thus, "B" is the correct answer. "A" is incorrect since the "many small pieces" would most likely not be something which could be repaired. "C" is incorrect since the specimen could not be processed. "D" is incorrect because the slide was called "Satisfactory" when it was really a rejected slide. There is a difference in the billing between slides which are examined and not processed and those which are processed, examined, and found to be unsatisfactory. The laboratory policy should attempt to define which slides could be repaired (e.g., broken into two pieces) and those which must be rejected in the laboratory policy for specimen rejection.

A-31. **(b) Are HIV positive, transplant patients, or on chemotherapy**
Patients who are HIV positive, on immunosuppressive therapy for organ transplant, or on chemotherapy are at a higher risk for the development of cervical carcinoma than patients whose immune status is intact. Thus, these patients should be on a more frequent screening surveillance than that dictated by their age. Patients older than 65 and post-hysterectomy for a noncancerous condition are at lower risk for cervical carcinoma. Patients who are younger than age 21 and have had HPV vaccination do not need to have additional screening compared to their peers. Patients between the ages of 21 and 29 have many HPV infections, but these are usually cleared by the patient's immune system, and they do not need a higher level of surveillance.

A-32. **(a) Refrain from douching or use of spermicides within 48 h of exam**.
The use of douching or spermicides may interfere with the accuracy of the cytologic examination. Therefore, the patient should refrain from their use for 48 h prior to the exam. The Pap test should not be canceled in the case of noncyclic bleeding, which is one of the most frequent symptoms of premalignant or malignant lesions. Patient preparations for the test should not include the restriction of fluids nor food as these do not make a difference in the findings.

A-33. **(a) ASC-US**
The only ASC-US cases which should be referred to colposcopy are those which are HR HPV positive. Only about one-third of ASC-US cases show HPV positivity for one or more of the high-risk types of HPV. By triaging the cases referred to colposcopy in this manner, substantial savings are created which offset the cost of testing all ASC-US for HR HPV. ASC-H, LGSIL, and ASC-US with + HR HPV results should all be referred for colposcopically directed biopsy.

A-34. (**b**) **Count the cells in 10 fields at 10× objective across the center to determine mean number of cells per field.**

Determining an average of the number of cells by counting the cells in 10 fields and comparing that to the minimum cellularity for the specific type of liquid-based preparation is the usual method of determining adequacy. It should be noted that in order to meet the minimum of at least 5,000 cells per slide, SurePath preparations need to have at least 118.3 cells per 10× objective (FN20), while ThinPrep preparations need to have 50.0 cells per 10× objective (FN20). Usually, cases are straightforward in this regard, and only borderline cases need to be counted to determine cellularity. Counting all of the cells on the slide is too time-consuming. Only conventional slides should be compared to the reference images, and using a digitalized image analysis device is unnecessary.

A-35. (**a**) **NILM, reactive cellular changes associated with radiation**

Radiation effect should be noted under reactive cellular change associated with radiation. These cells will often display cytomegaly without an increase in the nuclear/cytoplasmic ratio. Nuclear and cytoplasmic vacuolization are often seen, and the nuclei may also display nucleoli if repair coexists with the radiation effect. Polychromasia of the cytoplasm is also often seen. ASC-US is not often used along with radiation changes as slight nuclear enlargement is often seen as a result of the radiation changes. LGSIL is not properly defined as being caused by radiation, although the two interpretations might coexist. LGSIL does have an increase in nuclear/cytoplasmic ratio and thus does not fit into the interpretation of radiation effect.

A-36. (**a**) **The ability to test the remaining material in the vial for HR HPV**

One of the advantages of utilizing liquid-based preparations includes being able to test the remaining specimen in the vial for HR HPV without the patient having to return for another visit. Additionally, since the specimen is being co-tested, variances between specimens collected on different dates should be eliminated. The liquid-based preparations do not place more cells on the slide than conventional slides. Also, LBP does not eliminate organisms from the slide. HGSIL cases are not usually reduced, but often are increased to some degree with LBP. Thus, "a" is the correct answer.

A-37. (**d**) **p16**

p16(INK4a) is a staining methodology which uses monoclonal antibodies and stains neoplastic and carcinoma cells positively while not staining normal tissue. It has been used by some researchers as an adjunct to cytologic examination. Some cases of dysplasia and even carcinoma may not stain positive with this marker so negativity does not ensure a negative interpretation. Oil red O is used to detect lipids. Methyl green pyronin is used to detect RNA, and mucin stain is used to detect mucinous secretions. These histologic stains are not as useful as p16 in detecting neoplastic cells.

A-38. (**c**) **Performing colposcopy if the 16/18 result is positive**

In the case in which a patient who is older than 30 has a positive HR HPV test but the cytology is negative, a subtyping procedure to identify 16/18 subtypes may be performed. Since these are the two most common and significant subtypes in cervical neoplasia, a positive result would indicate the need for immediate colposcopic examination. This would triage the highest risk patients for an immediate biopsy under colposcopy and delay repeat co-testing for 1 year in those patients whose high-risk subtype was less likely to be involved in a neoplastic process. "A" would be the choice only if the 16/18 test were negative. "B" is incorrect since this would delay diagnosis and treatment in a high-risk group of patients. "D" is incorrect since this would delay diagnosis and treatment for 3 years in a high-risk group of patients.

A-39. (**c**) **50–75 %**

The criterion for the percentage of obscured cells to be interpreted as satisfactory but qualified by partially obscuring inflammation is between 50 and 75 %. Lower percentages of obscured cells such as 5–25 % or 25–50 % are not qualified, but the inflammation may be reported as "present" in such cases. Slides with greater than 75 % of the cells obscured are considered unsatisfactory.

A-40. (**d**) "**Unsatisfactory for evaluation. Specimen processed and examined, but unsatisfactory for evaluation because of… (specify reason)**"

A distinction should be made between those slides which are not processed but are rejected and those which are processed and examined but determined to be unsatisfactory after microscopic evaluation. Additionally, the reason for the unsatisfactory condition of the slide must be included (obscuring inflammation, air drying, etc.). The most complete comment therefore is "d."

1.5 Answers and Discussion of Image-Based Questions 41–70

A-41. (**b**) **Reactive cellular changes associated with radiation**

"Reactive cellular changes associated with radiation" is the correct terminology for this lesion. Note the enlarged cells which do not have an increased N/C ratio. Additionally, the cells show cytoplasmic vacuolization consistent with treatment by ionizing radiation therapy. These changes may last for decades after treatment. The other choices would not be suitable. Both LGSIL and post-radiation dysplasia are not warranted by the minimal changes in N/C ratio seen in this image. The cells are also not consistent with squamous metaplasia (being too large to be metaplastic) or repair (which has nucleoli and streaming cytoplasm unlike the cells seen here). Thus, b is the best answer.

A-42. (**a**) **Negative for intraepithelial lesion or malignancy**. **Atrophy**.

These cells are showing a marked immaturity consistent with an atrophic pattern seen in postmenopausal women. Many of the cells are small and rounded, and some are slightly polygonal and slightly increased in size. These correspond to parabasal cells and some lower level intermediate cells. There are no cells with the features of repair: nucleoli, cytoplasmic streaming, and hypochromatic nuclei. Although there is one cell which is quite small and a deep pink color, this cell is not diagnostic of parakeratosis (PK). For PK, one would expect to see more PK cells, a more thin transparent squamous type cytoplasm, and these cells are often found in plaques. Atrophic slides may show occasional small deep pink cells which are actually immature squamous cells which have not matured appropriately. Hyperkeratosis is the presence of large numbers of annucleated squamous cells which generally stain pink, light orange, or yellow. Like PK, HK occurs on the uppermost surface of the tissue and is considered a benign protective response.

A-43. (**e**) **LSIL**

"LSIL" stands for "low-grade squamous intraepithelial lesion" and is the preferred term to use when reporting. All of the other choices – HPV, mild dysplasia, CIN I, and slight dysplasia – are roughly equivalent terms and have all been consolidated into the term "LSIL" by the newest Bethesda System reporting terminology.

A-44. (**e**) **Cellular changes consistent with herpes simplex virus**

The appropriate terminology to use for the reporting of herpes according to the newest Bethesda System is "e." Although choice "C" is also a virus, CMV or cytomegalovirus is usually not multinucleated and usually has a very large intranuclear body which takes up the entire area of the nucleus. The large inclusion body gives the cell the appearance of an "owl's eye," and this description does not match the multinucleated, ground glass nuclei seen in the images. Thus, the only correct response which matches the reporting terminology given by the Bethesda System is "e."

A-45. (**d**) **Fungal organisms morphologically consistent with Candida species**

The Bethesda System of reporting uses the above terminology to indicate one of the several types of Candida species that may be present on Pap smears. As can be seen in this image, the common way for Candida to present is as an eosinophilic to indeterminate staining parallel strand which often pierces the squamous cells. This can give the appearance seen here, sometimes called "strand of pearls" or "shish kabob." On electron microscopy, the cells are actually pierced by the fungus. In addition to this pattern, other *Candida* species may show differing patterns. *Geotrichum candidum* shows a 90° branching angle; *Torulopsis glabrata* shows only the spore form without hyphae. The other terms used in this question do not follow the suggested terminology given by TBS.

A-46. (**b**) **Location B**

The exact anatomic site of the transformation zone varies between women, and varies over the course of a woman's lifetime, depending on hormonal states, pregnancy, etc. However, of the choices given, the external opening of the endocervical canal is the most likely site of the squamocolumnar junction. The sampling of this site is important as it is the most likely location for the development of squamous neoplasia. "A" indicates the vaginal canal, and the transformation zone is almost never seen in this area. "C" is the vaginal fornix which is actually a rather poor site from which to collect a Pap sample since the cells collected are often degenerated. Additionally, endocervical or squamous metaplastic cells usually do not originate in this site. "D" shows the internal endocervical os. Samples from this area would include endocervical epithelium and possibly lower uterine segment tissue, but would not include squamous mucosa. In order to be an ideal sample, the Pap sample should include well-preserved adequate numbers of squamous cells and endocervical and/or squamous metaplastic cells.

A-47. (**c**) **Image C (The image in C displays *Trichomonas*.)**
The colposcopic view of the cervix is pathognomonic for infection with *Trichomonas*. These organisms are usually found in abundance and may be accompanied by marked inflammation or, occasionally, with only a few inflammatory cells. Their presence on liquid-based preparations is often accompanied by a "busy" background, and Leptothrix may occasionally accompany the organism. The typical appearance on colposcopy, "strawberry cervix," is caused by the occurrence of many small red hemorrhages on the cervix and is accompanied by a thin greenish discharge. The other images are "A," chronic follicular cervicitis; "B," herpes simplex; and "D," HPV infection (LSIL).

A-48. (**d**) **Hyperkeratosis**
The colposcopic image displays a whitish, irregular, raised area. Areas such as this seen during colposcopy and prior to the application of an acetic acid solution are often associated with hyperkeratosis (HK), a benign protective reaction of the cervical epithelium. In this reaction, annucleated squamous cells accumulate on the surface of the cervix and provide additional protection for the underlying tissue. HK may be accompanied by parakeratosis (PK) which is also a benign protective reaction. However, these two conditions may also accompany underlying neoplastic lesions. Trichomonas infection will display a strawberry cervix (see previous question), *Candida* infection may display a whitish thick discharge and general reddening of the cervix, and follicular cervicitis has no particular colposcopic appearance. Areas of leukoplakia (white appearing prior to use of acetic acid) may be associated with HK and/or PK, condyloma, LSIL, or even a keratinizing squamous cell carcinoma may be found underlying the leukoplakia.

A-49. (**a**) **HSIL**
Of the answers given, HSIL is the most likely choice. The area seen on colposcopy is bright white with a distinct raised edge. The acetowhite area is denser appearing than in LSIL lesions, and the surface appears a duller white than LSIL due to the increased numbers of nuclei present in HSIL. Atrophy would appear as thin, friable epithelium without acetowhitening or punctation. Normal epithelium should be pink, smooth, glistening, and without acetowhitening. Cervicitis would be indicated by a reddening of the epithelium without acetowhite areas.

A-50. (**d**) **Parakeratosis**
Of the choices given, whitish plaques appearing on colposcopy prior to the application of acetic acid would most likely correspond to parakeratosis. This benign protective reaction cytologically appears as miniature superficial squamous cells: small cells with polygonal thin cytoplasm, small pyknotic nuclei, and pink or orange cytoplasm. Although HSIL might appear as whitish plaques on colposcopy, the cells seen do not correspond with HSIL, being too small without a high N/C ratio. Squamous metaplasia is not a reason for white plaques, and the cells are too small with small nuclei inconsistent with squamous metaplasia. Endocervical mucosa also does not show white plaques and endocervical cells are not seen.

A-51. (**b**) **Image B (image of invasive squamous cell carcinoma)**
The colposcopic image shows a cervix with an exophytic mass protruding from the external cervical os. This would be most consistent with the cytologic image of hyperchromatic, high N/C ratio cells with very irregular chromatin. Some blood is also visible in the background. Image A is showing infection by *Actinomyces* with starburst rays extending from a mass of bacteria. C shows the typical double contoured mass of endometrial cells common during the "exodus" of menses. D illustrates "shift in vaginal flora" with many coccobacilli in the background and coating the cells. Thus, the best answer is b.

A-52. (**c**) **This image displays the most frequent site of lesions found on the cervix.**
This histologic picture shows the squamocolumnar junction, the site of the most common squamous neoplastic lesions in the cervix. This junction may be quite well defined or may be the site of squamous metaplastic cells forming a transition between the highly protective layered squamous epithelium and the single layer of endocervical cells. Deeper areas of the endocervical glands are commonly noticed in this junction, as seen here. Dysplasia is not noted in this biopsy. Invasive squamous cell carcinoma is also not present. The typical back-to-back glands of adenocarcinoma are not present. Thus, the best answer is C.

A-53. (**d**) **The transformation zone, at arrow, is seen in its entirety.**
When performing a colposcopic examination, the clinician should make sure that the border area between the endocervical epithelium and the squamous epithelium can be completely visualized (transformation

zone – TZ). If a portion of the junction is not visible because it goes into the endocervical canal, the clinician may have to try to visualize it using instruments or the exam may not be considered satisfactory. Lesions may occur within the canal at the TZ and, thus, this area must be completely examined. The squamous mucosa of the cervix is found at this border, but cannot be entirely visualized, since it extends outward and down into the fornices and the vagina. Additionally, mature squamous epithelium is not as frequent a site of neoplasia as the TZ. The endocervical epithelium also cannot be completely visualized as it extends up to the internal cervical os. Also that area is not as frequent a site of neoplasia as the TZ. Finally, the vaginal epithelium is not usually entirely observed on colposcopy and is not the most frequent site of squamous neoplasia.

A-54. (**d**) **A cocklebur**

This deep reddish, starburst-like structure, often seen surrounded by inflammatory cells, is most frequently found in the gynecologic samples of pregnant women. However, it has not been shown to be diagnostic of any condition or associated with loss of the pregnancy. These usually measure from 50 to 100 μm in diameter and can occasionally be found in nonpregnant patients. As noted, this does not have an association with impending miscarriage. It is not a syncytiotrophoblast, which is a multinucleated cell derived from placental tissue and which may indicate loss of a pregnancy. The image is not of a small cell carcinoma which would have hyperchromatic nuclei, irregular chromatin patterns, and show very high N/C ratios.

A-55. (**d**) **Suture contaminants**

These linear, rectangular structures are rarely found in gynecologic samples but might be found in a postoperative situation. Note that the width of these structures is uniform, but their length is not. Often, as here, they may be seen in association with inflammatory cells. These structures are too uniform and rectangular to be considered for a diagnosis of *Candida*. The pseudohyphae of *Candida* are usually light pink, have small oval spore forms, and resemble "balloon dogs" with a pinching in of the outer wall of the pseudohyphae adjacent to branching. *Actinomyces* is much thinner than these structures and presents with a lavender starburst effect radiating out of a colony of dusty gray coccobacilli. Muscle fibers can occasionally be seen but are generally bright orange or deep pink, show cross striations, and have nuclei. These structures do not have cross striations.

A-56. (**d**) **10 endocervical and/or metaplastic cells must be present in any configuration**.

The criteria above were put into place with the latest Bethesda System reporting guidelines. A, adequate numbers of squamous cells present, is a criteria for adequacy but is not directly related to sampling the TZ. Choice B, endocervical cells, does not also mention the presence of squamous metaplastic cells which may also be used to determine TZ sampling. Squamous metaplastic cells alone are mentioned in C, and the presence of endocervical cells is omitted. Only answer D fulfills the correct criteria.

A-57. (**d**) **Satisfactory for evaluation**. **Epithelial cell abnormality**. **LSIL**. **A more serious lesion cannot be ruled out**.

Even at low power, several highly atypical cells with increased N/C ratio, hyperchromatic nuclei, and neoplastic features can be identified in the slide. While the suboptimal situation with the "holes" in the filter would normally exclude this ThinPrep from being adequate, the presence of these clearly abnormal cells creates a situation in which the abnormality must be reported. Thus, the most appropriate diagnosis is D. If it were not for the abnormal cells, A would be the best answer. Since abnormal cells are on the slide, B cannot be the correct answer. C is incorrect also since it does not mention the abnormal cells. If there are abnormal cells, even if they cannot be entirely specifically diagnosed due to lack of cells or obscuring factors, the slide can never be called unsatisfactory.

A-58. (**d**) **Satisfactory**. **Quality indicator**: **Blood obscuring from 50 to 75 % of the cells**. **HSIL**.

The cells seen in the image at about 1:00 show enlarged nuclei, coarse chromatin, and an increased N/C ratio. Thus, even though otherwise this case would be called unsatisfactory, the abnormal cells preclude reporting it as unsatisfactory. Unsatisfactory due to blood obscuring more than 75 % of the cells is incorrect due to the abnormal cells present. B, C, and E are also incorrect for the same reason.

A-59. (**c**) **Satisfactory for evaluation**. **Other**: **Endometrial cells in a woman over 40**

These cells are endometrial cells. The inset shows a compact cluster and the larger image shows endometrial stromal cells. Individually, stromal cells cannot be differentiated from small histiocytes, but finding a loose cluster of them in a patient with the appropriate history can lead to the appropriate diagnosis. Additionally, the clinical history of this woman is important since being over forty qualifies her for the diagnosis of "endometrial cells in a woman over 40." This addition to the Bethesda System reporting was made to help identify women who may be at risk for endometrial abnormalities, even if the shed cells appear normal. A and B do not mention the endometrial cells which is incorrect in this case. D is incorrect since this finding requires that the slide be sent to the pathologist for evaluation, which excludes the slide from being called unsatisfactory.

A-60. (**a**) **Satisfactory for evaluation. NILM.**
This image contains many more than the minimum 50 squamous cells, making the slide numerically adequate for evaluation. Thus, B is not correct. C mentions endocervical and metaplastic cells which would not be expected since the woman is post-hysterectomy. D is also incorrect since the circle contains more than 50 squamous cells.

A-61. (**b**) **Treat with a 1:4 solution of 3% glacial acetic acid and CytoLyt, centrifuge, decant, rerun.**
This image displays the so-called rusty ring which may be present in ThinPrep slides if there is a large amount of blood in the specimen. The hemosiderin and blood tends to gather around the outer edge of the filter and clog the central portion of the filter, resulting in inadequate cellularity in the center of the slide. Grossly bloody specimens may be centrifuged with a 1:4 solution of glacial acetic acid and CytoLyt, decanted, resuspended in CytoLyt, and rerun on the processor. This will complete the lysing of the blood and can convert an inadequate specimen into one that is sufficiently cellular. None of the other selections will remedy this appearance.

A-62. (**c**) **HMB-45**
The appearance of these cells, along with the dark pigment, suggests a melanoma. The best stain of those listed would be HMB-45, which is an immunohistochemical stain showing both sensitivity and specificity for melanomas. Only a few other rare tumors showing evidence of melanogenesis, such as pigmented schwannoma and clear cell sarcoma, are known to stain positively for HMB-45. Mucicarmine stain would be useful in cases of mucin-producing adenocarcinoma. The pigmentation present does not suggest an adenocarcinoma. Hale's colloidal iron has been used to differentiate chromophobe renal cell carcinoma as it reacts positively for acid mucopolysaccharides. Again the pigmentation argues against this diagnosis. pCEA is positive for many colorectal cancers and other tumors of the GI tract, as well as tumors of the lung, ovary, and pancreas. Again the morphology of these cells does not suggest any of these primaries. CD117 is often used as a special stain to detect the c-kit gene, found in some leukemias and gastrointestinal stromal tumors. Thus, the best answer is c.

A-63. (**a**) **Lobular carcinoma of the breast**
These cells are small, with high N/C ratios and nuclear molding. The additional information about the "targetoid" mucin droplets in some cells also helps to confirm a metastatic lesion derived from a lobular carcinoma of the breast. Colonic adenocarcinoma often shows much larger cells with an elongated cytoplasmic and nuclear shape. A squamous cell carcinoma of the lung also would not likely have the nuclear molding seen in these images. Finally, a serous cystadenocarcinoma of the ovary most likely would have very large cells, with large clear cytoplasmic vacuoles and macronucleoli.

A-64. (**d**) **Cotton fibers**
These fibers, most likely from a cotton-tipped collection device, are occasionally found as contaminants in a gynecologic slide. The fibers are not of fungal origin, being much wider than *Candida* pseudohyphae would be. Although mucormycosis can display very large and variable hyphae, these structures are not consistent with the extremely variable width and curvilinear appearance of that group of fungi. This leaves a nonbiologic origin for the structures. Cytobrush fibers may occasionally be found in a smear, but they are of a uniform size and do not have the tapering ends and slightly varying widths seen here. Finally, mucous stands have areas of thick and thin widths even dissipating out into the background and are not as well defined as these images appear. Thus, "cotton fibers" is the best answer.

A-65. (**d**) **Lubricant artifact**
The abundant areas of purplish amorphous material are lubricant artifact. As can be seen, sometimes these areas might be so numerous or thick as to interfere with the interpretation of the slide. Lysed blood will usually have a light blue or pinkish granular appearance. Mucinous discharge would usually stain pinkish on Pap stain and would not show the dense, thick purplish appearance seen here. While *Actinomyces* can have a purplish appearance, there is no starburst appearance of the organisms protruding from colonies of coccobacilli. A rectovaginal fistula might have a variety of appearances including contaminating fecal material (vegetable cells, meat fibers, inflammation,

etc.) as well as any abnormal cells that might be the cause of the fistula. Thus, the homogenous, amorphous purplish appearance seen here is most consistent with lubricant artifact.

A-66. (**d**) **Unsatisfactory, over 75 % of the cells are obscured by inflammation**.
This very thick, obscured slide is the result of severe inflammation in a conventional preparation. The correct reporting method is to mention the cause of the lack of adequacy, as well as the percentage (25–50 % obscured is quality indicator, and over 75 % obscured is unsatisfactory) of the cells which are unable to be adequately evaluated. Thus, this specimen is not adequate for evaluation, eliminating answers a and b. Answer c is incorrect since it is not blood but inflammation which is obscuring the cells. Additionally, the format of answer c is incorrect.

A-67. (**c**) **Part of a plant**
This puzzle-shaped, orange-staining structure is consistent with the appearance of a plant astrosclereid. These structures are derived from the sclerenchyma of plants and give rigidity to the mature plant parts. They are occasionally seen in conventional slides and should not be confused with human cells. Pollen varies somewhat depending on the plant from which it originates, but it is most usually rounded, often with dimpling or protrusions on its surface. Staining varies from yellow to orange. Ova are usually oval in shape, not the peculiar interlocking puzzle shape seen here. Fungi are usually smaller, show hyphae and or spores, and also do not have this particular shape.

A-68. (**d**) **Glove powder**
Starch crystals such as these are not infrequently seen in cytology specimens. They show somewhat refractile irregular small structures which, when viewed under polarized light, display a distinctive Maltese cross appearance. The variation in size and the central star-like pattern are not consistent with any of the fungal organisms listed (*Blastomyces dermatitidis*, *Cryptococcus neoformans*, or *Coccidioides immitis*). Psammoma bodies are calcified, concentrically laminated structures which may occur in benign conditions but which have also been associated with carcinomas of the ovary and thyroid. They generally stain reddish and they may vary somewhat in size, being generally larger than the starch crystals seen here.

A-69. (**c**) ***Enterobius vermicularis* ova**
The ova of *Enterobius vermicularis* may occasionally be seen in gynecologic specimens, and it represents a contaminant from the intestine. The ova are generally oval in shape with an asymmetric flattening at the smaller end of the egg. Sometimes the embryonic organism may be visible in the egg, as seen here. This organism should not be confused with a keratinized squamous cell, as the shape is not round to polygonal. Also, squamous metaplasia is usually not keratinized. Pollen is usually reddish to orange and is generally more round. A plant cell would show the cell walls characteristic of cells of this origin.

A-70. (**c**) **Pseudoparakeratosis (microglandular hyperplasia**)
This finding is composed of streams of degenerated endocervical cells usually seen within areas of endocervical mucous. Since these cells may often stain pink to orange and the degenerated cuboidal cells are quite small, they slightly resemble parakeratotic (PK) cells and have been called pseudoparakeratosis. Unlike true PK, however, the cells often have an eccentric nucleus, which is dark but not truly pyknotic. Also, they lack the polygonal cell shape and thin transparent cytoplasm of true PK. Hyperkeratosis is also not a good choice as HK cells have no nucleus unlike those seen here. Dyskeratosis is a feature associated with HPV infection. The cells are small but usually stain bright orange, have dense rounded cytoplasm, and have opaque, enlarged pyknotic nuclei. Squamous metaplasia is also not a good choice as those cells are derived from squamous epithelium, are round to polygonal, and have slightly enlarged nuclei. The degeneration apparent in these cells is quite characteristic of microglandular hyperplasia, and the condition is associated with both oral contraception and pregnancy.

Reading List

American Society for Colposcopy and Cervical Pathology. Practice management – cervix – colposcopy, Originally developed 2002-2004, most recent update, 2010 [online]. Available from: http://www.asccp.org/practicemanagement/cervix/colposcopy/tabid/7506/default.aspx. [cited 1 May 2012].

Clinical and Laboratory Standards Institute (formerly NCCLS). Cervicovaginal cytology based on the Papanicolaou technique; approved guideline. 3rd ed. CLSI document GP15-A3, Clinical and Laboratory Standards Institute, Wayne, PA. 2008; 28(28).

College of American Pathologists. Cytopathology Checklist. 2010; CYP.07439.

Cytyc. ThinPrep 2000 operators manual. Boxborough: 1995.

DeMay TM. Hyperchromatic crowded groups. Am J Clin Pathol. 2000;114 Suppl 1:S36–43.

DeMay RM. The Pap test. Chicago: ASCP Press; 2005.

DeMay RM. The art & science of cytopathology. 2nd ed. Chicago: ASCP Press; 2012.

Saslow D, Solomon D, Lawson HW, Killackey M, Kulasingam SL, Cain J, et al. American Cancer Society, American Society for Colposcopy and Cervical Pathology, and American Society for Clinical Pathology screening guidelines for the prevention and early detection of cervical cancer. CA Cancer J Clin. 2012; 62(3):147–72.

Solomon D, Nayar R. The Bethesda system for reporting cervical cytology. 2nd ed. New York: Springer; 2004.

SurePath® Collection Product Insert [online] Burlington: TriPath Imaging. 2011. Available from: http://www.bd.com/tripath/downloads/surepath_ctgc/779-07084-00_Rev_B_PI_SP.pdf. [cited 5 July 2012].

Wilbur DC, Henry MR. College of American pathologists practical guide to gynecologic cytopathology: morphology, management, and molecular methods. Northfield: CAP Press; 2008.

2 Human Papillomavirus (HPV) Infection and Cervical Lesions

Chengquan Zhao, Huaitao Yang, Marilee Means, and Walid E. Khalbuss

Contents

2.1 Tables and Summary

Table 2.1 HPV infection

The most common sexually transmitted disease (STD) in the USA estimated 20 million currently infected and > 6 million new infections per year. Approximately 12,710 women were diagnosed with and 4,290 women died of cervical cancer in 2011.
Both women and men can acquire HPV infection by genital contact.
Most women clear their HPV infection within 1–2 years.
HPV is also associated with squamous cell carcinoma of the anogenital region and head and neck region.
LSIL is related to a transient HPV infection with little risk for oncogenesis, whereas most HSILs are associated with HPV persistence and hence significant potential for progression to invasive cervical carcinoma.
HPV testing was introduced in the screening and management guidelines for cervical carcinoma as a primary test with Pap test cytology (co-testing for woman 30 years and oldest) or as a reflex test in cases with atypical squamous lesion of undermined significance (ASC-US).

C. Zhao, MD (✉)
Department of Pathology, Magee-Womens Hospital,
University of Pittsburgh Medical Center,
300 Halket Street, Pittsburgh, PA 15213, USA
e-mail: zhaoc@upmc.edu

H. Yang, MD, PhD
Department of Pathology, University of Pittsburgh Medical Center,
200 Lothrop Street, Pittsburgh, PA 15213, USA
e-mail: yangh2@upmc.edu

M. Means, PhD, SCT(ASCP)
School of Health Professions, University of Kansas Medical Center,
3901 Rainbow Blvd., Mail Stop 4048,
Kansas City, KS 66160, USA
e-mail: mmeans@kumc.edu

W.E. Khalbuss, MD, PhD, FIAC
Director of Cytology and Cytopathology Fellowship Program,
University of Pittsburgh Medical Center Shadyside Hospital,
5150 Centre Avenue, 2, Suite 201,
Pittsburgh, PA 15232, USA
e-mail: khalbussw2@upmc.edu

W.E. Khalbuss, M. Means (eds.), *Gynecological and Breast Cytopathology Board Review and Self-Assessment*,
DOI 10.1007/978-1-4614-7270-4_2,

Table 2.2 Molecular details of HPV

It is a non-enveloped, non-encapsulated icosahedral 55-nm DNA virus.
It consists of a circular double-stranded DNA genome of 7,900 base pairs.
HPV has coding regions (8 early and 2 late) and noncoding regions.
Six early genes that are associated with DNA replication regulatory functions and activation of the lytic life cycle (E1, E2, E4, E5, E6, and E7).
Late (L) genes that code for capsule proteins are L1 (90 %, major protein) and L2 (10 %, minor protein).
More than 150 HPV types gf more than 40 types can infect the genitical area of males and females.
HPV types with anogenital infection are divided into two groups low-risk HPV (LR HPV) and oncogenic or high-risk HPV (HR HPV).
HR HPV types are associated with cervical cancer squamous cell carcinoma adenocarcinoma.
Most LSIL (70–80 %) and almost all HSIL (> 90 %) are positive for HR HPV testing.
More than a dozen of HPV types can cause cervical cancers with type 16 and 18 together accounting for about 70 % of cervical cancer.

Table 2.3 Schematic of HPV

HPV DNA genome of HPV is divided into three major regions: early (E), late (L), and a long control region or noncoding region (LCR)
Genes for early viral function (E1, E2, E4, E5, E6, E7) code for viral replication processes
Genes for late viral function (L1 and L2) code for capsid proteins
E1 involves in DNA replication and maintenance of the viral episome
E4 involves in assembly of virus and cytokeratin interactions (causes halo morphology)
E6 binds and degrades p53 (oncogenic) and causes immortalization of cells
E7 binds and deregulates pRb (oncogenic) and causes immortalization of cells
Only E6 and E7 are oncogenic

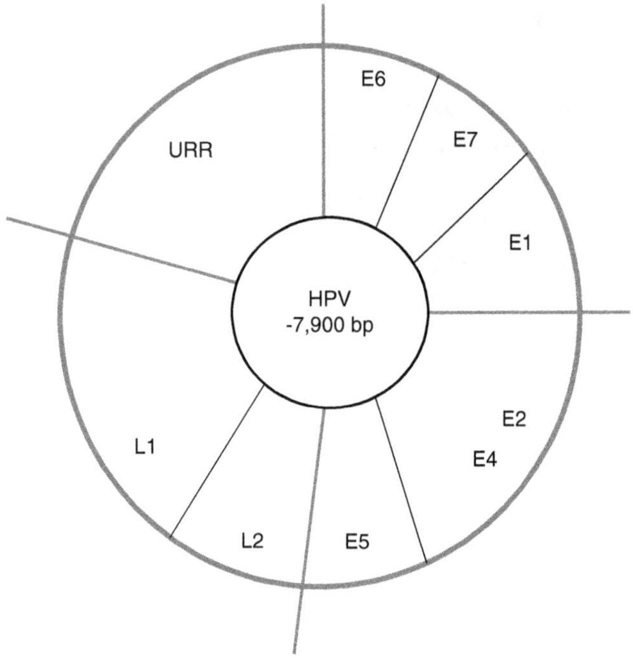

2.2 Text-Based Questions 1–43

Q-1. Which of the following statements is correct about koilocytes?
- (a) Koilocytes are pathognomonic of a permissive human papillomavirus (HPV) infection.
- (b) Koilocytes are mature squamous cells, usually of the intermediate type.
- (c) The nuclei of koilocytes contain mature viral particles.
- (d) Halos are due to a collapse of the cytoplasmic filaments or cytoplasmic necrosis.
- (e) All of the above.

Q-2. All of the following are true about human papillomavirus (HPV) except:
- (a) The HPVs are small, circular, double-stranded DNA viruses.
- (b) Open reading frames (ORF) E6 and E7 play a role in cell transformation. Their products regulate events in the cell cycle.
- (c) E6 protein reacts with p53.
- (d) E7 protein reacts with the p16 gene.
- (e) All of the above.

Q-3. Which is NOT correct about the role of HPV in the carcinogenesis of cervical lesions?
- (a) In most young women, the presence of the virus is transient.
- (b) In most pregnant women, the presence of the virus is not transient.
- (c) Only persisting infections with viruses of HR HPV type lead to precancerous lesions.
- (d) In the USA, the presence of HPV, mainly of high-risk type, could be documented in nearly half of precancerous lesions.
- (e) All of the above.

Q-4. Which is NOT true about HR & HPV infection?
- (a) Only a small percentage of the women with persisting infection develop precancerous lesions.
- (b) The frequency of documented viral presence is not related to age.
- (c) The presence of HPV in sexually active young women increases with the number of sexual partners.
- (d) A nonsexual mode of viral infection may exist.
- (e) The carcinogenic role of HR HPVs can only take place under certain conditions, such as immunodeficiency/immunosuppression.

Q-5. Which statement about LSIL is *not* correct?
- (a) LSIL is encountered in approximately 2–3 % of all Pap samples in liquid-based cytology.
- (b) LSIL is caused by a large number of different HPVs, which include low-risk and high-risk HPVs.
- (c) More than 70 % cervical LSIL Pap samples are HR HPV positive.
- (d) More than 10 % HR HPV-positive cervical LSILs have a follow-up biopsy diagnosis of CIN2/3.
- (e) None of the above.

Q-6. Which of the following statements is correct about HSIL?
- (a) HSIL is an intraepithelial lesion that is encountered in about 0.5 % of all Pap samples.
- (b) HR HPV is found in >90 % of women with cervical HSIL.
- (c) HR HPV is found in >80 % of women with vaginal HSIL.
- (d) More than 60 % of HR HPV-positive cervical HSIL cases have a follow-up biopsy diagnosis of CIN2/3.
- (e) All of the above.

Q-7. Which is correct about US women with negative imaged liquid-based cytology and positive HR HPV results?
- (a) CIN1 is seen in histopathologic follow-up in about 5 % of patients.
- (b) CIN3 is seen in histopathologic follow-up in about 5 % of patients.
- (c) CIN1 is seen in histopathologic follow-up in about 30 % of patients.
- (d) CIN2+ is seen in histopathologic follow-up in about 2 % of patients.
- (e) None of the above.

Q-8. Which is correct in women with ASC-US cytology results?
- (a) The overall prevalence rates of HR HPV are 30–50 %.
- (b) The overall prevalence rates of HPV 16 and HPV 18 are about 10 %.
- (c) Genotypes 16 and/or 18 are detected in 8 % of women without CIN.
- (d) Genotypes 16 and/or 18 are detected in 61 % of women with CIN3 or worse.
- (e) All of the above.

Q-9. Which is correct about ASC-H and HR HPV?
- (a) HR HPV is detected in 5 % of patients with ASC-H.
- (b) HR HPV is detected in 10 % of patients with ASC-H.
- (c) HR HPV is detected in 30 % of patients with ASC-H.
- (d) HR HPV is detected in 50 % or more of patients with ASC-H.
- (e) None of the above.

Q-10. Which is correct about ASC-H and HR HPV DNA testing?
(a) The HR HPV-positive rate in women <40 years is about 30 %.
(b) The HR HPV-positive rate in women <40 years is higher than in women 40 years and older.
(c) The HR HPV-positive rate in women <40 years is lower than in women 40 years and older.
(d) The HR HPV-positive rate in women <40 years is equal to that in women 40 years and older.
(e) None of the above.

Q-11. Which is correct about ASC-H histopathologic follow-up?
(a) CIN2/3 is identified in 0–10 % of HR HPV-positive women.
(b) CIN2/3 is identified in 10–20 % of HR HPV-positive women.
(c) CIN2/3 is identified in 20–30 % of HR HPV-positive women.
(d) CIN2/3 is identified in 30–50 % of HR HPV-positive women.
(e) None of the above.

Q-12. What percentage of women in the US will have HPV infection during their lifetime?
(a) 10–20 %
(b) 20–40 %
(c) 30–50 %
(d) 70–80 %
(e) 90–100 %

Q-13. All of the following are true about precancerous lesions induced by HR HPV of uterine cervix except:
(a) They display predictable behavior.
(b) They may vanish without treatment.
(c) They may persist without major changes for many years.
(d) Invasive cancer may follow any type of precursor lesion.
(e) Most invasive cancers are derived from a high-grade lesion.

Q-14. Which of the following are correct about HPV infection and men?
(a) HPV is passed on through genital contact—most often during vaginal and anal sex.
(b) HPV may also be passed on during oral sex.
(c) Most men who get HPV (of any type) never develop any symptoms or health problems.
(d) About 1 % of sexually active men in the US have genital warts at any one time.
(e) Gay and bisexual men (who have sex with other men) are about 17 times more likely to develop anal cancer than men who only have sex with women.
(f) All are correct.

Q-15. "Karyomegaly" is an indication of HPV infection. It is one of the classification and morphologic features of neoplastic cells in cervicovaginal smears. All of the following are true about karyomegaly *except*:
(a) It is the enlargement of nuclei occurring in superficial, intermediate, or parabasal squamous cells with morphologically normal cytoplasm.
(b) The cytoplasm may show cytolysis during the second half of the menstrual cycle.
(c) It is not seen in inflammatory and regenerative processes.
(d) Karyomegaly with significant nuclear hyperchromasia is seen in dysplastic (dyskaryotic) cells.
(e) The increase in nuclear sizes is best verified by comparing the nuclear size between an atypical cell and adjacent normal cells.

Q-16. Which of the following is true about HPV clearance?
(a) 100 % of HPV infections will be cleared at 5 years.
(b) 50–60 % of HPV infections will be cleared at 2 years.
(c) 80–90 % of HPV infections will be cleared at 2 years.
(d) 50 % of HPV infections will be cleared at 1 year.
(e) None of the above.

Q-17. All of the following are true about koilocytes except:
(a) Koilocytosis is HPV-type dependent.
(b) Nuclei are enlarged, hyperchromatic, single, double, or, rarely, multiple.
(c) Nuclei are surrounded by large, sharply demarcated perinuclear clear zones or halos.
(d) Nuclei are usually smudged and homogeneous.
(e) Koilocytes are mature squamous cells, usually of the intermediate type.

Q-18. Which cancer is not HPV-related?
(a) Vaginal
(b) Vulvar
(c) Anal
(d) Penile
(e) Oropharyngeal
(f) All of the above cancers are HPV related

Q-19. What are the risk factors for cervical cancer?
(a) HPV infection
(b) Other STDs
(c) Smoking
(d) Multiparity
(e) All of the above

Q-20. Which is correct about HR HPV testing and a Pap test finding of AGC (atypical glandular cells)?
(a) HR HPV + rates are highest in women with coexisting ASC-US and AGC.
(b) HR HPV + rates are highest in women with coexisting AGC and HSIL.
(c) HR HPV + rates are highest in women with AGC-EC (endocervical).
(d) HR HPV + rates are highest in women with AGC-EM (endometrial).
(e) HR HPV + rates are highest in women with AGC-NOS.

Q-21. Which one is not an FDA-approved HPV detection method?
(a) Hybrid Capture 2 HPV test
(b) Cervista HPV 16/18 test
(c) Cervista HPV HR test
(d) Cobas 4,800 HPV test
(e) APTIMA HPV assay
(f) All above tests are FDA approved

Q-22. In what circumstance(s) is high-risk (oncogenic) HPV DNA testing appropriate based on the ASCCP guidelines?
(a) Routine cervical cancer screening in conjunction with cervical cytology (dual testing or co-testing) for women aged 30 years
(b) Initial triage management of women aged 21 years or older with a cytological result of atypical squamous cells of undetermined significance (ASC-US)
(c) Initial triage management of postmenopausal women with a cytological result of low-grade squamous intraepithelial lesion (LSIL)
(d) Post-colposcopy management of women aged 21 years or more with initial cytological results of ASC-US or LSIL (when the initial colposcopy does not identify a high-grade lesion)
(e) All of the above

Q-23. All of the following are true about LSIL except:
(a) Squamous cell carcinoma may develop in less than 0.3 % of women with LSIL.
(b) 70 to 80 % women with LSIL Pap tests are HR HPV positive.
(c) 5 % have CIN2–3 on subsequent biopsy.
(d) Spontaneous regression is seen in approximately 80 % of cases.
(e) Progression to CIN2–3 is seen in 10–20 % of cases.

Q-24. Which is *not* true about HPV vaccine?
(a) Cervarix is made by GlaxoSmithKline.
(b) Gardasil is made by Merck.
(c) Both vaccines are very effective against diseases caused by HPV types 16 and 18.
(d) Both vaccines are very effective against diseases caused by HPV types 6 and 11.

Q-25. All of the following are true about the cytomorphological features of HSIL except:
(a) Cells appear singly, in sheets, or in syncytial aggregates.
(b) Cells are of parabasal, basal, or metaplastic type.
(c) Chromatin may be fine or coarsely granular and evenly distributed.
(d) Marked irregular contour of the nuclear membrane and prominent indentations.
(e) Nuclei are two to five times the size of intermediate cell nuclei. There is variation in the size and the shape of the nuclei.
(f) All of the above.

Q-26. According to the "2006 Consensus Guidelines for the Management of Women with Abnormal Cervical Screening Tests," all of the following are true except:
(a) The median reporting rate of ASC-US in US laboratories is 4.7 %.
(b) The median rate of ASC-H is 0.4 %.
(c) The rate of HR HPV DNA positivity is from 40 to 51 % among women with ASC-US but 74–88 % among women with ASC-H.
(d) The rate of high-risk HPV DNA positivity is from 74 to 88 % among women with ASC-H.
(e) The rate of HR HPV DNA positivity is 76.6 % among women with LSIL.
(f) All of the above.

Q-27. Which of the following is *not* true?
(a) Cytological LSIL is not equivalent to histological CIN1.
(b) Cytological HSIL is not equivalent to histological CIN2 and CIN3.
(c) FDA-approved HPV DNA tests are restricted to low-risk (oncogenic) HPV types.
(d) "HPV testing" referred to in the guidelines applies only to testing for high-risk (oncogenic) HPV types.
(e) A single HPV test identifies 92 % of CIN3 lesions.

Q-28. According to the "2006 Consensus Guidelines for the Management of Women with Abnormal Cervical Screening Tests," which of the following is not considered as a special population for the purposes of management of abnormal Pap results?
(a) An 18-year-old woman
(b) A 21-year-old woman

(c) Postmenopausal women
(d) 18 weeks pregnant women
(e) 38 weeks pregnant women

Q-29. According to the "2006 Consensus Guidelines," which of the following is NOT considered an adolescent woman?
(a) Aged 17 and younger
(b) Aged 18 and younger
(c) Aged 19 and younger
(d) Aged 20 and younger
(e) Aged 21 and older

Q-30. According to the "2006 Consensus Guidelines," which management approach is preferred for ASC-US in a 21-year-old woman at the initial screening visit?
(a) Repeat cytology at 6- and 12-month intervals
(b) "Reflex" HPV testing
(c) "Reflex" HPV testing and repeat cytology at 6- and 12-month intervals
(d) Single colposcopy
(e) Single colposcopy and "reflex" HPV testing

Q-31. According to the "2006 Consensus Guidelines," which management approach is recommended for ASC-US in a 20-year-old woman at the initial screening visit?
(a) Repeat cytology at 6- and 12-month interval
(b) Repeat cytology at 12-month interval
(c) "Reflex" HPV testing
(d) Single colposcopy
(e) None of the above

Q-32. According to the "2006 Consensus Guidelines," which management approach is recommended for ASC-US in a 21-year-old woman who is HPV DNA negative?
(a) Repeat cytological testing at 6 months
(b) Repeat cytological testing at 12 months
(c) Repeat cytological testing at 6 and 12 months
(d) Single colposcopy
(e) None of the above

Q-33. According to the "2006 Consensus Guidelines," which management approach is preferred for ASC-US in a 21-year-old woman who is HPV DNA positive?
(a) Repeat cytological testing at 6 months
(b) Repeat cytological testing at 12 months
(c) Repeat cytological testing at 6 and 12 months
(d) Colposcopy
(e) None of the above

Q-34. A 21-year-old woman is diagnosed with ASC-US at the initial screening visit and follow-up HPV DNA test is positive. The subsequent colposcopy shows no CIN2 and CIN3 lesions. Which approach is acceptable for her post-colposcopy management, according to the "2006 Consensus Guidelines"?
(a) Repeat HPV DNA testing at 6 months
(b) Repeat HPV DNA testing at 12 months
(c) Repeat cytological testing at 12 months
(d) Repeat cytological testing at 6 and 12 months
(e) Repeat cytological testing at 6 and 12 months and HPV DNA testing at 12 months

Q-35. A 19-year-old woman is diagnosed as ASC-US at the initial screening visit. The follow-up cytology is performed at 12 months. Which of the following results of her 12-month cytology Pap test should trigger a referral to colposcopy, according to the "2006 Consensus Guidelines"?
(a) ASC-US
(b) ASC-H
(c) LSIL
(d) HSIL or greater
(e) Negative cytology

Q-36. A 21-year-old woman is diagnosed as ASC-H at the initial screening visit. She is referred for colposcopic evaluation, and CIN2 and CIN3 are not identified. Which recommendation is acceptable, according to the "2006 Consensus Guidelines"?
(a) HPV DNA testing at 6 months
(b) HPV DNA testing at 12 months
(c) Pap testing at 6 and 12 months
(d) HPV DNA testing at 12 months or Pap testing at 6 and 12 months
(e) None of the above

Q-37. Which of the following statements is *not* true?
(a) HPV DNA positivity among women with ASC-US is 70–80 %.
(b) In adolescents with LSIL, the cumulative regression rate is 90 % at 36 months.
(c) HPV DNA testing in adolescents with LSIL has limited value.
(d) In postmenopausal women with LSIL Pap test, triage using HPV testing may be an efficient alternative to colposcopy.
(e) None of the above.

Q-38. According to the "2006 Consensus Guidelines," what is an acceptable option(s) for the management of postmenopausal women with LSIL?
(a) Reflex HPV DNA testing
(b) Repeat cytological testing at 6 and 12 months
(c) Colposcopy
(d) All of the above
(e) None of the above

Q-39. Regarding subsequent evaluation or follow-up of atypical glandular cells (AGC), the recommended post-colposcopy management of women of known HPV status who do not have CIN2 and CIN3 or glandular neoplasia identified histologically is which of the following?
(a) If they are HPV DNA positive, repeat cytological testing combined with HPV DNA testing at 6 months.
(b) If they are HPV DNA negative, repeat cytological testing combined with HPV DNA testing at 12 months.
(c) If they are HPV DNA status unknown, repeat cytological testing at 6-month intervals.
(d) None of the above.
(e) All of the above.

Q-40. In cervical cancer screening testing, what does "reflex" HPV testing indicate?
(a) Test the residual specimen of original liquid-based cytology only.
(b) Test a separate co-collected sample at the initial screening visit only.
(c) Both a and b.
(d) Either a or b.
(e) None of the above.

Q-41. Hybrid Capture 2 (HC2) HPV DNA test is one of the FDA-approved assays for the detection of HR HPV types. Which one is true about HC2?
(a) It is an in vitro nucleic acid hybridization assay with signal amplification.
(b) It uses microplate chemiluminescence for the qualitative detection high-risk types of HPV DNA.
(c) It detects 13 high-risk types of HPV DNA.
(d) It cannot determine the specific HPV genotype.
(e) It is the most frequently used diagnostic HPV test worldwide.
(f) It lacks an internal control.
(g) All of the above are true.

Q-42. The APTIMA HPV assay from Gen-Probe of San Diego is the latest FDA-approved HPV test. Which statement is true about the APTIMA HPV assay?
(a) It detects the L1 region of 14 high-risk HPV types.
(b) This assay does determine the specific HPV genotype.
(c) The internal control is not used for quality control.
(d) Cervical specimens can be collected in PreservCyt solution.
(e) It shows cross-reactivity with rare HPV types.
(f) It shows cross-reactivity with some normal flora and opportunistic organisms.

Q-43. Which one is NOT true about the HPV life cycle?
(a) HPV infects superficial cells.
(b) E1, E2, E4, and E5 are viral replication proteins.
(c) E6 and E7 are oncoproteins.
(d) E4 protein persists in upper epithelial layers.
(e) L1 and L2 are capsid proteins and are found in upper epithelial layers.

2.3 Image-Based Questions 44–71

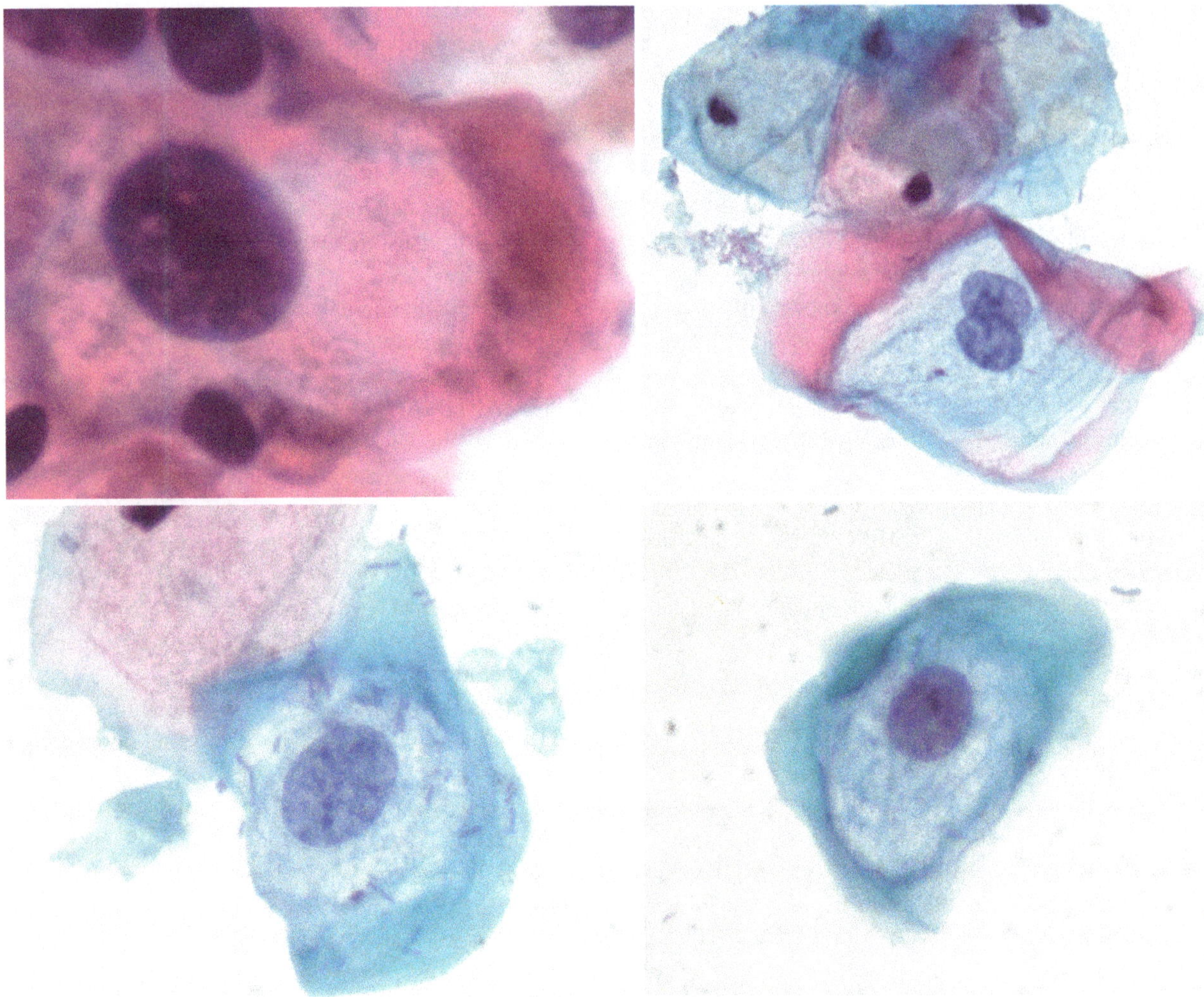

Fig. 2.44

Q-44. These images are from the cervical Pap test of 21-year-old woman. The cytoplasmic change is due to ____.

(a) Glycogen accumulated in the cytoplasm
(b) Lipid accumulated in the cytoplasm
(c) Viral particles accumulated in the cytoplasm
(d) Water accumulated in the cytoplasm
(e) Abundant expression of the HPV E4 protein which binds with cytoplasmic keratin
(f) None of the above

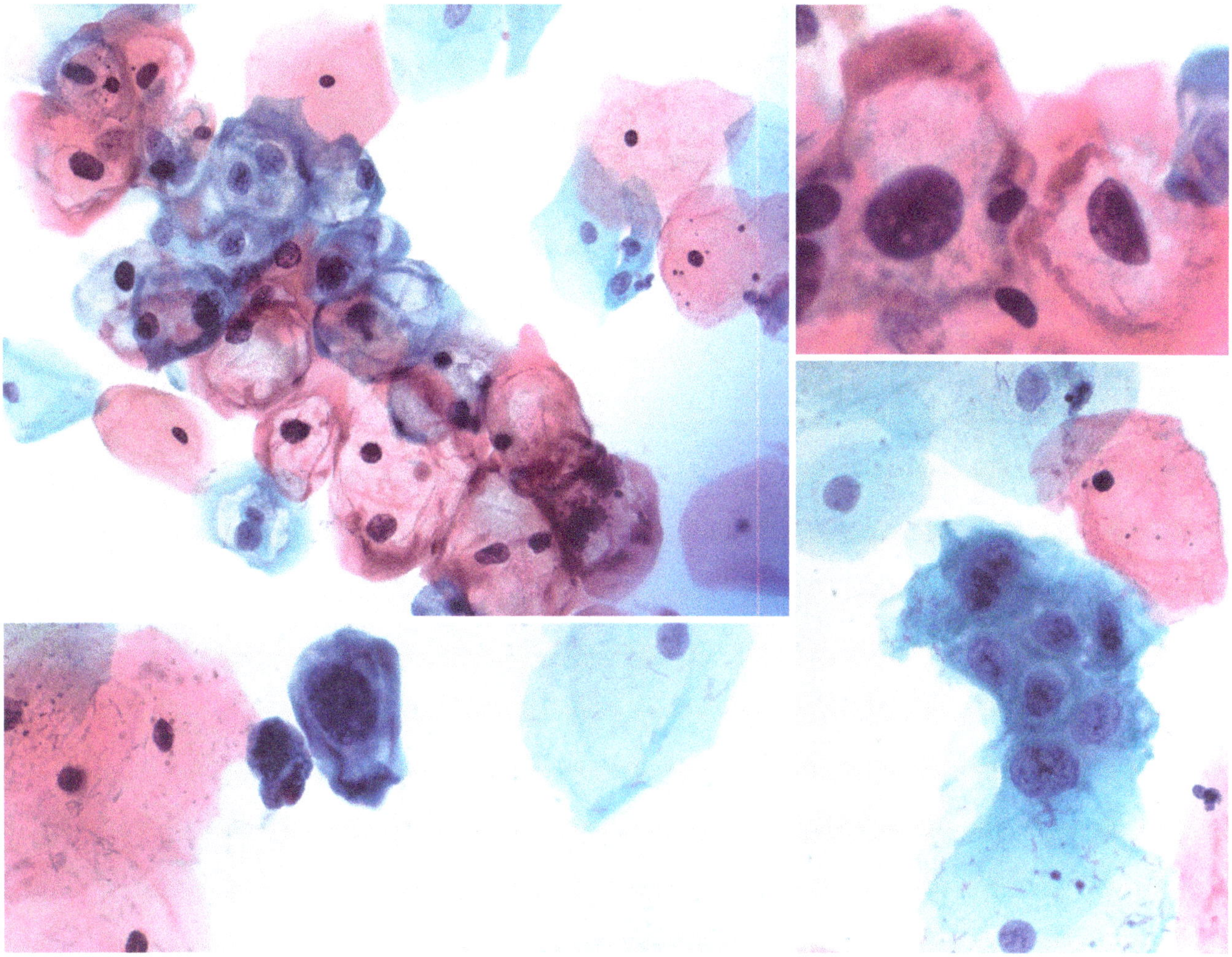

Fig. 2.45

Q-45. These images are from the cervical Pap test of 29-year-old woman. Which is correct about these cells and their causative agents?

(a) They are intermediate cells.
(b) They can be associated with HPV types 6 and 11.
(c) They can be associated with HPV types 16 and 18.
(d) They are seen in condyloma acuminatum.
(e) Approximately 21 % progress to HSIL.
(f) All of the above.

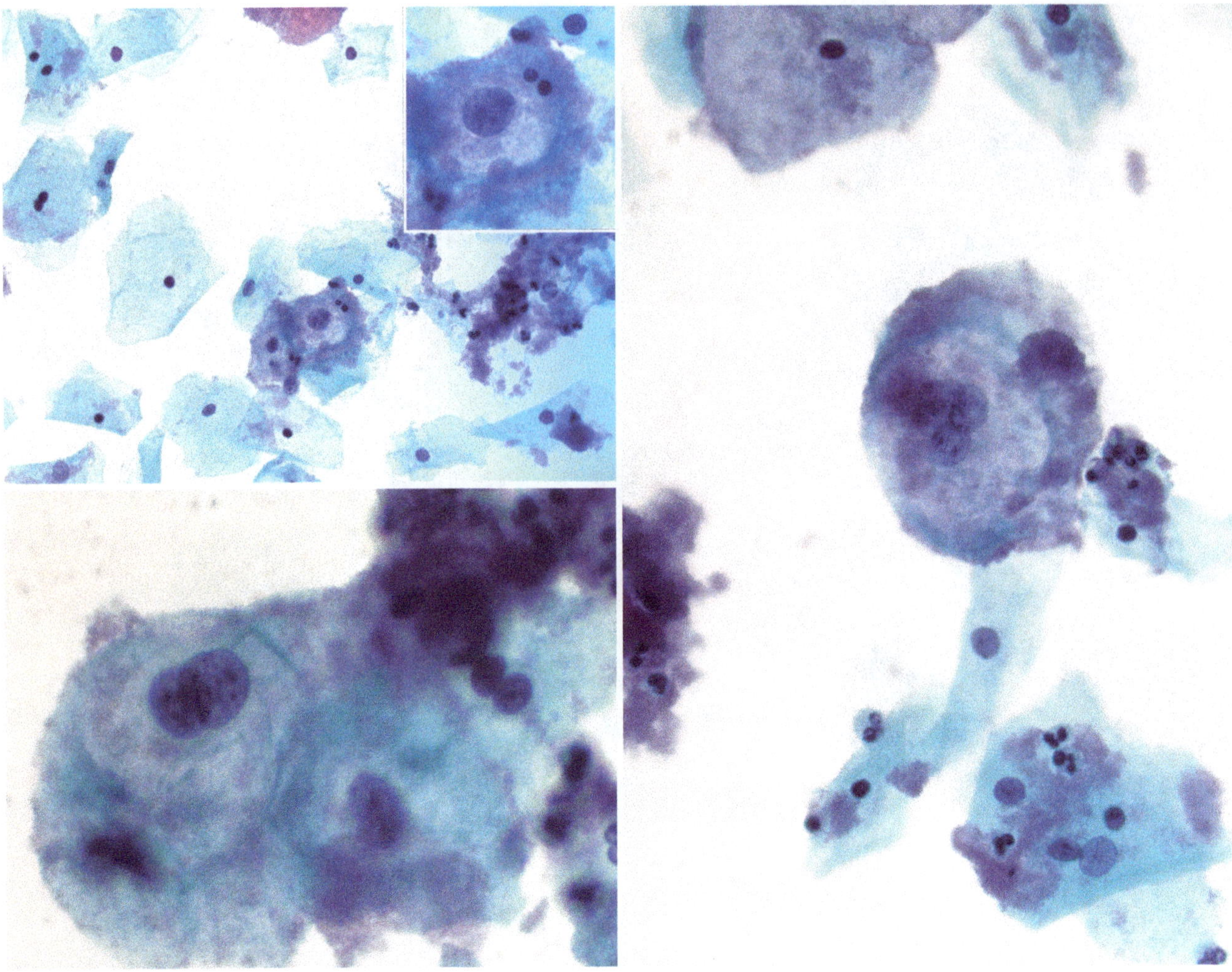

Fig. 2.46

Q-46. These images are from the cervical Pap test of 21-year-old woman. Which one is *not* correct about the causative agent?

(a) It is a double-stranded DNA virus.
(b) Its genome is approximately 8,000 base pairs in length.
(c) It has three functioning areas: early, late and noncoding.
(d) The vast majority of these viruses infect epithelial surfaces.
(e) The changes are mainly due to infection by LR HPV.

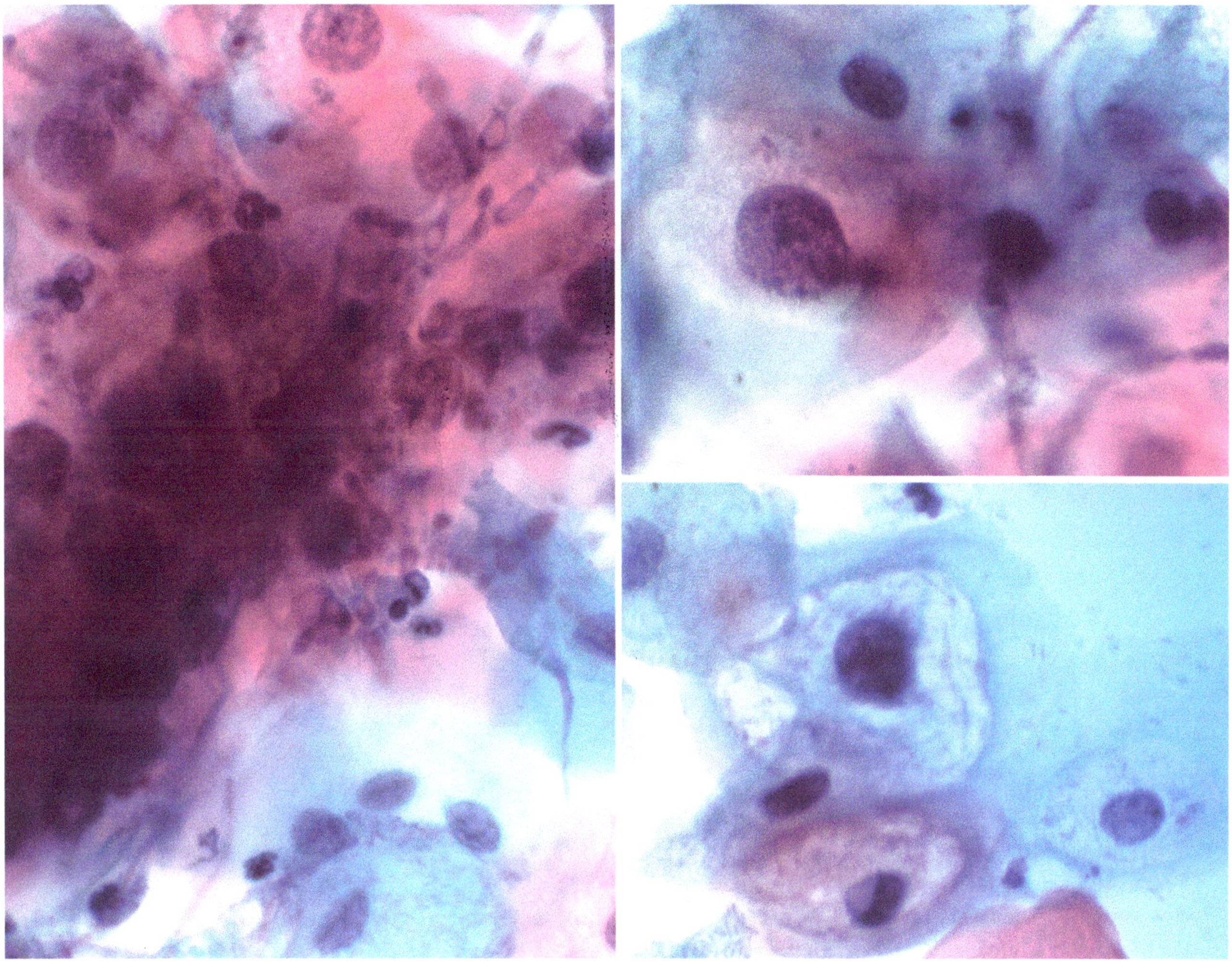

Fig. 2.47

Q-47. These images are from the cervical Pap test of 23-year-old woman. Which one is NOT true about these cells and their causative agents?

(a) The virus replicates in the nuclei of squamous epithelial cells.

(b) The virus reaches full maturity in the superficial squamous epithelium.

(c) The virus is latent in the basal layers of squamous cells.

(d) The virus is usually retained intact in an episomal form.

(e) The nuclear changes are due to *Candida albicans* infection.

(f) The viral DNA has not integrated into the host DNA.

Fig. 2.48

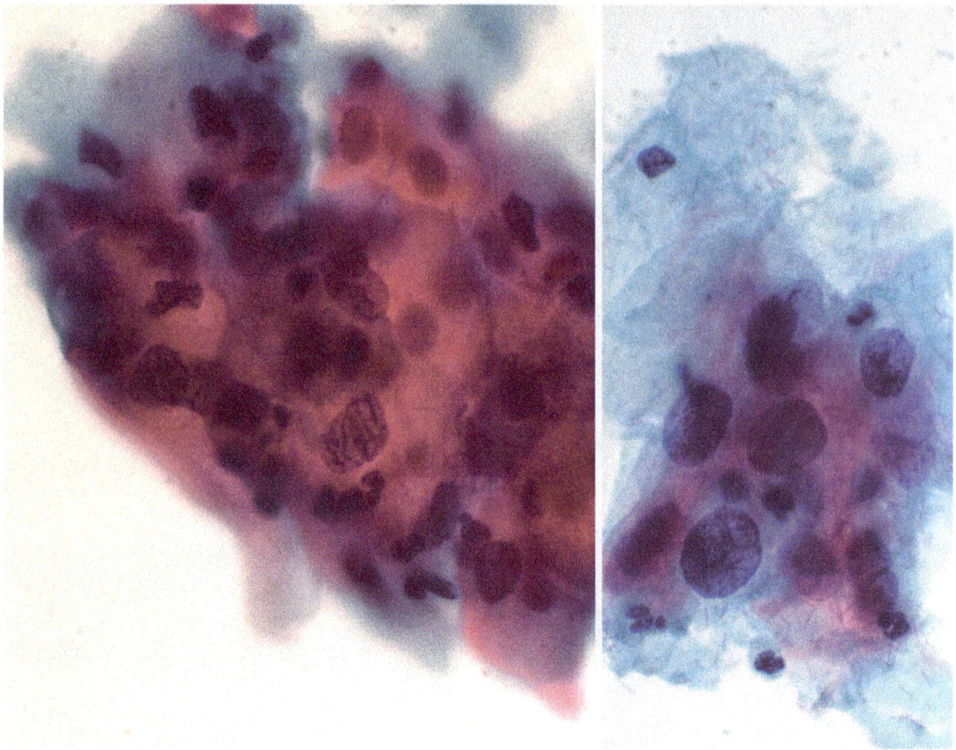

Q-48. These images are from the cervical Pap test. The most likely diagnosis is:

(a) Atypical squamous cells of undetermined significance (ASC-US)
(b) Atypical squamous cells cannot exclude high-grade squamous intraepithelial lesion (ASC-H)
(c) Low-grade squamous intraepithelial lesion (LSIL)
(d) High-grade squamous intraepithelial lesion (HSIL)
(e) Invasive squamous cell carcinoma (keratinizing or nonkeratinizing)
(f) None of the above

Fig. 2.49

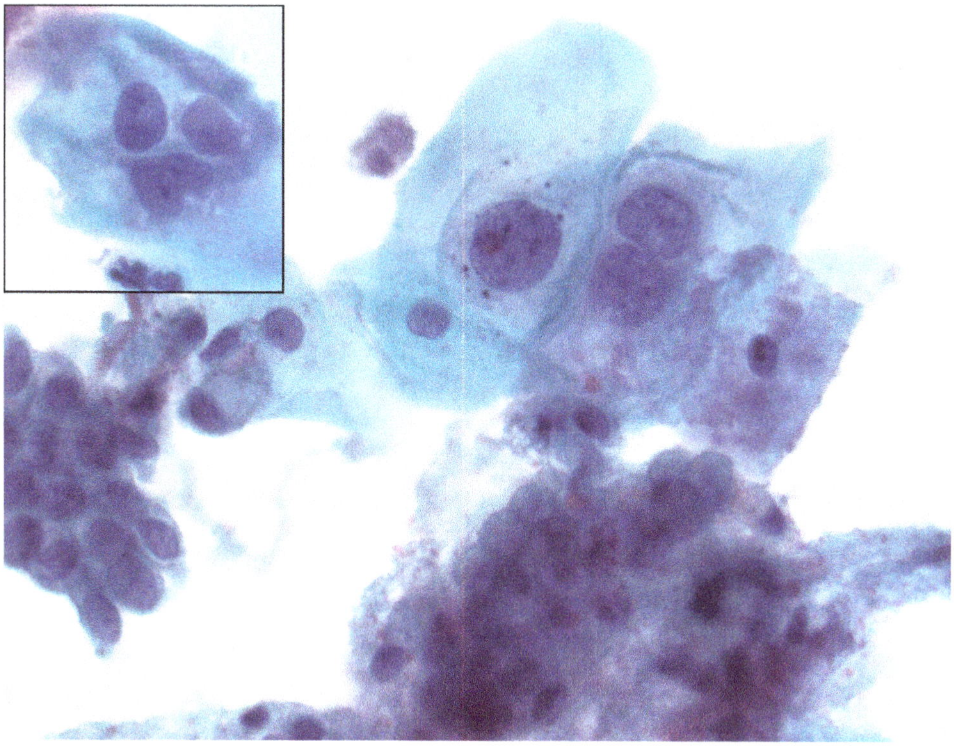

Q-49. These images are from a cervical Pap test. Which of the following is NOT correct about these cells and their causative agents?

(a) Approximately 80 % of high-risk HPV (+) women have CIN1 on subsequent biopsy.

(b) Approximately 25–50 % have CIN2–3 on subsequent biopsy.

(c) Progression to CIN2–3 is seen in 10 % of LSIL cases.

(d) Squamous cell carcinoma may develop in less than 0.3 % of women with LSIL.

(e) There is no reliable indicator of which women with CIN1 will progress to a higher grade lesion.

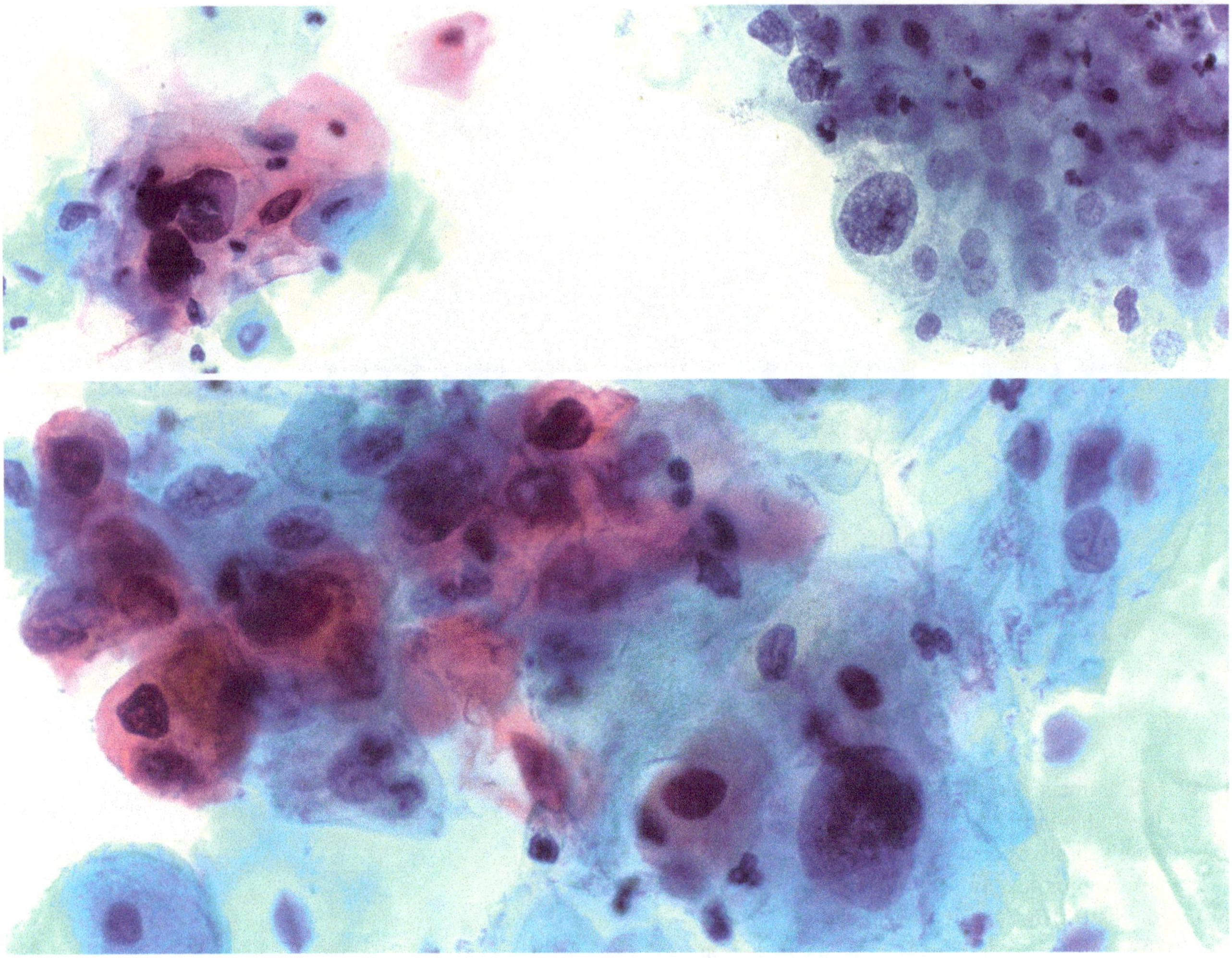

Fig. 2.50

Q-50. These images are from the cervical Pap test of a 35-year-old woman. Which of the following is the correct interpretation?

(a) Atypical squamous cells of undetermined significance (ASC-US)
(b) Atypical squamous cells cannot exclude high-grade squamous intraepithelial lesion (ASC-H)
(c) Low-grade squamous intraepithelial lesion (LSIL)
(d) High-grade squamous intraepithelial lesion (HSIL)
(e) Invasive squamous cell carcinoma (nonkeratinizing)

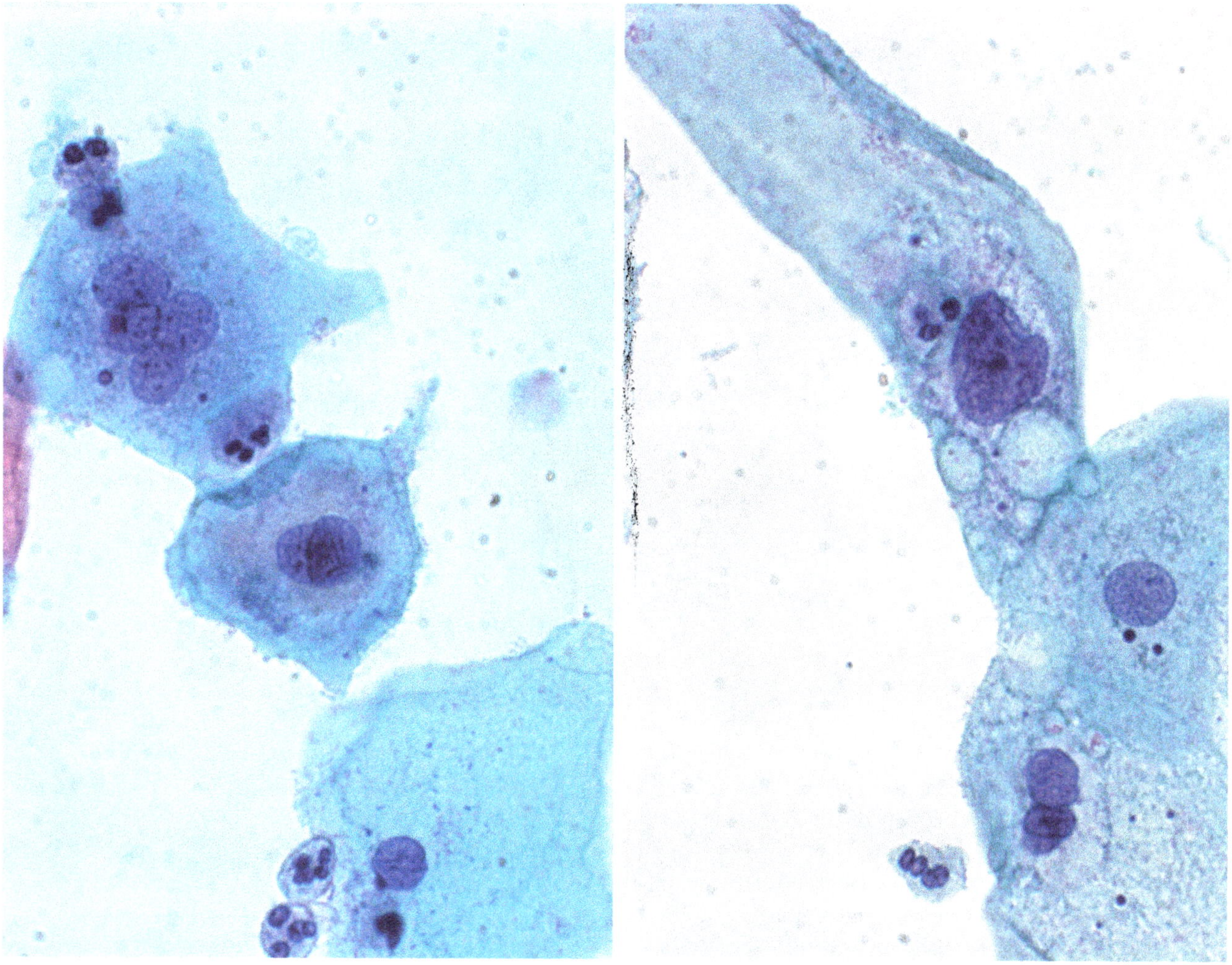

Fig. 2.51

Q-51. These images are from a cervical Pap test. Which of the following is *not* true about its causative agents?

(a) HR HPV is the main causative agent of invasive squamous cell carcinoma.
(b) HPV is detected in 5–40 % of asymptomatic reproductive women, and 50–75 % of them are HR HPV type.
(c) The majority of them are transient infections.
(d) Some infections may persist.
(e) More than 50 % of HPV infections persist for 2 years or more.

Fig. 2.52

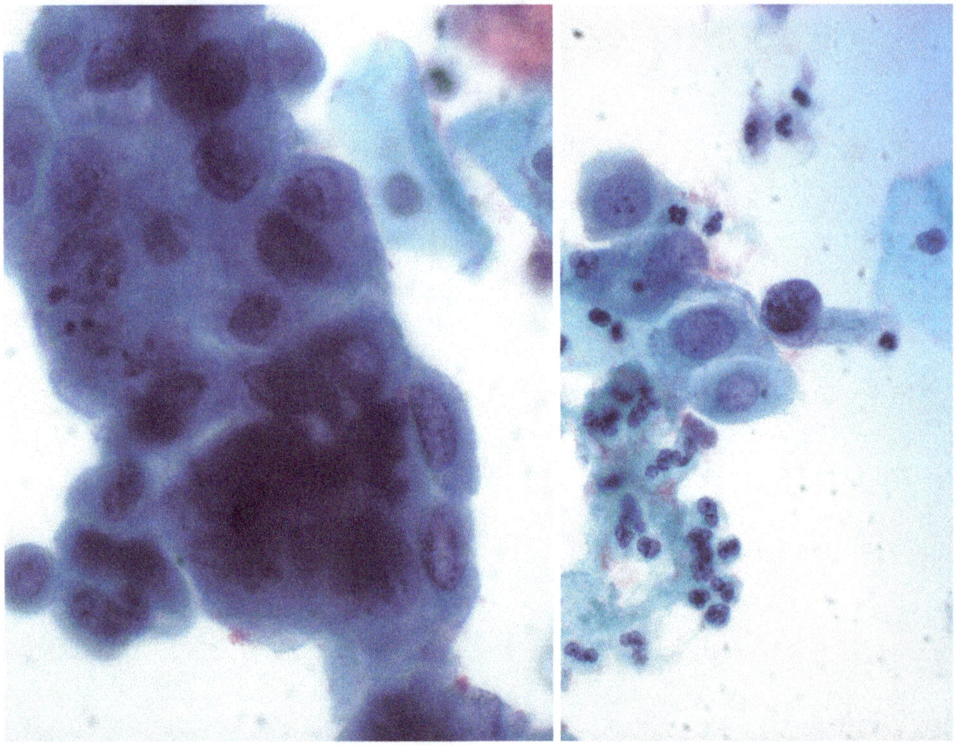

Q-52. These images are from the cervical Pap test of a 28-year-old woman. Which of the following is *not* true about its causative agents?

(a) It is divisible into three regions: an early region, a late region, and a noncoding region.
(b) E1 is the viral replication protein.
(c) E2 is the major viral regulator and controls the viral oncogenes.
(d) E6 and E7 are viral oncogenes.
(e) E6 binds p53.
(f) E7 binds to p16.

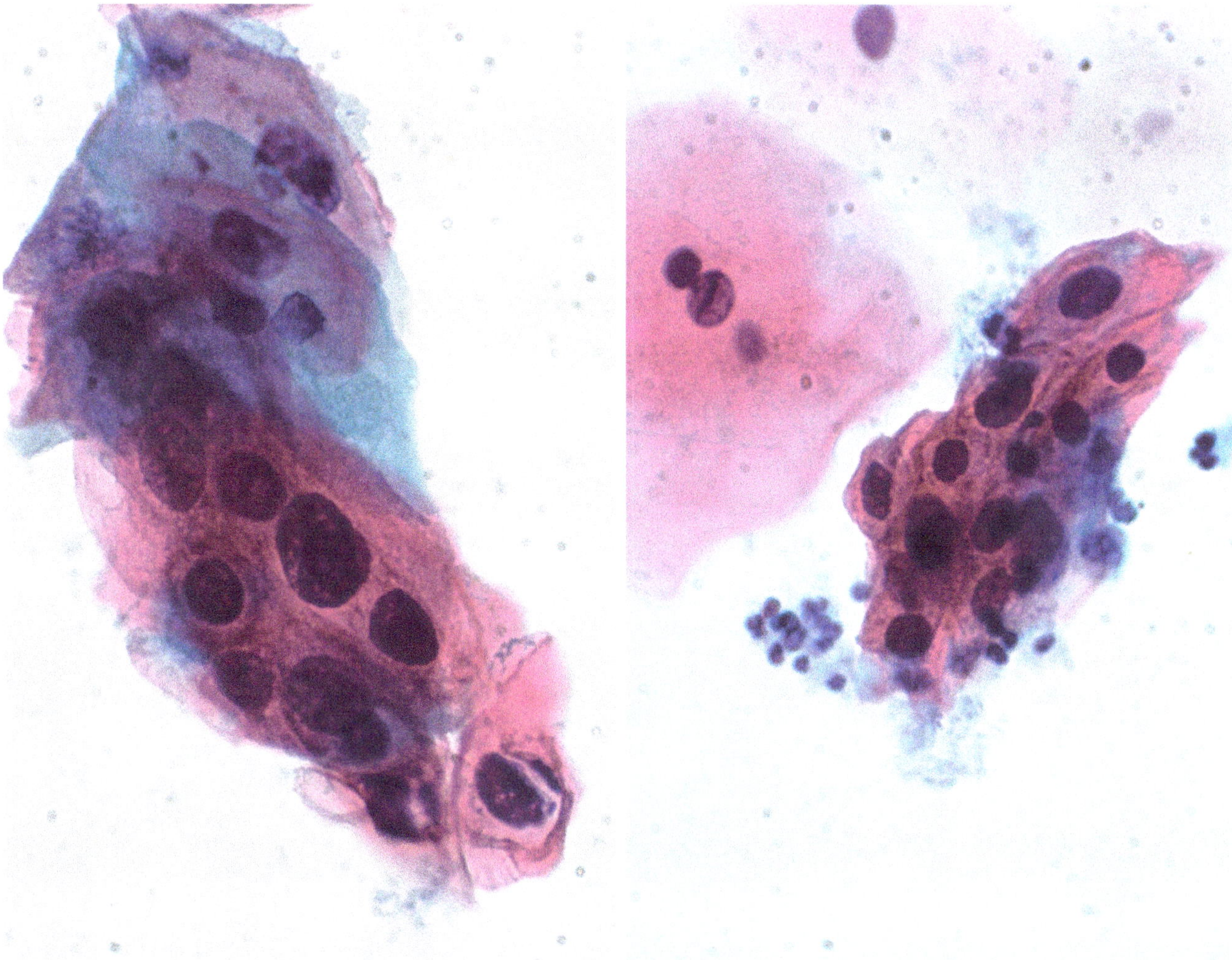

Fig. 2.53

Q-53. These images are from the cervical Pap test of a 35-year-old woman. Which of the following is *not* the FDA-approved assay for detection of its causative agents?

(a) Hybrid Capture 2 HPV DNA test
(b) Cervista HPV HR test and Cervista HPV 16/18 test
(c) APTIMA HPV assay
(d) Cobas 4,800 HPV test
(e) INFORM HPV (Ventana Medical Systems, Inc, Tucson, AZ, USA)

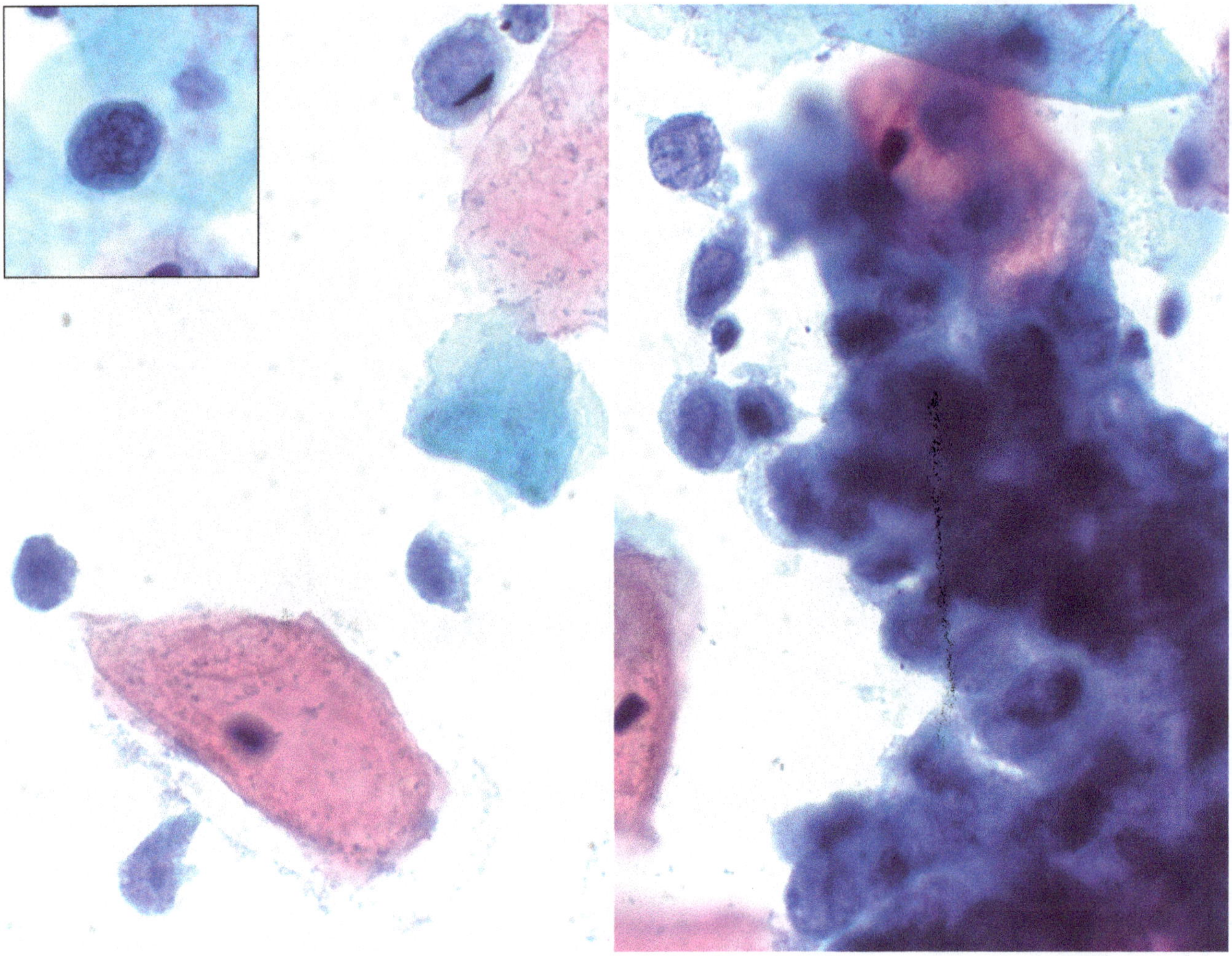

Fig. 2.54

Q-54. These images are from the cervical Pap test of a 24-year-old woman. Which of the following is the correct interpretation?

(a) Atypical squamous cells of undetermined significance (ASC-US)
(b) Atypical squamous cells cannot exclude high-grade squamous intraepithelial lesion (ASC-H)
(c) Low-grade squamous intraepithelial lesion (LSIL)
(d) High-grade squamous intraepithelial lesion (HSIL)
(e) Invasive squamous cell carcinoma (nonkeratinizing)

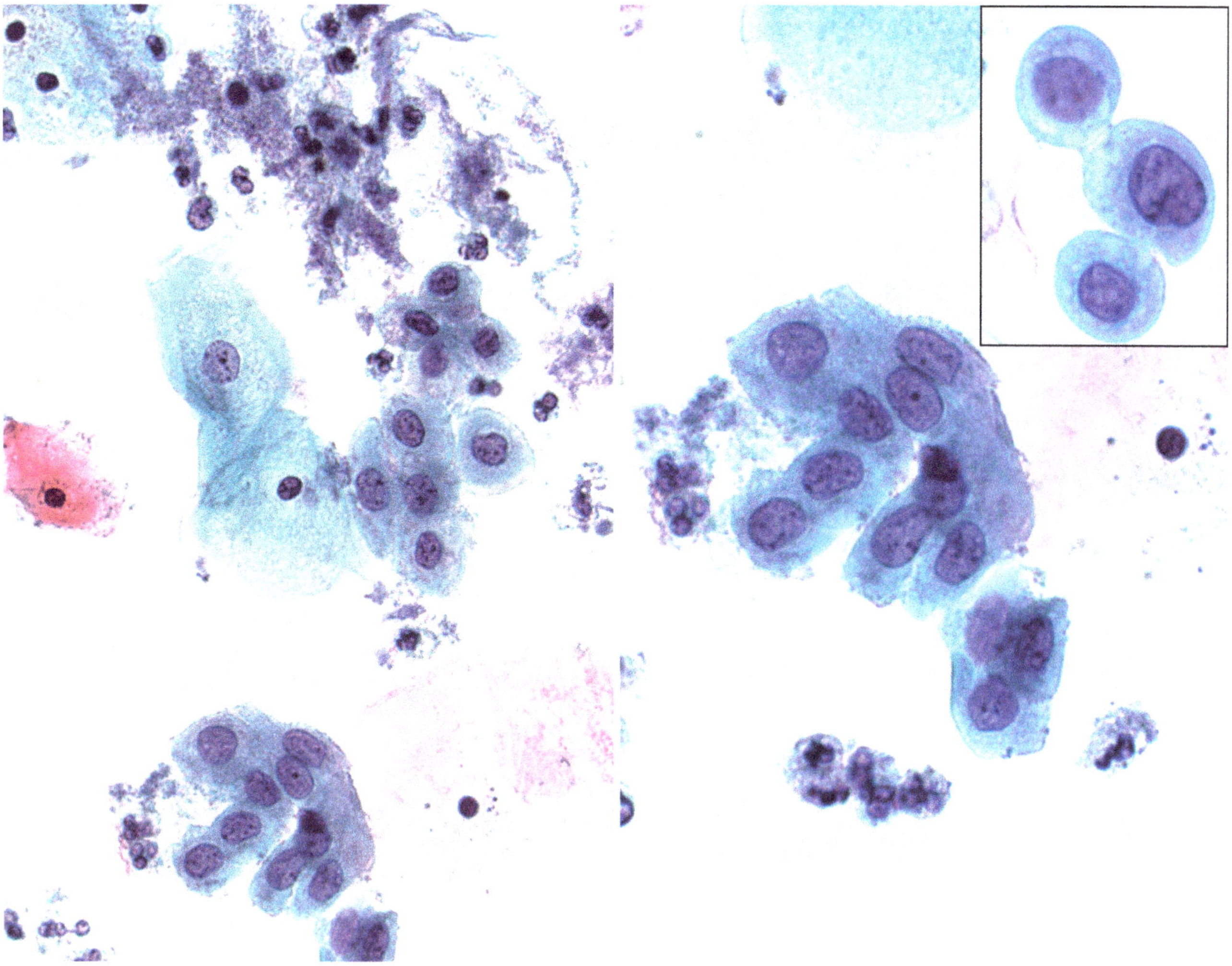

Fig. 2.55

Q-55. These images are from a cervical Pap test. The most likely diagnosis is:

(a) Atypical squamous cells of undetermined significance (ASC-US)
(b) Atypical squamous cells cannot exclude high-grade squamous intraepithelial lesion (ASC-H)
(c) Low-grade squamous intraepithelial lesion (LSIL)
(d) High-grade squamous intraepithelial lesion (HSIL)
(e) Invasive squamous cell carcinoma (keratinizing)
(f) None of the above

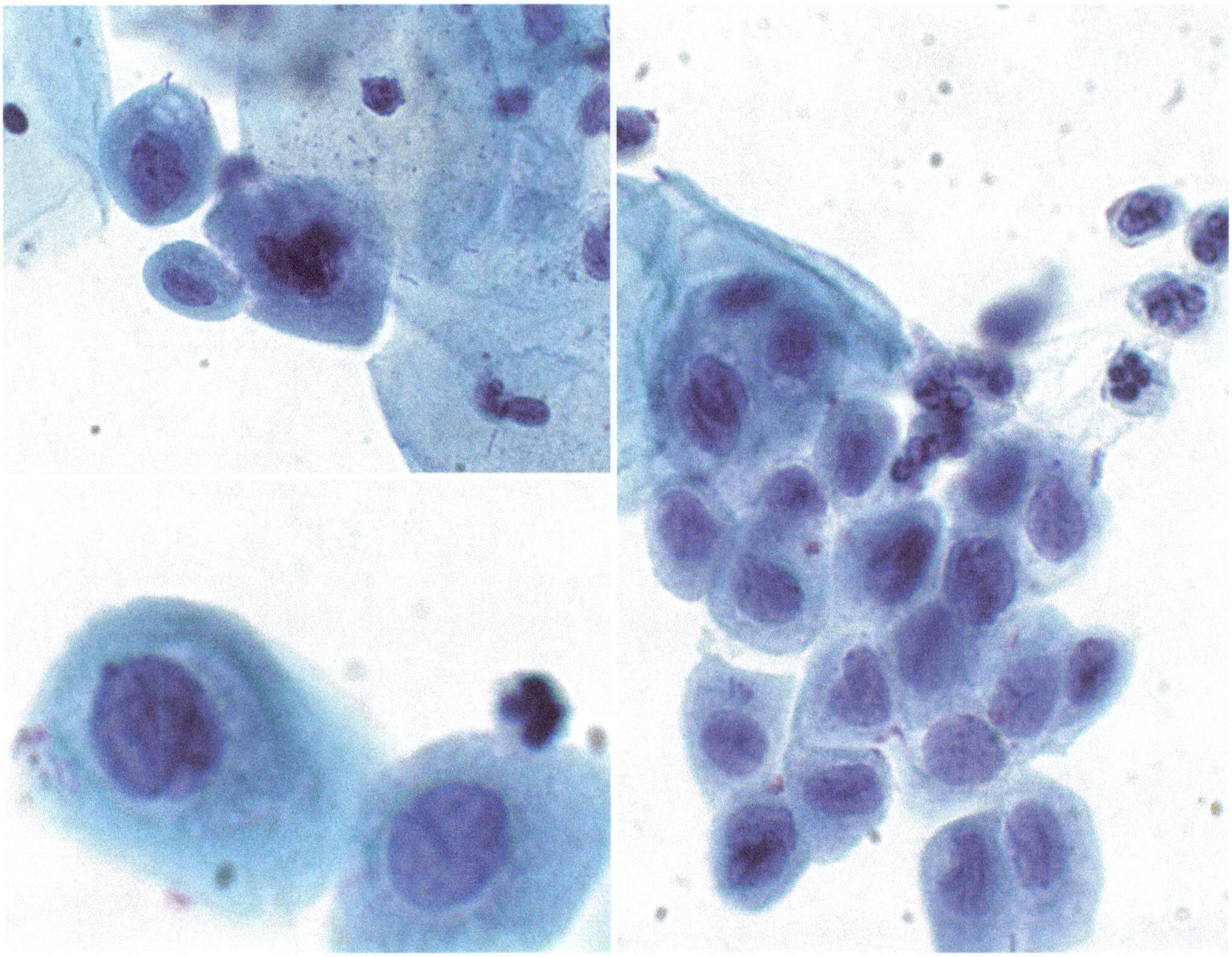

Fig. 2.56

Q-56. These images are from the cervical Pap test of a 23-year-old woman. Which of the following is *not* true about these cells and their causative agents?

(a) The virus replicates in the nuclei of squamous epithelial cells.
(b) The virus reaches full maturity in the superficial squamous epithelium.
(c) The virus is latent in the basal layers of squamous cells.
(d) The virus is usually retained intact in an episomal form.
(e) HR HPV is found in 95 % of women.

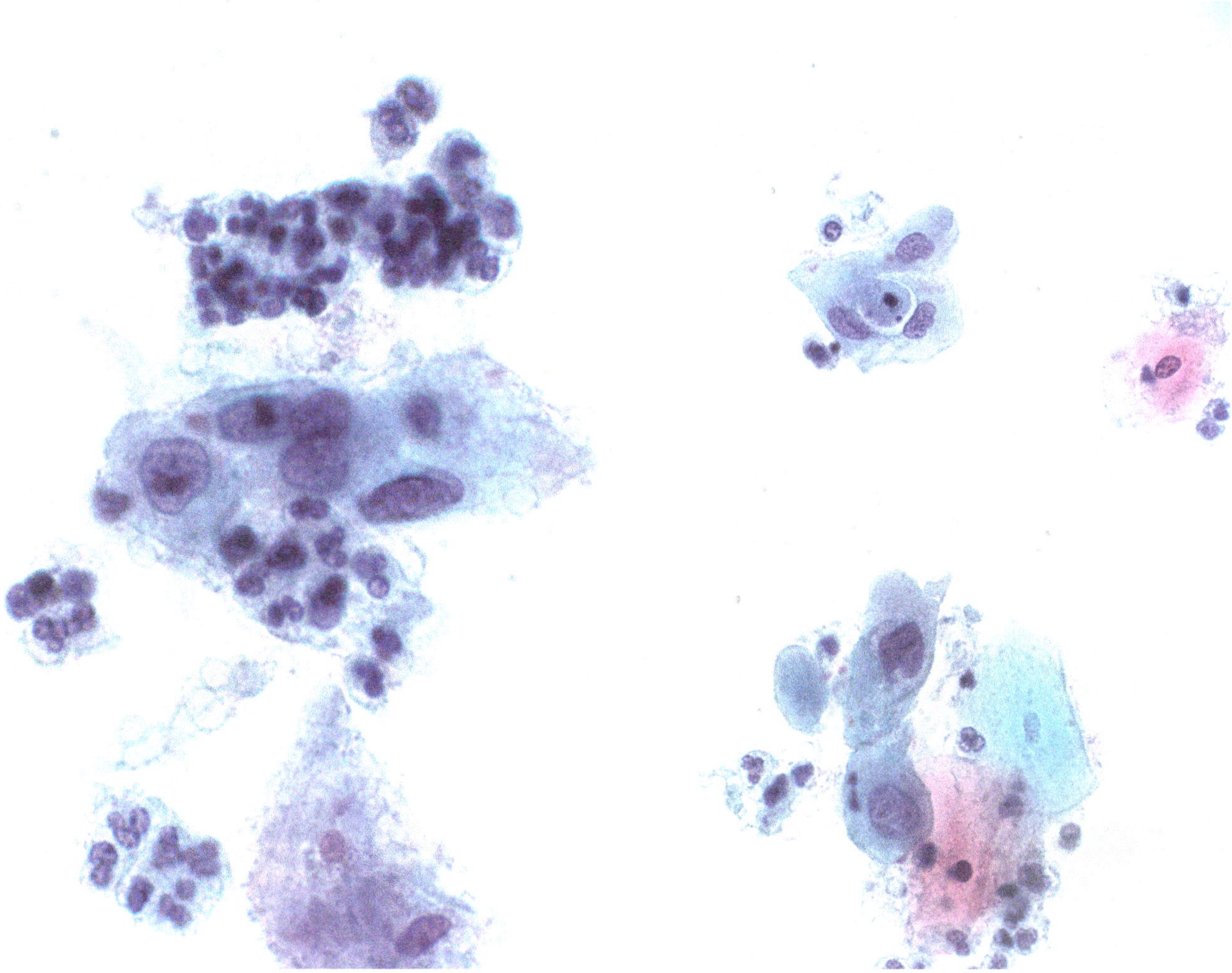

Fig. 2.57

Q-57. These images are from a cervical Pap test. Which of the following are correct interpretations?

(a) It is atypical squamous cells of undetermined significance (ASC-US).
(b) It is atypical squamous cells cannot exclude high-grade squamous intraepithelial lesion (ASC-H).
(c) It is low-grade squamous intraepithelial lesion (LSIL).
(d) It is high-grade squamous intraepithelial lesion (HSIL).
(e) It is suspicious for invasive squamous cell carcinoma.
(f) The lesion is LR HPV related.

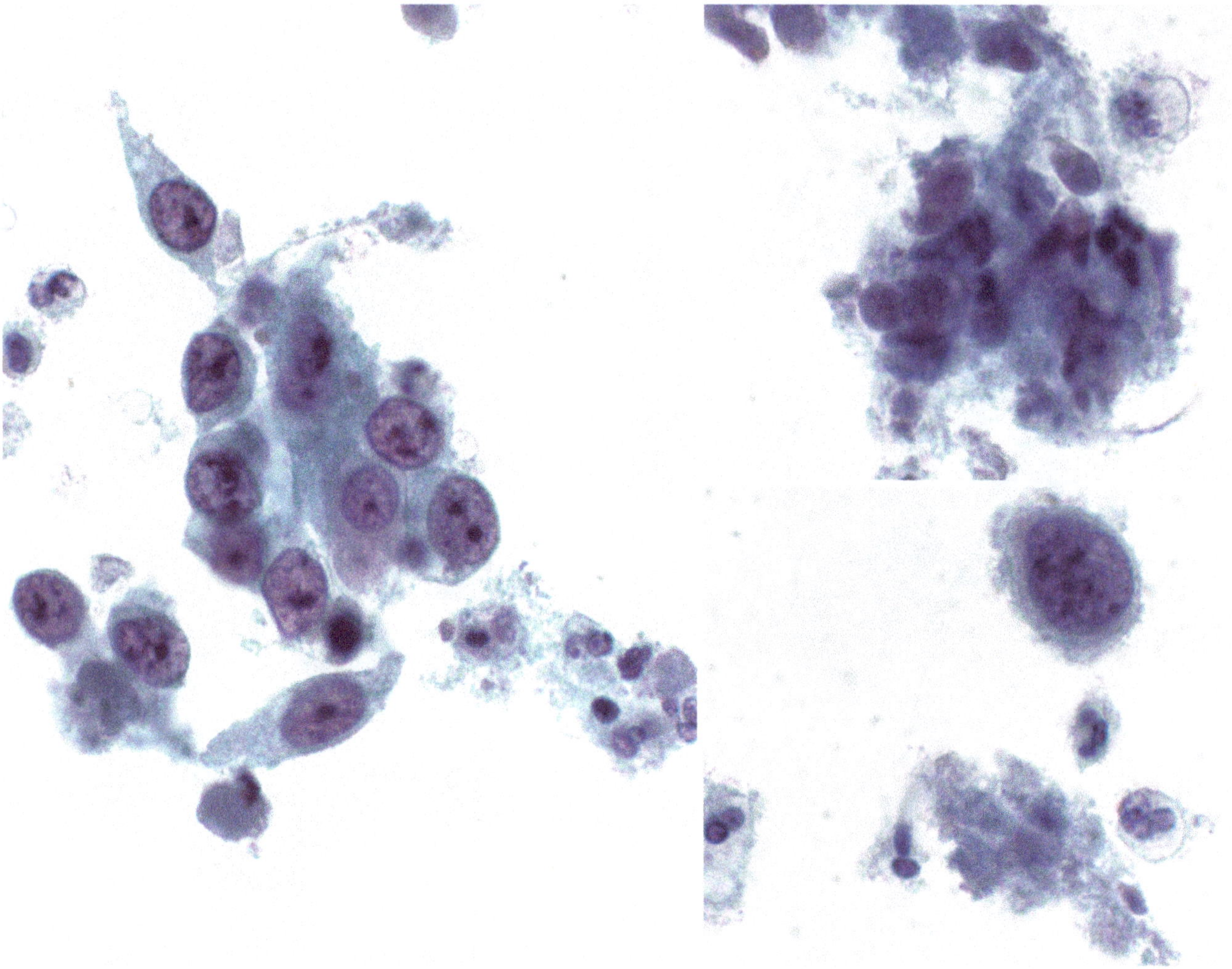

Fig. 2.58

Q-58. These images are from a cervical Pap test. The most likely diagnosis is:

(a) Atypical squamous cells of undetermined significance (ASC-US).
(b) Atypical squamous cells cannot exclude high-grade squamous intraepithelial lesion (ASC-H).
(c) Low-grade squamous intraepithelial lesion (LSIL).
(d) High-grade squamous intraepithelial lesion (HSIL).
(e) Invasive squamous cell carcinoma (nonkeratinizing).
(f) None of the above.

Fig. 2.59

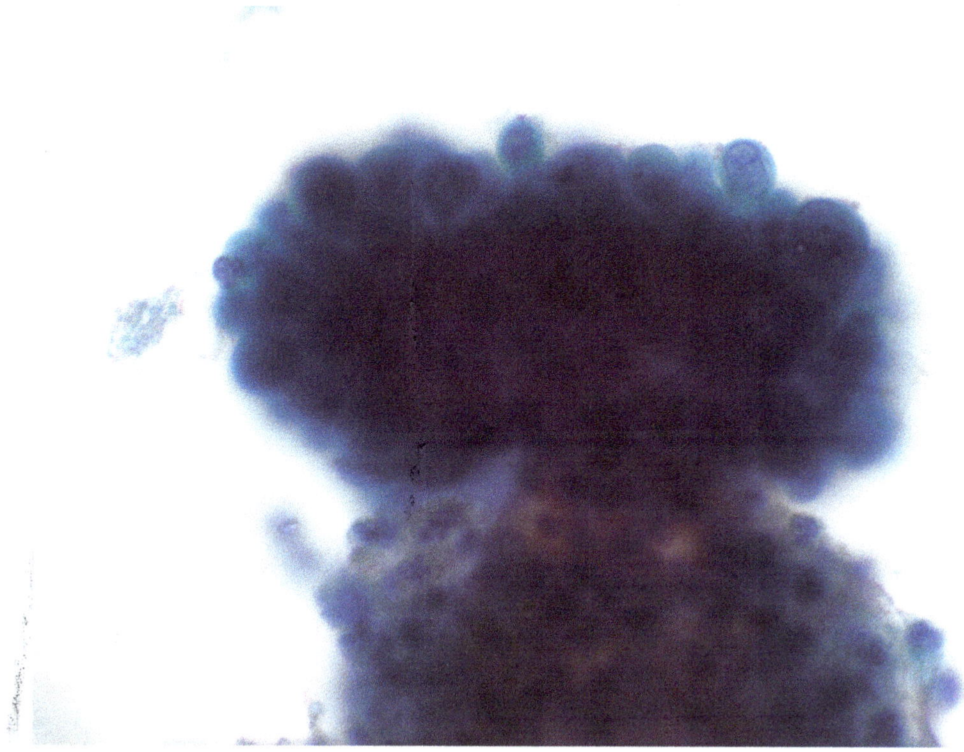

Q-59. This image shows the cervical Pap test from a 75-year-old woman with vaginal bleeding. Which one of the following interpretations is correct?

(a) It is atypical squamous cells of undetermined significance (ASC-US).
(b) It is reactive endocervical cells.
(c) It is low-grade squamous intraepithelial lesion (LSIL).
(d) It is high-grade squamous intraepithelial lesion (HSIL).
(e) It is not HPV related.

Fig. 2.60

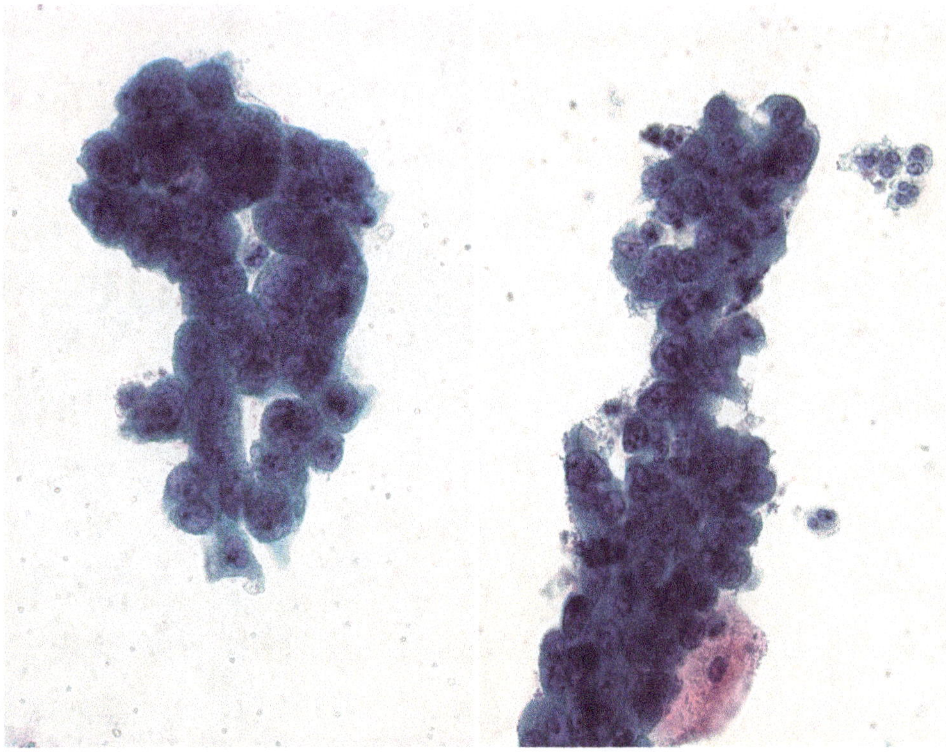

Q-60. These images are from a cervical Pap test. Which of the following interpretations is correct?
- (a) Atypical squamous cells of undetermined significance (ASC-US).
- (b) Atypical squamous cells cannot exclude high-grade squamous intraepithelial lesion (ASC-H).
- (c) Low-grade squamous intraepithelial lesion (LSIL).
- (d) High-grade squamous intraepithelial lesion (HSIL).
- (e) Invasive squamous cell carcinoma (nonkeratinizing).
- (f) HR HPV is often positive.
- (g) None of the above.

Fig. 2.61

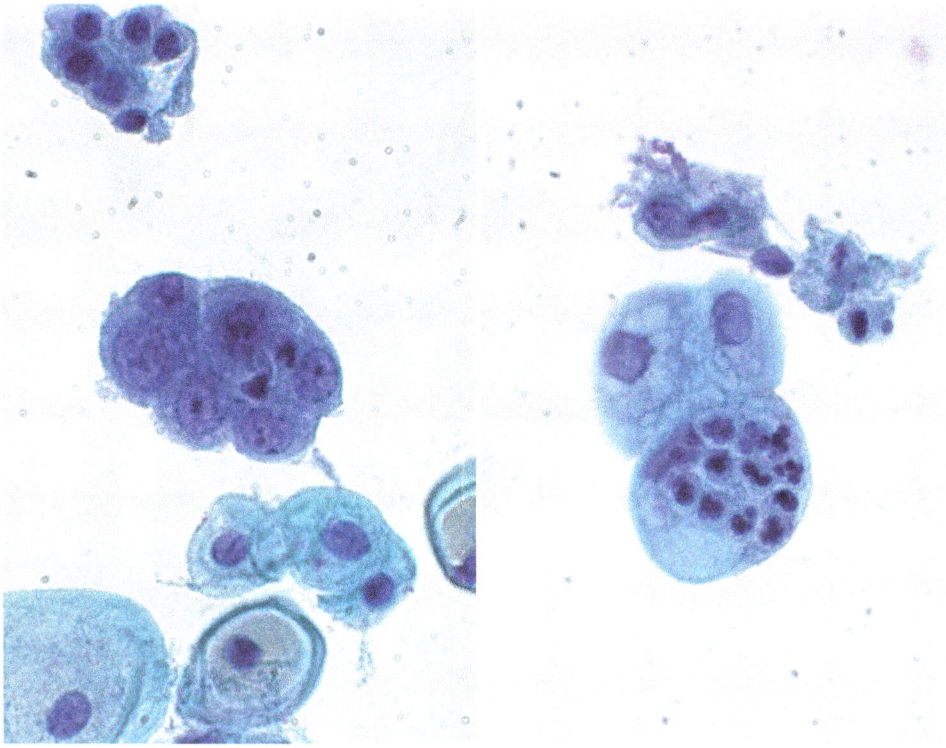

Q-61. These images are from a cervical Pap test. Which of the following is correct?
- (a) It is atypical glandular cells (AGC).
- (b) Atypical squamous cells cannot exclude high-grade squamous intraepithelial lesion (ASC-H).
- (c) It is adenocarcinoma in situ (AIS).
- (d) It is high-grade squamous intraepithelial lesion (HSIL).
- (e) It is endocervical adenocarcinoma.
- (f) Most likely the HPV test will be positive.

Fig. 2.62

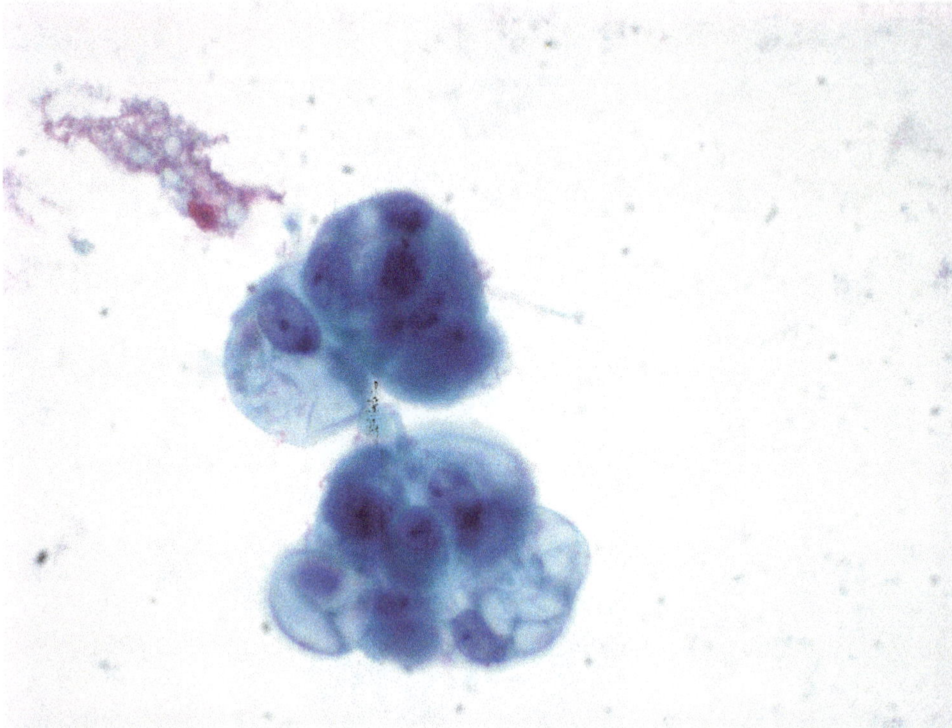

Q-62. These images are from a cervical Pap test. The most likely diagnosis is:
(a) Atypical glandular cells (AGC).
(b) Atypical squamous cells cannot exclude high-grade squamous intraepithelial lesion (ASC-H).
(c) Adenocarcinoma in situ (AIS).
(d) High-grade squamous intraepithelial lesion (HSIL).
(e) Endocervical adenocarcinoma.
(f) None of the above.

Fig. 2.63

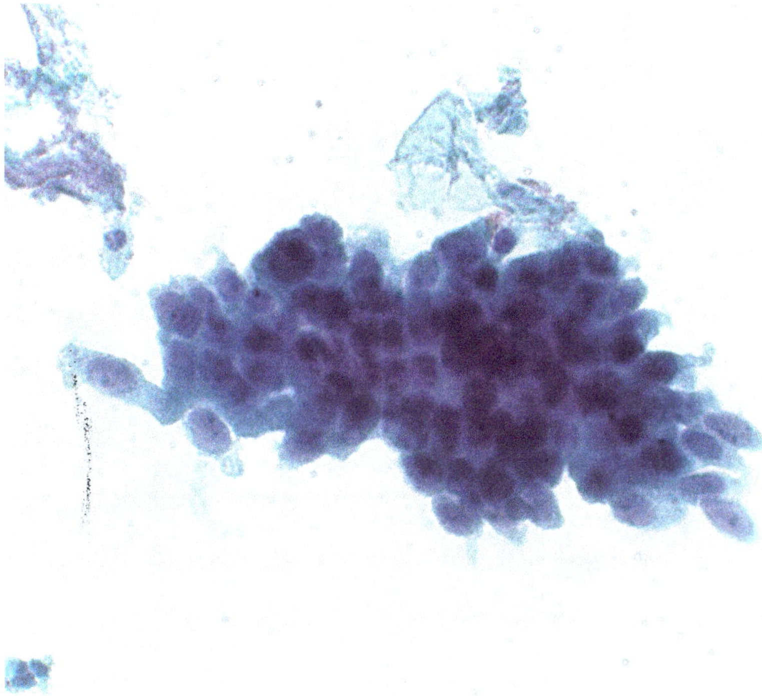

Q-63. These images are from a cervical Pap test. The most likely diagnosis is:
(a) Atypical glandular cells (AGC).
(b) Atypical squamous cells cannot exclude high-grade squamous intraepithelial lesion (ASC-H).
(c) Adenocarcinoma in situ (AIS).
(d) High-grade squamous intraepithelial lesion (HSIL).
(e) Endocervical adenocarcinoma.
(f) None of the above.

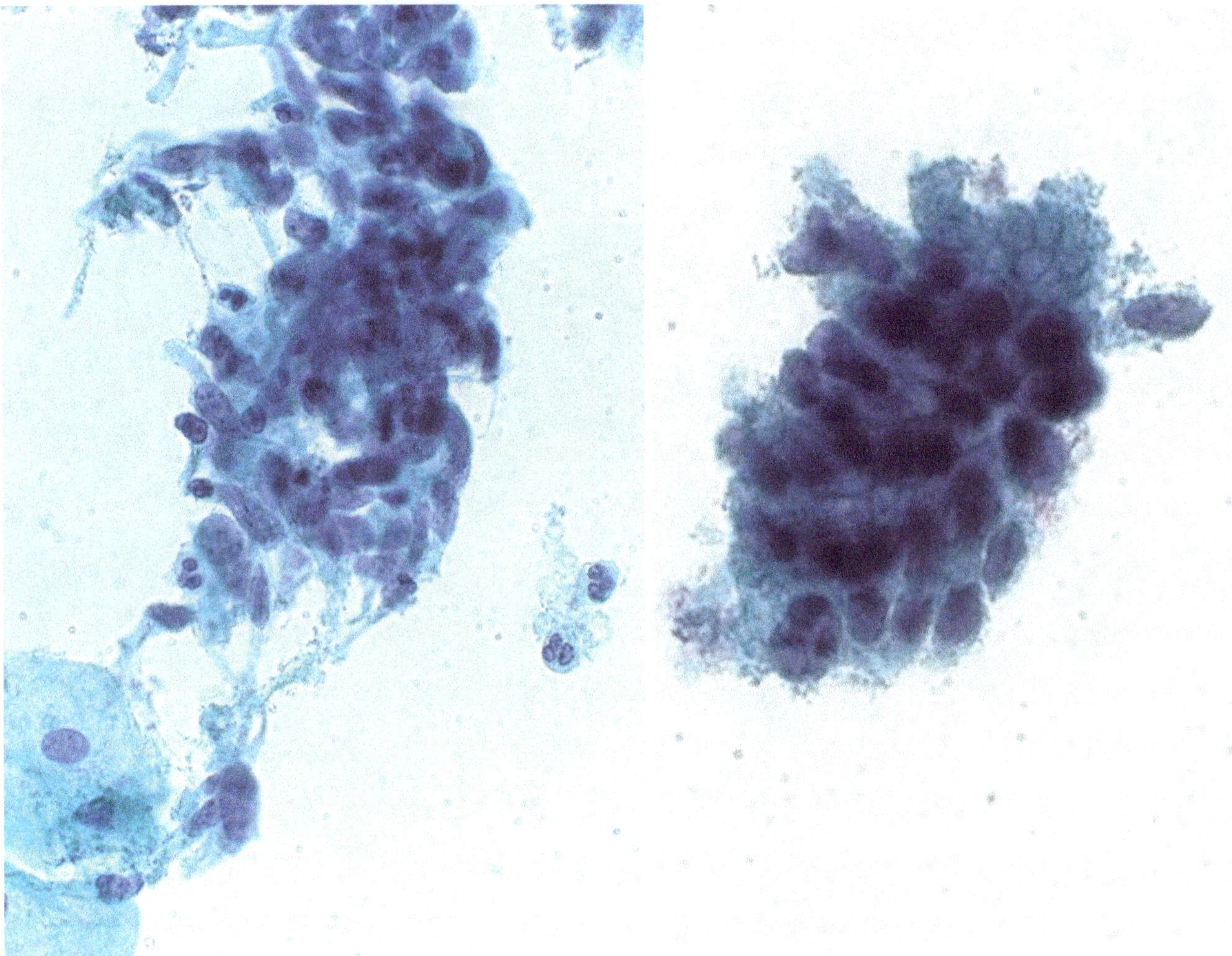

Fig. 2.64

Q-64. These images are from a cervical Pap test. Which statement is *not* true?

(a) It is a precursor lesion of invasive endocervical adenocarcinoma.
(b) It is associated with HPV in virtually all cases.
(c) Squamous dysplasias are a commonly identified association.
(d) It is most commonly associated with HPV 16/18 infection.
(e) It is not associated with HPV 18.
(f) None of the above.

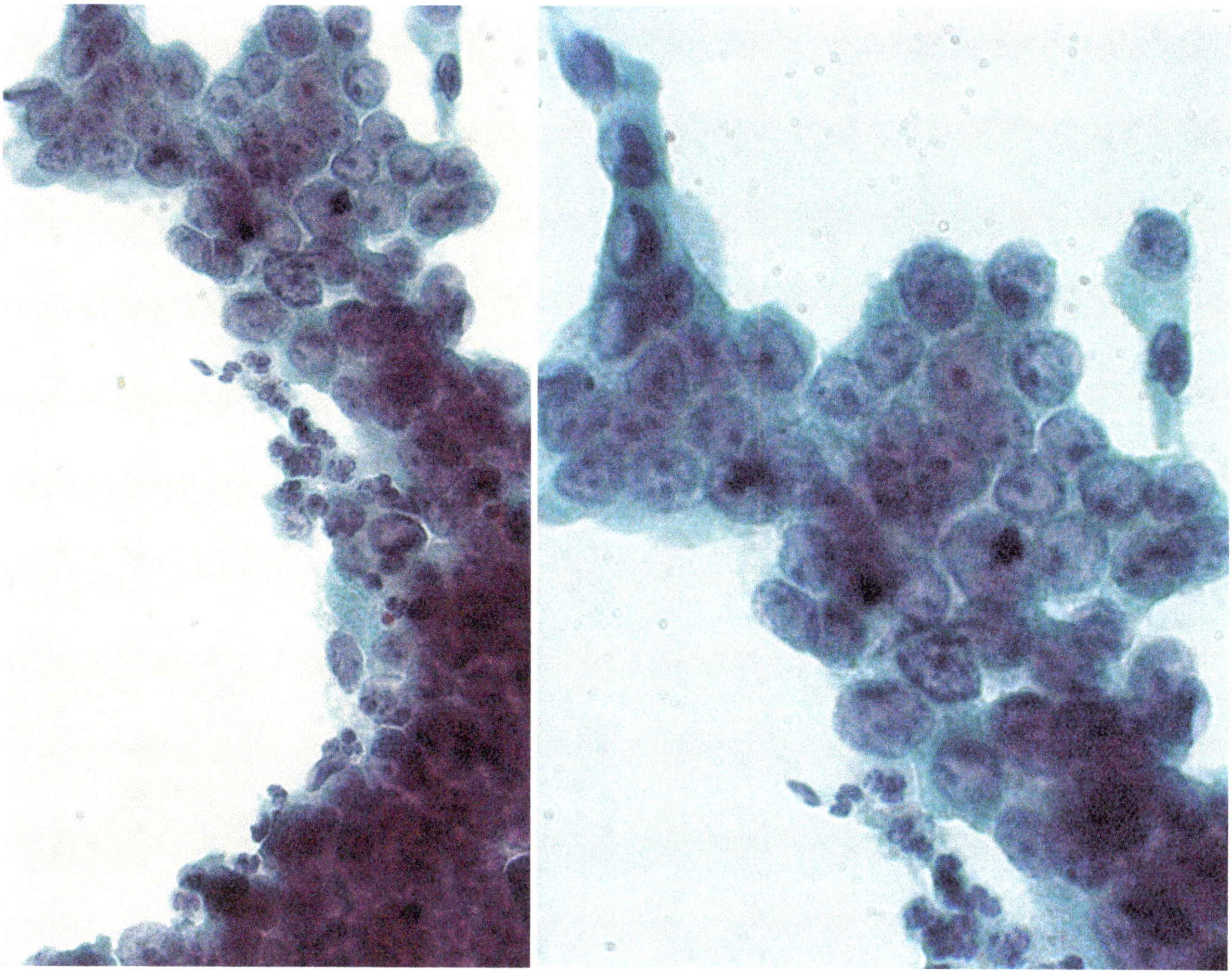

Fig. 2.65

Q-65. These images are from a cervical Pap test. Which one is NOT true about its epidemiology?
(a) Infection of HR HPV types.
(b) Nonsmokers.
(c) Lower parity.
(d) Hormone replacement therapy.
(e) It is a benign reactive process.

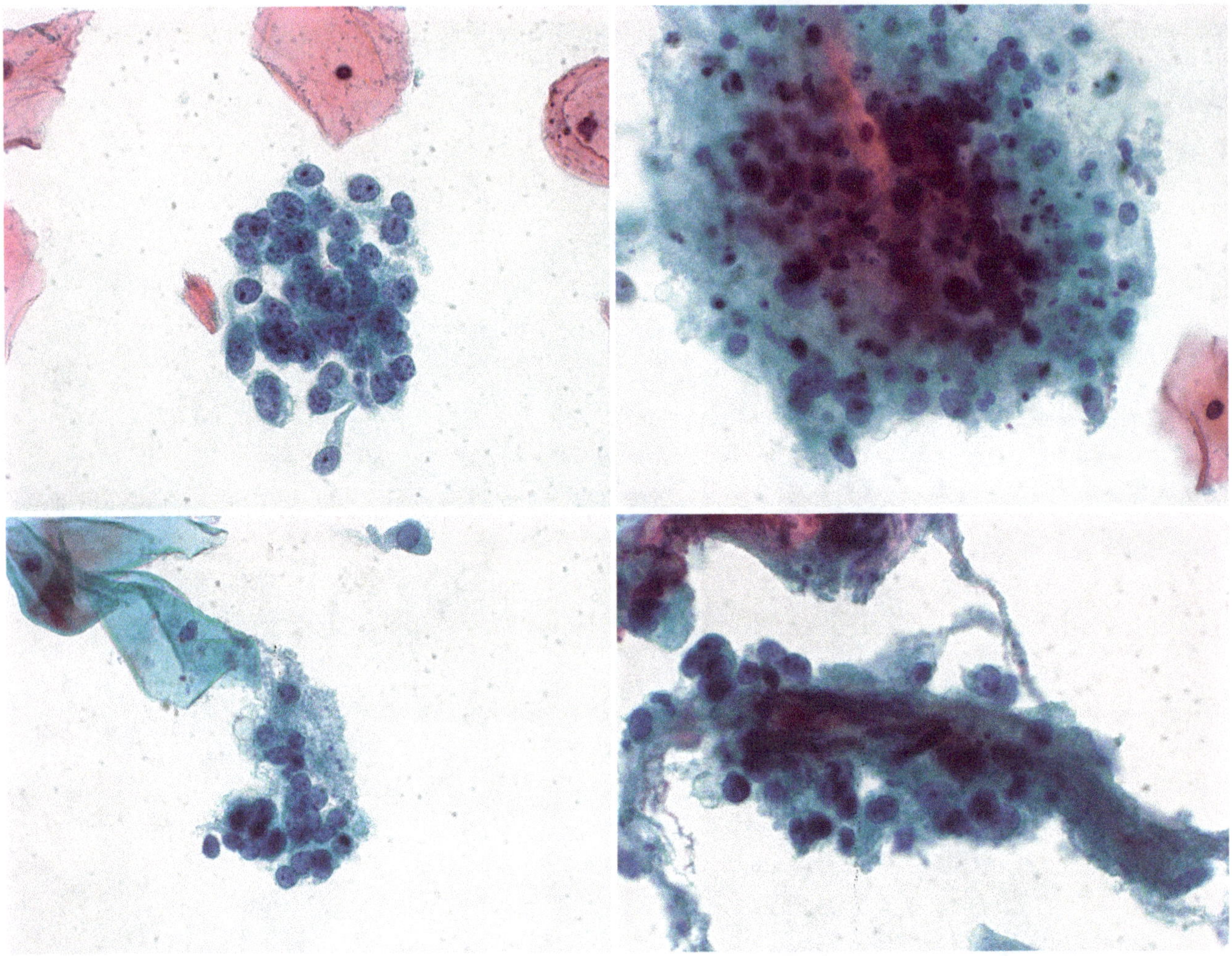

Fig. 2.66

Q-66. These images are from a cervical Pap test. The most likely diagnosis is:

(a) Malignant melanoma
(b) Malignant lymphoma
(c) Adenocarcinoma in situ (AIS)
(d) High-grade squamous intraepithelial lesion (HSIL)
(e) Endocervical adenocarcinoma
(f) Invasive squamous cell carcinoma

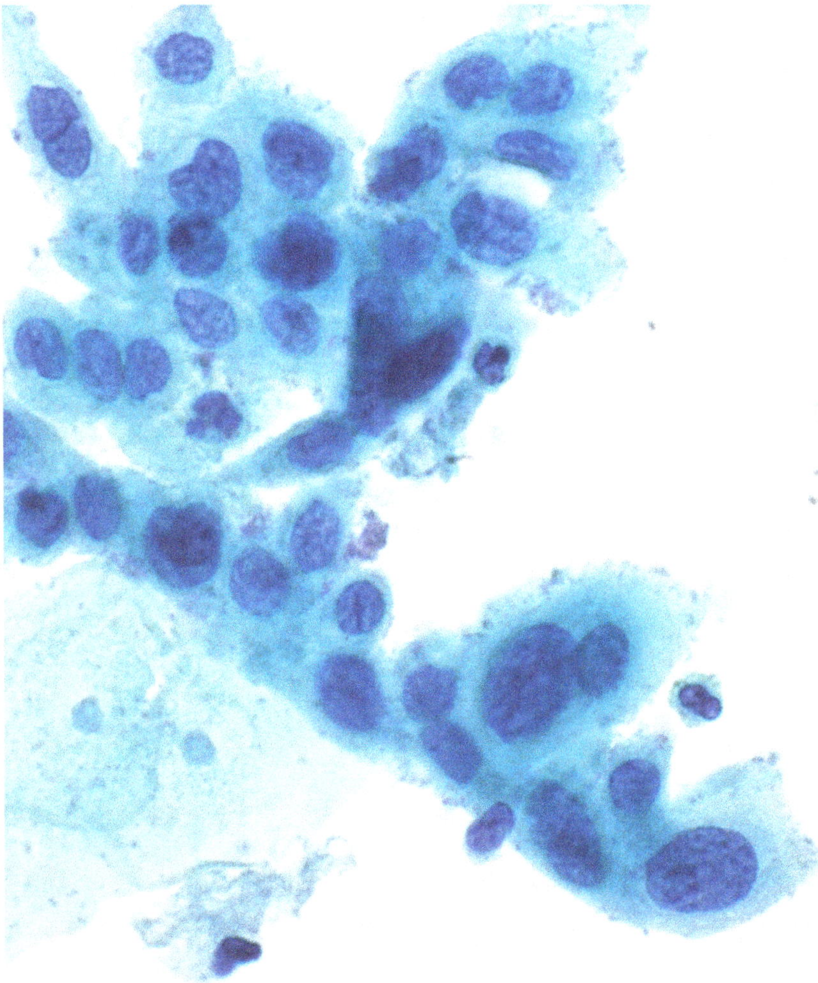

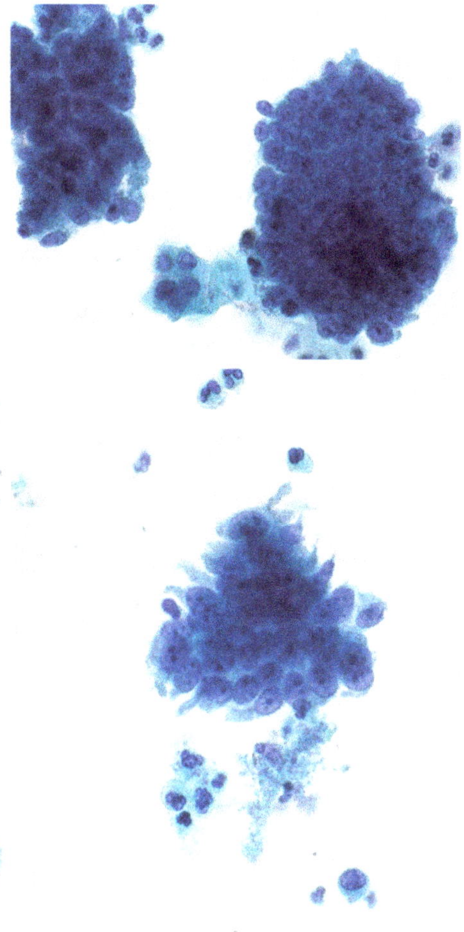

Fig. 2.67

Q-67. These images are from a cervical Pap test. Which of the following interpretations is correct?
(a) Atypical glandular cells (AGC) only.
(b) Atypical squamous cells cannot exclude high-grade squamous intraepithelial lesion (ASC-H) only.
(c) Reactive changes.
(d) AGC and ASC-H.
(e) Endometrial carcinoma.

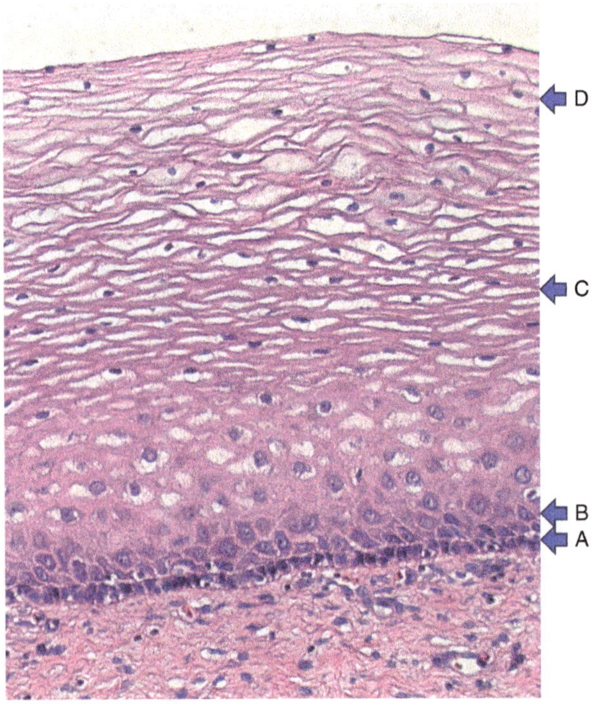

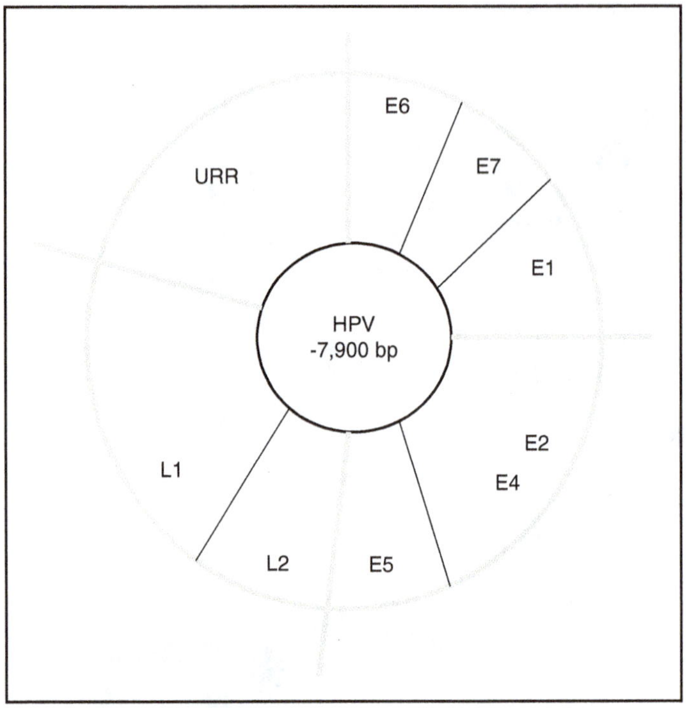

Fig. 2.68

Q-68. The left image is a biopsy from the ectocervix. What is the type of virus described at in the image on the right, and which layer of the epithelium does it infect?

(a) HSV, A
(b) CMV, B
(c) HPV, A
(d) HPV, B
(e) HPV, C
(f) HPV, D

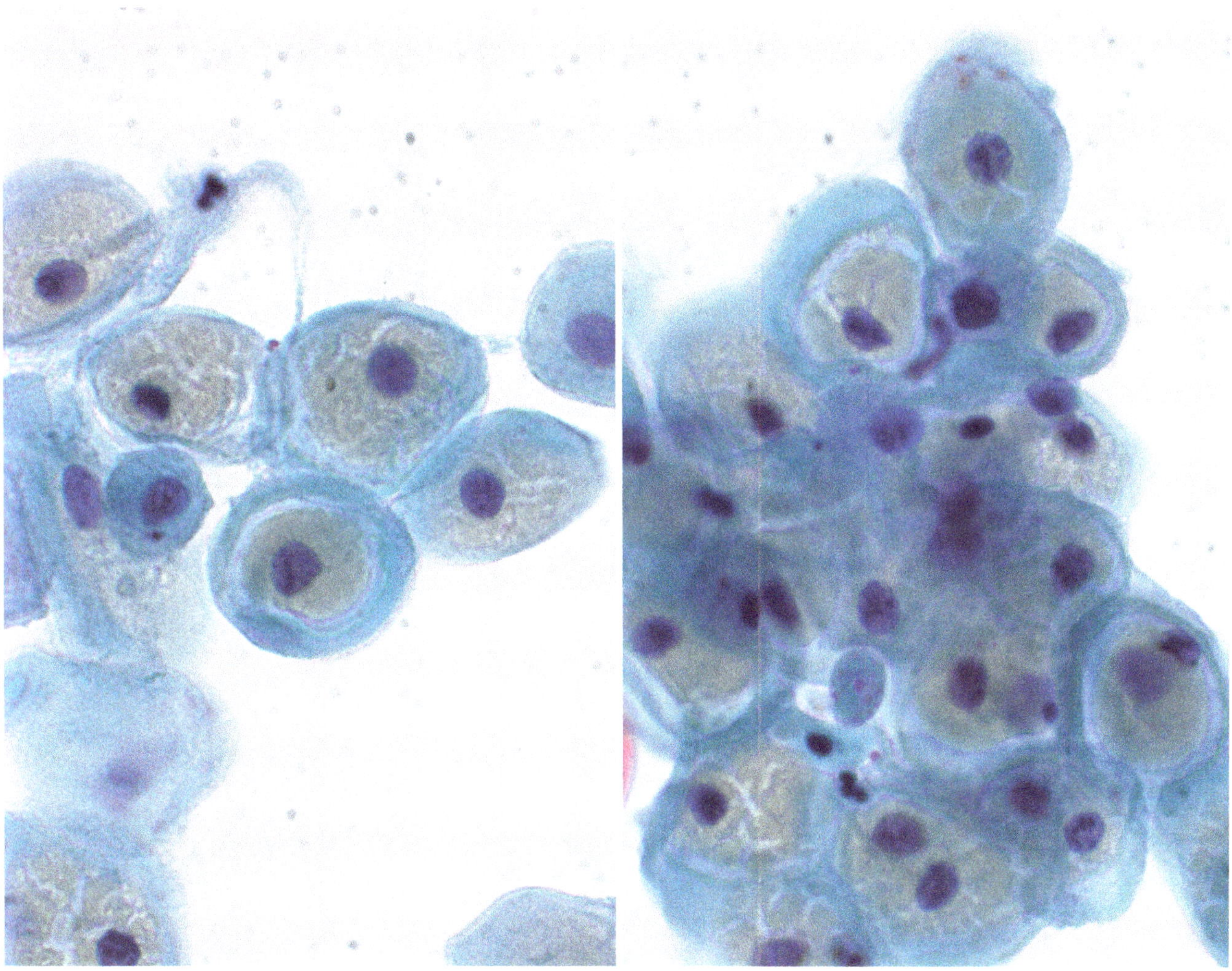

Fig. 2.69

Q-69. These images are from the cervical Pap test of a 50-year-old woman. The cytoplasmic change is due to:

(a) Glycogen accumulated in the cytoplasm
(b) Lipid accumulated in the cytoplasm
(c) Viral particles accumulated in the cytoplasm
(d) Water accumulated in the cytoplasm
(e) Abundant expression of the HPV E4 protein which binds with cytoplasmic keratin
(f) None of the above

Fig. 2.70

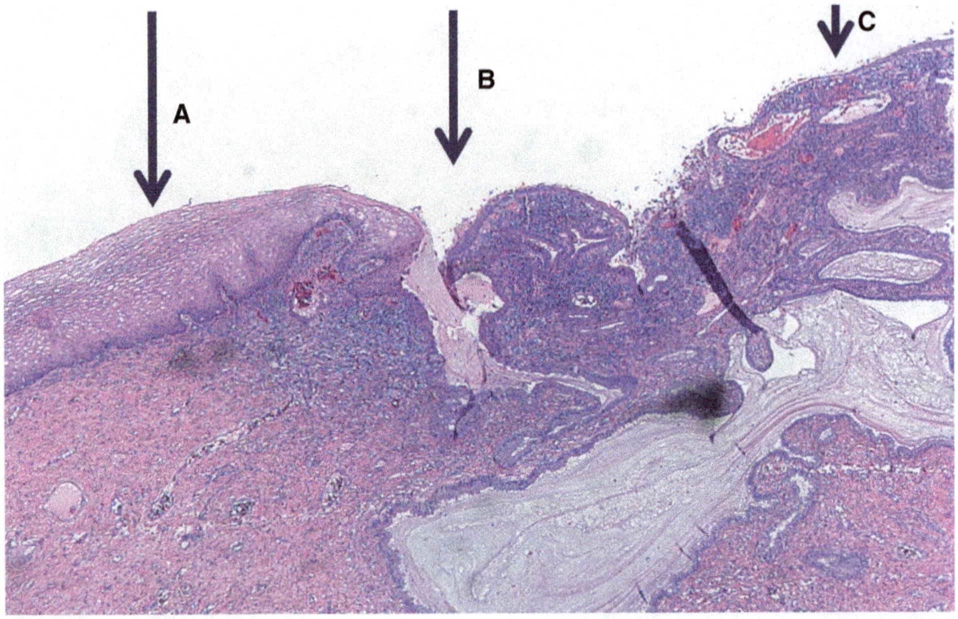

Q-70. This image is from a biopsy of the cervix. Which site is the most vulnerable area of HR HPV infection?

(a) Site A
(b) Site B
(c) Site C
(d) All of the above
(e) None of the above

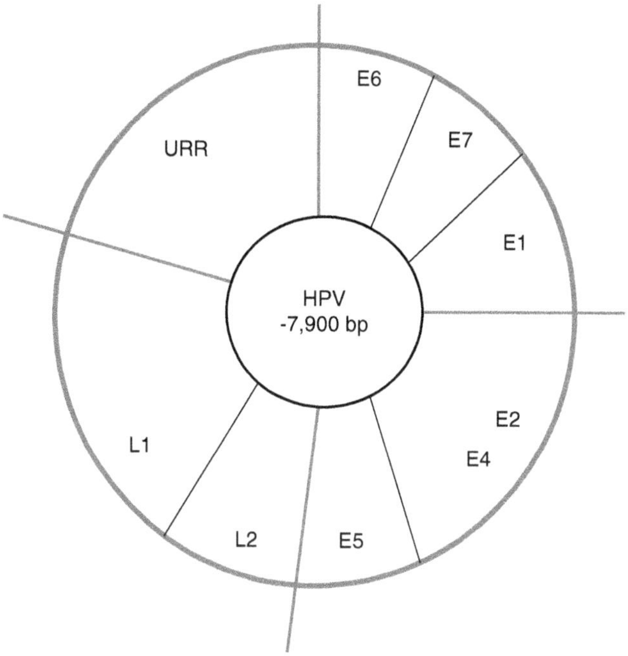

Fig. 2.71

Q-71. Gardasil (Merck & Co., Inc.) is a quadrivalent vaccine against HPV types 6, 11, 16, and 18. This vaccine consists of empty protein shells called virus-like particles. They are made up of the major HPV capsid protein ______.

(a) URR
(b) E6
(c) E7
(d) E2
(e) E5
(f) L1
(g) L2

2.4 Answers and Discussion of Text-Based Questions 1–43

A-1. **(e) All of the above.**

In 1956, Koss and Durfee named the term koilocytotic atypia. The term is derived from the Greek words koilos = a hollow and cytos = cell. Koilocytes are used to describe, in cervicovaginal smears, peculiar large squamous cells with enlarged, hyperchromatic nuclei and a large clear perinuclear clear zone or halo. The koilocytes are pathognomonic of a permissive human papillomavirus (HPV) infection. Electron microscopy demonstrates that the nuclei of koilocytes contain mature viral particles and the clear cytoplasmic zones (halos) represent a collapse of the cytoplasmic filaments or cytoplasmic necrosis caused by the viral infection.

A-2. **(d) E7 protein reacts with the p16 gene.**

The statement would be correct if it read "E7 protein reacts with the Rb gene."

HPV are small, circular, double-stranded DNA viruses, each strand being composed of approximately 7,900 nucleotides. The genetic organization of the HPV viruses is presented as a single strand of DNA in the form of "open reading frames" (ORFs) or genes, which contain messages for protein formation. These include early (E) and late (L) ORFs/genes. Early ORFs/genes ensure the replication of the genetic machinery of the virus. Two late ORFs/genes inscribe capsular proteins. The protein products of ORF 1 and 2 reproduce the viral genome. ORF 2 regulates the transcription of the viral genome. ORFs E6 and E7 play a role in cell transformation. Proteins of E6 and E7 from the HR HPV types 16 and 18 react with proteins regulating events in the cell cycle. E6 protein reacts with p53, which governs G1 phase of the cell cycle. E7 protein reacts with the Rb gene, which governs the orderly transition of cells from G1 to G2 phase.

A-3. **(b) In most pregnant women, the presence of the virus is not transient.**

In most young women, the presence of the virus is transient and of no apparent clinical significance. Normal pregnant women are frequent carriers of HPV. Depending on the trimester of pregnancy, 30–50 % of women show evidence of HPV infection. The presence of the virus in pregnant women is transient and is related to somewhat lowered immunity occurring during pregnancy.

A-4. **(b) The frequency of documented viral presence is not related to age.**

The correct statement is "The frequency of documented viral presence diminishes with age."

HPV infection rate is highest in teenagers and in women in the third decade of life. It becomes much lower in women in the fourth decade of life and older. Invasive cancer of the uterine cervix peaks in the fourth and fifth decades of life. HPV virus must remain latent for many years and remain active to induce the multiple molecular genetic and carcinogenic changes.

A-5. **(e) None of the above (i.e., all of the statements are correct).**

LSIL (low-grade squamous intraepithelial lesion) is a low-risk intraepithelial lesion. It is encountered in approximately 2–3 % of all Pap samples. LSIL is caused by a large number of different types of HPVs, including low-risk HPVs (LR HPVs) and high-risk HPVs (HR HPVs). Many LSILs regress spontaneously. However, some persist for long periods of time. Approximately 18–21 % of LISL cases progress to HSIL. Less than 1 % (0.15 %) of untreated LSIL cases progress to invasive cancer. More than 70 % of cervical LSIL Pap samples are HR HPV positive. More than 10 % of HR HPV-positive cervical LSIL cases have a follow-up biopsy diagnosis of CIN2/3.

A-6. **(e) All of the above.**

HSIL (high-grade squamous intraepithelial lesion) is an intraepithelial lesion that is encountered in about 0.5 % of all Pap samples. Virtually all women (97 %) with an HSIL Pap result test positive for high-risk HPV. If left untreated, it carries a significant risk of progression to cervical cancer. HR HPV is found in >95 % of women with cervical HSIL and in >80 % of women with vaginal HSIL. More than 60 % of HR HPV-positive cervical HSIL cases have a follow-up biopsy diagnosis of CIN2/3.

A-7. **(d) CIN2+ is seen in histopathologic follow-up in about 2 % of patients.**

A study of US women with negative computer-imaged liquid-based cytology (LBC) and positive HR HPV results found that both LSIL and LSIL + lesions were detectable in follow-up histological studies. Cervical intraepithelial neoplasia (CIN1) and low-grade squamous intraepithelial lesions (CIN1/LSIL) and more severe lesions (CIN1/LSIL+) were detected in more than 10 % of pap HR HPV + patients. CIN2+ was diagnosed in about 2 %.

A-8. **(e) All of the above.**
The 2011 ATHENA HPV study showed that the overall prevalence rates of HR HPV, HPV 16, and HPV 18 detected with the Cobas 4,800 HPV test were 32.6, 8.2, and 2.9 %, respectively. In women with ASC-US cytology results, biopsy-confirmed CIN1, CIN2, and CIN3 were seen in 10.0, 2.2, and 2.9 % of women, respectively. No cases of invasive cervical cancers or adenocarcinoma in situ were detected. The prevalence of CIN2 or worse was 5.1 %, and the prevalence of CIN3 or worse was 2.9 %. Genotypes 16 and/or 18 were detected in 8 % of women without CIN, 18 % of women with CIN1, 44 % of women with CIN2, and 61 % of women with CIN3 or worse.

A-9. **(d) HR HPV is detected in 50 % or more of patients with ASC-H.**
The reported incidence of cases interpreted as ASC-H varies significantly and ranges from 0.22 to 1.09 % of all Pap test results. The reported rate of subsequent histological diagnoses of CIN2/3 on follow-up tissue studies also varies in a wide range from 12.2 to 68.2 %. A recent study performed at the Magee-Womens Hospital/University of Pittsburgh Medical Center cytopathology laboratory, a large subspecialized academic hospital laboratory, showed that HR HPV was detected in 50 % (589 of 1,187) of women with ASC-H (ALTS data: 84 % women with ASC-H were reported positive for HR HPV).

A-10. **(b) The HR HPV-positive rate in women <40 years is higher than in women 40 years and older.**
The reported incidence of cases interpreted as ASC-H varies significantly, ranging from 0.22 to 1.09 % of all Pap test results. The reported rate of subsequent histological diagnosis of CIN2/3 on follow-up tissue studies also varies widely, ranging from 12.2 to 68.2 %.

The HR HPV-positive rate in women younger than 40 years is significantly higher than in women 40 years and older.

A-11. **(d) CIN2/3 is identified in 30–50 % of HR HPV-positive women.**
The reported incidence of cases interpreted as ASC-H varies significantly, ranging from 0.22 to 1.09 % of all Pap test results. The reported rate of subsequent histological diagnosis of CIN2/3 on follow-up tissue studies also varies widely, ranging from 12.2 to 68.2 %.

A recent study performed at the Magee-Womens Hospital/University of Pittsburgh Medical Center cytopathology laboratory showed that in histopathologic follow-up, CIN2/3 was identified in 32.7 % of HR HPV-positive women compared with 1.2 % in HR HPV-negative women. The accumulated mean risk of biopsy-proven CIN2/3 for HR HPV-positive ASC-H cases was 41.2 %, compared with 4.9 % for HR HPV-negative ASC-H cases.

A-12. **(d) 70–80 %**
Most women in the world are probably infected with at least one if not several types of HPV during their sexual life. Total exposure is difficult to measure because DNA detection is usually transient and serology is not accurate. It is estimated that about 70–80 % of sexually active women in the US will have HPV infection during their lifetime.

A-13. **(a) They display predictable behavior.**
The behavior of precancerous lesions of uterine cervix is unpredictable. Many of these lesions, particularly of the low-grade lesions, may vanish without treatment or after follow-up biopsies. In contrast, other precursor lesions may persist for many years without major changes or may undergo atrophy after the menopause. Although it is much more likely that invasive cancer of the uterine cervix develops from high-grade lesions, it is important to know that it may follow any type of precursor lesion.

A-14. **(f) All are correct.**
The same as women, most sexually active men in the USA will obtain HPV infection at some time during their lives. Although HPV-related penile cancers can occur, the cancer risk is lower than that for cervical cancer in women. Some men will get HPV-related anal cancers.

A-15. **(c) It is not seen in inflammatory and regenerative processes.**
In 1949, Papanicolaou proposed the term karyomegaly. It was defined as the nuclear enlargement of superficial, intermediate, or large parabasal cells with morphologically normal cytoplasm. The cytoplasm of the affected cells may show normal folding or cytolysis during the second half of the menstrual cycle. In the 2001 Bethesda System, karyomegaly is included in the category of epithelial cell abnormality. Nuclear enlargement of "two and a half to three times" above the size of normal nuclei of intermediate cells may qualify as karyomegaly or ASC-US. This definition is a necessary requirement because, in routine work, the sizes of the nuclei are not measured. Only conspicuous nuclear

enlargement may qualify as karyomegaly. In practice, the increase in nuclear sizes is best verified by comparing the nuclear size of an atypical cell with the nuclear size of adjacent normal cells. Karyomegaly can be seen in inflammatory and regenerative processes.

A-16. **(c) 80–90 % of HPV infections will be cleared at 2 years.**
Most cervical HPV infections (with cytological abnormality or not) are temporary and cleared or suppressed by cell-mediated immunity and have little long-term significance. Seventy percent of infections are gone in 1 year and 90 % in 2 years. Most of these genital infections are self-limiting. A small proportion (about 10 %) of carcinogenic infections persisting for several years is strongly linked to a high absolute risk of diagnosis of precancer. In fact, persistent HR HPV is the single most important risk factor for CIN3 or cervical cancer. It is not completely clear how long an infection must continue before affirmed persistence, but given an average duration of transient HPV of 6–9 months, persistence is usually defined as infections in which the same HPV type is identified in two genital samples taken over an interval at least 12 months apart. Of the various HPV types, infection with HPV 16 is more likely to persist.

A-17. **(a) Koilocytosis is HPV type dependent.**
Koilocytes are mature squamous cells. They are usually the intermediate type and are characterized by abnormal, enlarged and hyperchromatic, single, double or, rarely, multiple nuclei. Large, sharply demarcated perinuclear clear zones or halos surround the nuclei. The nuclei are usually smudged and homogeneous. The koilocytes are pathognomonic of a permissive HPV infection. However, koilocytosis is not HPV-type dependent, as any type of HPV may cause it, whether LR HPV or HR HPV.

A-18. **(f) All of the above**
Human papillomavirus (HPV) has been found to be associated with several types of cancer: cervical, vulvar, vaginal, penile, anal, and a few head and neck (oropharyngeal) cancers. Each year, more than 20,000 HPV-associated cancers occur in women; cervical cancer is the most common. More than 11,000 HPV-associated cancers occur each year in men; oropharyngeal cancers are the most common.

A-19. **(e) All of the above**
The risk of cervical cancer is mainly a function of HPV infection and lack of effective screening. It is clear that although HPV infection of the HR types is required for cervical carcinogenesis, it is not sufficient. Since only a low percentage of women with high-risk HPV develop cancer, host and environmental factors must play some role. Factors such as smoking, pregnancy, multiparity, and long-term use of oral contraceptives, micronutrients, and other STDs can be independently associated with an increased cervical cancer risk after adjustment for HPV infection.

A-20. **(b) HR HPV + rates are highest in women with coexisting AGC and HSIL.**
The HR HPV + rates are highest in women with AGC and HSIL (75.0 %), AGC and ASC-H (41.4 %), and AGC-EC (37.3 %) and lowest in the AGC-EM group (5.3 %).

A-21. **(f) All above tests are FDA approved**
Currently, there are five FDA-approved assays that can be used to detect high-risk HPV. These include the Hybrid Capture 2 HPV test and the Cervista HPV HR test, which are high-risk HPV DNA-based screening assays. The Cervista HPV 16/18 test, which is a high-risk HPV DNA-based genotyping assay, is approved for reflex testing of patients with positive high-risk HPV Cervista test results. The recently FDA-approved Cobas 4,800 HPV test is a high-risk HPV DNA-based PCR screening assay with capability for concurrent genotyping for HPV 16 and HPV 18 by real-time PCR. Most recently, the APTIMA HPV assay for the detection of E6 and E7 mRNA received FDA approval for detection of high-risk HPV.

A-22. **(e) All of the above**
Based on the ASCCP guidelines, the HPV test is appropriate in the following circumstances:

A. Routine cervical cancer screening in conjunction with cervical cytology (dual testing or co-testing) for women aged 30 years or more:
   (a) For women who are cytology negative but HPV positive, repeat both tests in 12 months.
   (b) For women who are both cytology and HPV-negative, repeat both tests only after a 3-year interval.
B. Initial triage management of women aged 21 years or older with a cytological result of atypical squamous cells of undetermined significance (ASC-US).
C. Initial triage management of postmenopausal women with a cytological result of low-grade squamous intraepithelial lesion (LSIL).
D. Post-colposcopy management of women of any age with an initial cytological result of atypical

glandular cells (AGC). [Note that for a finding of AGC, HPV testing is not to be used for triage to decide whether to refer for colposcopy; however, HPV testing may be performed at the time of colposcopy to guide post-colposcopy management.]

E. Post-colposcopy management of women aged 21 years with initial cytological results of ASC-US or LSIL (when the initial colposcopy does not identify a high-grade lesion).

F. Post-treatment surveillance.

A-23. (**c**) **5 % have CIN2–3 on subsequent biopsy**.
Low-grade squamous intraepithelial lesion (LSIL) encompasses both human papillomavirus (HPV) effects and mild dysplasia (cervical intraepithelial neoplasia [CIN] 1). Approximately 70–80 % women with LSIL Pap test are HR HPV-positive and 15–25 % have CIN2–3 on subsequent biopsy. Spontaneous regression is seen in approximate 80 % cases. Squamous cell carcinoma may develop in less than 0.3 % of women with CIN1.

A-24. (**d**) **Both vaccines are very effective against diseases caused by HPV types 6 and 11**.
Gardasil is the only cervical cancer vaccine that helps protect against four types of HPV: two high-risk types, HPV 16 and HPV 18, and also HPV 6 and HPV 11 that cause 90 % of genital warts cases. **Cervarix** is designed to prevent infection from HPV types 16 and 18. Additionally, some cross-reactive protection against virus strains 45 and 31 was shown in clinical trials. Both vaccines are given as shots and require three doses.

A-25. (**f**) **All of the above**.
Cytomorphological features of HSIL:

- Cells appear singly, in sheets, or in syncytial aggregates.
- Cells are of parabasal, basal, or metaplastic type.
- Nuclei are hyperchromatic with fine or coarse, evenly distributed chromatin.
- Nuclear membrane is markedly irregular.
- Nucleoli may be present.
- Cytoplasm is "immature," dense or lacy, and delicate.
- Cytoplasm is eosinophilic/orangeophilic in keratinizing dysplasia.
- High N:C ratio.

A-26. (**f**) **All of the above**.
The median reporting rate of ASC-US in US laboratories is 4.7 %, and the median rate of ASC-H is 0.4 %. The rate of high-risk HPV DNA positivity is from 40 to 51 % among women with ASC-US but 74–88 % among women with ASC-H. The rate of high-risk HPV DNA positivity is from 74 to 88 % among women with ASC-H. The rate of high-risk HPV DNA positivity is 76.6 % among women with LSIL.

A-27. (**c**) **FDA-approved HPV DNA tests are restricted to low-risk (oncogenic) HPV types**.
The histological classification used in cervical intraepithelial neoplasia is a three-tiered system: CIN1 and CIN2 and CIN3. However, it is important to note that cytological LSIL is not equivalent to histological CIN1 and cytological HSIL is not equivalent to histological CIN2 and CIN3. It is also important to stress that HPV DNA testing should be restricted to high-risk (i.e., oncogenic) HPV types (i.e., 16, 18, 31, 33, 35, 39, 45, 51, 52, 56, 58, 59, and 66). Therefore, whenever "HPV testing" is referred to in the 2006 guidelines, it applies only to testing for high-risk (oncogenic) HPV types. Single HPV testing can identify 92 % of CIN3 lesions.

A-28. (**b**) **A 21-year-old woman**
Adolescent women, pregnant women, postmenopausal women, and immunosuppressed women all belong to special populations according to the "2006 Consensus Guidelines for the Management of Women with Abnormal Cervical Screening Tests."

A-29. (**e**) **Aged 21 and older**
Adolescent women are defined as aged 20 and younger according to the "2006 Consensus Guidelines for the Management of Women with Abnormal Cervical Screening Tests."

A-30. (**b**) **"Reflex" HPV testing**
All three management approaches (two repeat cytology exams at 6- and 12-month intervals, "reflex" testing for HPV, and single colposcopic examination) are considered acceptable for managing women with ASC-US in general populations. Although all three are considered acceptable, "reflex" HPV testing is preferred. Reflex testing refers to testing either the residual specimen of original liquid-based cytology or a separate co-collected sample at the initial screening visit. It is preferred because "reflex" HPV testing eliminates the need for women to return for repeat testing, rapidly reassures many patients that they do not have a significant lesion, and spares 40–60 % of women from undergoing colposcopy.

A-31. **(b) Repeat cytology at 12-month**
Management Approach of ASC-US in Special Populations

A 20-year-old woman belongs to a special population, according to the "2006 Consensus Guidelines." In adolescents with ASC-US, follow-up with annual cytological testing is recommended.

A-32. **(b) Repeat cytological testing at 12 months**
Recommended Management of Women with ASC-US—general management approaches:

Women with ASC-US who are HPV DNA negative can be followed up with repeat cytological testing at 12 months.

A-33. **(d) Colposcopy**
Recommended Management of Women with ASC-US—general management approaches:

Women with ASC-US who are HPV DNA negative can be followed up with repeat cytological testing at 12 months. Women who are HPV DNA positive should be managed in the same fashion as women with LSIL and be referred for colposcopic evaluation. Endocervical sampling is preferred for women in whom no lesions are identified and those with an unsatisfactory colposcopy but is acceptable for women with a satisfactory colposcopy and a lesion identified in the transformation zone.

A-34. **(e) Repeat cytological testing at 6 and 12 months and HPV DNA testing at 12 months**
A 21-year-old woman is regarded as a member of the general population. For a woman with ASC-US and a positive HPV DNA test, if CIN is not identified in her post-colposcopy management, an acceptable option for her is HPV DNA testing at 12 months and repeat cytological testing at 6- and 12-month intervals. It is recommended that HPV DNA testing not be performed at intervals less than 12 months.

A-35. **(d) HSIL or greater**
In adolescents with ASC-US, recommended follow-up is annual cytological testing. At the 12-month follow-up, only adolescents with HSIL or greater on the repeat cytology should be referred to colposcopy.

A-36. **(d) HPV DNA testing at 12 months or Pap testing at 6 and 12 months**
The recommended management of women in the general population with ASC-H is referral for colposcopy. If CIN2 and CIN3 are not identified in the colposcopy, follow-up with HPV DNA testing at 12 months OR cytological testing at 6 and 12 months is acceptable. In women in whom the subsequent HR HPV DNA test at 12 months is positive or their repeat cytological test is ASC-US or greater, colposcopy is recommended.

A-37. **(a) HPV DNA positivity among women with ASC-US is 70–80 %.**
HPV DNA positivity among women with LSIL is 70–80 %. Among women with ASC-US, the rate of HR HPV DNA positivity is from 30 to 50 %.

Most adolescents with HPV infection will be completely recovered with 2–3 years.

Both HPV DNA positivity and CIN2 and CIN3 decline with age which suggests that postmenopausal women with LSIL can be managed less aggressively than premenopausal women. Triage using HPV testing may be an efficient alternative to colposcopy.

A-38. **(d) All of the above**
According to the "2006 Consensus Guidelines," acceptable options for the management of postmenopausal women with LSIL include:

1. Reflex HPV DNA testing
2. Repeat cytological testing at 6 and 12 months
3. Colposcopy

If the HR HPV DNA test is negative or if CIN is not identified at colposcopy, repeat cytology in 12 months is recommended. In postmenopausal women in whom subsequent HR HPV DNA test at 12 months is positive or their repeat cytological test is ASC-US or greater, colposcopy is recommended.

A-39. **(e) All of the above**.
Subsequent Evaluation or Follow-Up of Atypical Glandular Cells (AGC):

The recommended post-colposcopy management of women of known HPV status with either atypical endocervical, endometrial, or glandular cells NOS who do not have CIN2, CIN3, or glandular neoplasia identified histologically is as follows:

1. If they are HPV DNA positive, repeat cytological testing combined with HPV DNA testing at 6 months.
2. If they are HPV DNA negative, repeat cytological testing combined with HPV DNA testing at 12 months.
3. If they are HPV DNA status unknown, repeat cytological testing at 6-month intervals.

The next step in management depends on the results of HPV DNA testing and cytology: Colposcopy is recommended for the women who subsequently test positive for HR HPV DNA or who are found to have ASC-US or greater on the repeat Pap tests. If both the HPV DNA and Pap tests are negative, women can return to routine cytological testing. In the women whose HPV DNA status is unknown, repeat cytological testing at 6-month intervals is recommended. After 4 consecutive negative results are obtained, women are allowed to return to annual cytological testing.

A-40. (**d**) **Either a or b**.
According to the "2006 Consensus Guidelines," in cervical screening testing, reflex testing refers to testing <u>either</u> the residual specimen of original liquid-based cytology <u>or</u> a separate co-collected sample at the initial screening visit.

A-41. (**g**) **All of the above are true**.
The HC2 HPV DNA test is an in vitro nucleic acid hybridization assay. The assay signal is amplified using microplate chemiluminescence for the qualitative detection of 13 high-risk types of HPV DNA 16, 18, 31, 33, 35, 39, 45, 51, 52, 56, 58, 59, and 68. In March 2003, the FDA approved its use in conjunction with routine Pap testing of women over age 30. The HC2 High-Risk HPV DNA test is the most frequently used diagnostic HPV test worldwide. The main problems with the current version of HC2 are cross-reactivity of its probe cocktail with untargeted HPV types 11, 53, 54, 55, 66, MM4, MM7, MM8, or MM9.39 and the lack of an internal control.

A-42. (**d**) **Cervical specimens can be collected in PreservCyt solution**.
The APTIMA HPV assay (Gen-Probe, San Diego, CA) is the latest FDA-approved HPV test. It was approved on October 31, 2011. The APTIMA HPV assay is a transcription-mediated amplification-based assay, which allows the detection of E6/E7 mRNA transcripts of 14 high-risk HPV types (16, 18, 31, 33, 35, 39, 45, 51, 52, 56, 58, 59, 66, 68). However, this assay does not discriminate between the 14 high-risk HPV types. The internal control is used for the quality control. Cervical specimens are collected in either ThinPrep Pap test vials containing PreservCyt solution or the APTIMA Cervical Specimen Collection and Transport Kit. It does not show cross-reactivity with any tested high-risk HPV types or with normal flora and opportunistic organisms that may be found in cervical samples.

A-43. (**a**) **HPV infects superficial cells**.
After HR HPV infects basal cells, they mature up to the surface of the epithelium. Upon infection, the viral genome is maintained as a low copy number in the form of episomes. During epithelial differentiation, the p97 promoter directs expression of E6 and E7 oncoproteins for S-phase entry and subsequent increase in the abundance of viral replication proteins (E1, E2, E4, E5) and facilitates amplification of viral genomes. E4 persists in the upper epithelial layers where viral capsid proteins are found.

2.5 Answers and Discussion of Image-Based Questions 44–71

A-44. (e) **Abundant expression of the HPV E4 protein which binds with cytoplasmic keratin**

The "koilocyte" is an intermediate cell. It has a prominent cytoplasmic perinuclear space around an atypical nucleus. The halo has a sharp edge. The cytoplasmic change is thought to be due to the abundant expression of the HPV E4 protein which binds with cytoplasmic keratin. The nuclei are irregular, hyperchromatic, and may show a wrinkled nuclear membrane. Koilocytotic atypia is considered a SIL under the Bethesda classification.

A-45. (f) **All of the above**.

These cells are LSIL. Low-risk types of HPV (most commonly types 6 and 11) have essentially no risk association for invasive cervical carcinoma but tend to cause condyloma acuminatum, flat condyloma, and some LSIL (cervical intraepithelial neoplasia CINI). The high-risk HPV types (16, 18, 31, 33, 35, 39, 45, 51, 52, 56, 58, 59, 66, 68, 73, and 82) are often found in HSIL (CIN2 and 3), cervical carcinoma in situ (CIS), invasive squamous cell carcinoma, cervical AIS, and adenocarcinoma. High-risk HPV types are also commonly seen in CIN1 (LSIL) lesions. It is true that approximately 21 % of LSIL progress to HSIL.

A-46. (e) **The changes are mainly due to infection of LR HPV**.

The images show LSIL cells and coexisting clue cells which may be seen with Gardnerella vaginalis.

HPVs consist of double-stranded DNA and which is approximately 8,000 base pairs in length. It has three functioning areas: early viral function, late region containing genes for viral structural proteins, and a noncoding regulatory region. The vast majority of these viruses infect epithelial surfaces of either the skin or mucosa. Both LR HPV and HR HPV are associated with LSIL, but most cases of LSIL are related to HR HPV.

A-47. (e) **The nuclear changes are due to *Candida albicans* infection**.

The images show LSIL coexisting with *Candida albicans* infection. HPV replicates in the nuclei of squamous epithelial cells. In the superficial squamous epithelium, the virus reaches full maturity. In the basal layers of squamous cells, the virus is latent, and its DNA can only be detected by molecular techniques. In many low-grade precancerous lesions, HPV DNA is usually retained intact in an episomal form. In contrast, in invasive cancers and some high-grade precancers such as HSIL, CIS, and invasive squamous cell carcinoma, viral DNA is integrated into the host DNA.

With *Candida albicans* infections, squamous cells often exhibit increased evidence of maturation, with parakeratosis and hyperkeratosis. Occasionally, mature squamous cells can show prominent perinuclear halos which are degenerative vacuolar change and can be mistaken for koilocytosis. In addition, some intact squamous cells may show nuclear enlargement that can prompt an interpretation of atypical squamous cells of undetermined significance.

A-48. (c) **Low-grade squamous intraepithelial lesion (LSIL)**

The images show a sheet of LSIL cells with parakeratosis.

The nuclei are more than three times the size of a normal intermediate cell nucleus with hyperchromatic, finely granular chromatin, and irregular nuclear membranes.

Cytomorphology of LSIL, Mild Dysplasia

- Mature squamous cells, superficial or intermediate cell type.
- Single or in sheets.
- Nuclei are more than three times the size of a normal intermediate cell nucleus.
- Hyperchromatic with finely granular chromatin.
- Irregular nuclear membrane.
- Nucleoli rare and inconspicuous.
- Nuclear-to-cytoplasmic ratio is relatively high.
- Better detection of LSIL on liquid-based preparations has reduced the atypical squamous cell to squamous intraepithelial lesion ratio.

A-49. (b) **Approximately 25–50 % have CIN2–3 on subsequent biopsy**.

The upper field and insert show LSIL. The enlarged nuclei are more than three times a normal intermediate cell nucleus with hyperchromatic, finely granular chromatin, and irregular nuclear membranes. The lower field shows normal endocervical cells.

Approximately 80 % of high-risk HPV (+) women have CIN1 on subsequent biopsy and 15–25 % have CIN2–CIN3 on subsequent biopsy. Progression to CIN2 and CIN3 is seen in 10–20 % of LSIL cases. Squamous cell carcinoma may develop in less than 0.3 % of women with LSIL. There is no reliable indicator of which women with CIN1 will progress to a higher grade lesion.

A-50. (c) **Low-grade squamous intraepithelial lesion (LSIL)**

The images show LSIL.

Cytomorphology of LSIL, Mild Dysplasia

- Mature squamous cells, superficial or intermediate cell type.
- Single or in sheets.
- Nuclei are more than three times a normal intermediate cell nucleus.
- Hyperchromatic with finely granular chromatin.
- Irregular nuclear membrane.
- Nucleoli rare and inconspicuous.
- Nuclear-to-cytoplasmic ratio is relatively high.
- Better detection of LSIL on liquid-based preparations has reduced atypical squamous cell: squamous intraepithelial lesion ratio.

Most cases of LSIL are caused by high-risk HPV.

A-51. (e) **More than 50 % of HPV infections persist for 2 years or more**.

The images show ASC-US cells with enlarged nuclei more than 2.5–3 times the area of the nucleus of a normal intermediate cell nucleus, hyperchromatic, finely granular chromatin, and slight irregular nuclear membrane.

High-risk human papillomavirus (HPV) is the main causative agent of invasive squamous cell carcinoma. Cervical HPV is detected in 5–40 % of asymptomatic reproductive women. Fifty to seventy-five percent of them are high-risk HPV type. The majority of them are transient infections with the changes of koilocytes or LSIL. However, some infections may persist and ultimately progress to CIN3/carcinoma in situ. Less than 50 % of HPV infections persist for 2 years or more. Persistent infections are defined as amounts of HPV DNA sufficient enough to be detected using standard molecular assays.

A-52. (f) **E7 binds to p16**.

The images show LSIL.

The HPV cells circular genome consists of 8,000 base pairs, encodes eight viral proteins, and is divisible into three regions: an early (E) region, a late (L) region, and a noncoding region. E1 is the viral replication protein. E2 is the major viral regulator and controls the viral oncogenes. E6 and E7 are viral oncogenes and encode proteins capable of inducing cellular proliferation.

Loss of E2 function leads to overexpression of E6 and E7 which disrupt the cell cycle by promoting the degradation of tumor suppressor genes p53 and retinoblastoma gene (pRb). E6 binds to p53. E7 binds to the pRb. These directly stimulate and maintain cell division, thus causing genomic instability that may lead to HSIL and cancer.

A-53. (e) **INFORM HPV**

The images show LISL. The causative agents are both low-risk and high-risk HPVs. Low-risk HPVs include HPV 6, 11, 40, 42–44, 53, 54, 61, 72, 73, and 81, and high-risk HPVs are 16, 18, 31, 33, 35, 39, 45, 51, 52, 56, 58, 59, 68, and 82.

Currently, there are five (5) FDA-approved assays for HPVs detection:

Hybrid Capture 2 HPV DNA test (Digene Corporation, Gaithersburg, MD, USA), Cervista HPV HR test and Cervista HPV 16/18 test (Hologic, Bedford, MA), Cobas 4,800 HPV test (Roche Molecular Diagnostics, Pleasanton, CA), and APTIMA HPV assay (APTIMA; Gen-Probe, San Diego, CA, USA).

A-54. (d) **High-grade squamous intraepithelial lesion (HSIL)**

The images show HSIL and trichomonas. The HSIL cells are arranged singly and in syncytial fragments with high N:C ratios and enlarged hyperchromatic nuclei. Chromatin is coarse and evenly distributed. The nuclear membrane is markedly irregular.

Cytomorphology of HSIL

- Cells appear singly, in sheets, or in syncytial fragments.
- Cells are of parabasal, basal, or metaplastic type.
- Nuclei are three times the size of intermediate cell nuclei. However, there is variation in the size and the shape of the nuclei.
- Nuclei are hyperchromatic with coarse, evenly distributed chromatin.
- Nuclear membrane is markedly irregular.
- Nucleoli may be present.
- Cytoplasm is "immature," dense or lacy, and delicate.
- Cytoplasm maybe eosinophilic/orangeophilic in keratinizing dysplasia.
- High nuclear-to-cytoplasmic (N:C) ratios.

A-55. (d) **High-grade squamous intraepithelial lesion (HSIL)**

Images show HSIL in a background of inflammation. The HSIL cells are arranged in syncytial fragments with enlarged hyperchromatic nuclei. Chromatin is coarse and evenly distributed. Nuclear membranes are markedly irregular. Some cells show nucleoli. The nuclear-to-cytoplasmic ratio is increased, both by nuclear enlargement and by reduction of the cytoplasmic volume. The nucleus generally occupies less than half of the total area of the cell.

A-56. (d) **The virus is usually retained intact in an episomal form**.

The images show HSIL.

HPV replicates in the nuclei of squamous epithelial cells. In the superficial squamous epithelium, the virus reaches full maturity. In the basal layers of squamous cells, the virus is latent and its DNA can only be detected by molecular techniques. In many low-grade precancerous lesions, HPV DNA is usually retained intact in an episomal form. In contrast, in invasive cancers and some high-grade precancers such as HSIL, CIS, and invasive squamous cell carcinoma, viral DNA is integrated into the host DNA. HR HPV is found in 95 % of women with HSIL.

A-57. (e) **It is suspicious for invasive squamous cell carcinoma**.

The follow-up on this case shows invasive squamous cell carcinoma.

Key Features of Nonkeratinizing Squamous Cell Carcinoma

- Round-to-oval cells predominantly arranged in syncytial aggregates.
- Cyanophilic cytoplasm with relative increase in cytoplasmic volume.
- Round-to-oval nuclei with considerable variation in size.
- N/C is lower than in carcinoma in situ due to larger volume of cytoplasm.
- Unevenly distributed, coarsely granular hyperchromatic nuclear chromatin.
- Irregularly shaped micronucleoli are present, and macronucleoli are frequently found.
- Possible association with unsatisfactory specimens due to tissue necrosis and bleeding.

Almost all cervical squamous cell carcinomas are HPV-associated.

A-58. (e) **Invasive squamous cell carcinoma (nonkeratinizing)**

The images show invasive nonkeratinizing squamous cell carcinoma

Key Features of Nonkeratinizing Squamous Cell Carcinoma

- Round-to-oval cells predominantly arranged in syncytial aggregates.
- Cyanophilic cytoplasm with relative increase in cytoplasmic volume.
- Round-to-oval nuclei with considerable variation in size.
- N/C is lower than in carcinoma in situ due to larger volume of cytoplasm.
- Unevenly distributed, coarsely granular hyperchromatic nuclear chromatin.
- Irregularly shaped micronucleoli are present, and macronucleoli are frequently found.
- Possible association with unsatisfactory specimens due to tissue necrosis and bleeding.

A-59. (a) **It is not HPV-related**.

The image shows endometrial adenocarcinoma. Almost all cervical squamous cell carcinomas and adenocarcinomas are associated with HR HPV infection, but endometrial carcinoma is not HPV related.

A-60. (g) **None of the above**.

The images show reactive endocervical cells with microacinar architecture—microglandular hyperplasia. It is a benign alteration of endocervical epithelium associated with oral contraceptive use. Cytological changes range from entirely normal endocervical cells to marked nuclear enlargement, prominent nucleoli, and cytoplasmic vacuolization. It is a diagnostic pitfall of HSIL. However, the presence of isolated diagnostic HSIL cells is virtually always noted in HSIL. Microglandular hyperplasia is not HPV related.

A-61. (a) **It is atypical glandular cells (AGC)**.

The images show AGC of hyperchromatic groups with enlarged nuclei, hyperchromasia, and small nucleoli. Cytoplasm is moderate to scant with engulfed neutrophils. Most women with AGC Pap test will have a negative HR HPV test.

In Bethesda 2001, atypical glandular cells are classified as:

- Atypical glandular cells (AGC)
  - Atypical endocervical cells (EC)
  - Atypical endometrial cells
  - Not otherwise specified (NOS)
- AGC
  - Atypical endocervical cells, favor neoplastic
  - AGC favor neoplastic
- Endocervical adenocarcinoma in situ (AIS)
- Adenocarcinoma
  - Endocervical
  - Endometrial
  - Extrauterine
  - NOS

Cytological Features of AGC, AGC-NOS

- Cells occur in hyperchromatic groups, sheets, or strips.
- Nuclei are enlarged, three to five times larger than normal endocervical cell nuclei, and variable.
- Slight contour irregularity and hyperchromasia.
- Nucleoli may be present.

- Cytoplasm is moderate to scant.
- Relatively high nuclear-to-cytoplasmic (N:C) ratio.

A-62. (a) **Atypical glandular cells** (**AGC**)
The images show atypical endometrial cells (AGC). Cells occur in small groups with 3-dimentional arrangement. Nuclei are enlarged with small nucleoli. The cytoplasm is scant with occasional vacuolation, and ill-defined cell border.

A-63. (c) **Adenocarcinoma in situ** (**AIS**)
The images show AIS.

Key features of endocervical adenocarcinoma in situ (AIS):

- Hyperchromatic crowded groupings of cells
- Pseudostratified strips of columnar cells
- Epithelial rosettes (gland formations)
- Nuclear and cytoplasmic "feathering"
- Nuclear size twofold greater than normal endocervical nuclei
- N:C ratio increased beyond normal endocervical cells
- Coarsely granular, evenly distributed hyperchromatic chromatin
- Possible presence of small nucleoli
- Presence of mitotic figures and apoptotic bodies
- Not associated with a background "tumor" diathesis

A-64. (e) **It is not associated with HPV 16/18 infection**.
The images show AIS.

AIS is a precursor lesion of invasive endocervical adenocarcinoma. AIS shares many of the same epidemiologic risk factors as invasive endocervical adenocarcinoma and is associated with HPV in virtually all cases. Squamous dysplasias are commonly identified in association with AIS (more than 50 %). HR HPV types 16 and 18 are the most prevalent oncogenic viruses found in AIS, the ratio of HPV 18/HPV 16 in cervical glandular is higher than that in squamous neoplasia.

A-65. (e) **It is benign reactive process**.
The images show AGC, endocervical. The F/U biopsy shows AIS (Images A, B, C).

Both squamous and glandular neoplastic lesions of the cervix are thought to be derived from a common progenitor cell, the undifferentiated reserve cells. Infection of HR HPV types of these cells is thought to be the primary and necessary event. For glandular lesions such as AIS, in addition to HPV association, there are distinctly identified risk factors associated with the development of glandular lesions. They are more highly associated with nonsmokers and lower parity than are squamous carcinomas. They are also associated with hormonal factors, such as use of oral contraceptives and hormone replacement therapy.

A-66. (e) **Endocervical adenocarcinoma**
The images show endocervical adenocarcinoma. The F/U biopsy (See images below) shows cervical adenocarcinoma with neuroendocrine features.

Malignant neoplasms, other than conventional squamous carcinoma and adenocarcinoma, may be seen in cervical cytological preparation. Familiarity with cytological features of these entities is useful when an unusual tumors morphology is encountered.

A-67. (d) **AGC and ASC-H**
The images show the coexistence of AGC and ASC-H. This set of images consists of two lesions. The first lesion is exhibited at left image. There is a single syncytial two-dimensional cluster, hyperchromatic crowded group, with nuclear enlargement, variable nuclear size and shape, nuclear hyperchromasia, abnormal chromatin pattern with nuclear membrane irregularity, metaplastic cytoplasm, and high nuclear-to-cytoplasmic ratio. Nucleoli are absent. The findings are consistent with ASC-H. The second lesion is exhibited at right the images on the right. The glandular cells are arranged in sheets, clusters, and rosettes with variable nuclear enlargement, nuclear hyperchromasia, evenly dispersed coarsely chromatin, and nuclear elongation. Nuclear crowding and overlap are present. Some cells demonstrate conspicuous nucleoli. Neoplastic cells have increased nuclear-to-cytoplasmic ratio. These changes are characteristics of atypical glandular cells (AGC), favor neoplastic.

The f/u endocervical biopsy (see below) shows two lesions: CIN3 involving cervical gland and intestinal type AIS. It is not uncommon to find the coexistence of squamous dysplasia with atypical glandular cells.

A-68. (c) **HPV**, **A**
The image on the right is a depiction of HPV DNA. HR HPVs infect the basal cell layer, which is indicated as A in the left image. A productive infection of HR HPV leads to the production of whole infectious virions, which are limited to epithelia that will undergo maturation. Cervical epithelial maturation is a process that occurs under the influence of estrogen and progesterone. In basal cells, HPV replication is limited by E2.

A-69. (**a**) **Glycogen accumulated in the cytoplasm**

The images show parabasal cells with glycogen accumulated in the cytoplasm, which look like koilocytes.

Koilocytes are the pathognomonic change of infection with HPV. Koilocytes have distinct cytomorphological features. They are superficial or intermediate squamous cells. Koilocytic cells display a large perinuclear halo with irregular, clear-cut edges, and a dense, often amphophilic, sometimes almost hyaline cytoplasm in the area surrounding the perinuclear cavity. Glycogen often displays the yellowish appearance seen here.

A-70. (**b**) **Site B**

The image shows squamous metaplasia.

The arrow B in the image is the ectocervical–endocervical interface, i.e., transformation zone or squamocolumanar junction. The ectocervical–endocervical interface is the most vulnerable area, situated between the squamous-lined ectocervix and the columnar-lined endocervix. It is also referred to as the transformation zone or squamocolumnar junction. HPV infection is believed to originate in this zone. Once the infection is established, it may move proximally or distally and affect the adjacent epithelial cells, i.e., the squamous cells and columnar cells. Ectocervical involvement by HPV results in infected cells presenting as dyskeratosis. When the infection is situated in the transformation zone, parakeratotic- and metaplastic-type cells may predominate in the Pap smear. When HPV infection involves the transformation zone or the endocervical canal, the infected cells may show immature, metaplastic-type cells (atypical repair-type cells) in the Pap smear.

A-71. (**f**) **L1**

There are two recently developed prophylactic HPV vaccines. Both vaccines consist of empty protein shells called virus-like particles that are made up of the major HPV capsid protein L1. They contain no DNA and therefore are not infectious. One of the vaccines, Gardasil (Merck & Co., Inc.), is a quadrivalent vaccine against HPV types 6, 11, 16, and 18. The other, Cervarix (GlaxoSmithKline), is a bivalent vaccine that protects against HPV 16 and HPV 18.

Reading List

Bandyopadhyay S, Austin RM, Dabbs D, Zhao C. Adjunctive human papillomavirus DNA testing is a useful option in some clinical settings for disease risk assessment and triage of females with ASC-H Papanicolaou test results. Arch Pathol Lab Med. 2008;132(12): 1874–81.

Cibas ES. Cervical and vaginal cytology. In: Cibas ES, Ducatman BS, editors. Cytology diagnostic principles and clinical correlates. Philadelphia: Saunders/Elsevier; 2009.

Gao FF, Austin RM, Zhao C. Histopathologic follow-up and human papillomavirus DNA test results in 290 patients with high-grade squamous intraepithelial lesion Papanicolaou test results. Cancer Cytopathol. 2011;119(6):377–86.

Heider A, Austin RM, Zhao C. HPV test results stratify risk for histopathologic follow-up findings of high-grade cervical intra-epithelial neoplasia in women with low-grade squamous intra-epithelial lesion Pap results. Acta Cytol. 2011;55(1):48–53.

Hoda RS, Hoda SA. Low-grade squamous intra-epithelial lesion. In: Fundamentals of Pap test cytology. Totowa: Humana Press; 2007.

Koss LG, Melamed MR. Squamous carcinoma of the uterine cervix and its precursors. In: Koss LG, Melamed MR, editors. Koss' diagnostic cytology and its histopathologic bases. Philadelphia: Lippincott Williams and Wilkins; 2005.

Solomon D, Nayar R. Bethesda system for reporting cervical cytology: definitions, criteria, and explanatory notes. 2nd ed. New York: Springer; 2004.

Wright Jr TC, Massad LS, Dunton CJ, Spitzer M, Wilkinson EJ, Solomon D, et al. 2006 consensus guidelines for the management of women with abnormal cervical screening tests. J Low Genit Tract Dis. 2007;11(4):201–22.

Zhao C, Florea A, Austin RM. Clinical utility of adjunctive high-risk human papillomavirus DNA testing in women with Papanicolaou test findings of atypical glandular cells. Arch Pathol Lab Med. 2010;134(1):103–8.

Zhao C, Chen X, Onisko A, Kanbour A, Austin RM. Follow-up outcomes for a large cohort of US women with negative imaged liquid-based cytology findings and positive high risk human papillomavirus test results. Gynecol Oncol. 2011;122(2):291–6.

3 Normal, Infectious, and Reactive Changes in the Pap Test

Marilee Means and Walid E. Khalbuss

Contents

M. Means, PhD, SCT(ASCP) (✉)
School of Health Professions,
University of Kansas Medical Center,
3901 Rainbow Blvd., Mail Stop 4048,
Kansas City, KS 66160, USA
e-mail: mmeans@kumc.edu

W.E. Khalbuss, MD, PhD, FIAC
Director of Cytology and Cytopathology Fellowship Program,
University of Pittsburgh Medical Center Shadyside Hospital,
5150 Centre Avenue, 2, Suite 201,
Pittsburgh, PA 15232, USA
e-mail: khalbussw2@upmc.edu

3.1 Tables and Summary

Table 3.1 Normal epithelial cells in the Pap test

Epithelial cells	Size	Nucleus	Cytoplasm
Superficial cells	45–50 μm in diameter	Smallest, dark, pyknotic	Polygonal
	~1,600 μm²	5–6 μm in diameter	Eosinophilic
		Centrally located	Occasionally basophilic
			Thin, transparent
Intermediate cells	35–50 μm in diameter	Small, bland, vesicular	Polygonal to slightly rounded
	~1,200–1,600 μ²	7–8 μm in diameter	Usually basophilic
		Centrally located	Thin, transparent
Parabasal cells	15–30 μm in diameter	Larger, vesicular	Slightly polygonal to rounded
		8–9 μm in diameter	Basophilic
		Centrally located	Denser appearing, transparent
Basal cells	10–12 μm in diameter	Larger, vesicular	Round to oval
		Slightly smaller than cell	Basophilic
		Centrally located	Densest appearing, scant
Endocervical cells	188 ± 40 μm²	Variably sized, vesicular	Columnar, 2-D picket fence or honeycomb arrangement
		55–82 μm²	Usually basophilic
		Eccentrically located	Vacuolated, may rarely be ciliated
		Micronucleoli may be present	

(continued)

W.E. Khalbuss, M. Means (eds.), *Gynecological and Breast Cytopathology Board Review and Self-Assessment*, DOI 10.1007/978-1-4614-7270-4_3, © Springer Science+Business Media New York 2013

Table 3.1 (continued)

Epithelial cells	Size	Nucleus	Cytoplasm
Endometrial cells	45–72 μm^2	7–8 μm in diameter (equals intermediate cell nucleus)	Cuboidal, 3-D arrangements
	8–10 μm in diameter	No nucleoli	Scant, delicate, poorly staining
	SS – occurs in clusters or singly	SS – oval to bean shaped	May have delicate vacuolization
	DS – occurs in clusters	DS – oval to spindle	SS – more abundant, finely vacuolated
			DS – spindle, very scanty

SS superficial stromal, *DS* deep stromal

Table 3.2 Normal non-epithelial cells in the Pap test

Non-epithelial cells	Cytoplasm	Nucleus	Other
Histiocytes	Abundant, finely vacuolated, amphophilic staining	Vesicular, centrally located	Small histiocytes may be morphologically identical to endometrial superficial stromal cells
Mean 21 μm diameter	Range from small to large multinucleated forms	Oval to bean shaped	Chronic inflammation
Variable	May contain ingested debris		Associated with exodus, foreign bodies, radiation, and surgery
Lymphocytes	Very scanty, basophilic staining	Small, round, and pyknotic in mature cells to slightly larger and vesicular in more immature cells	Variably sized lymphs may be seen in pools with tingible body macrophages in chronic follicular cervicitis
7–8 μm diameter			Chronic inflammation
Polymorphonuclear leukocytes	Scanty, delicately staining	Three to four lobes of the very small nucleus	Most frequently seen inflammatory cell
8–12 μm diameter			Acute inflammation
Plasma cells	Lightly basophilic	Eccentrically located	Not frequently seen
8–10 μm diameter	Egg shaped	"Clockface" chromatin	Chronic inflammation
		Perinuclear "hof"	Associated with antibody production
Eosinophils	Pale with orange granules	Bilobed nuclei	Not frequently seen
10 μm diameter			Chronic inflammation
			Associated with allergic reactions

Table 3.3 Common viral infectious agents in the Pap test

Viral	Morphology	Differential Dx.	Clinical symptoms
Herpes	Multinucleation, molding, ground-glass nuclei, margination of the chromatin	Multinucleated endocervical cells – *no molding*	Blisters, ulceration, recurrent outbreaks
	May have eosinophilic intranuclear inclusions	Mononuclear forms may resemble HSIL – *no hyperchromatic clumpy chromatin*	
	Early changes may be mononuclear		
HPV	Koilocytes, dyskeratocytes	Dysplasia – *insufficient N:C ratio* (*LSIL includes HPV and dysplasia*)	Flat or warty growth pattern, causative factor for CA if high-risk type (16 and 18 most often)
		Keratinizing dysplasia – *DK is too small*	

(continued)

Table 3.3 (continued)

Viral	Morphology	Differential Dx.	Clinical symptoms
CMV	Large basophilic intranuclear inclusion "Owl-eye" appearance Small cytoplasmic inclusions Mononuclear cells Markedly enlarged	Herpes – *multinucleation is not present in CMV, no cytoplasmic inclusions in herpes*	May be asymptomatic, usually a transient infection if immunocompetent Associated with immunosuppression (HIV, transplant)
Molluscum contagiosum	Large eosinophilic or basophilic inclusions in squamous cells Nucleus is often inconspicuous as it is pushed to the side by the large cytoplasmic inclusion	May resemble CMV	Pubic area but also in vagina and cervix, dome-shaped vesicles with centralized crater, occurs after trauma Inclusions are called molluscum bodies

Table 3.4 Common bacterial infectious agents in the Pap test

Bacterial agent	Morphology	Differential Dx.	Clinical symptoms
Leptothrix	Long filamentous bacteria most often seen with Trichomonas; however, trich occurs frequently by itself Much thinner than Candida Often curves	Candida – *too thick and usually stains pink while Leptothrix is bluish* Doderlein bacilli – *usually shorter and do not loop and curve*	No symptoms by itself; however, it usually occurs with Trichomonas which has a greenish discharge
Actinomyces	Higher-order bacteria which are found in colonies of mixed bacteria. Actinomyces shows lavender, starburst arrangements of the thin bacilli, "dust bunnies"	Doderlein bacilli – *do not occur in starburst arrangement mixed with other bacteria*	Associated with IUD or other foreign object such as pessary, may be an incidental finding and removal of IUD may not be necessary if asymptomatic
Bacterial vaginosis	Clue cells with bacteria coating squamous cells, and in the background, normal bacilli are absent, filmy look to the preparation	Doderlein (lactobacilli) – *do not coat the squamous cells and are longer than normal*	Thin, milky vaginal discharge, KOH test for amine odor ("whiff test") is positive
Chlamydia trachomatis	Targetoid cytoplasmic inclusions, nuclear enlargement, increased N:C ratio, multinucleation, and hyperchromasia. Inclusions should be in endocervical and metaplastic cells but not in mature squamous cells	Innumerable reasons for cytoplasmic vacuoles – *cannot distinguish reliably on cytology*	Common infection leading to infertility, cannot be accurately diagnosed on cytology, yellowish vaginal discharge, may be asymptomatic, obligate intracellular organism, needs culture or molecular methods to diagnose

Table 3.5 Common fungal and parasitic infectious agents in the Pap test

Agent	Morphology	Differential Dx.	Clinical symptoms
Candida sp. (fungal)	Pink, branching pseudohyphae with oval buds, often found extending from cellular clusters, may pierce cells to form a "string of pearls" pattern. *Torulopsis* has the yeast form without the hyphae; *Geotrichum* has 90° branching without the oval yeast forms. Often seen with increased staining and/or small perinuclear halos	Bacilli – *much thinner than Candida* Mucous strands – *vary in width, thick to thin and back again, and may fade into the background*	Whitish vaginal discharge, irritation, pruritus Associated with antibiotic use, pregnancy, and diabetes May have few neutrophils to a great many
Trichomonas vaginalis (parasitic)	Oval- to pear-shaped 8–30 μm organism with eccentric, pale oval nucleus. The nucleus must be identified. Red granules may be present in the grayish to lavender cytoplasm. Flagella may occasionally be identified in LBP. "Busy" background on LBP	Degenerated cytoplasmic debris or cells – *do not have the eccentric nucleus of Trichomonas*	Frothy, yellow-green vaginal discharge with strong odor. Cervix is inflamed with small hemorrhages described as a "strawberry" cervix. May have intense inflammatory response to virtually none

Table 3.6 Repair vs. invasive squamous cell carcinoma

	Repair	Carcinoma
Arrangement of cells	Cohesive, retained polarity Rare single cells	Discohesive, syncytial, frequent single cells
Background of the slide	Clean background, no necrosis	Dirty background, necrosis, blood
Nuclei	Enlarged, hypochromatic, finely granular chromatin pattern Smooth membranes	Enlarged, hyperchromatic Irregular coarse chromatin pattern, anisonucleosis, irregular nuclear membranes
Nucleoli	Almost 100 % of the cells	Variable in percentage May have perinucleolar halos
Cytoplasm	N:C ratio not highly abnormal Streaming Nonkeratinized	Increased N:C ratio Scanty cytoplasm May be keratinized
Architecture	Orderly	Disorderly

Table 3.7 Benign proliferative conditions

Condition	Morphology	Differential Dx.	Clinical information
Squamous metaplasia	Resembles parabasal cells – *SM usually occurs in limited specific places on the slide in a background of normal hormonal effect* Dense round to polygonal cytoplasm. May have fine vacuolization. Central oval nucleus that is larger than intermediate cell nucleus	Parabasal cells – *usually occur all over the slide in response to decreased estrogen*	SM is the replacement of normal endocervical epithelium with the more protective layers of squamous epithelium. Very common in Pap samples. Finding either endocervical cells or SM in the slide is an indication of T-zone sampling
Hyperkeratosis	Yellow to pink anucleated squamous cells. May have an empty space where nucleus should normally be – "ghost nucleus"	To diagnose, should see multiple plaques of HK or an allover pattern. Cells derived from handling the slides without gloves usually only show anucleated squamous cells on edges of the slide	This causes whitish plaques on the surface of the vagina and/or cervix – "leukoplakia" HK and/or PK may overlie a more serious dysplastic lesion
Parakeratosis	Small, polygonal, pink to orange cells with a very small, dark, pyknotic nucleus "miniature superficial squamous cells." PK cells are often only about 20–25 % of the size of normal squamous cells. N:C ratio is not significantly abnormal	To diagnose, should see several areas of the miniature superficial squamous cells. Review the rest of the slide carefully for a coexisting HK or neoplastic lesion Dyskeratosis – *difficult differential but note any enlargement of the nucleus with increased N:C ratio for DK. Also, irregular, smudgy, or enlarged nuclei in small, orangeophilic cells may indicate DK*	May coexist with HK and overlie a more serious lesion. Usually found on the topmost surface of the epithelium

3.2 Text-Based Questions 1–30

Q-1. The two most common types of squamous epithelial cells found in the gynecologic sample of a normal woman of childbearing years are:
(a) Basal and parabasal
(b) Parabasal and intermediate
(c) Intermediate and superficial
(d) Superficial and parabasal

Q-2. Architectural features of normal endocervical cells that may be identified in gynecologic samples include:
(a) Three-dimensional cell groups
(b) Palisading two-dimensional groups
(c) Cytoplasmic ribboning
(d) Syncytial groups

Q-3. Normal parabasal cells most resemble which of these benign cellular changes?
(a) Hyperkeratosis
(b) Parakeratosis
(c) Inflammatory cell changes
(d) Squamous metaplasia

Q-4. The most likely days of the menstrual cycle to detect an endometrial cell ball are:
(a) 1–4
(b) 5–10
(c) 11–20
(d) 21–28

Q-5. The area of intermediate cell nuclei is normally:
(a) 5–10 μm^2
(b) 35 μm^2
(c) 50 μm^2
(d) 100 μm^2

Q-6. A large multinucleated cell with frothy cytoplasm is seen in the gynecologic sample of a patient who has received radiation to the cervix for squamous cell carcinoma. The nuclei of this cell are similar in size to one another and have finely granular chromatin and occasional small chromocenters and nucleoli. The most likely diagnosis is:
(a) Recurrent squamous cell carcinoma
(b) Radiation effect
(c) Multinucleated histiocyte
(d) Herpes simplex

Q-7. Patients with severe atrophy may also display:
(a) Vacuolization of superficial cell cytoplasm
(b) Small orangeophilic cells with dark, pyknotic nuclei
(c) A balanced pattern of equal numbers of parabasal, intermediate, and superficial cells
(d) Feathering of endocervical cells

Q-8. A patient presented to the gynecologist with complaints of a greenish discharge. The cervix appeared reddened and the gynecologic sample revealed cells with small perinuclear halos and a slightly intensified cytoplasmic stain. The slide should be carefully examined for the likely presence of:
(a) Candida
(b) Trichomonas
(c) Herpes simplex
(d) Aspergillus
(e) HPV

Q-9. The most likely organism to coexist with Trichomonas is:
(a) Leptothrix
(b) Aspergillus
(c) Candida
(d) Entamoeba histolytica

Q-10. Which of the following is the most likely to occur in women who are pregnant, diabetic, or taking oral antibiotics?
(a) Trichomonas
(b) Actinomyces
(c) Herpes simplex
(d) Candida

Q-11. The yeast forms of Candida can best be differentiated from spermatozoa by:
(a) Size
(b) Shape
(c) Staining characteristics
(d) Distribution in the slide

Q-12. Pseudohyphae which pierce the epithelial cells causing a cytologic pattern in which the cells line up along the length of the organism is most suggestive of infection with:
(a) Candida
(b) Actinomyces
(c) Aspergillus
(d) Nocardia

Q-13. A gynecologic sample containing colonies of bacteria which have radiating filamentous projections giving a characteristic "fuzzy" appearance is the most likely to be associated with a patient with a history of:
(a) Pregnancy
(b) Radiation

(c) IUD
(d) Candida

Q-14. The cytologic finding of multinucleation, nuclear molding, and margination of the chromatin is most associated with infection by:
(a) Cytomegalovirus
(b) Herpes simplex
(c) Trichomonas
(d) Candida

Q-15. Cells containing large intranuclear inclusions and occasional cytoplasmic inclusions are most likely caused by:
(a) HIV
(b) Herpes simplex
(c) Cytomegalovirus
(d) HPV

Q-16. Cells which have large, distinct perinuclear halos, increased nuclear size, and hyperchromasia are most likely showing the effects of infection with:
(a) Candida
(b) Trichomonas
(c) HPV
(d) Cytomegalovirus

Q-17. The most likely subtype of HPV found in cells of LGSIL is:
(a) 5
(b) 11
(c) 16
(d) 31

Q-18. A number of cells from the gynecologic sample of a 28-year-old female were found to have the following abnormalities: increased nuclear size, hyperchromatic nuclei, slightly increased N:C ratio, smudgy chromatin, and large perinuclear halos. The most likely cause is:
(a) Infection with Candida
(b) Infection with HPV
(c) Infection with Trichomonas
(d) Infection with CMV

Q-19. Abnormal keratin pearls, atypical parakeratosis, and hyperkeratosis may all be associated with:
(a) Candida
(b) Trichomonas
(c) Repair
(d) HPV

Q-20. These bacteria help to maintain the normal pH of the vagina.
(a) Doderlein (lactobacilli)
(b) Actinomyces
(c) Leptothrix
(d) Gardnerella vaginalis
(e) Aspergillus

Q-21. Bacilli, cytoplasmic debris, and naked nuclei are consistent with a finding of:
(a) Gardnerella vaginalis
(b) Hyperkeratosis
(c) Cytolysis
(d) Actinomyces

Q-22. Multinucleated cells with dense, tapering cytoplasm and dark, degenerating nuclei associated with pregnancy, postpartum, or postabortion states are most likely:
(a) Decidual cells
(b) Syncytial trophoblasts
(c) Microglandular hyperplasia
(d) Endocervical polyps

Q-23. Glycogen-filled intermediate cells common in the latter half of the menstrual cycle and in the second to third trimesters of pregnancy are often referred to as:
(a) Navicular cells
(b) Syncytial trophoblasts
(c) Decidual cells
(d) Arias-Stella change

Q-24. The clinical finding of white plaques in the vaginal canal and cervix corresponds to the cytologic finding of ______ and is often associated a clinical history of __________.
(a) Microglandular hyperplasia; oral contraceptive use
(b) Candida; radiation
(c) Hyperkeratosis; uterine descensus
(d) Arias-Stella change; pregnancy

Q-25. The finding of parakeratosis in a gynecologic sample is significant due to the fact that:
(a) These cells might be confused with squamous cell carcinoma.
(b) These cells may overlie a more serious lesion.

(c) These cells may cause bleeding and ulceration.
(d) These cells are associated with IUD effect.

Q-26. Dense cyanophilic cytoplasm in round to oval or slightly polygonal cells, combined with a nuclear size of about 100 μm^2, is most frequently found in cells from which of the following benign protective reactions:
(a) Hyperkeratosis
(b) Parakeratosis
(c) Squamous metaplasia
(d) Repair

Q-27. The best cytologic criteria to use in differentiating IUD effect from endometrial adenocarcinoma is that in IUD effect:
(a) The cells are too big for adenocarcinoma, unless there were also macronucleoli consistent with Grade 3–4 endometrial adenocarcinoma.
(b) The clusters are entirely made up of cells with vacuoles, macronucleoli, and powdery chromatin.
(c) A watery tumor diathesis is present.
(d) The cells are in a palisading two-dimensional arrangement.

Q-28. A 28-year-old female with no previous abnormal history returns to her gynecologist for a routine checkup. Her history is significant for placement of an IUD 1 year ago and a previous normal pregnancy and delivery (G1, P1) 14 months earlier. Occasional cells were found in the slide which were small, rare, and isolated, had very high N:C ratios, and had dark smudged chromatin. The most likely explanation for these cells is:
(a) IUD effect
(b) Carcinoma in situ
(c) Repair
(d) Decidual cells

Q-29. In the gynecologic sample of a 39-year-old woman, cells were found which had the following characteristics: enlarged nuclei and cytoplasm, finely granular chromatin, frequent macronucleoli, smooth nuclear borders, and ribbonlike arrangement. The most likely diagnosis is:
(a) Microglandular hyperplasia
(b) Tubal metaplasia
(c) Nonkeratinizing squamous cell carcinoma
(d) Repair

Q-30. Cells with the following characteristics were found in the smear of a 32-year-old woman: polychromasia, pale finely granular chromatin, slightly enlarged nuclei, and ill-defined small perinuclear halos. These changes are most consistent with:
(a) Repair
(b) HGSIL
(c) Inflammatory cell changes
(d) HPV

3.3 Image-Based Questions 31–90

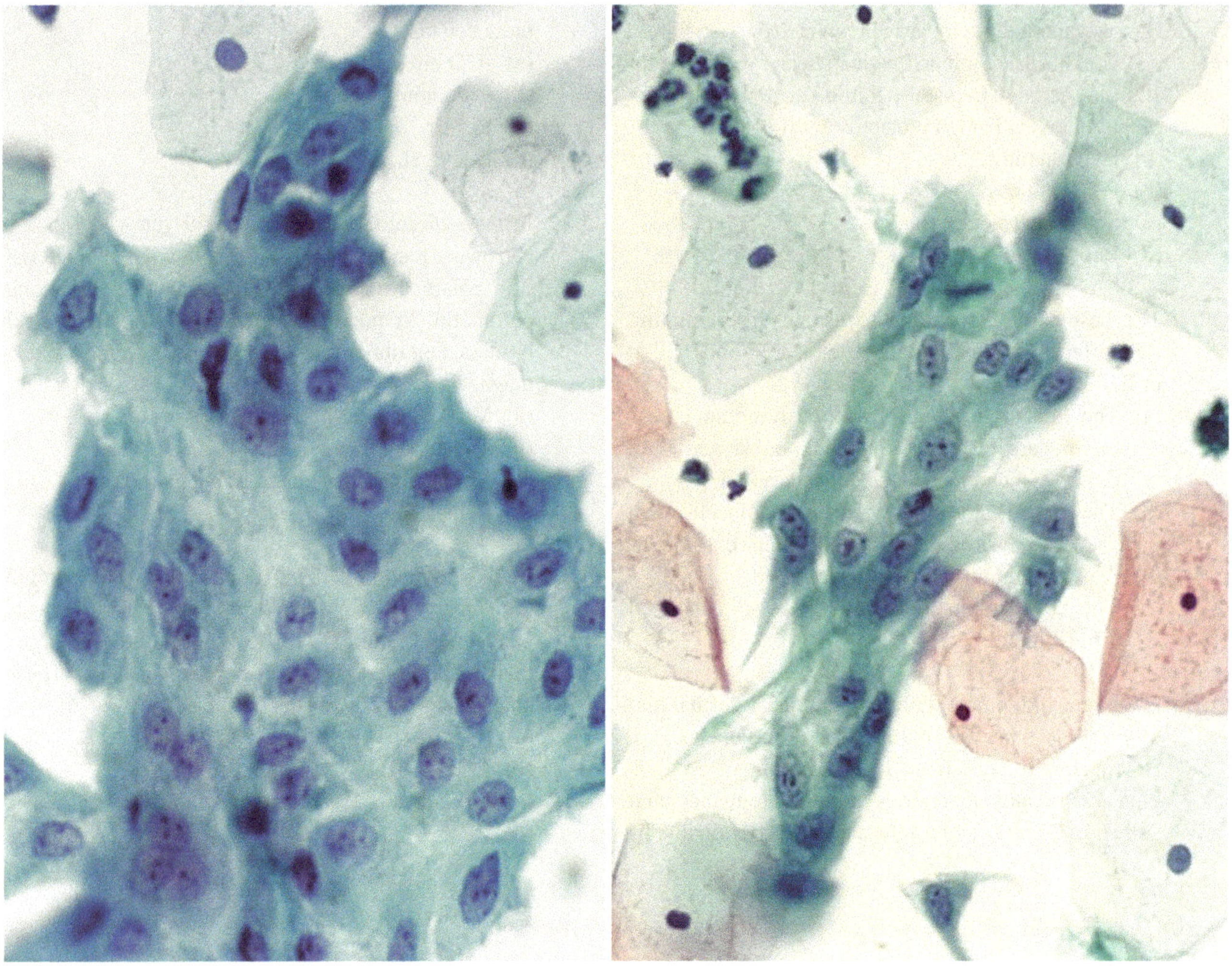

Fig. 3.31

Q-31. Cells such as these were found in the gynecologic sample of a 42-year-old woman (SurePath, left and right, medium magnification). The most likely diagnosis is:

(a) Repair
(b) Squamous metaplasia
(c) Squamous cell carcinoma
(d) Hyperkeratosis
(e) Endocervical cells

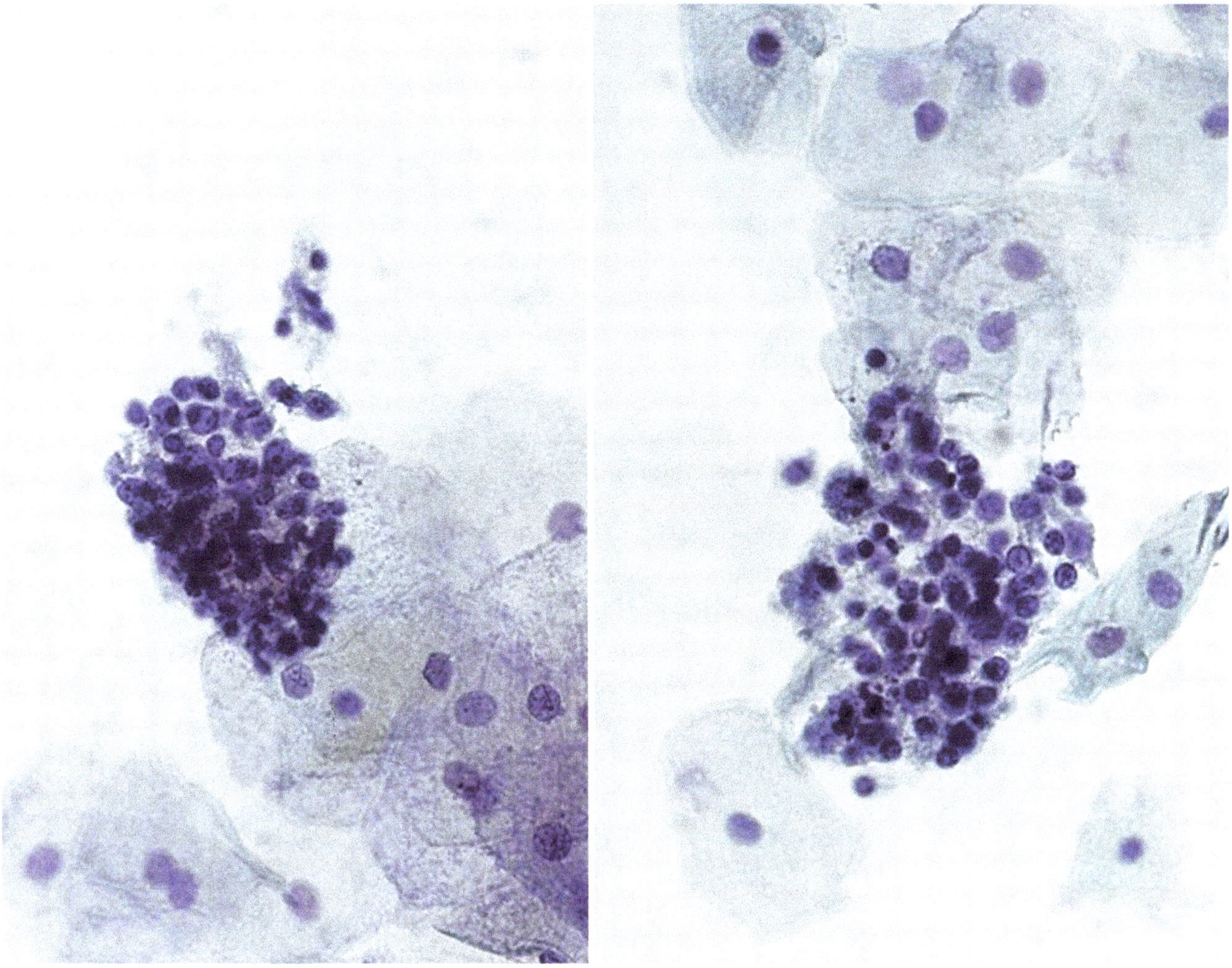

Fig. 3.32

Q-32. These cells (ThinPrep, medium magnification, right and left) are indicative of which of the following:
- (a) Acute inflammation
- (b) Endocervical cell component
- (c) Chronic follicular cervicitis
- (d) Lymphoma
- (e) Small cell carcinoma of the cervix

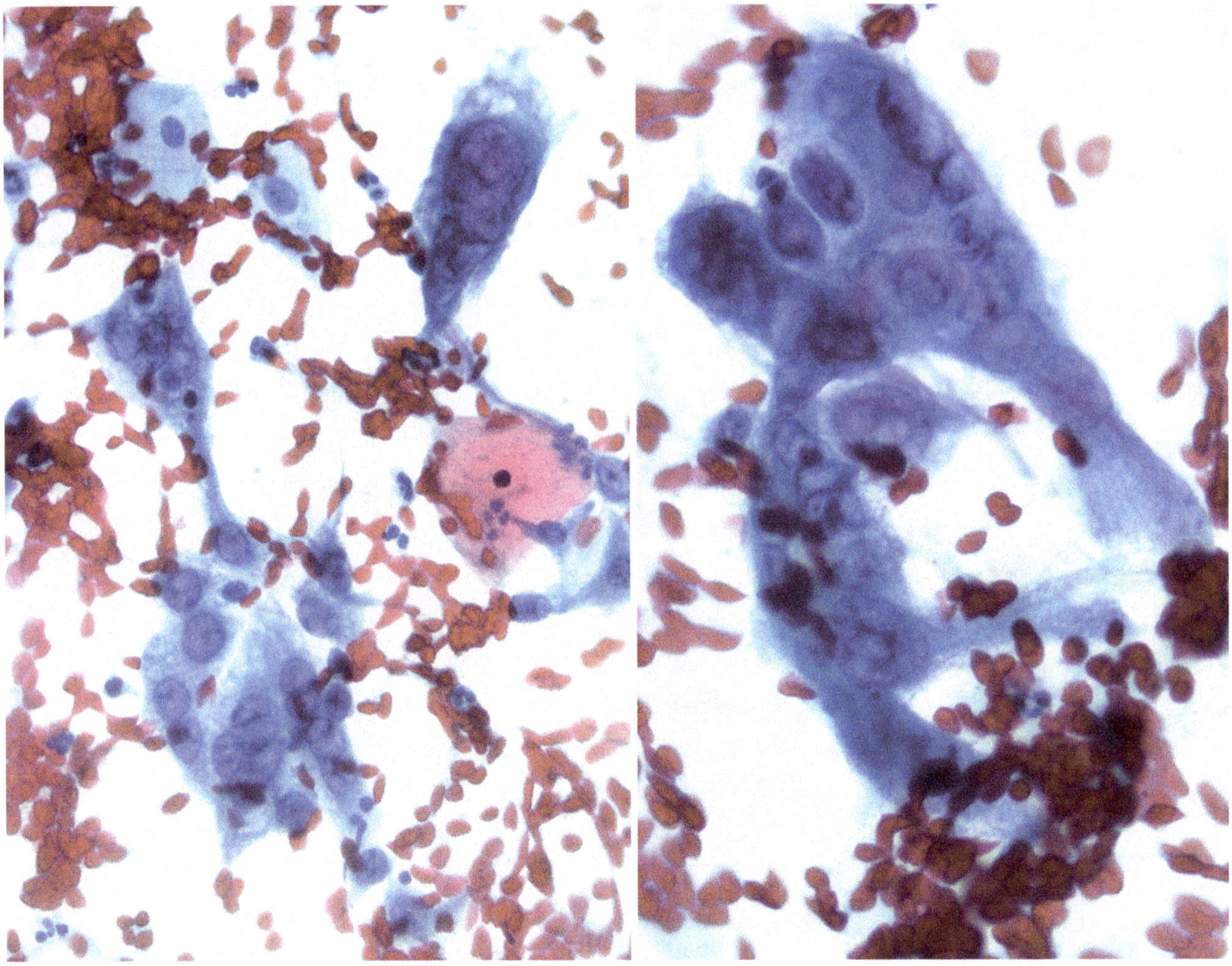

Fig. 3.33

Q-33. These cells were found in the gynecologic sample of a 32-year-old female (conventional, right and left, medium magnification). These cells are most consistent with which of the following:

(a) Repair
(b) Herpes
(c) Cytomegalovirus
(d) HGSIL
(e) Adenovirus

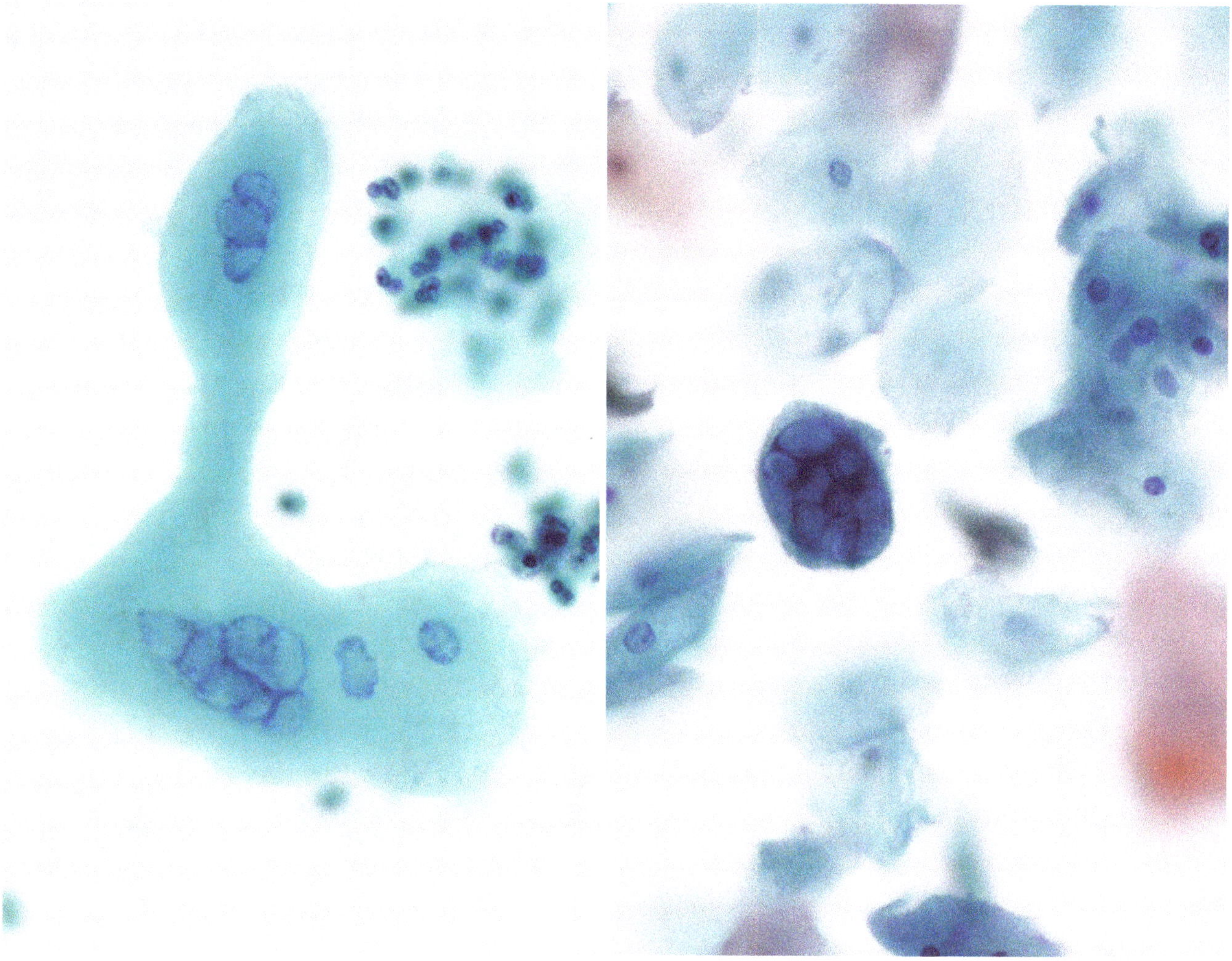

Fig. 3.34

Q-34. The most significant clinical history when treating a patient with these types of cells (SurePath, medium magnification, right and left) is which of the following:
(a) Previous history of HGSIL
(b) Second trimester pregnancy
(c) Postmenopausal
(d) Day 6 of a normal menstrual cycle
(e) IUD placement

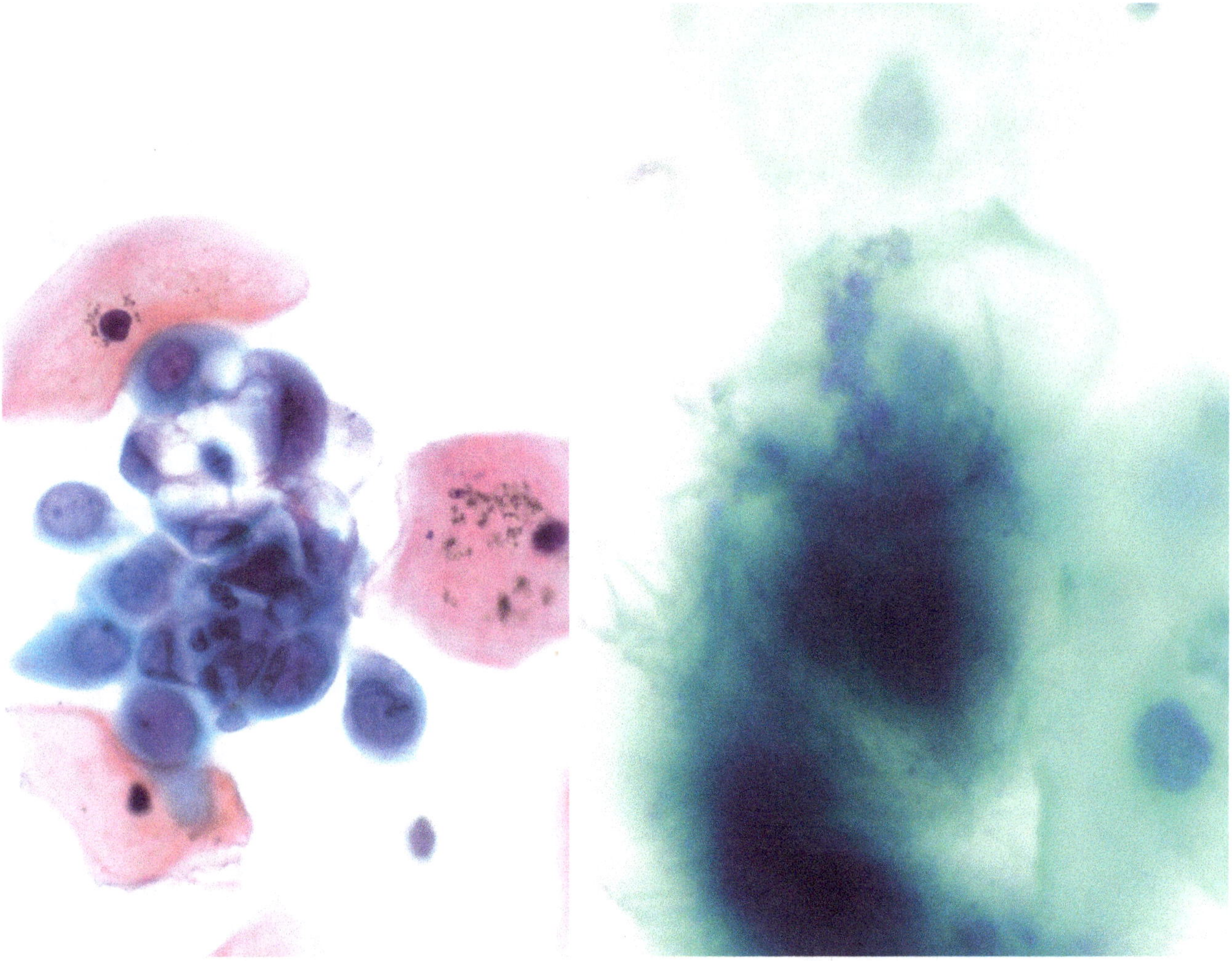

Fig. 3.35

Q-35 The findings illustrated here (conventional, medium, left; ThinPrep, high, right) are most consistent with a patient with a clinical history of which of the following?

(a) Postradiation
(b) Adenovirus
(c) Repair
(d) IUD wearer
(e) Herpes

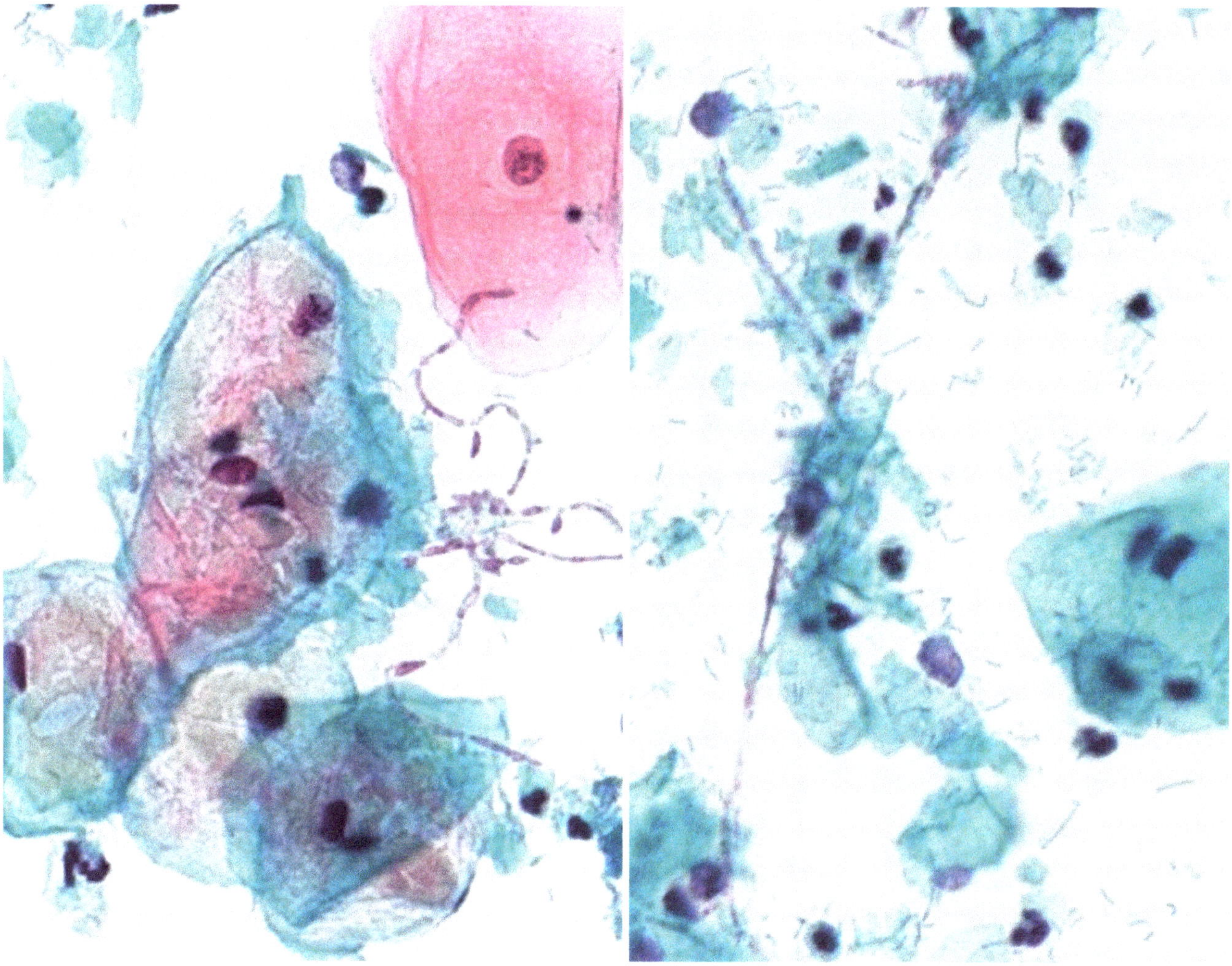

Fig. 3.36

Q-36. A risk factor for this finding (ThinPrep, high, right and left) is:
(a) Previous history of herpes simplex
(b) Pregnancy
(c) Previous history of HGSIL
(d) HPV infection
(e) IUD use

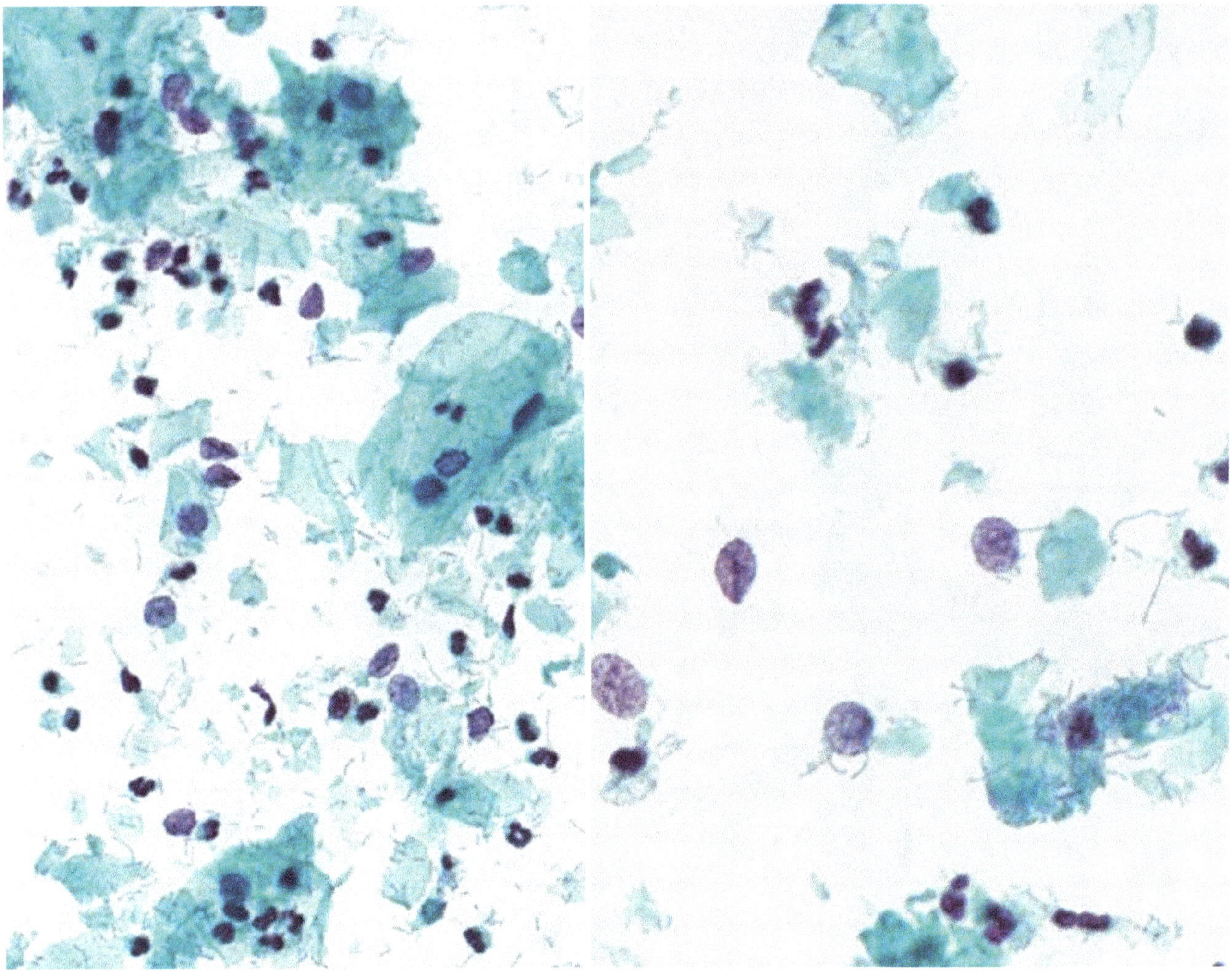

Fig. 3.37

Q-37. This pattern seen in a ThinPrep sample from a 29-year-old woman (ThinPrep, medium, left; ThinPrep, high, right) is most often seen in which of the following days of the cycle?
(a) Days 1–6
(b) Days 7–11
(c) Days 12–16
(d) Days 17–21
(e) Days 22–28

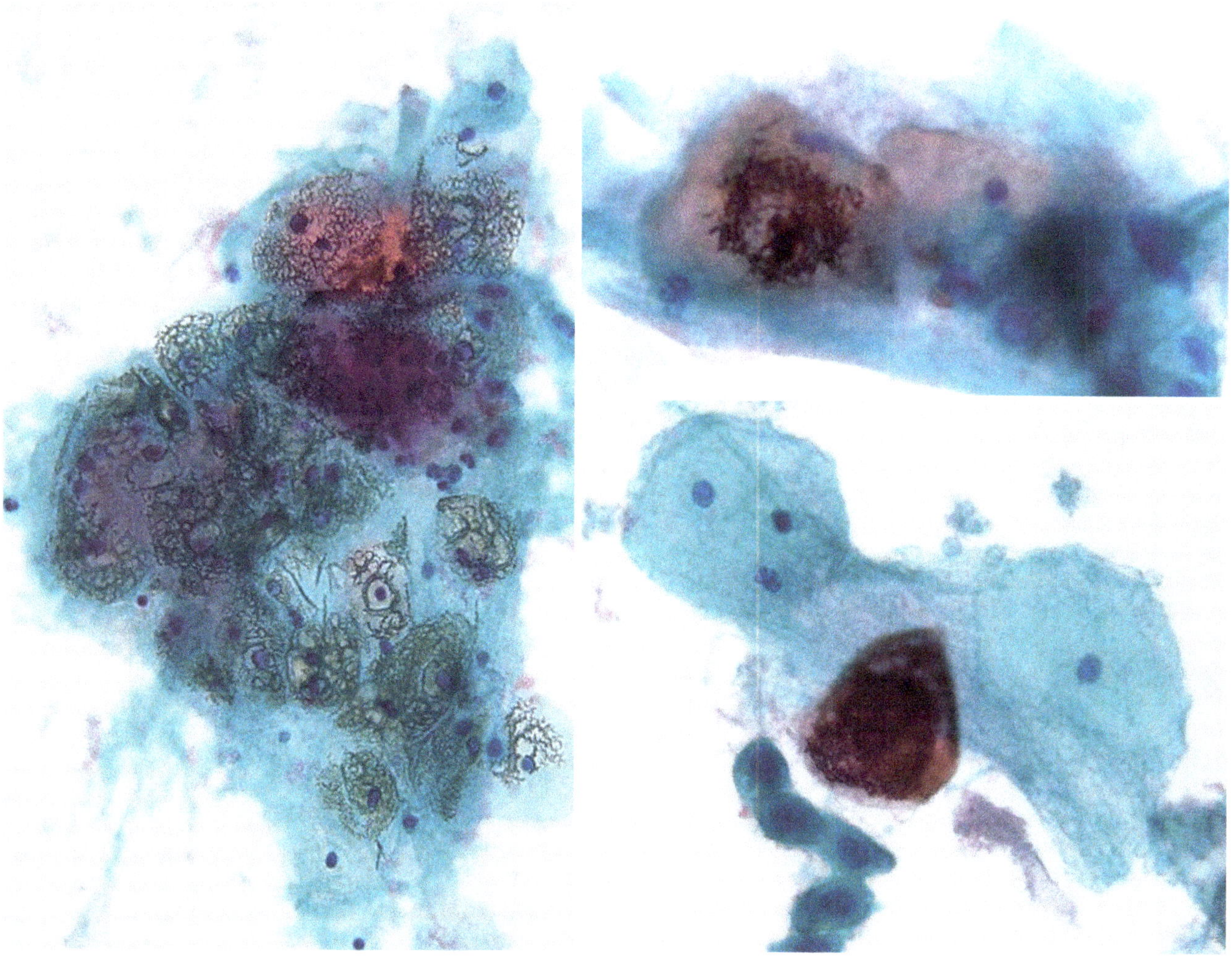

Fig. 3.38

Q-38. This appearance of this slide (ThinPrep, medium, left; high, upper and lower right) is most likely due to:
(a) Melanin
(b) Hemosiderin
(c) Glycogen
(d) Lipofuscin
(e) Trapping of air under the coverslip

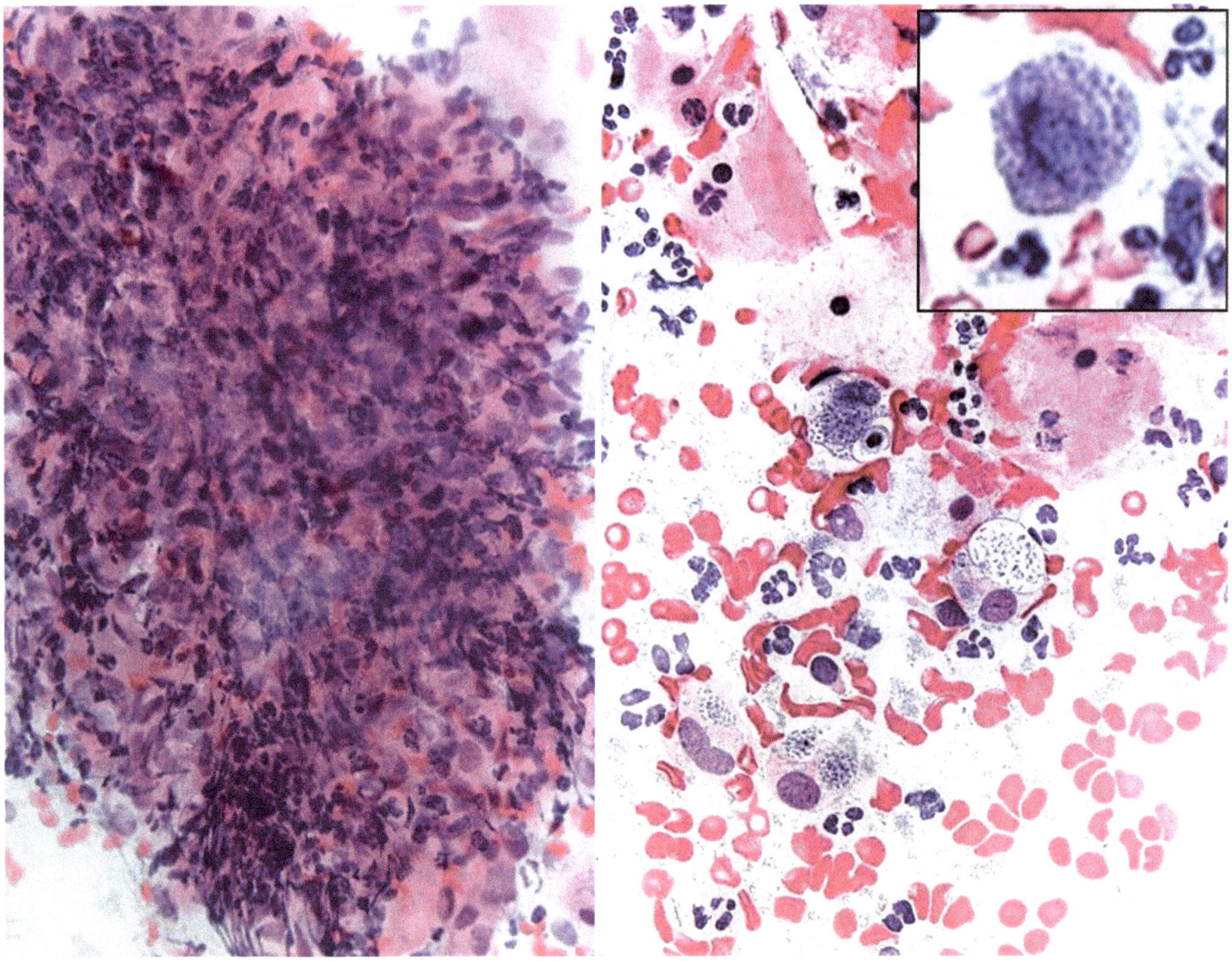

Fig. 3.39

Q-39. The structure on the left, combined with the finding on the right of small safety pin-shaped inclusions within histiocytes, is most compatible with a diagnosis of which of the following (conventional, medium, left; medium, lower right; oil, inset upper right)?

(a) Tuberculosis
(b) Sarcoidosis
(c) Chlamydia
(d) Granuloma inguinale
(e) Coccidioides immitis

Fig. 3.40

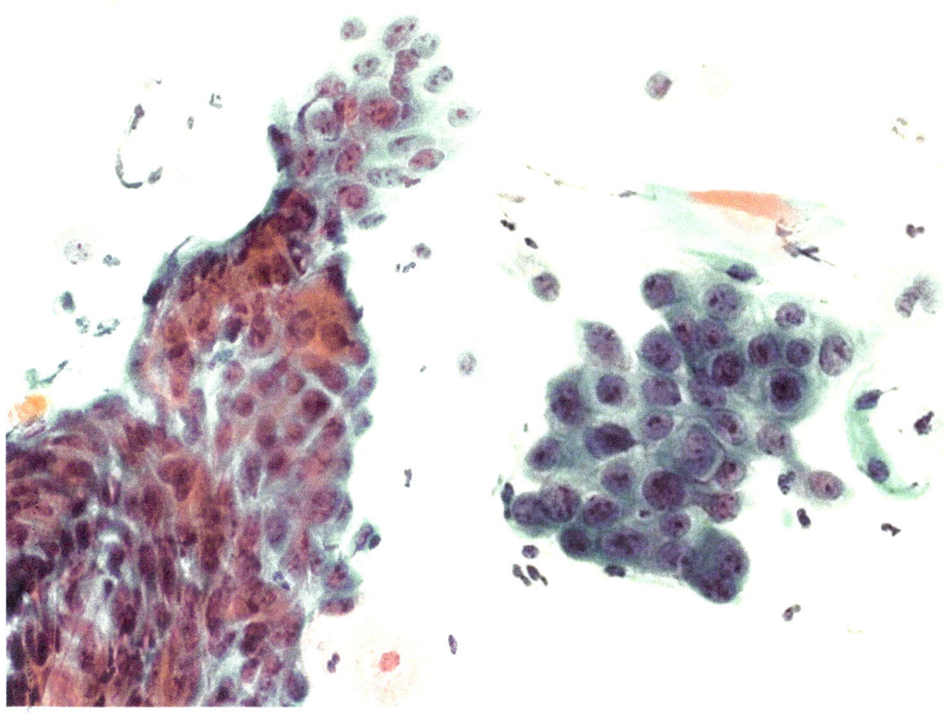

Q-40. Several groups of cells such as these with abundant cytoplasm, nucleoli, and finely granular chromatin patterns were found in the gynecologic sample from a 28-year-old woman on her postpartum checkup (conventional, medium, right and left). These cells are most consistent with a diagnosis of:

(a) LGSIL
(b) HGSIL
(c) Squamous cell carcinoma
(d) Choriocarcinoma
(e) Repair

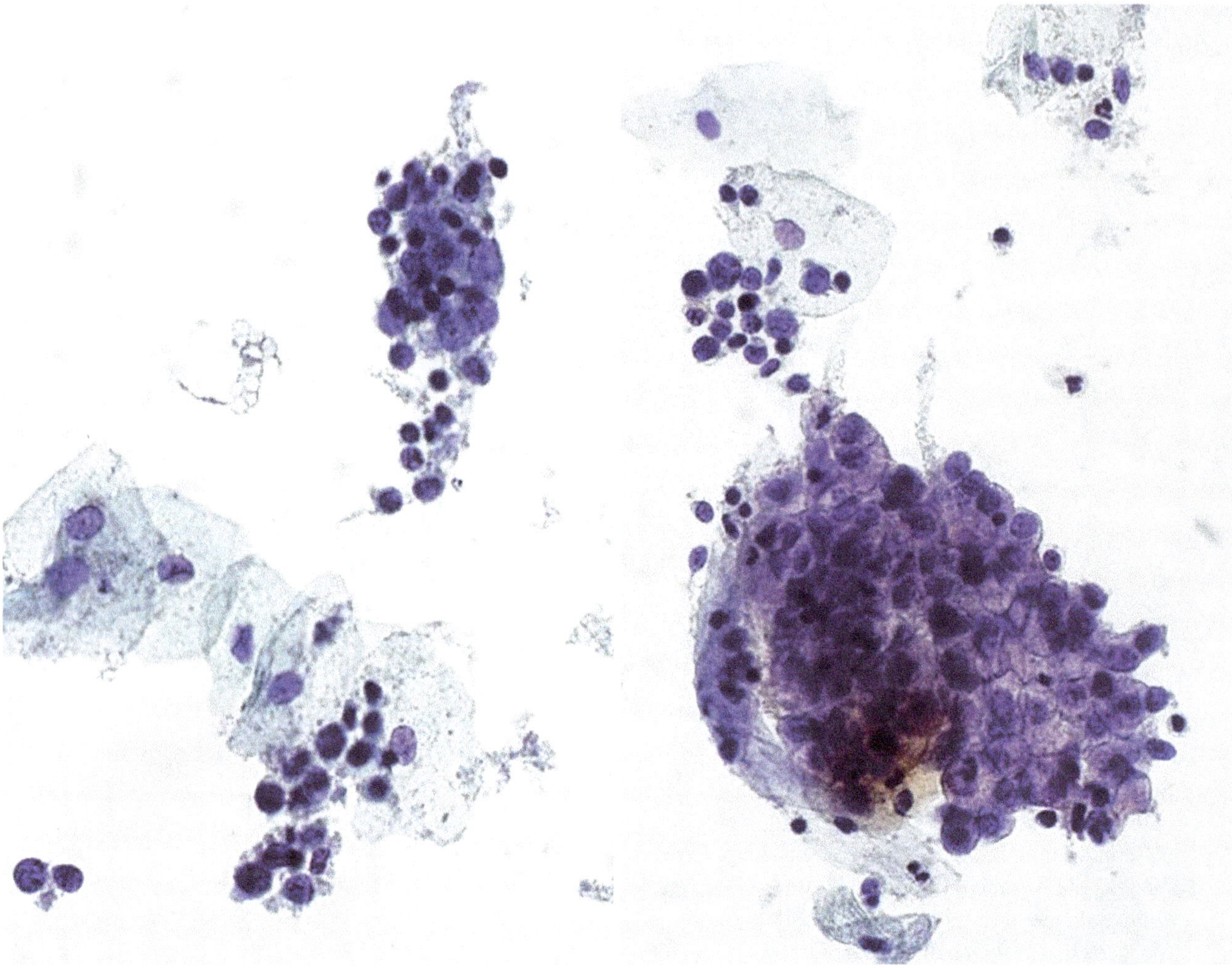

Fig. 3.41

Q-41. The next immediate step in the appropriate follow-up and treatment of this patient (ThinPrep, medium, right and left) should be which of the following?
(a) High-risk HPV testing
(b) Colposcopically directed biopsy of cervix
(c) Repeat Pap in 4 weeks
(d) Repeat Pap in 1 year
(e) Hysterectomy

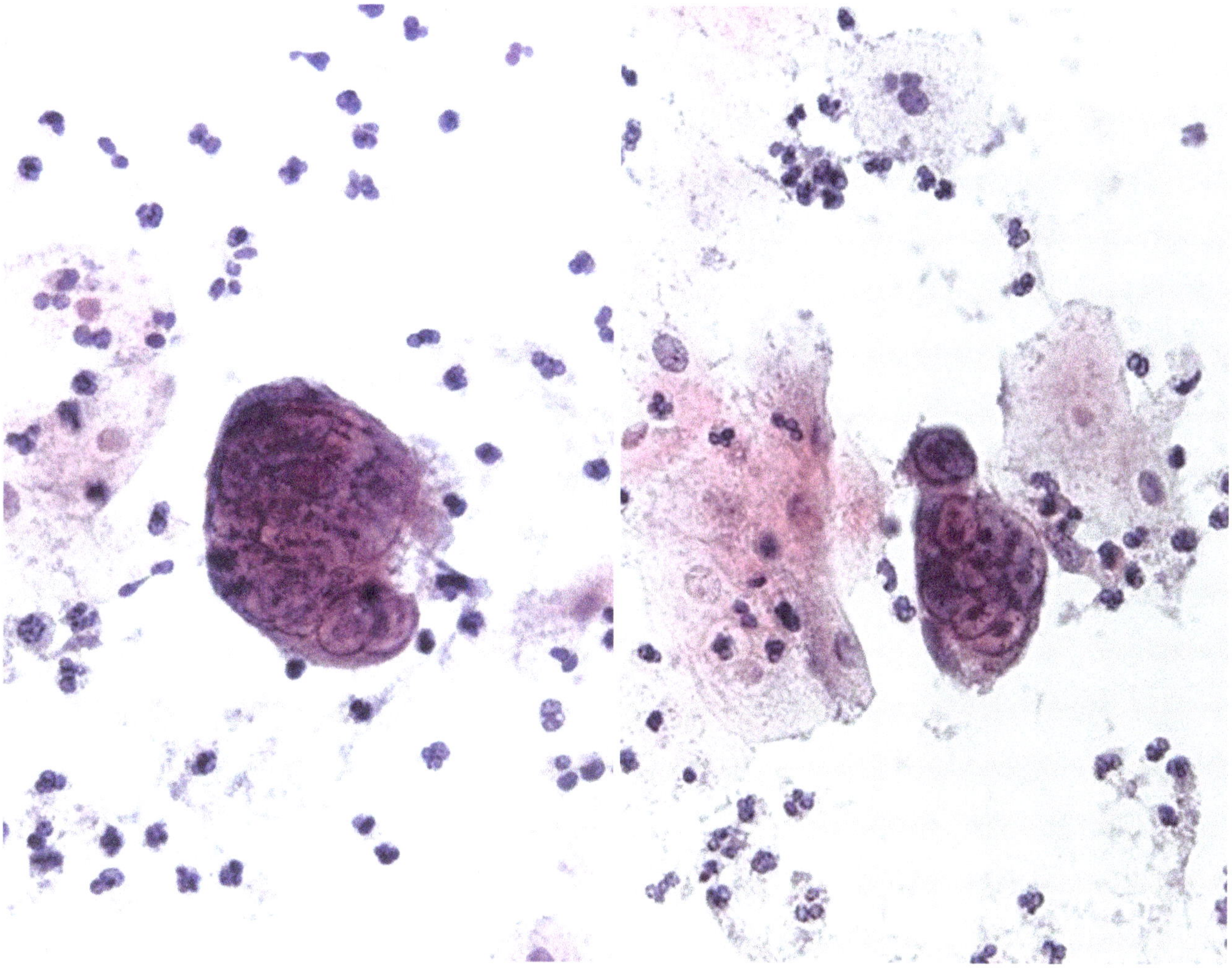

Fig. 3.42

Q-42. These findings (conventional, medium, right and left) are most consistent with a diagnosis of which of the following?
(a) Repair
(b) Endocervical adenocarcinoma
(c) HGSIL
(d) HPV
(e) Herpes

Fig. 3.43

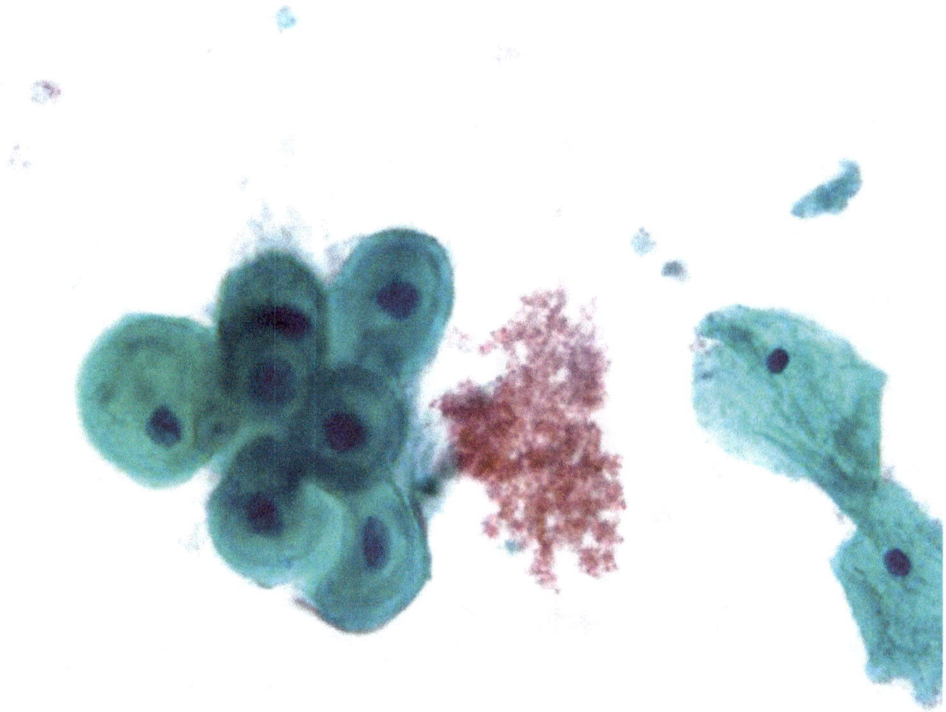

Q-43. (ThinPrep, medium) The pinkish granular substance in the center of this slide is most likely which of the following?

(a) Doderlein bacilli
(b) Gardnerella vaginalis
(c) Coccobacilli
(d) Blood
(e) Candida spores

Fig. 3.44

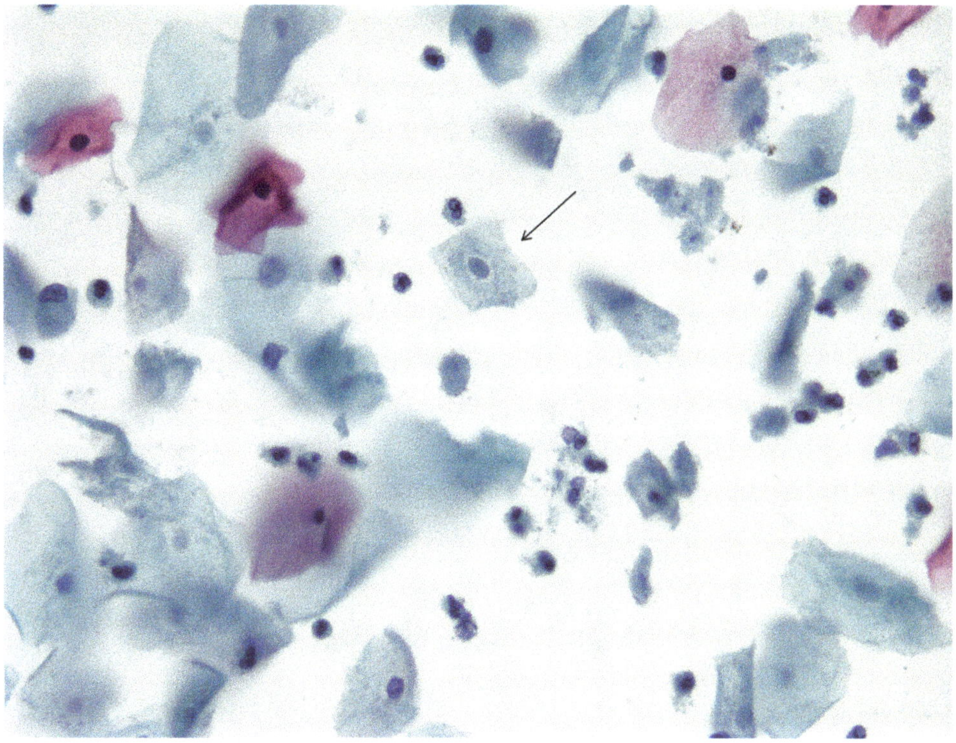

Q-44. The perinuclear halo in the cell near the center of the image is most likely caused by which of the following (SurePath, medium)?

(a) HPV
(b) Candida
(c) Trichomonas
(d) Nonspecific inflammatory cell changes
(e) Herpes

Fig. 3.45

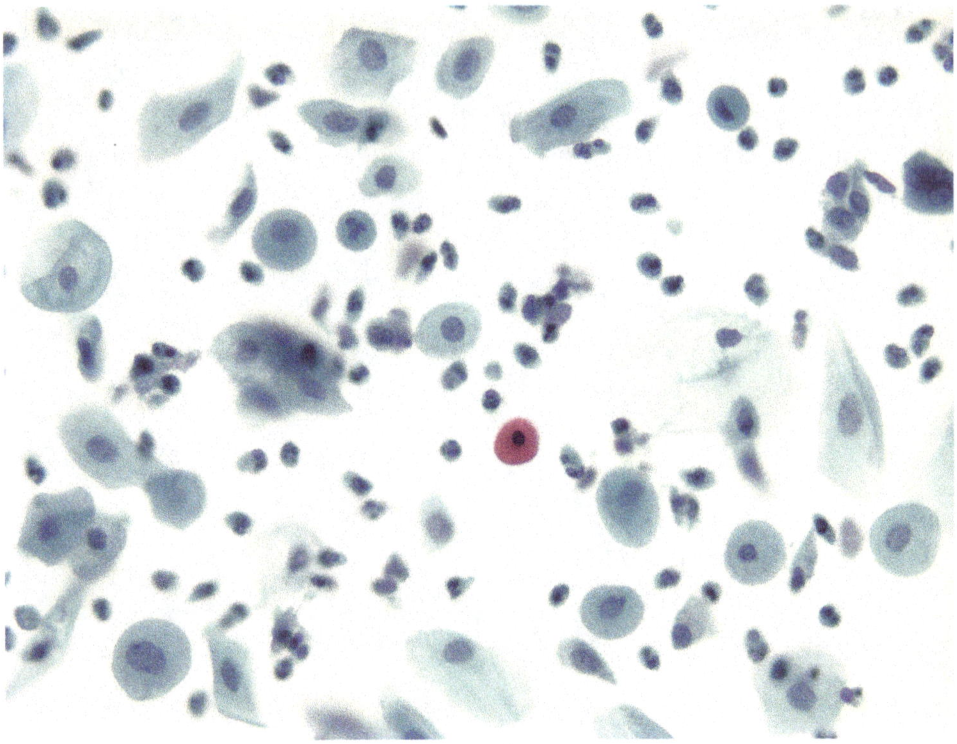

Q-45. This gynecologic sample was taken from a 59-year-old female (SurePath, medium). The small pinkish cell in the middle of the image is most likely representative of which of the following?

(a) Parakeratosis
(b) Hyperkeratosis
(c) HPV effect
(d) Degenerated parabasal cell
(e) LGSIL

Fig. 3.46

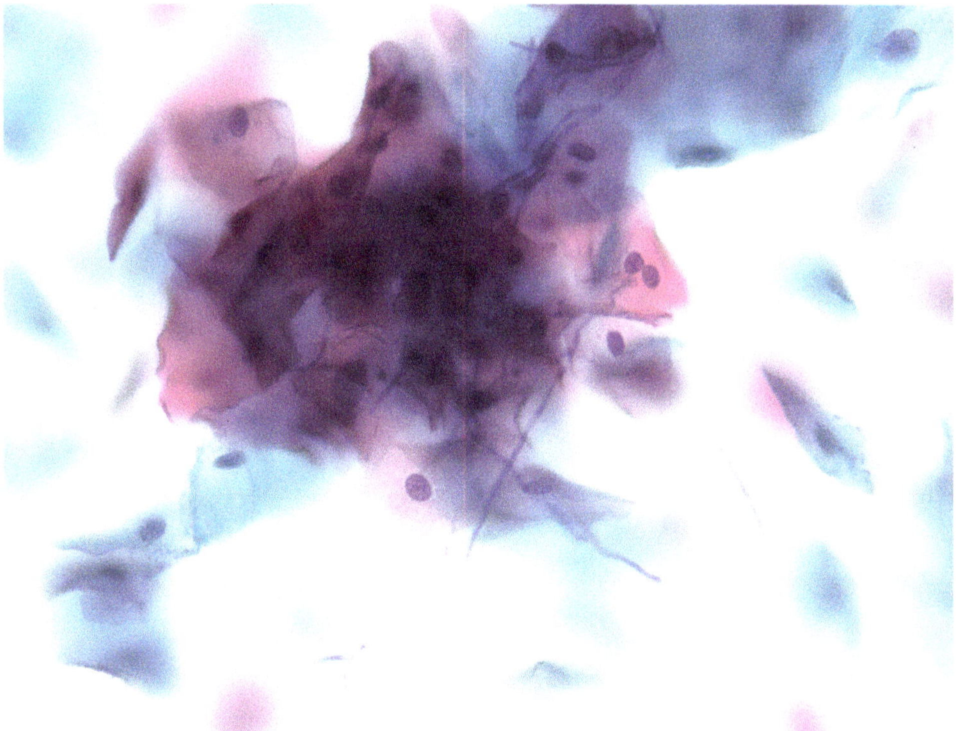

Q-46. This finding is most consistent with which of the following (SurePath, medium)?
(a) Actinomyces
(b) Mucin strands
(c) IUD effect
(d) Candida
(e) Leptothrix

Fig. 3.47

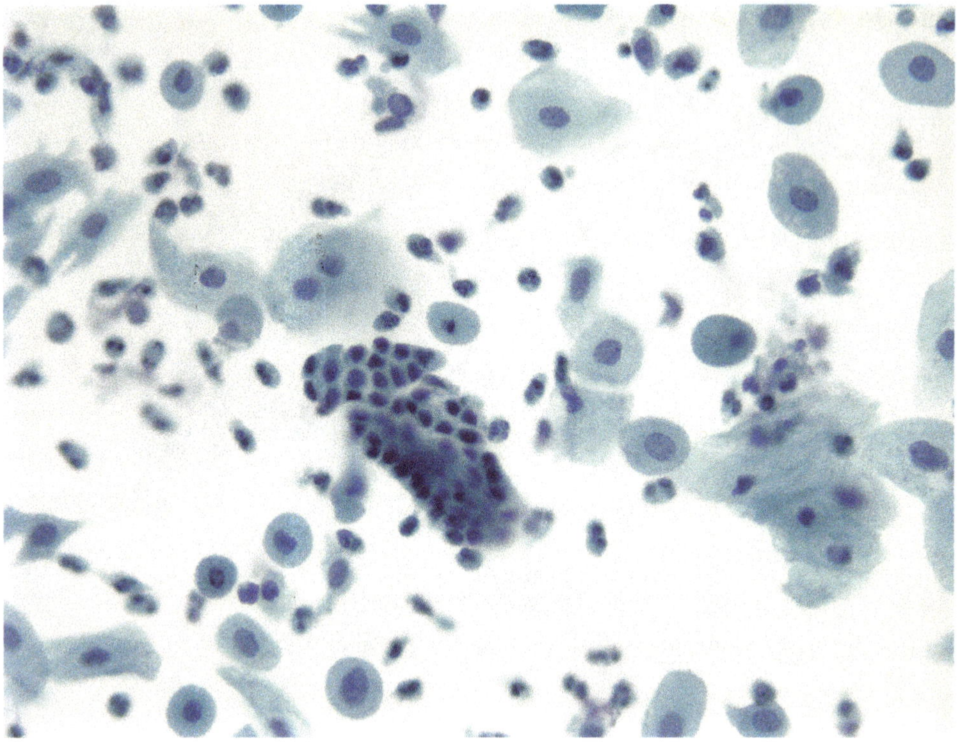

Q-47. The most likely clinical history for this patient, given the appearance of this sample (SurePath, medium power), is which of the following?

(a) Day 2, 18-year-old nonpregnant woman
(b) Day 13, 29-year-old nonpregnant woman
(c) Day 28, 32-year-old nonpregnant woman
(d) Second trimester, 33-year-old pregnant woman, normal pregnancy
(e) 64-year-old postmenopausal woman, no hormone use

Fig. 3.48

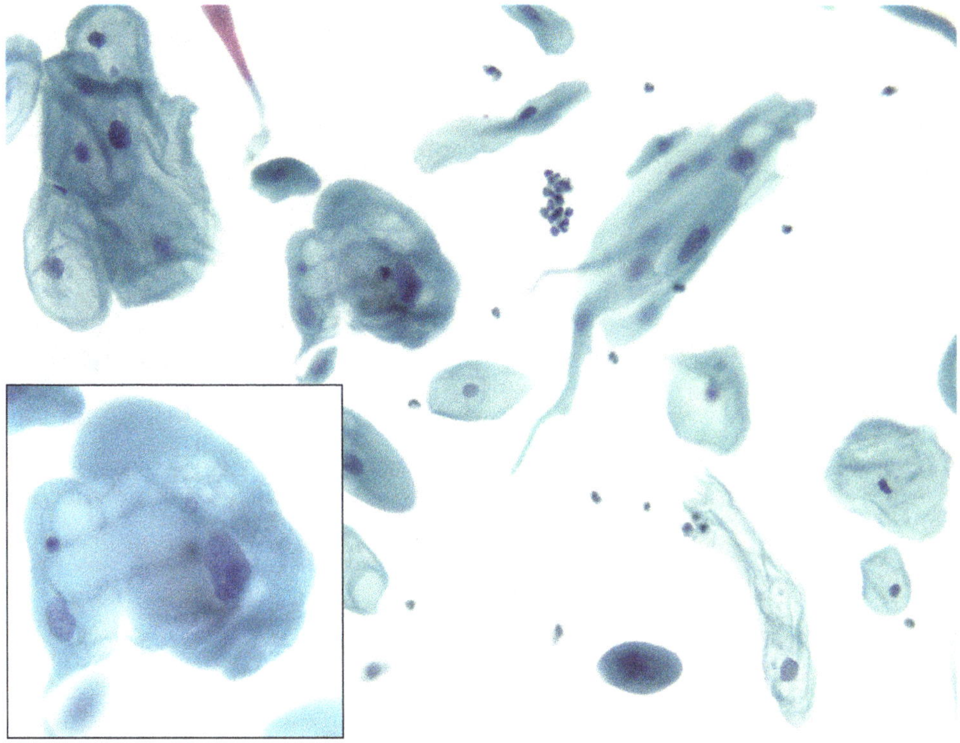

Q-48. Cells such as these were found in the gynecologic sample from a 64-year-old patient who had received a hysterectomy and radiation therapy for squamous cell carcinoma (SurePath, medium power; inset, high power). The most likely diagnosis of these cells is:
(a) Repair
(b) Recurrent squamous cell carcinoma
(c) Radiation effect
(d) Mixed Müllerian tumor
(e) Endometrial adenocarcinoma

Fig. 3.49

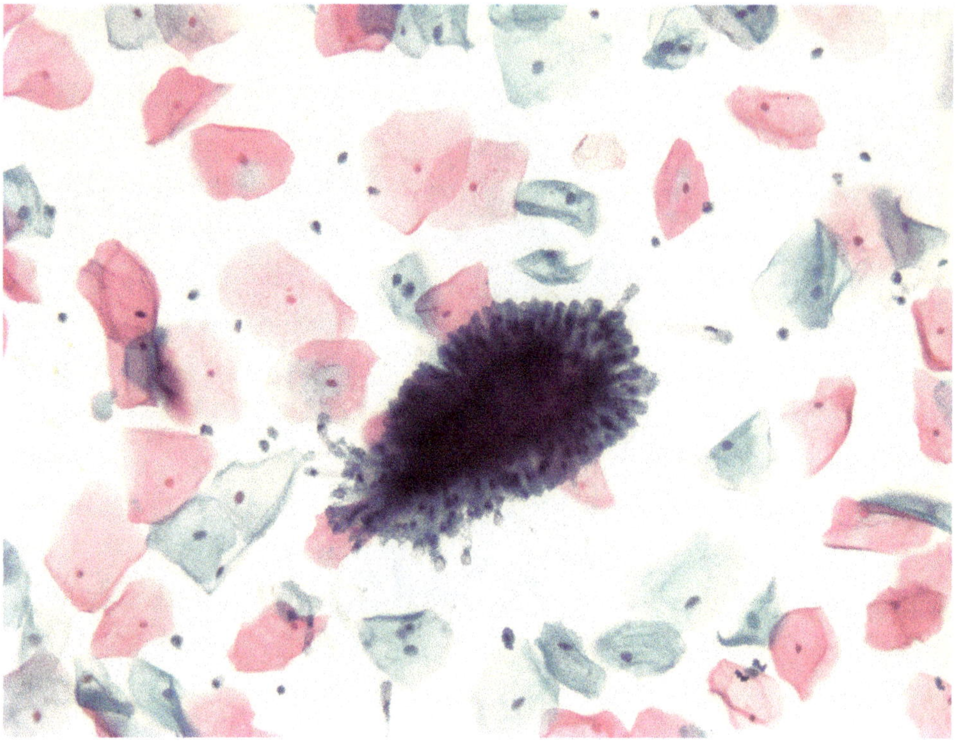

Q-49. The cellular material in the center of this image (SurePath, medium) from a 26-year-old patient is most likely:

(a) Endometrial cells
(b) Endocervical cells
(c) Colonic adenocarcinoma
(d) Fibroblasts
(e) Granuloma

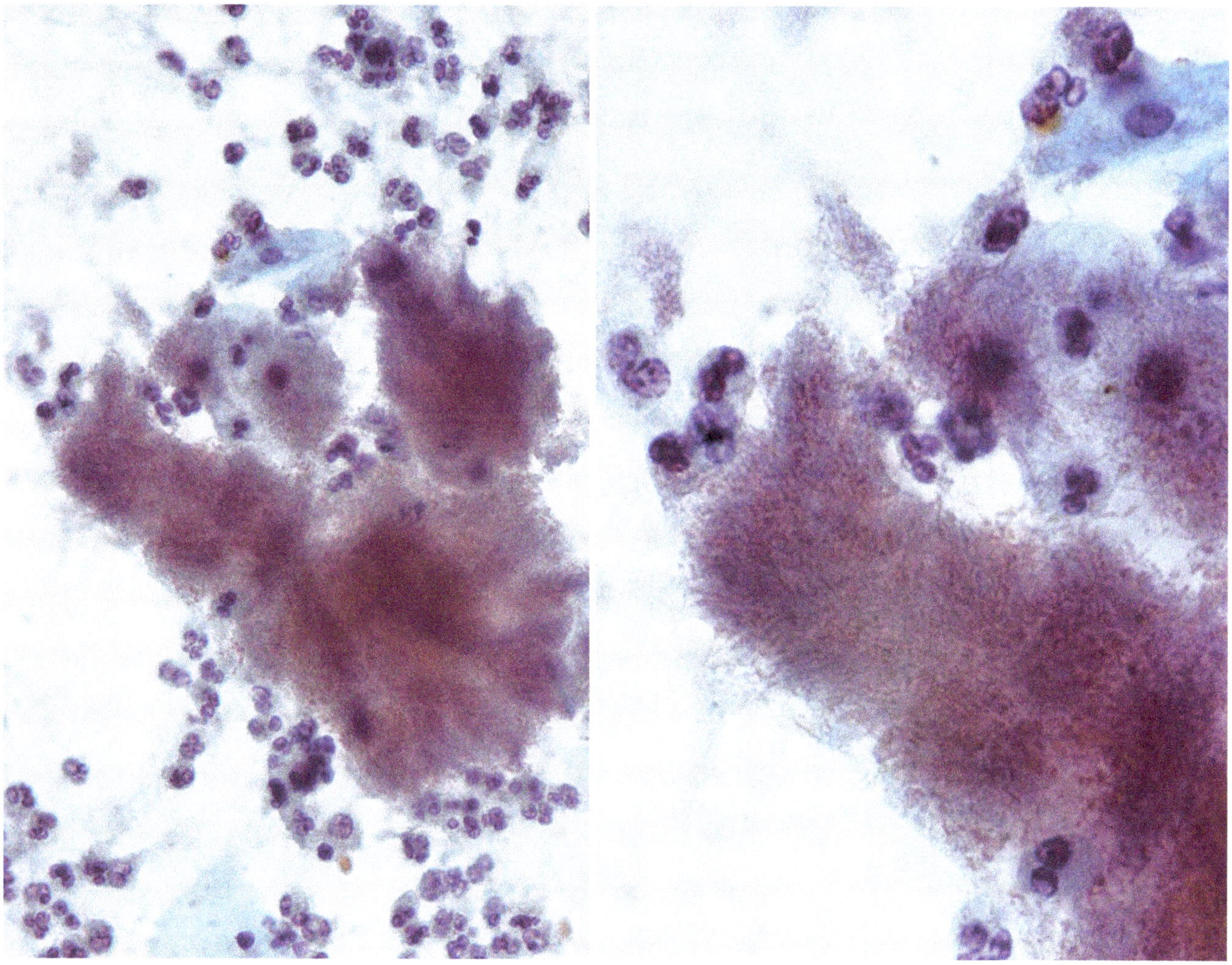

Fig. 3.50

Q-50. These findings (left, high, ThinPrep; right, medium, ThinPrep) may be associated with which clinical history?
(a) Vaginal pessary use
(b) Condom use
(c) Oral contraception
(d) Coexisting HPV infection
(e) Radiation effect

Fig. 3.51

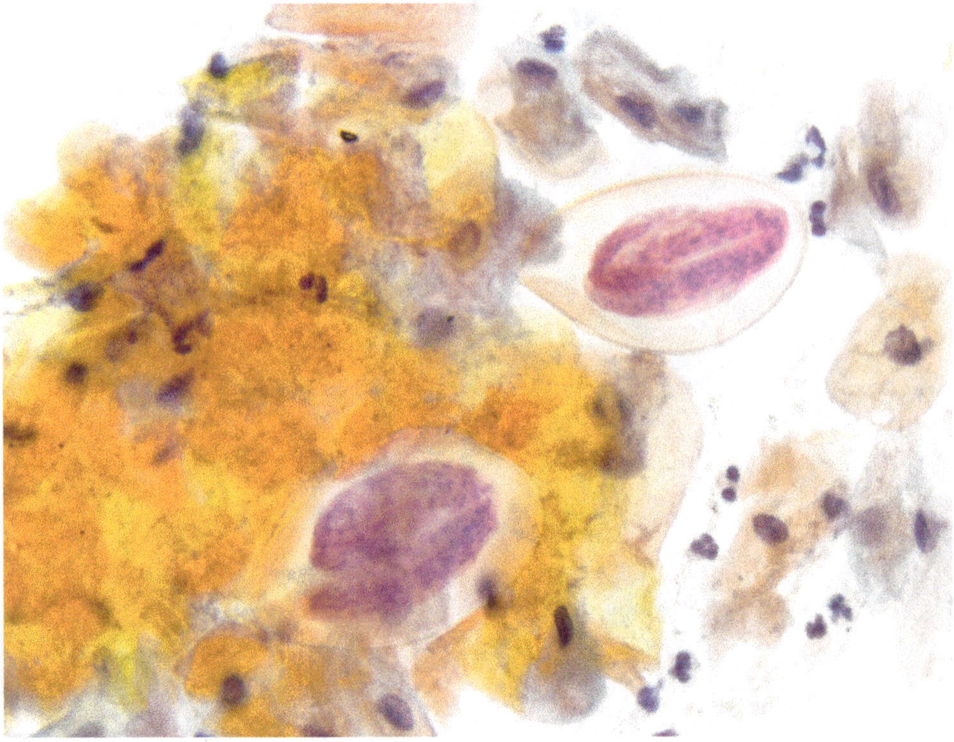

Q-51. This finding from a gynecologic sample (conventional, high magnification) is most likely which of the following?
(a) Psammoma body
(b) Cholesterol crystal
(c) Vegetable contaminant
(d) Ova of Enterobius vermicularis
(e) Suture contaminant

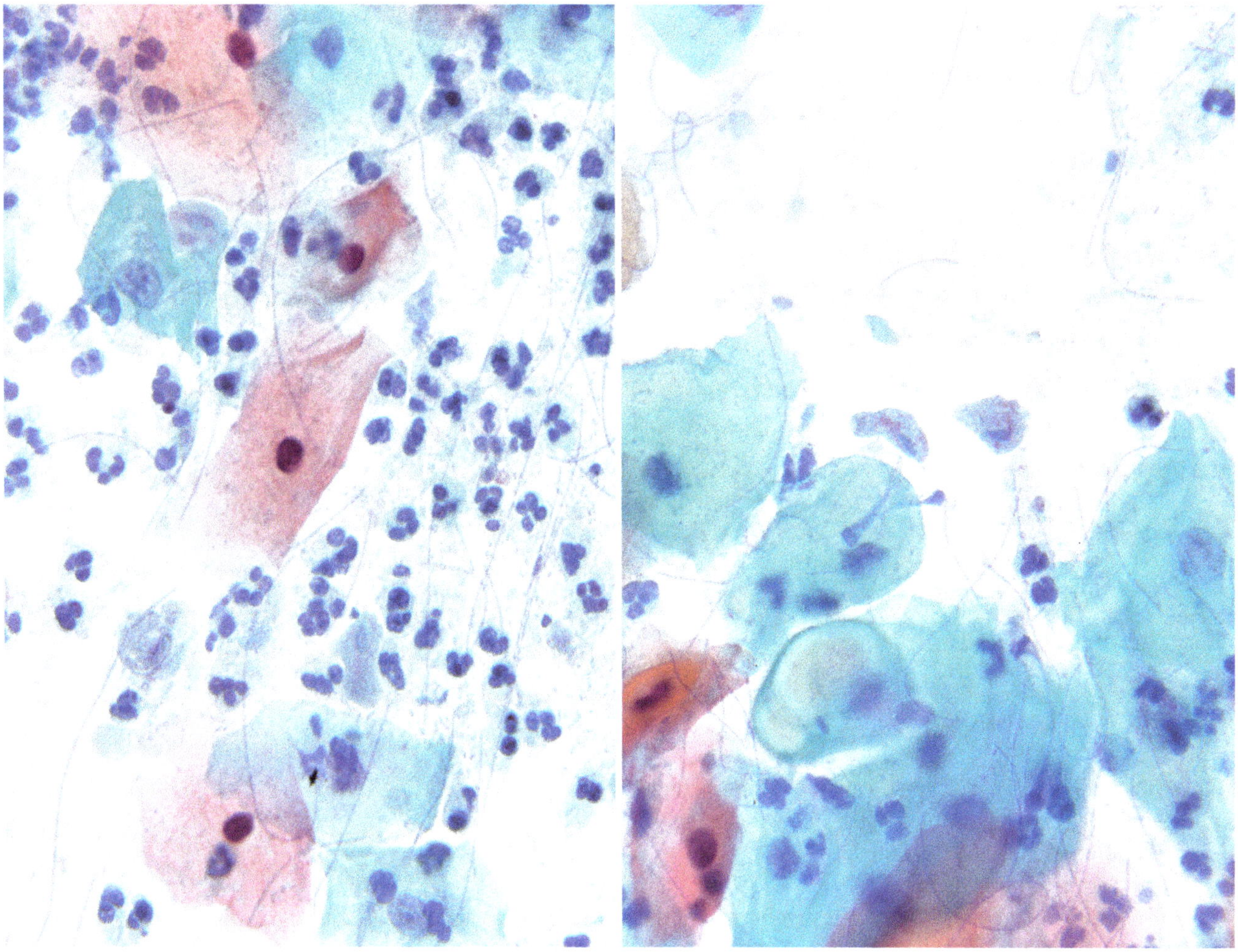

Fig. 3.52

Q-52. These findings in the gynecologic sample from a 27-year-old woman (conventional, right and left, high magnification) most likely represent which of the following?

(a) Candida and Trichomonas
(b) Actinomyces and IUD effect
(c) Leptothrix and Trichomonas
(d) Aspergillus and Entamoeba histolytica
(e) Lactobacillus and Giardia lamblia

Fig. 3.53

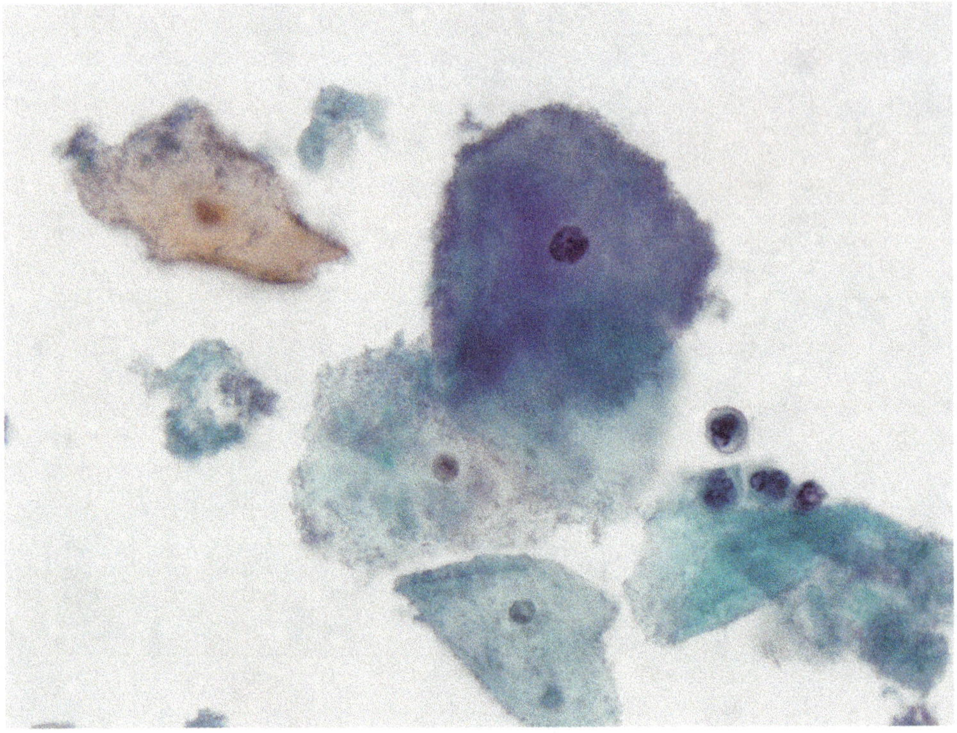

Q-53. This finding in a gynecologic sample (ThinPrep, high) would be reported as which of the following using the 2001 Bethesda System terminology?

(a) Gardnerella vaginalis
(b) Shift in vaginal flora suggestive of bacterial vaginosis
(c) Coccobacilli
(d) Lactobacilli consistent with Doderlein bacilli
(e) Bacteria morphologically consistent with Actinomyces

Fig. 3.54

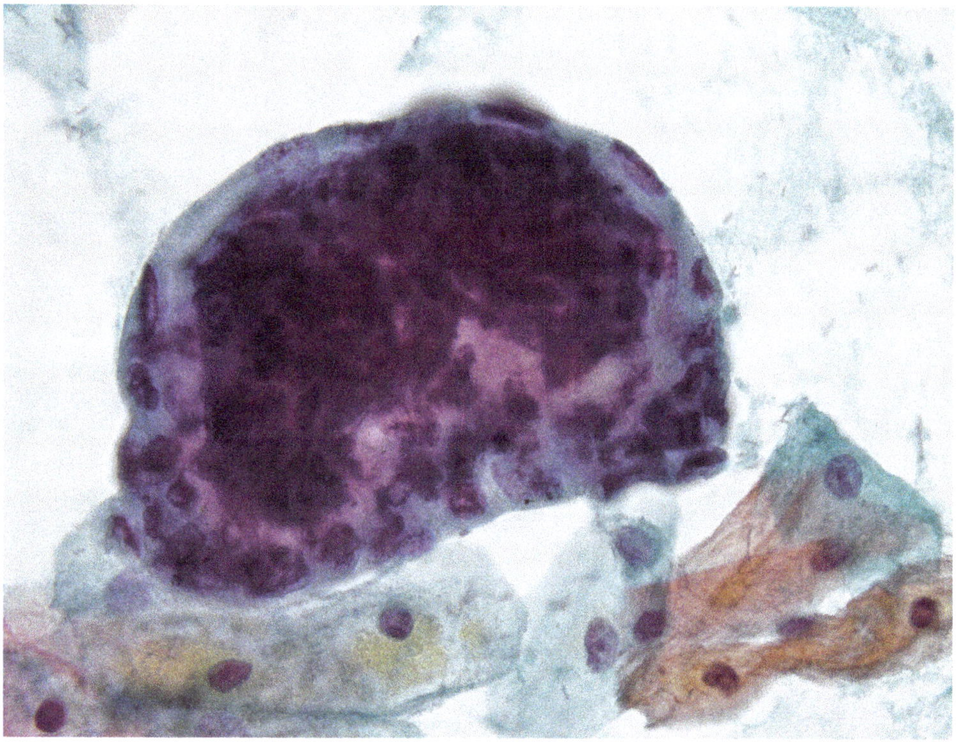

Q-54. This image is from the conventional smear of a 28-year-old woman (conventional, high magnification). The cells seen here are most consistent with which of the following?

(a) Normal endometrial cells during exodus
(b) Endocervical cells
(c) Inflammatory cell balls
(d) HGSIL

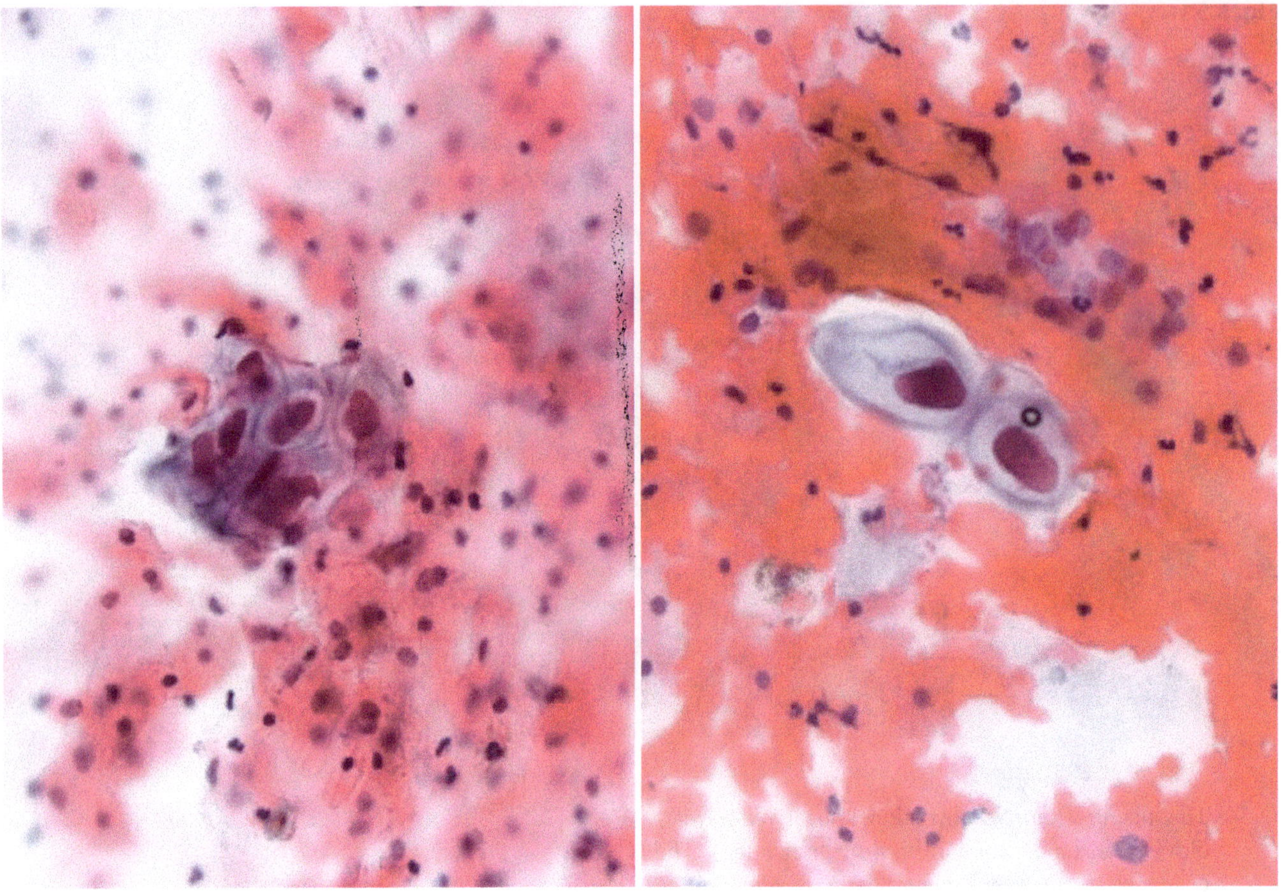

Fig. 3.55

Q-55. These squamous cells have prominent eosinophilic inclusions (vulvar scrape, conventional, medium). The most likely clinical presentation in this patient is:

(a) Postcoital bleeding
(b) Dome-shaped nodules with umbilicated margins
(c) Widespread reddish rash
(d) Draining groin lymph nodes

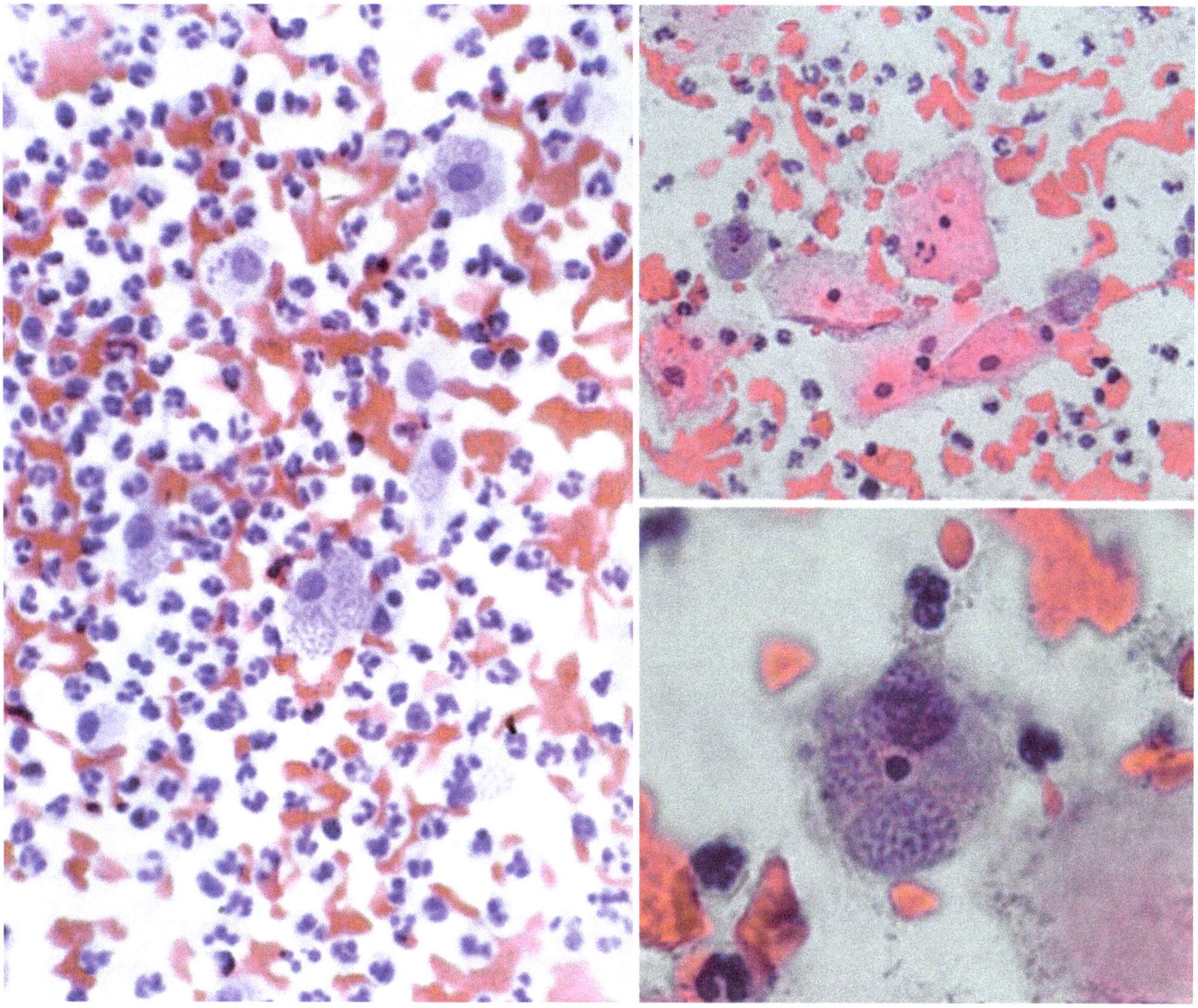

Fig. 3.56

Q-56. These small safety pin-shaped inclusions found within the macrophages are called by which of the following (conventional, left, high magnification; right upper, low magnification; right lower, oil immersion):

(a) Schaumann bodies
(b) Donovan bodies
(c) Histoplasma capsulatum
(d) Torulopsis glabrata
(e) Coccidioides immitis

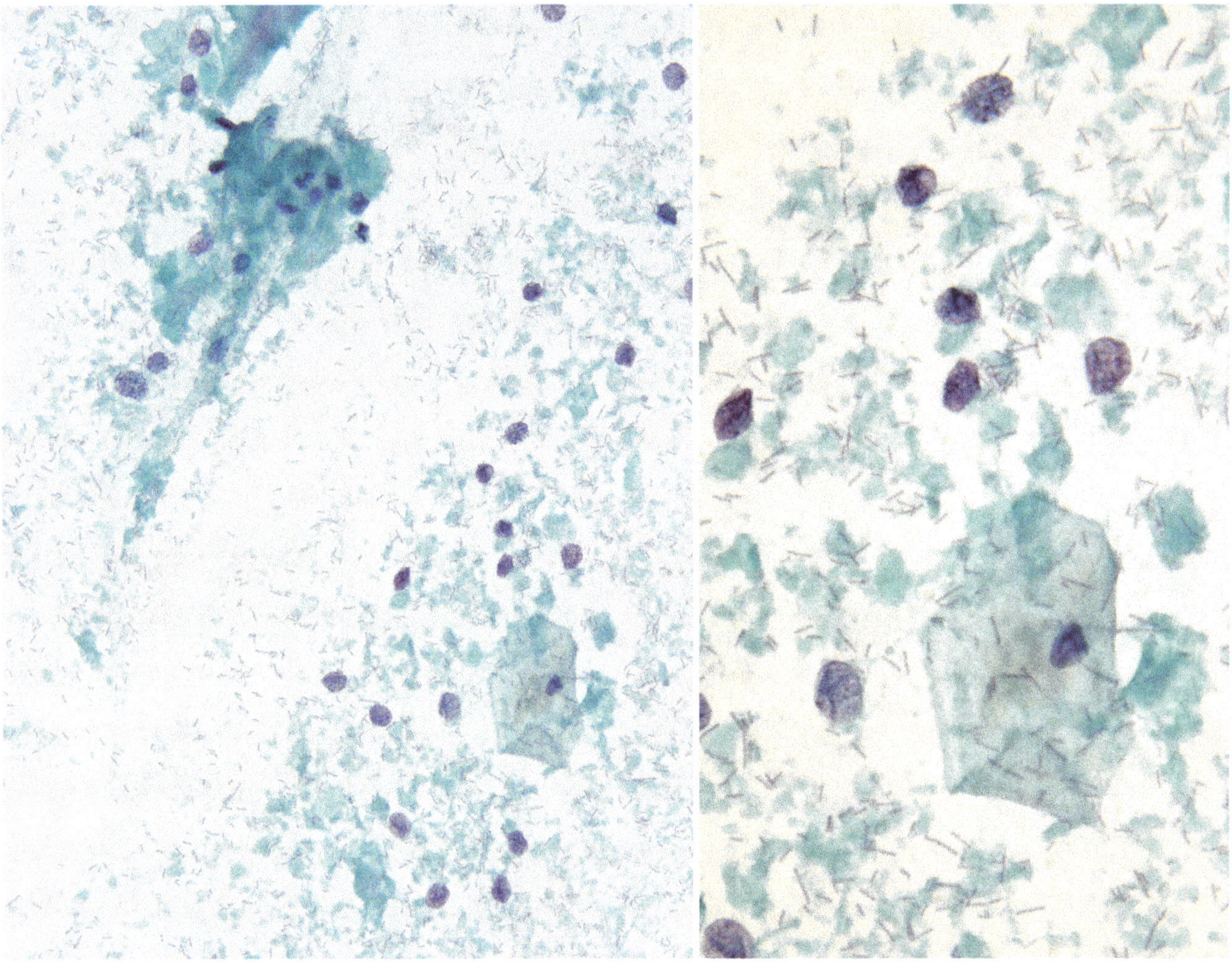

Fig. 3.57

Q-57. The three elements seen here, naked nuclei, lactobacilli, and cytoplasmic debris, are consistent with a diagnosis of which of the following (conventional, left, low magnification; right, conventional, high magnification)?

(a) Cytolysis
(b) Tumor diathesis
(c) Shift in vaginal flora suggestive of bacterial vaginosis
(d) Degenerative changes consistent with atrophy

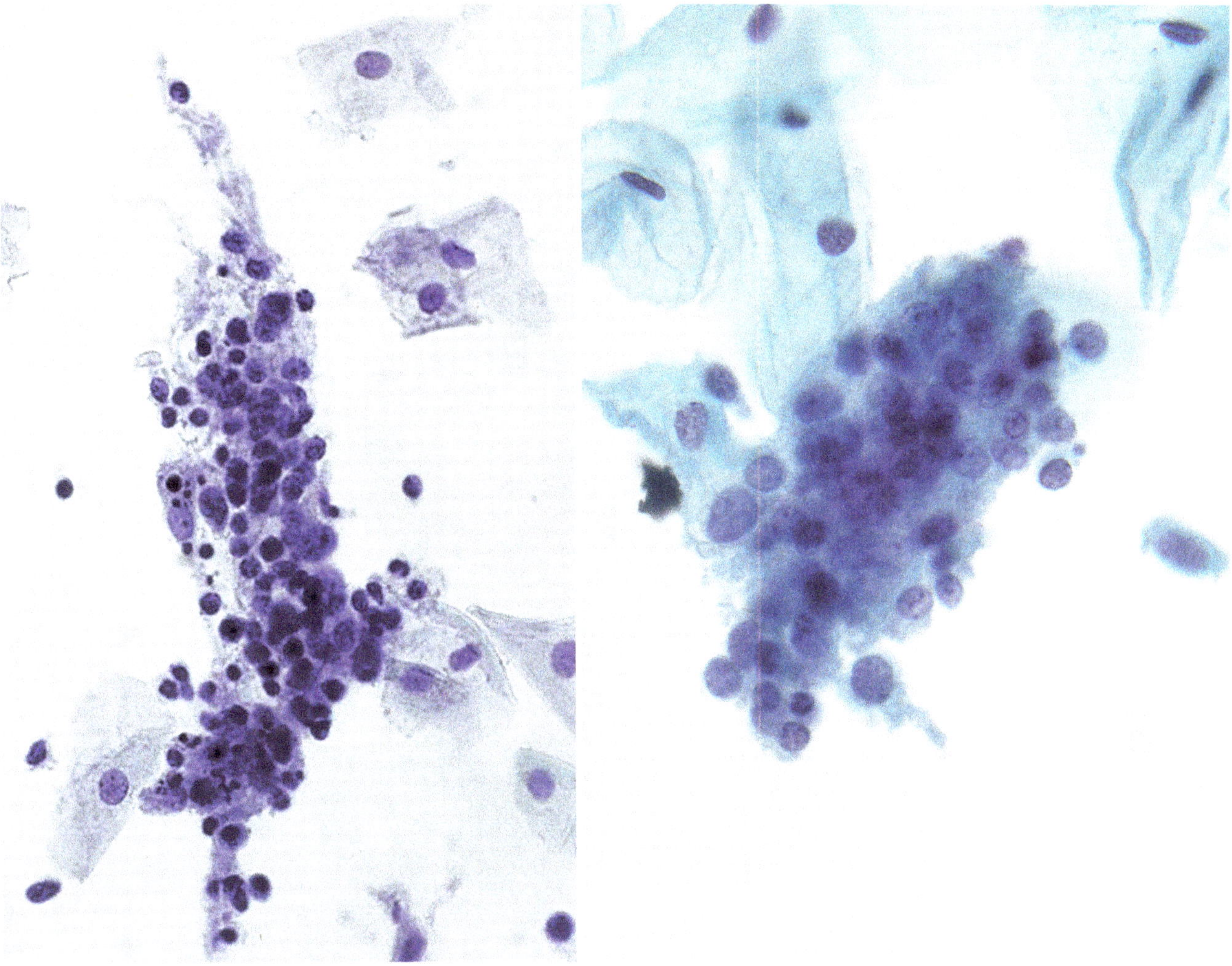

Fig. 3.58

Q-58. These findings (ThinPrep, medium magnification, left; ThinPrep, medium magnification, right) are indicative of which of the following?

(a) Acute inflammatory response
(b) Lymphoma
(c) ALL
(d) Chronic follicular cervicitis
(e) Small cell carcinoma of the cervix

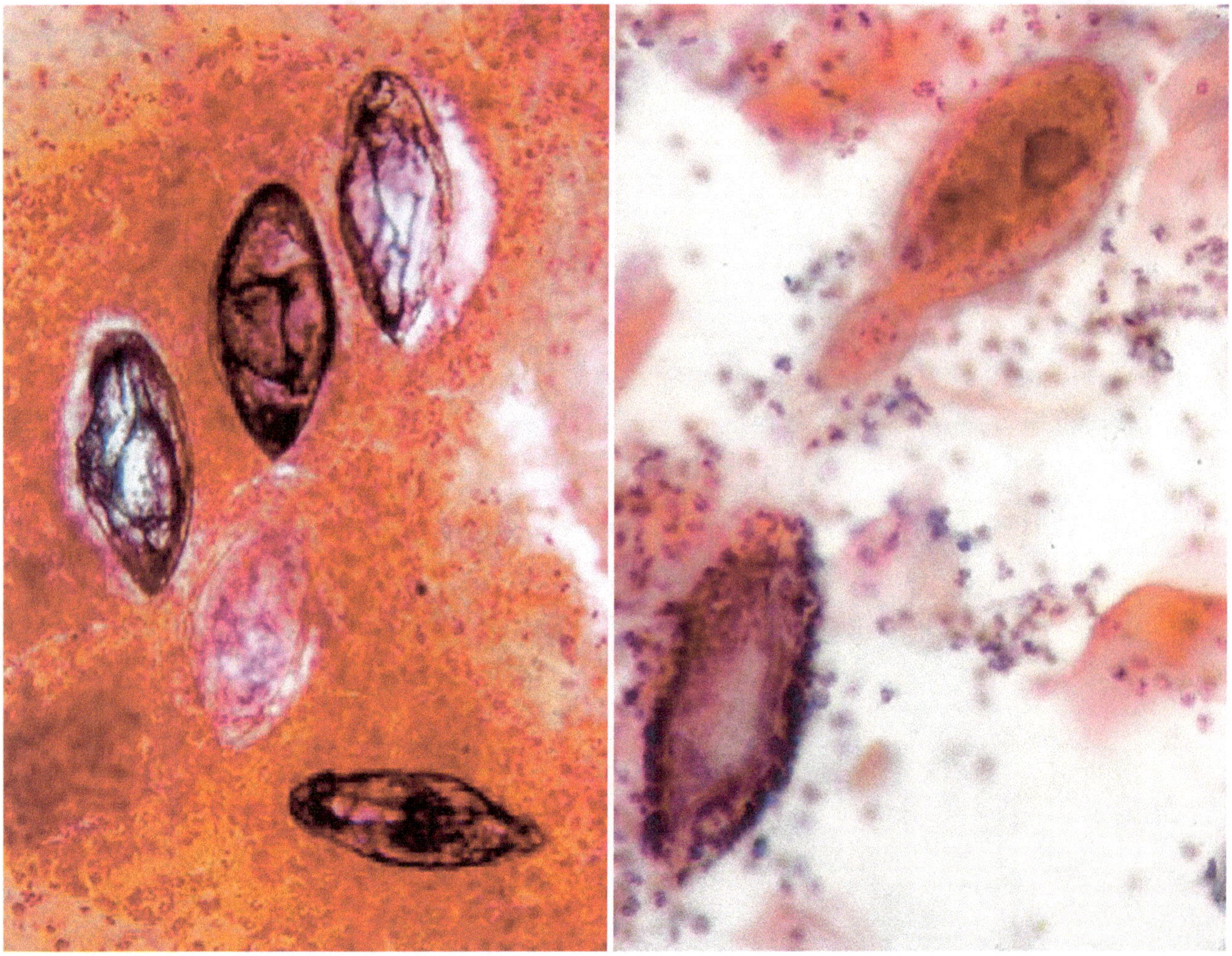

Fig. 3.59

Q-59. This finding from the cervical sample of a 42-year-old female (conventional, medium magnification, right and left) is most consistent with:
(a) Enterobius vermicularis
(b) Schistosoma haematobium
(c) Vegetable contaminant
(d) Lubricant artifact

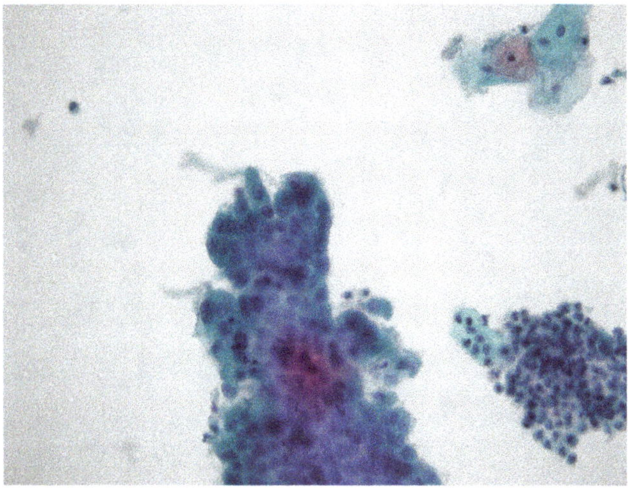

Fig. 3.60

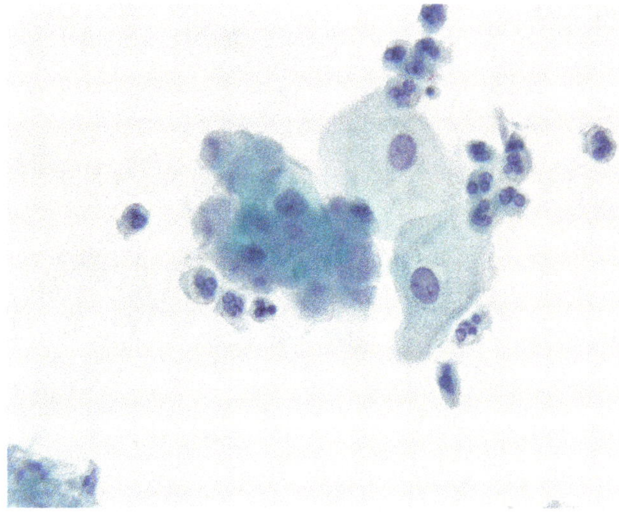

Fig. 3.61

Q-60. This finding in the conventional smear of a 45-year-old woman (conventional, medium magnification) is consistent with which of the following?
(a) Squamous metaplasia
(b) Endocervical cells
(c) Endometrial cells
(d) HGSIL

Q-61. This finding is from the gynecologic sample of a 27-year-old female (ThinPrep, high magnification). It is most likely to be found with which of the following?
(a) HPV changes
(b) Adenovirus
(c) Leptothrix
(d) Molluscum contagiosum
(e) Actinomyces

Fig. 3.62

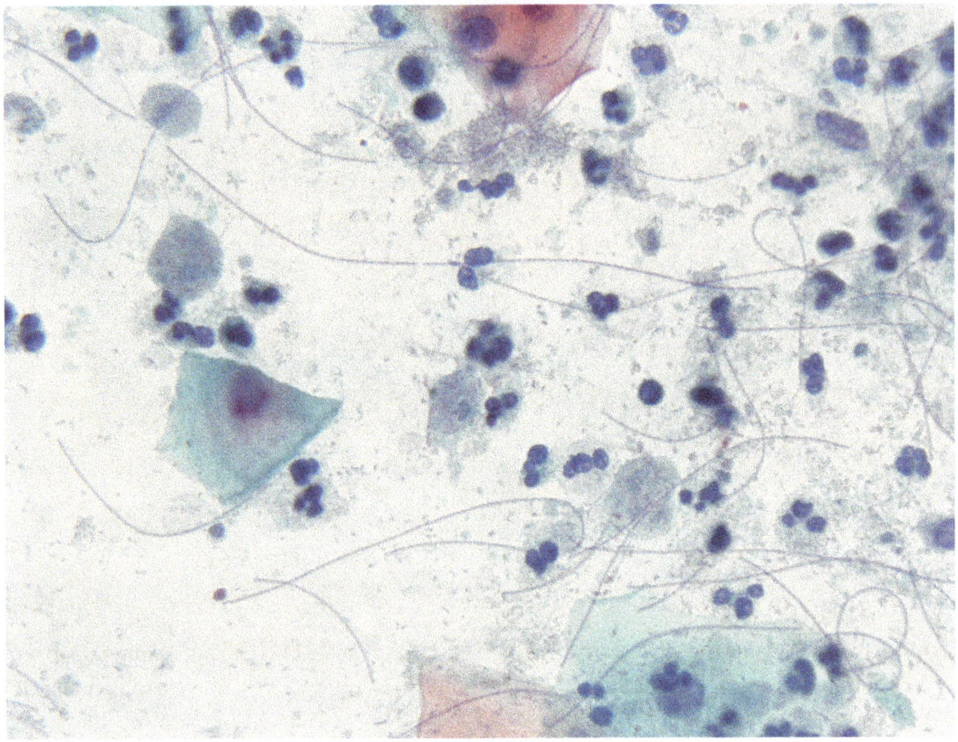

Q-62. This image is from the gynecologic sample of a 24-year-old female (conventional, high magnification). The curving structures noted are most likely:

(a) Actinomyces
(b) Doderlein bacilli
(c) Flagella from Trichomonas
(d) Leptothrix
(e) Aspergillus

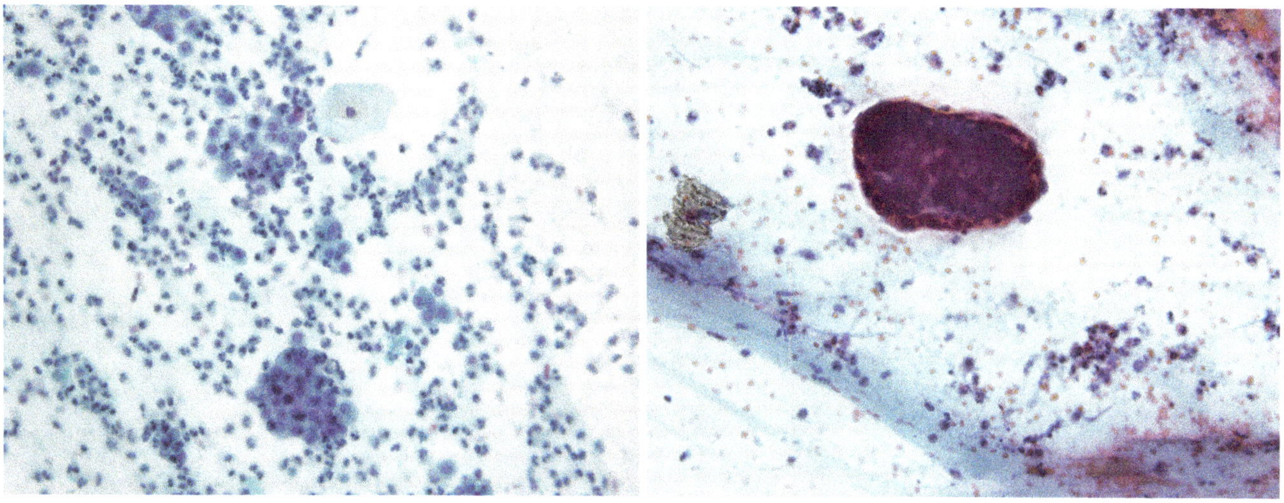

Fig. 3.63

Q-63. This finding is from the gynecologic sample of a 29-year-old woman (conventional, medium magnification). The most likely clinical symptoms accompanying this finding are:

(a) Watery discharge with "fishy" odor
(b) White thick discharge with pruritus
(c) Abnormal bleeding, abdominal cramping
(d) Greenish discharge with skin irritation

Fig. 3.64

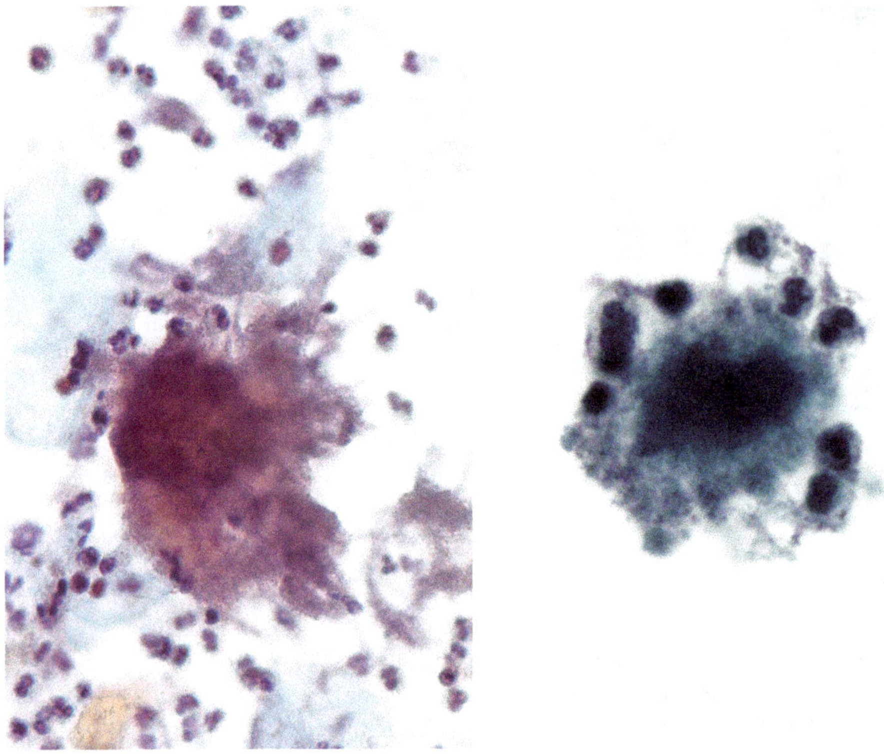

Q-64. These images are from a 32-year-old female G1P1 (conventional slide, left, medium magnification; right upper, high magnification; right lower, medium magnification). This is most likely which of the following?

(a) Actinomyces
(b) Aspergillus
(c) IUD effect
(d) Trichomonas and Leptothrix
(e) Cytolysis

Fig. 3.65

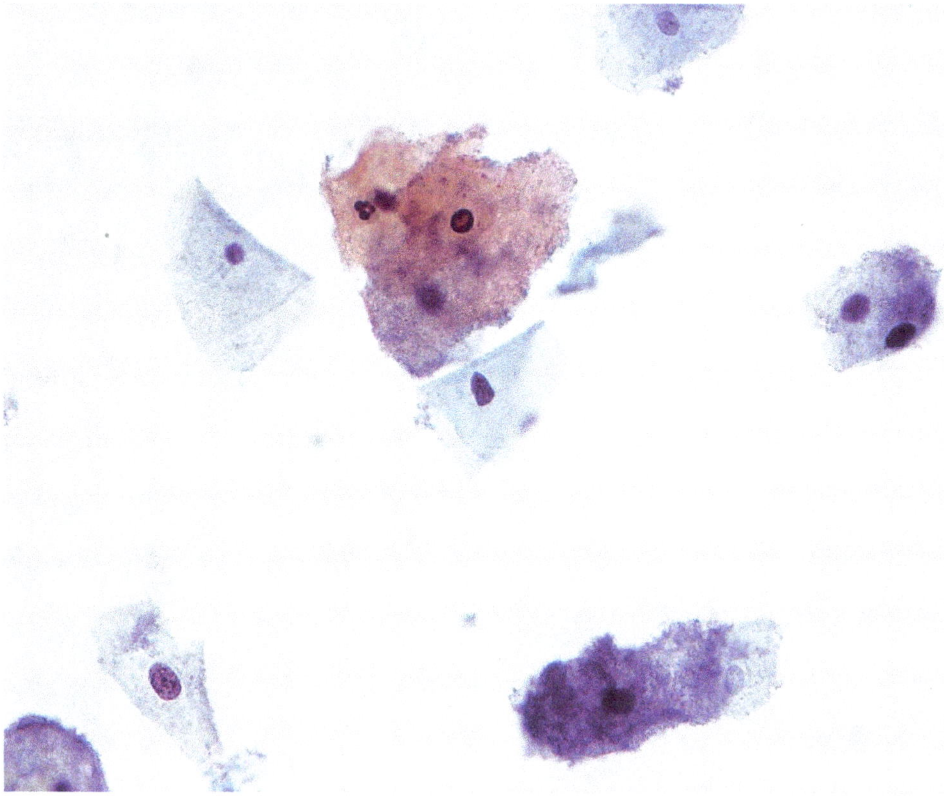

Q-65. A conventional Pap smear was done on a 32-year-old female and many fields such as the one illustrated were seen (conventional, medium magnification). The most likely diagnosis for this case is which of the following?

(a) Trichomonas vaginalis
(b) Doderlein bacilli
(c) Actinomyces
(d) Candida species
(e) Shift in vaginal flora suggestive of bacterial vaginosis

Fig. 3.66

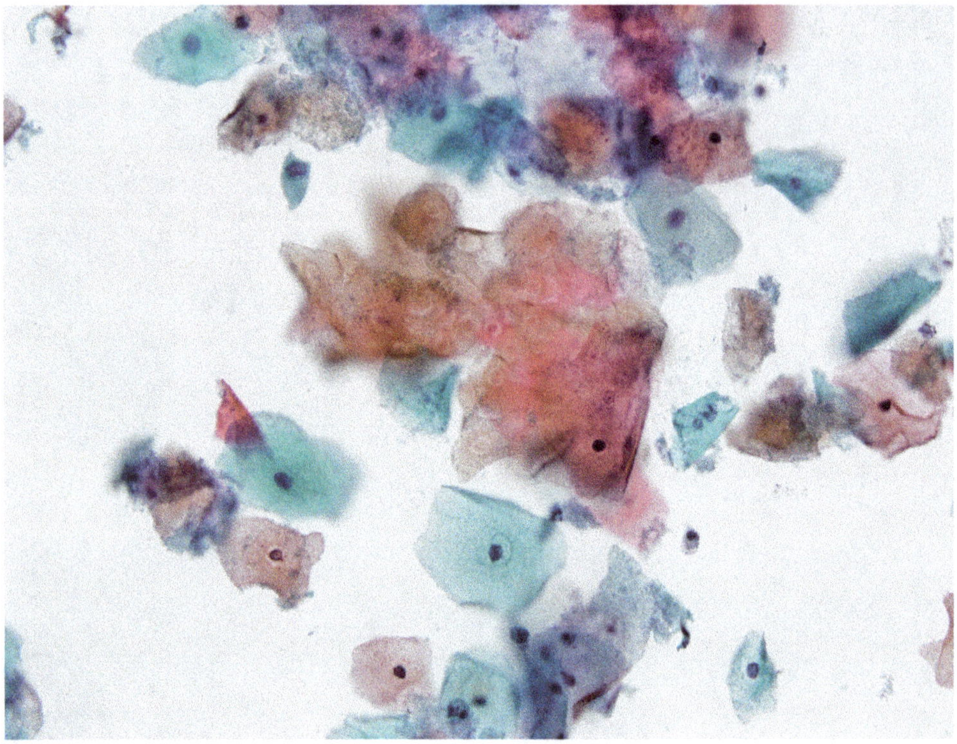

Q-66. This finding in a 32-year-old non-gravid female would be most consistent with a diagnosis of which of the following (conventional, medium magnification)?

(a) HPV
(b) LGSIL
(c) Hyperkeratosis
(d) Parakeratosis
(e) Shift in vaginal flora suggestive of bacterial vaginosis

Fig. 3.67

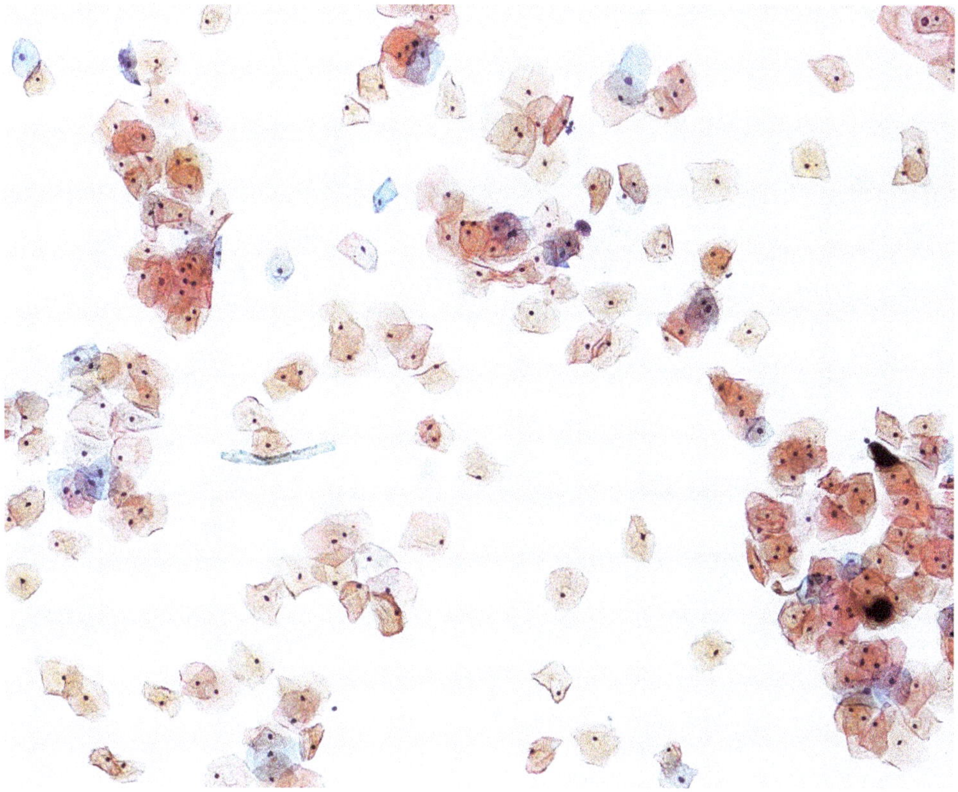

Q-67. This overall pattern is most consistent with which day of the menstrual cycle (ThinPrep, low magnification)?
(a) Days 0–5
(b) Days 6–11
(c) Days 12–16
(d) Days 17–21
(e) Days 22–28

Fig. 3.68

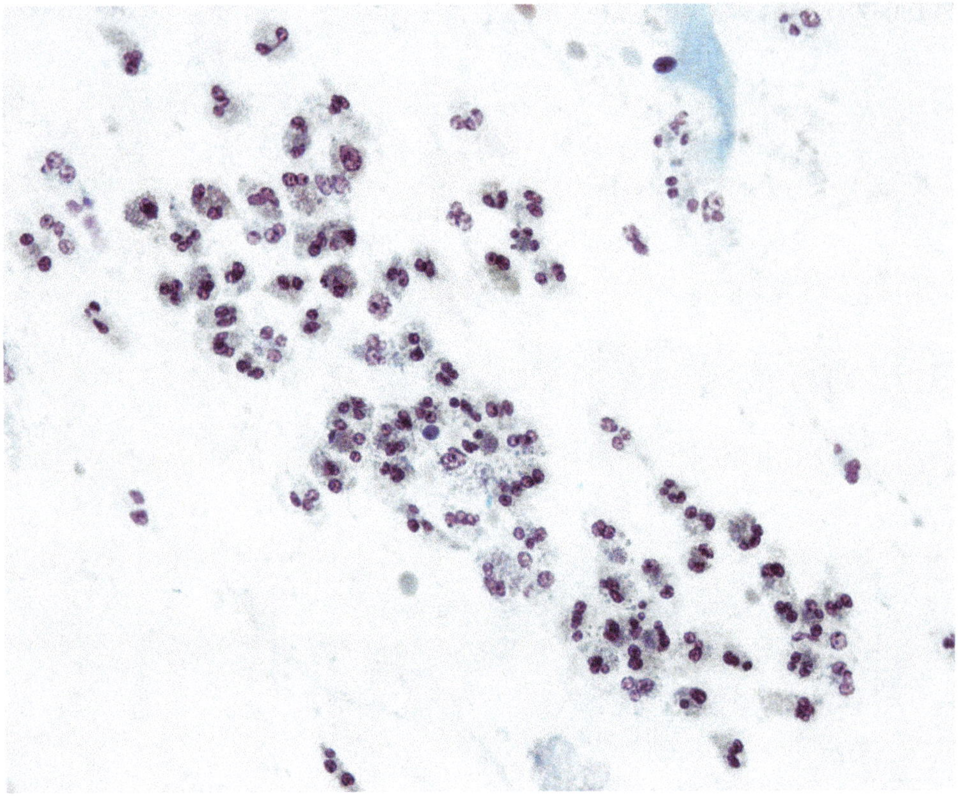

Q-68. Most of the cells seen in this image (conventional, high magnification) are:

(a) Lymphocytes
(b) Plasma cells
(c) Histiocytes
(d) Polymorphonuclear leukocytes
(e) Eosinophils

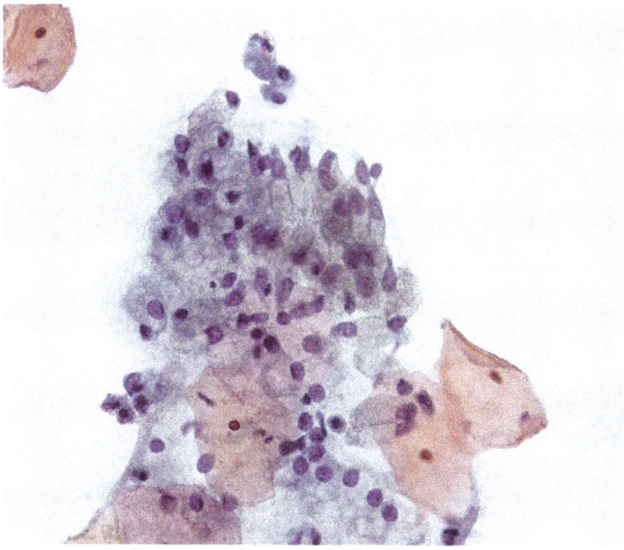

Fig. 3.69

Q-69. The yellowish material seen in the cytoplasm of these elongated cells is most likely (ThinPrep, medium magnification):
(a) Glycogen
(b) Mucin
(c) Lipofuscin
(d) Melanin
(e) Hemosiderin

Fig. 3.70

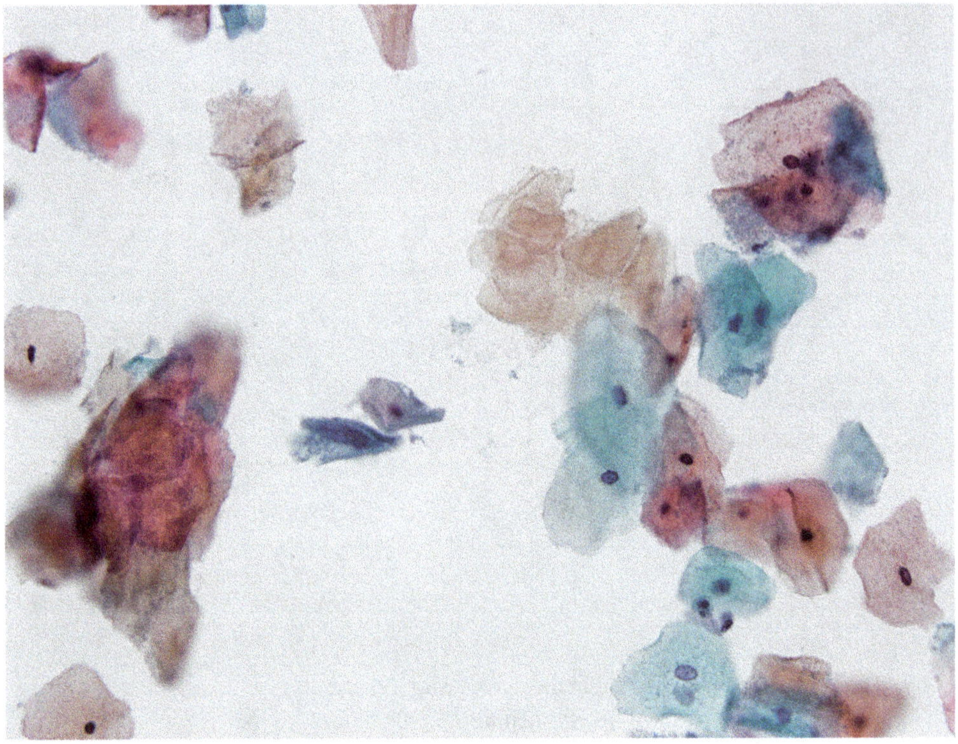

Q-70. These cellwere frequently found in the gynecologic sample of a 48-year-old woman (ThinPrep, medium magnification). The most likely diagnosis of these cells is:

(a) Normal superficial and intermediate cells
(b) Squamous metaplasia
(c) Inflammatory cell changes
(d) Hyperkeratosis
(e) Pseudoparakeratosis

Fig. 3.71

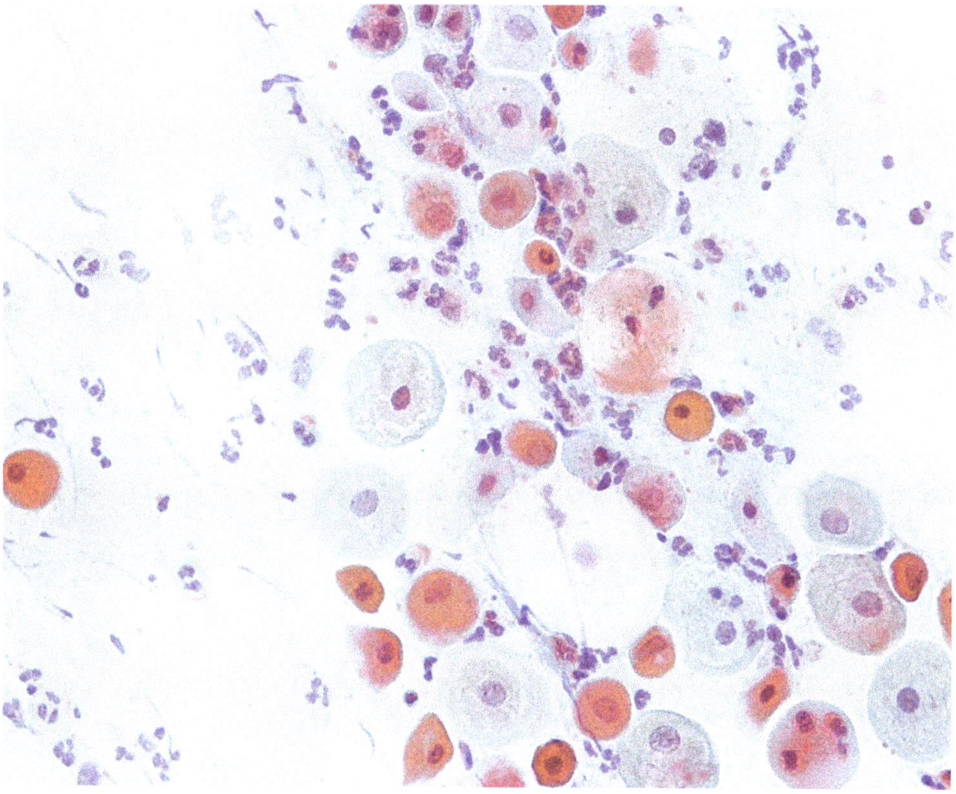

Q-71. Many cells such as these were found in the gynecologic sample from a 62-year-old woman with no history of hormone use or previous abnormality (conventional, low magnification). The most likely diagnosis of these cells is:

(a) Squamous metaplasia
(b) Parakeratosis
(c) Atrophy
(d) Keratinizing LGSIL

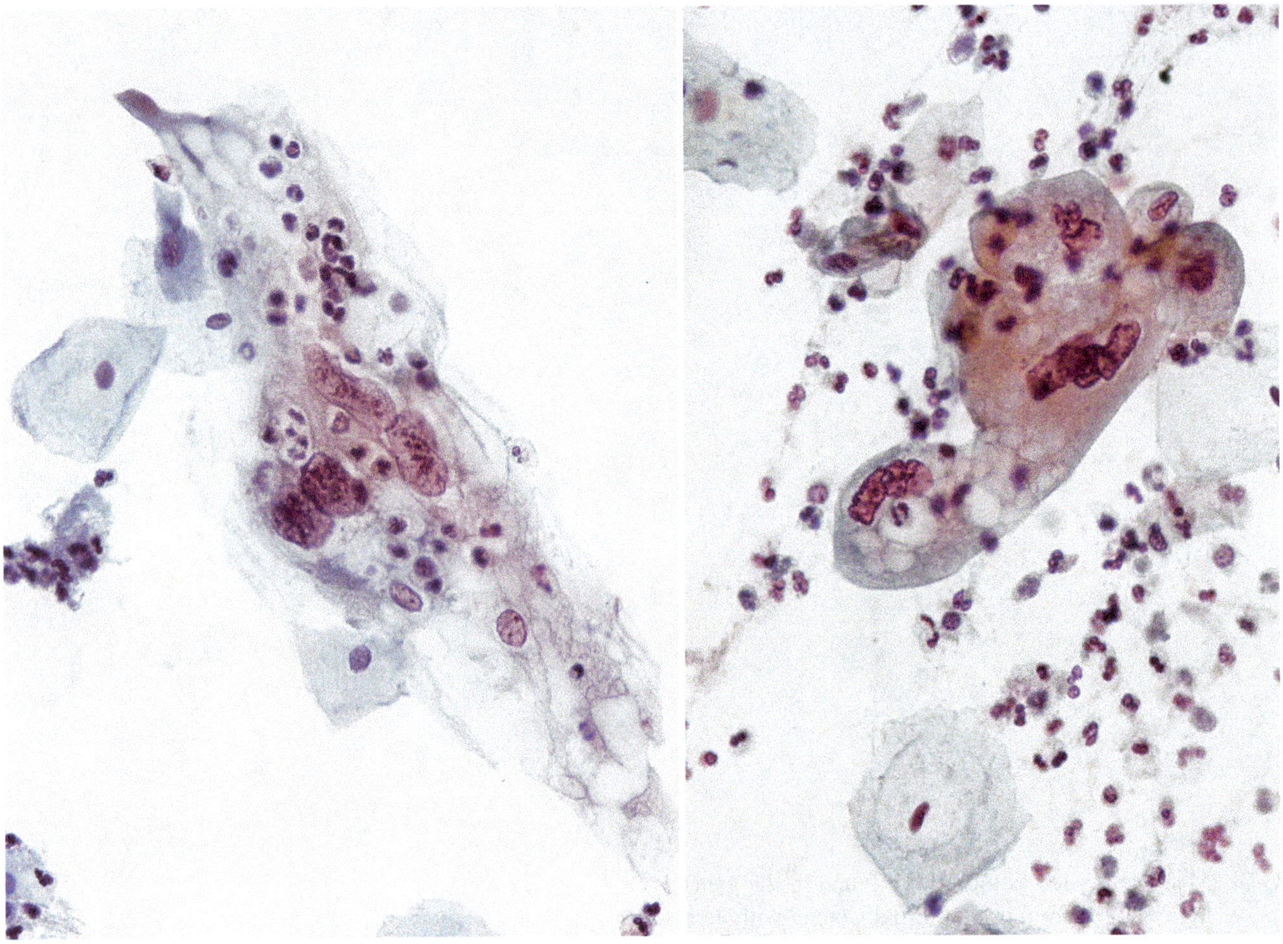

Fig. 3.72

Q-72. Cells such as these were seen in the Pap sample (ThinPrep, medium magnification) from a 49-year-old woman, status post hysterectomy and radiation for squamous cell carcinoma of the cervix 10 years ago. The correct interpretation of these cells is most likely:

(a) Repair
(b) Recurrent squamous cell carcinoma
(c) Normal superficial and intermediate cells
(d) Radiation effect
(e) Atypical endocervical cells

Fig. 3.73

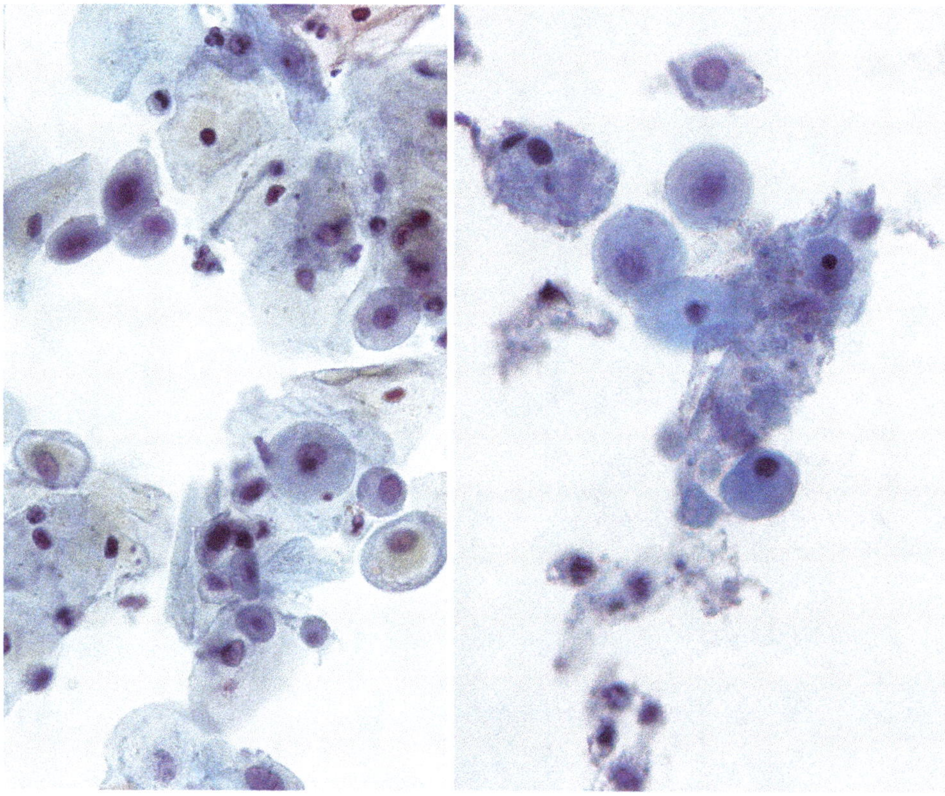

Q-73. Cells such as these were seen occasionally in a ThinPrep slide (medium magnification) from a 28-year-old female, G0P0. The smaller, more rounded cells are most consistent with which of the following?

(a) Squamous metaplasia
(b) Atrophy
(c) Inflammatory cell changes
(d) LGSIL
(e) Navicular cells

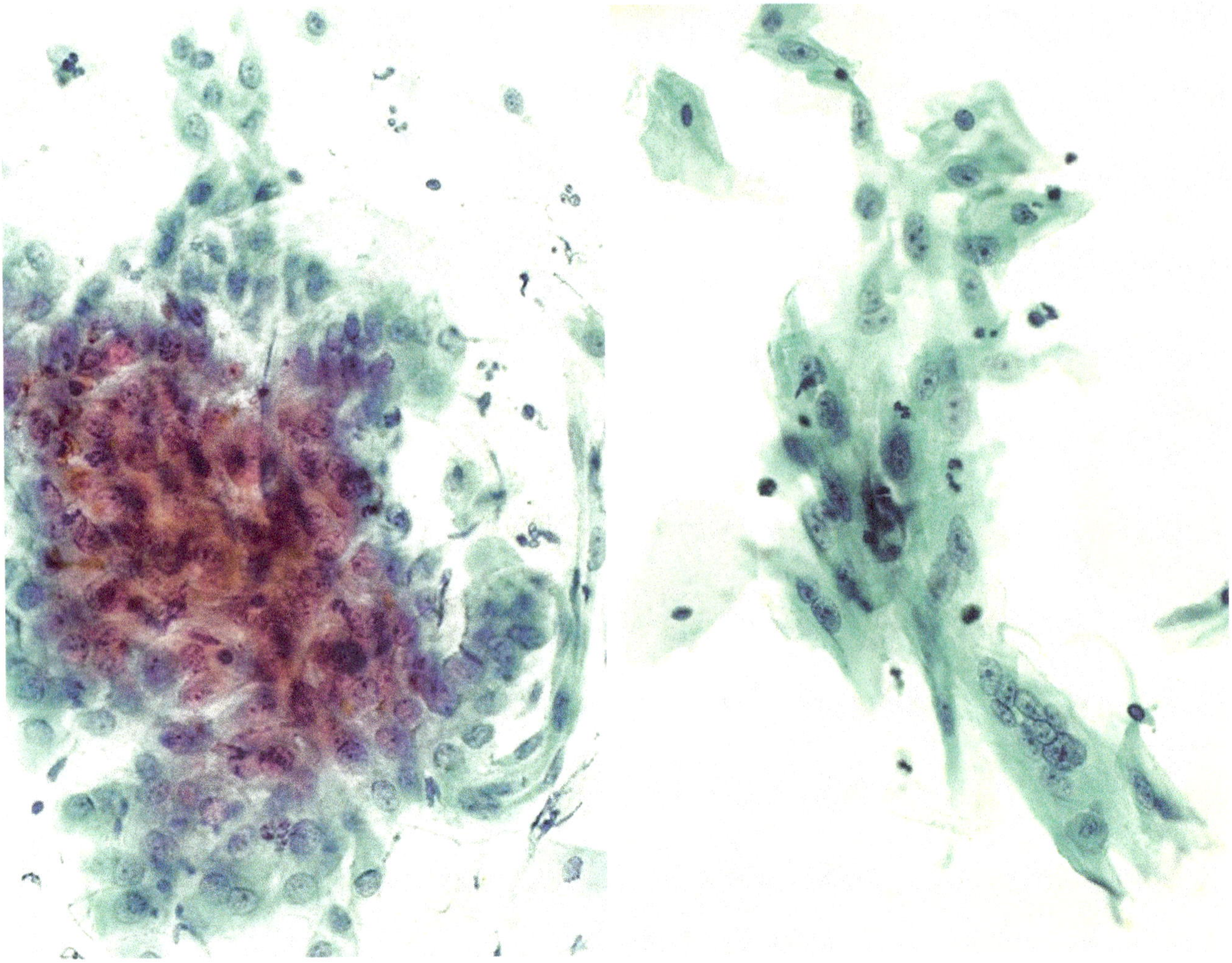

Fig. 3.74

Q-74. These cells were found in the gynecologic sample from a 48-year-old female (SurePath, medium magnification, left and right). The most likely interpretation of these cells is:

(a) Endocervical adenocarcinoma
(b) Endometrial adenocarcinoma
(c) Endocervical AIS
(d) HGSIL
(e) Repair

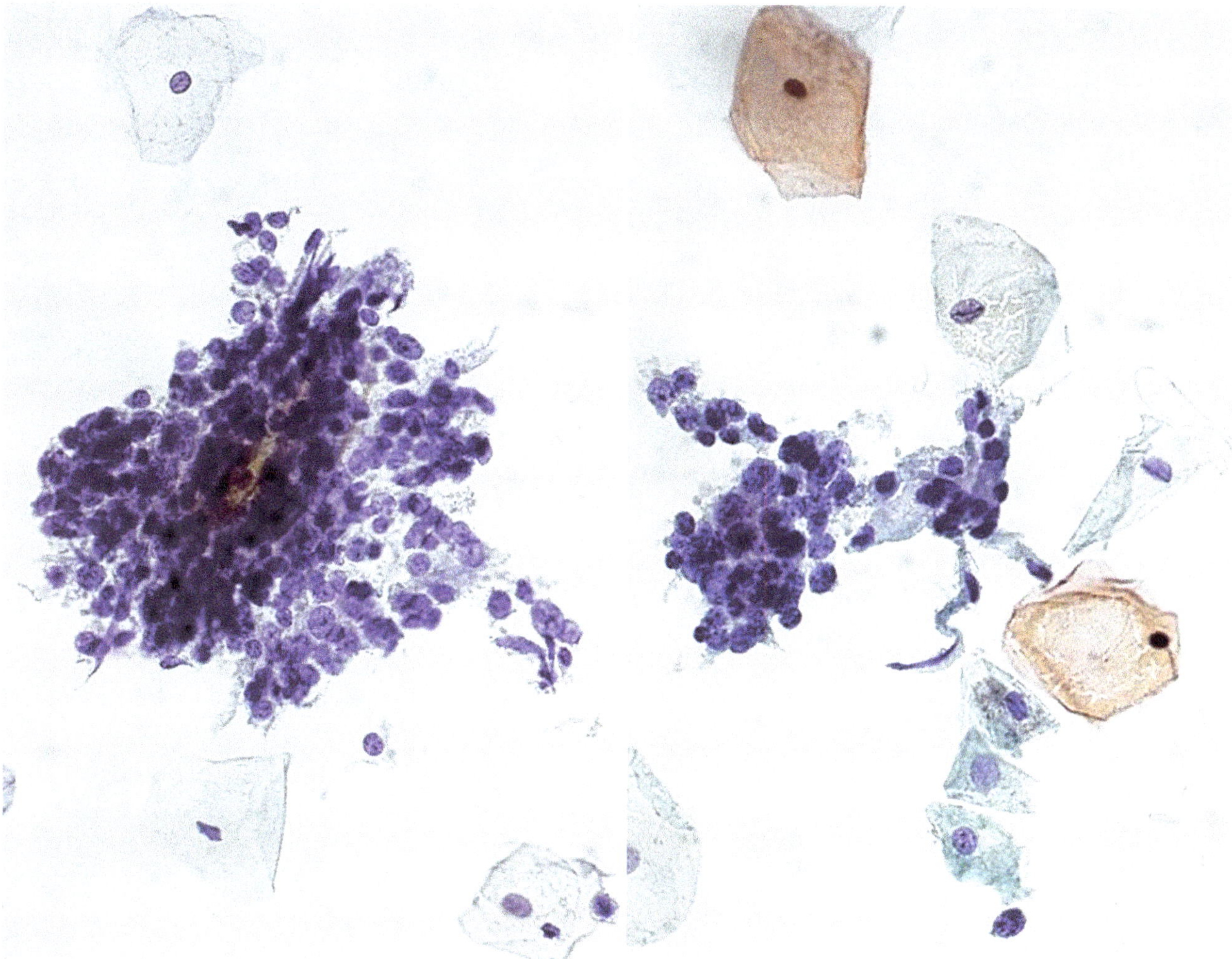

Fig. 3.75

Q-75. The most likely interpretation for cells such as these found in the gynecologic sample (ThinPrep, medium magnification) from a 39-year-old woman would be:
(a) Chronic follicular cervicitis
(b) Poly balls suggestive of Trichomonas
(c) Small cell carcinoma of the cervix
(d) HGSIL
(e) Suggestive of lymphoma

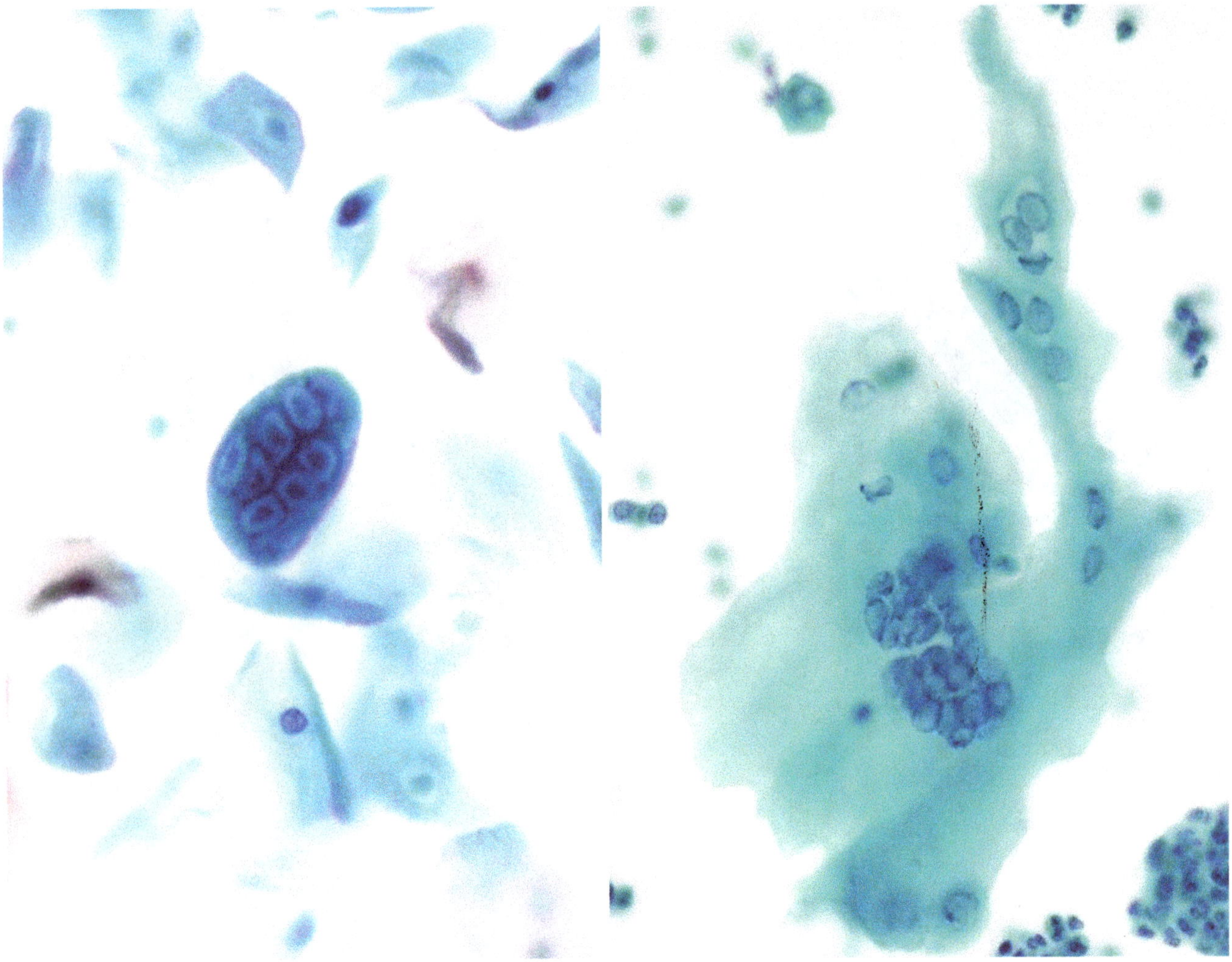

Fig. 3.76

Q-76. The most likely interpretation of these cells is (ThinPrep, medium magnification):

(a) Adenovirus
(b) CMV
(c) Herpes
(d) HGSIL
(e) LGSIL

Fig. 3.77

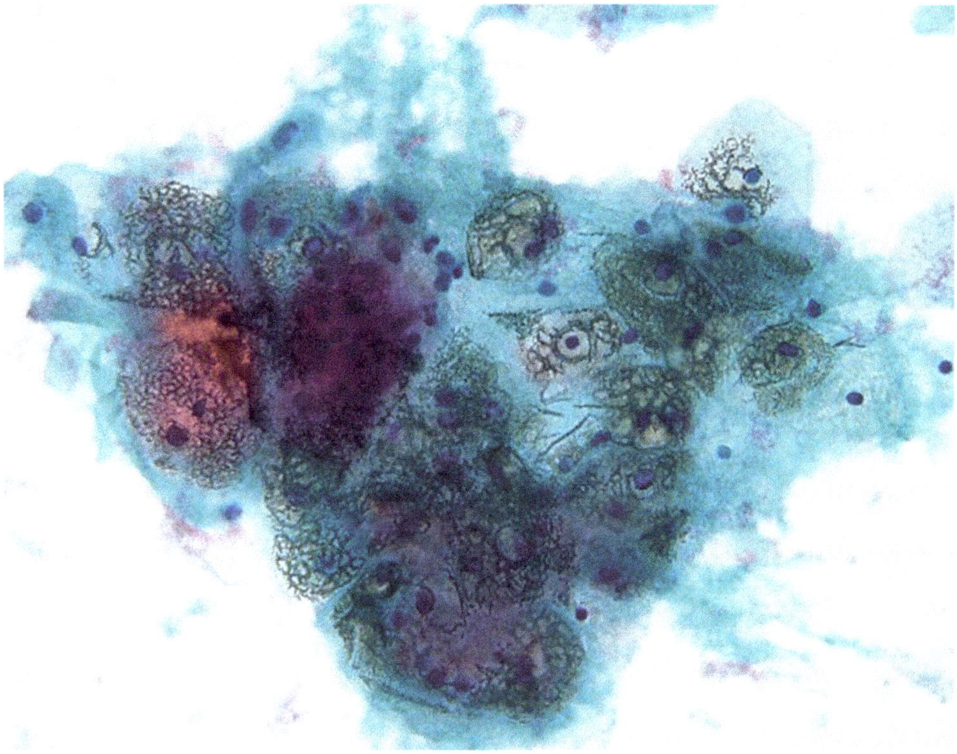

Q-77. This artifact, if extensive, can interfere with the interpretation of the slide. The best method to remove it is to remove the coverslip and the mounting media in xylene and then:

(a) Soak in glycerin for 30 min; restain.
(b) Restain and extend the time in the hematoxylin stain by 5 min.
(c) Restain and extend the time in the EA 65 by 5 min.
(d) Restain and shorten the time in the OG6 stain.
(e) Restain and use a mixture of 50 % ETOH and xylene immediately prior to coverslipping.

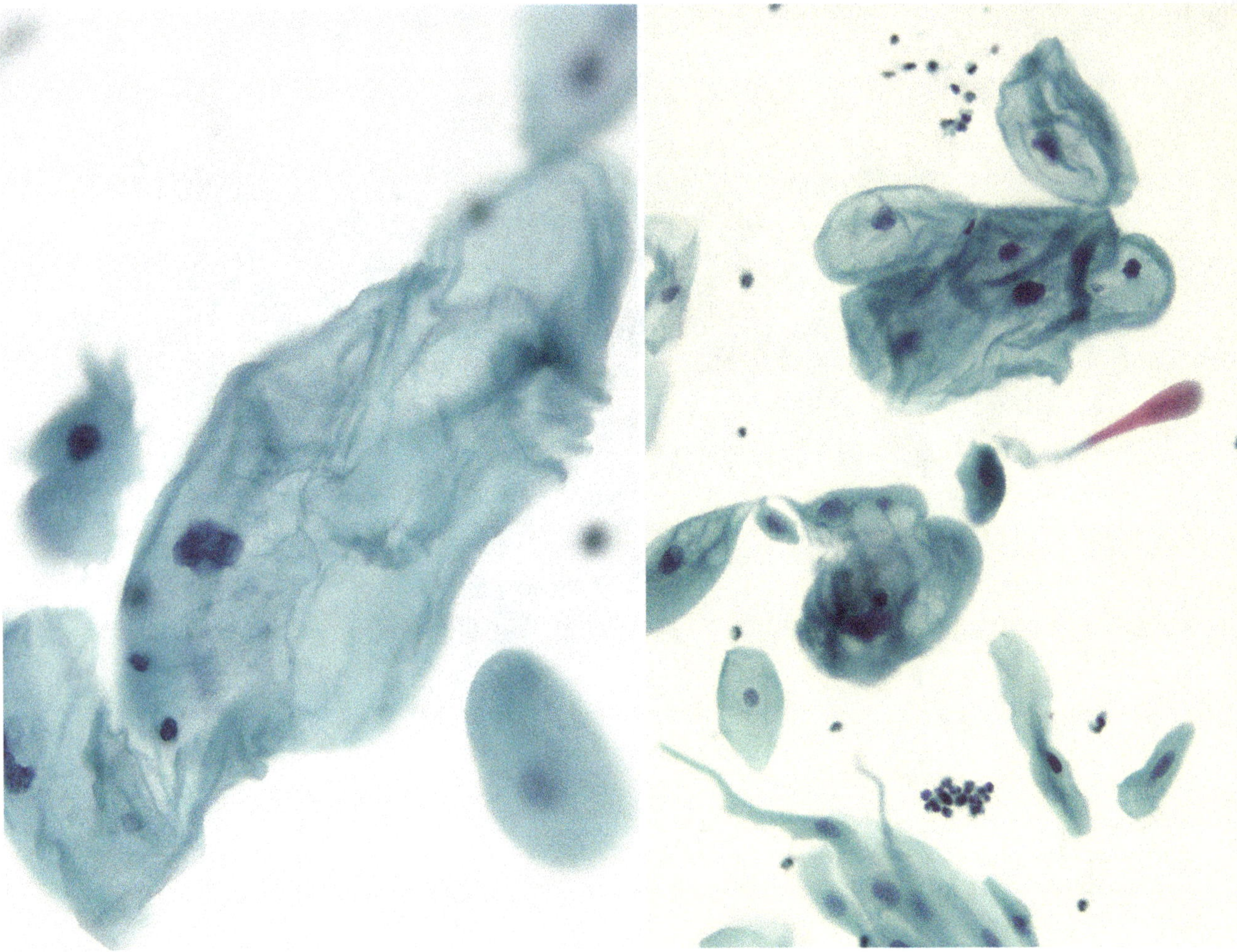

Fig. 3.78

Q-78. This patient is status post hysterectomy and therapy for squamous cell carcinoma of the cervix 5 years ago (SurePath, medium magnification, right and left). A number of cells with cytomegaly, cytoplasmic vacuolization, and bizarre shapes such as these were found on the slide. The most likely interpretation is:

(a) Inflammatory cell changes
(b) Radiation effect
(c) Repair
(d) LGSIL
(e) Recurrent squamous cell carcinoma

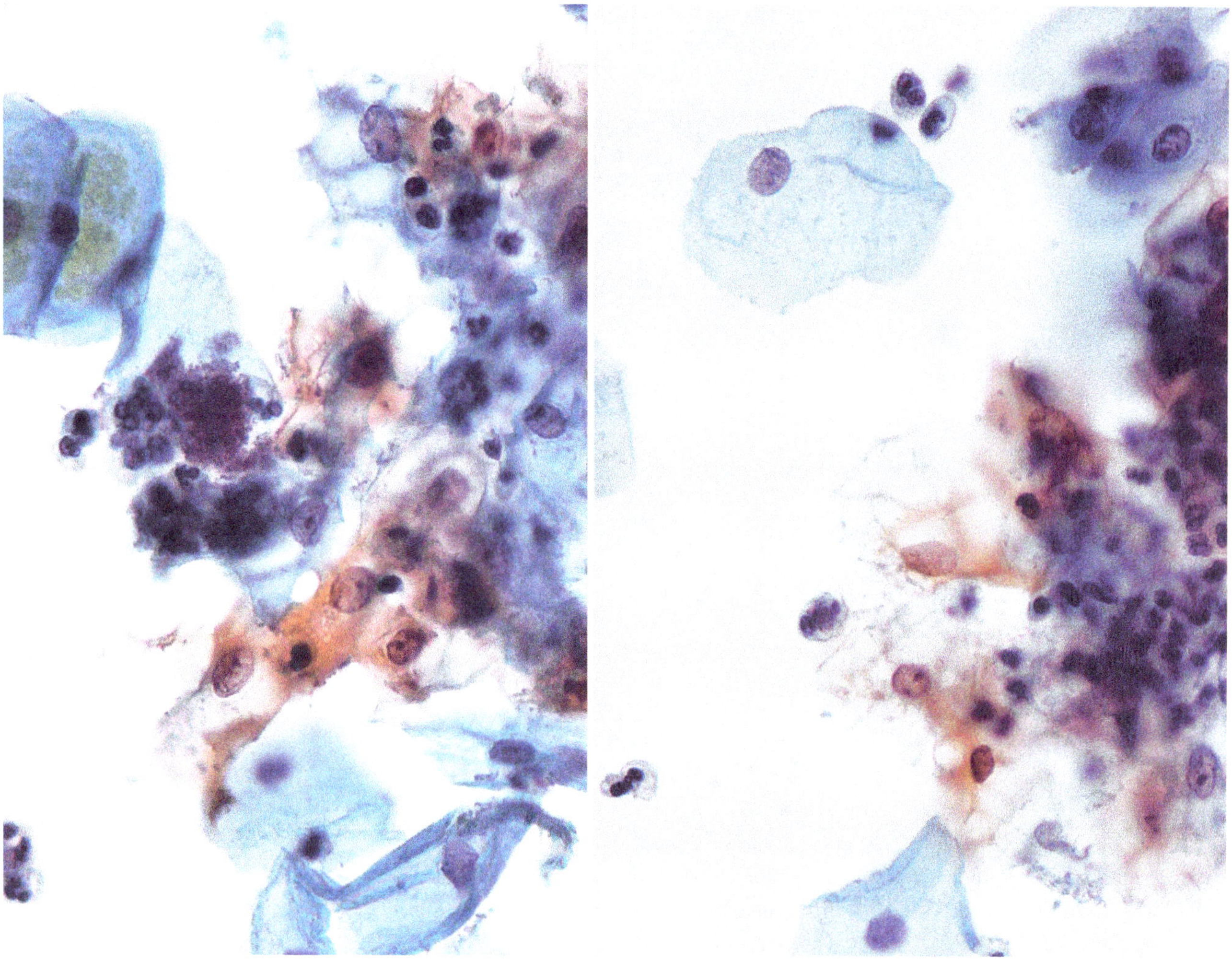

Fig. 3.79

Q-79. Many clusters of cells such as these were found in the gynecologic sample (ThinPrep, medium magnification) from a 27-year-old woman in her second trimester of a normal pregnancy. The squamous cells with the "moth-eaten" appearance to the cytoplasm are a clue to look carefully for which of the following likely organisms?

(a) CMV
(b) Herpes
(c) Actinomyces
(d) Candida
(e) Chlamydia

Fig. 3.80

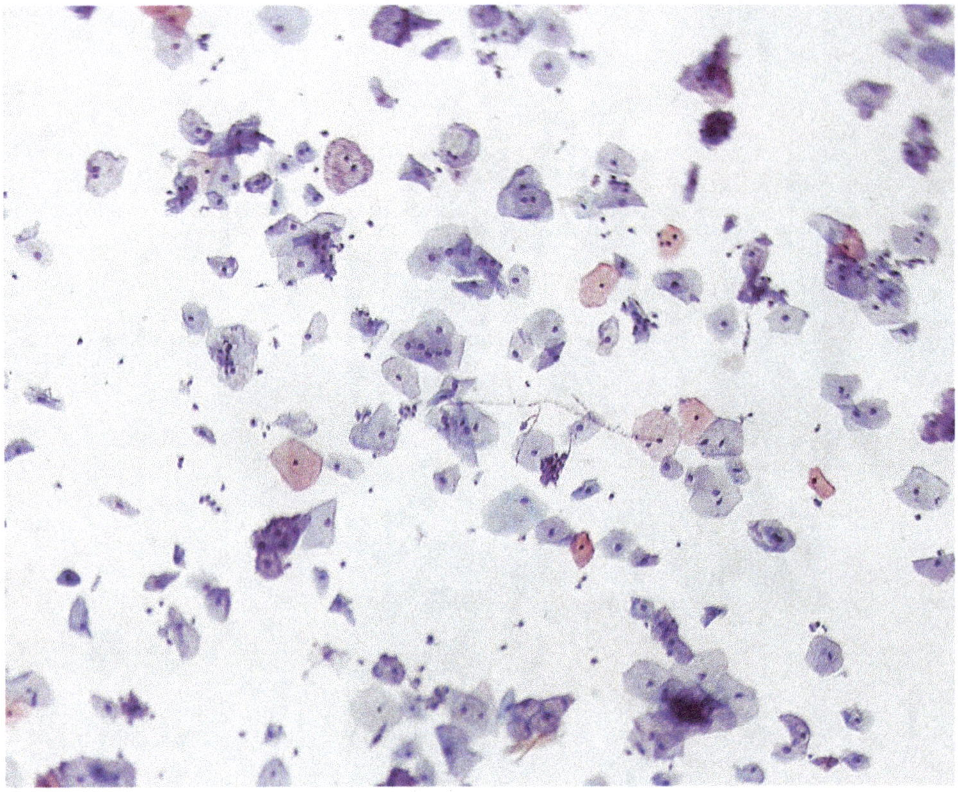

Q-80. This appearance in a gynecologic sample processed on a ThinPrep slide (low magnification) gives an important clue in searching for organisms, cytolysis, atrophy, or possible cancer. This appearance is called:

(a) Busy background
(b) Tumor diathesis
(c) Increased stain intensity
(d) Endometrial cell balls
(e) Estrogen effect

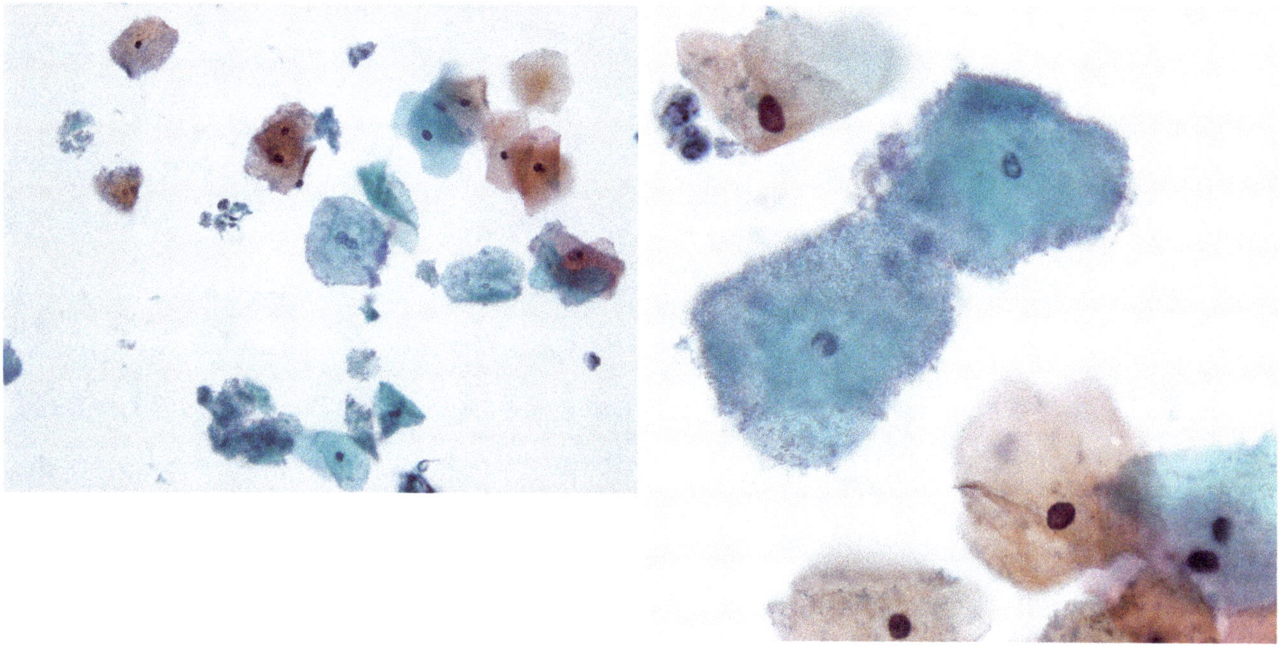

Fig. 3.81

Q-81. Cells such as these (ThinPrep, medium magnification, left; high magnification, right) are now referred to in the Bethesda System 2001 terminology as:
   (a) Clue cells
   (b) Shift in vaginal flora suggestive of bacterial vaginosis
   (c) Gardnerella vaginalis
   (d) Coccobacilli
   (e) Actinomyces

Fig. 3.82

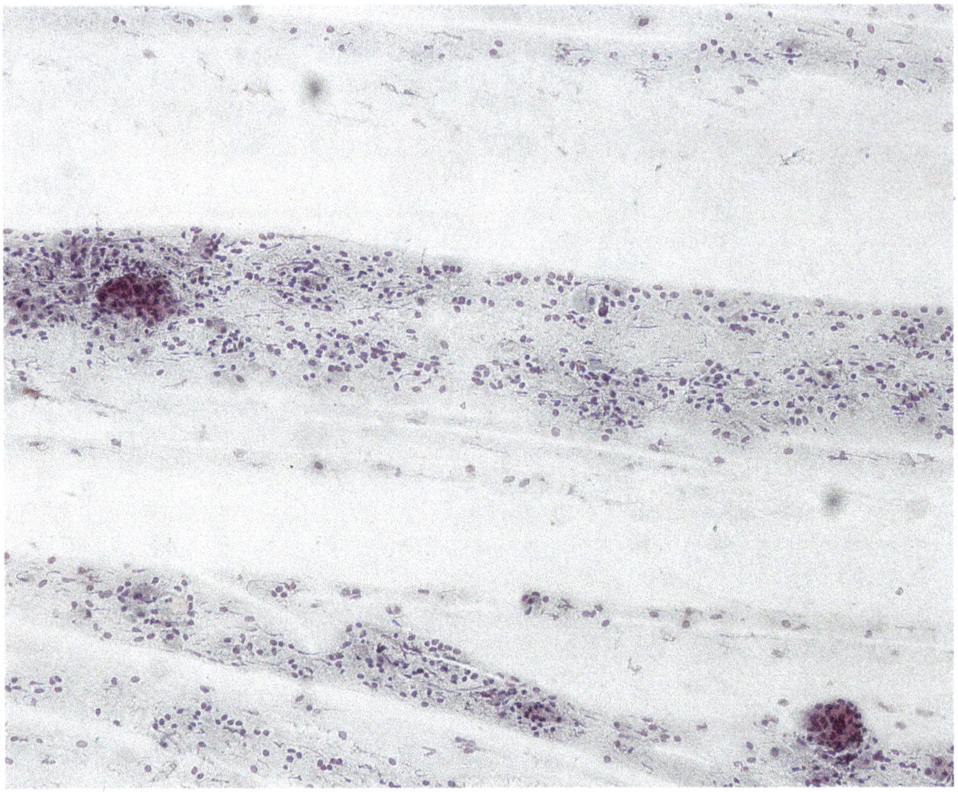

Q-82. This gynecologic sample (conventional, low magnification) would be most consistent with which of the following clinical histories?

(a) 17-year-old patient, day 5
(b) 25-year-old patient, third trimester of a normal pregnancy
(c) 32-year-old patient with testicular feminization
(d) 69-year-old patient with no exogenous hormone use

Fig. 3.83

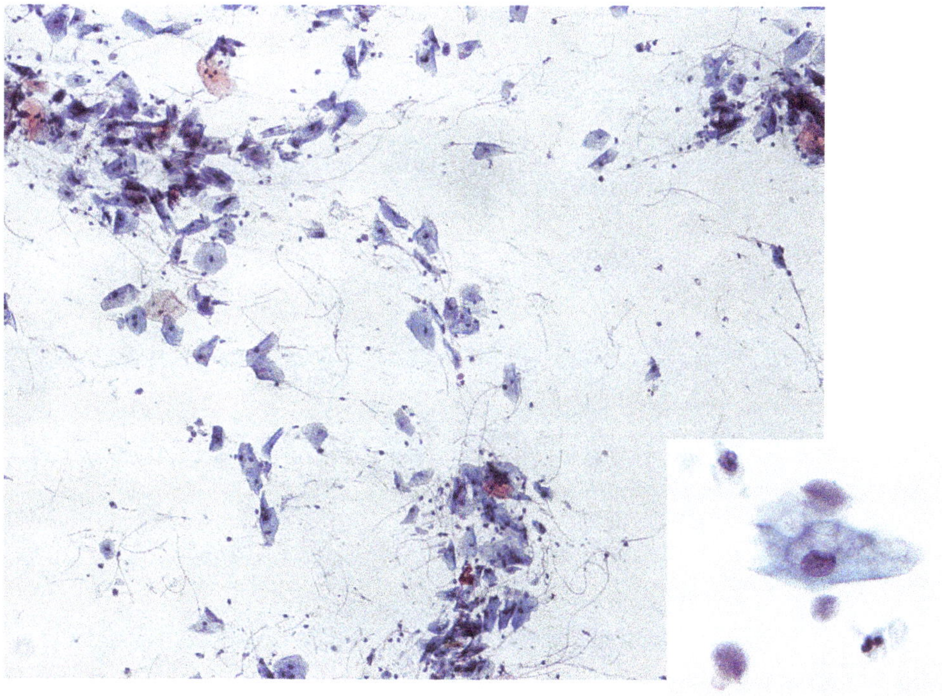

Q-83. This sample is from the gynecologic smear of a 32-year-old female (conventional, low magnification, left; high magnification, right inset). The best interpretation of these findings is:

(a) Doderlein bacilli and Trichomonas
(b) Actinomyces and shift in vaginal flora suggestive of bacterial vaginosis
(c) Candida and Trichomonas
(d) Entamoeba histolytica and Doderlein bacilli
(e) Leptothrix and Trichomonas

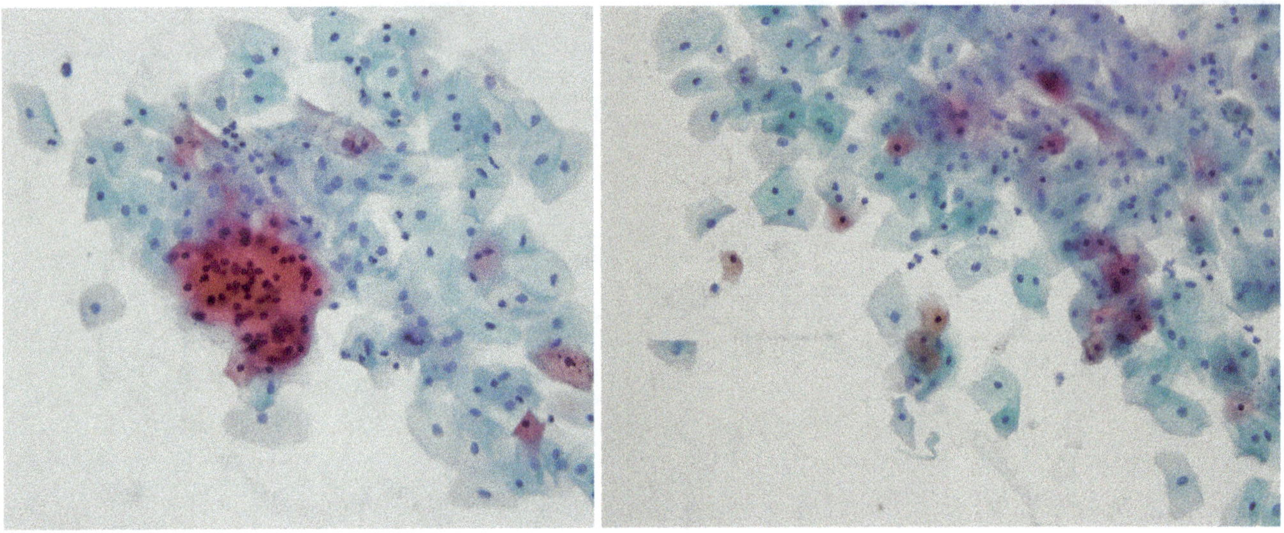

Fig. 3.84

Q-84. Small, pink to orange cells such as these were found throughout the gynecologic sample from a 42-year-old female (ThinPrep, right and left, medium magnification). The best diagnosis is:

(a) Normal squamous cells
(b) Parakeratotic cells
(c) Hyperkeratosis
(d) Squamous cell carcinoma
(e) Repair

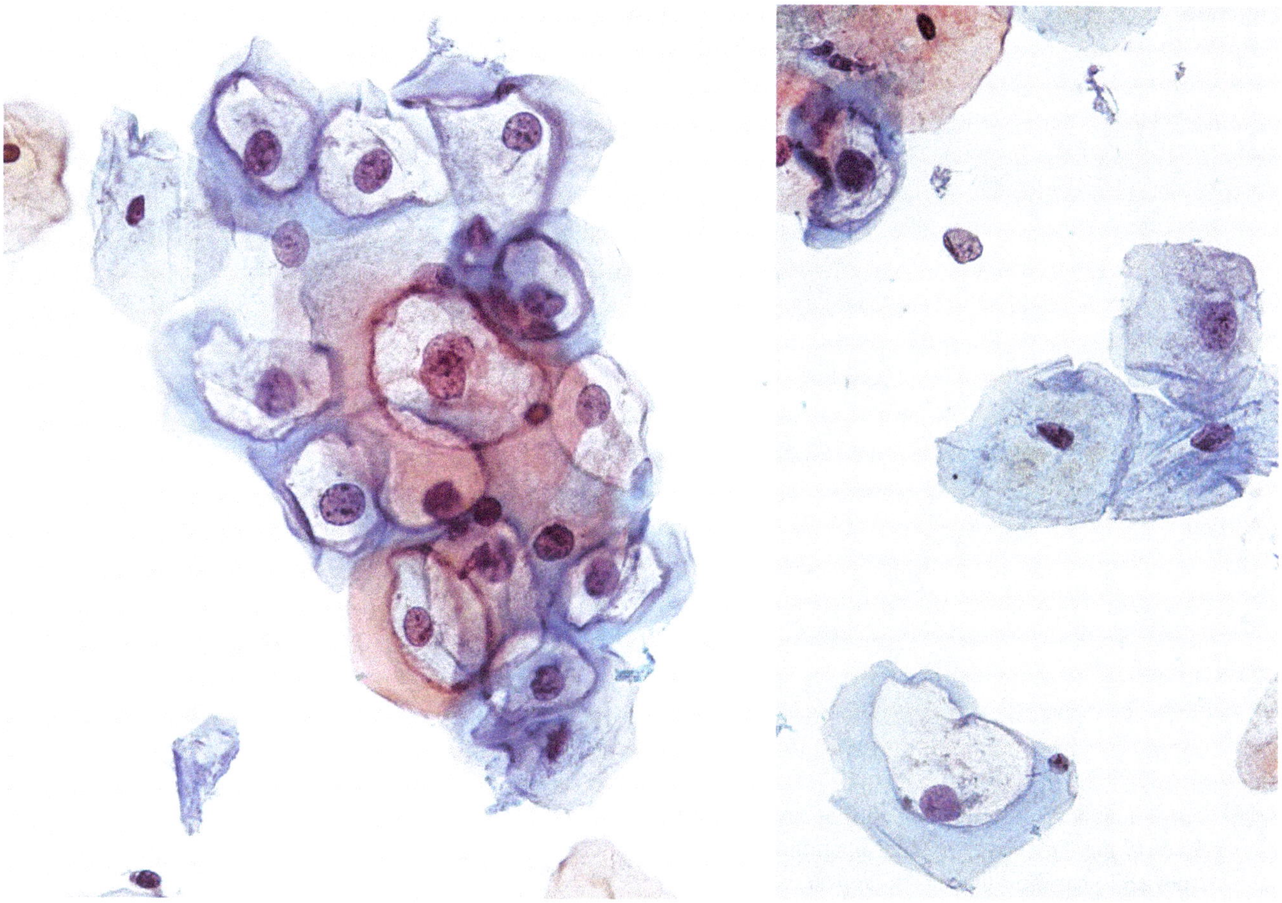

Fig. 3.85

Q-85. In the Bethesda System 2001, cells such as these found in the ThinPrep slide (right and left, medium magnification) of a 36-year-old woman would be interpreted as:
(a) ASC-US
(b) ASC-H
(c) LGSIL
(d) HGSIL
(e) Glycogenated squamous cells

Fig. 3.86

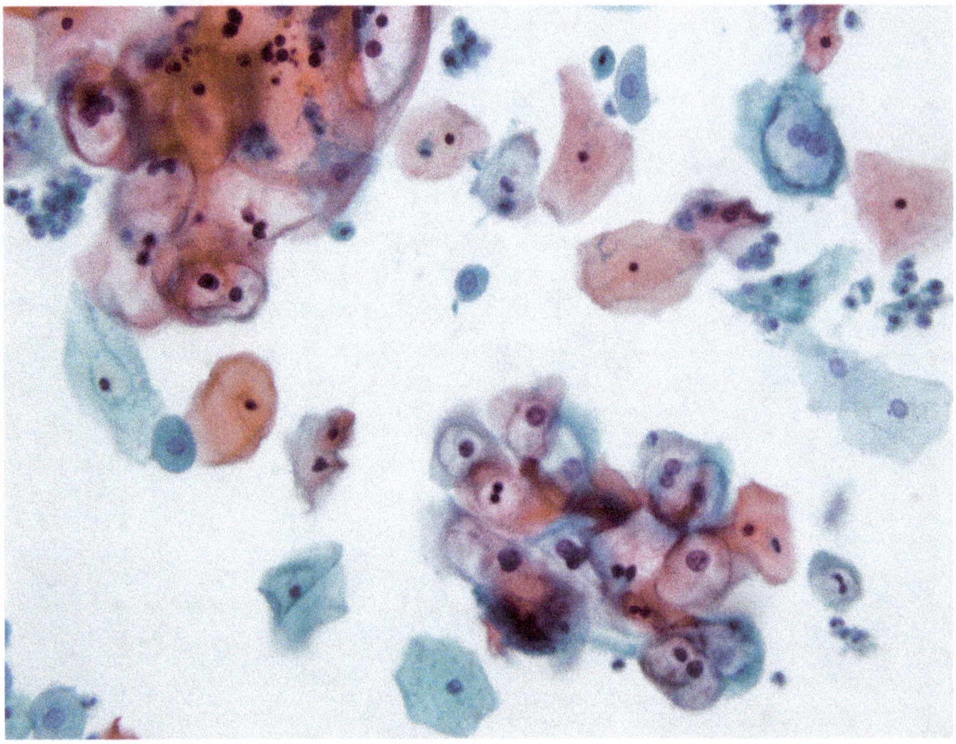

Q-86. Large numbers of cells with this appearance were seen on the ThinPrep (medium magnification) slide from a 32-year-old woman. This appearance is consistent with infection with:

(a) Herpes simplex
(b) CMV
(c) HPV
(d) HIV
(e) HBV

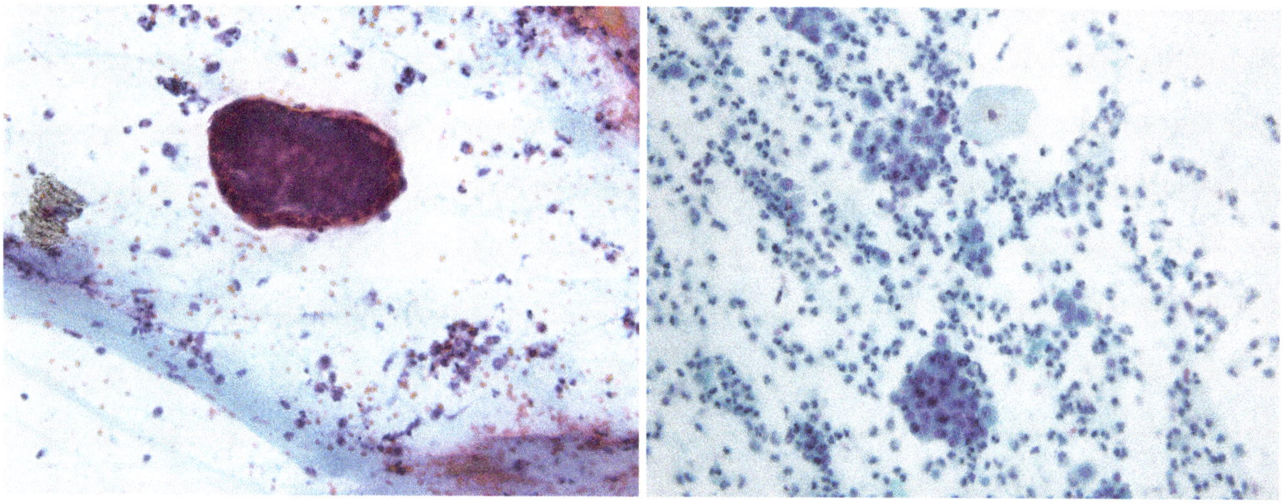

Fig. 3.87

Q-87. This slide (conventional, left and right, medium magnification) shows cells taken from a 36-year-old female. This appearance is most consistent with:

(a) Endometrial cells
(b) Endocervical cells
(c) Syncytiotrophoblasts
(d) Multinucleated histiocytes
(e) Severe chronic inflammation

Fig. 3.88

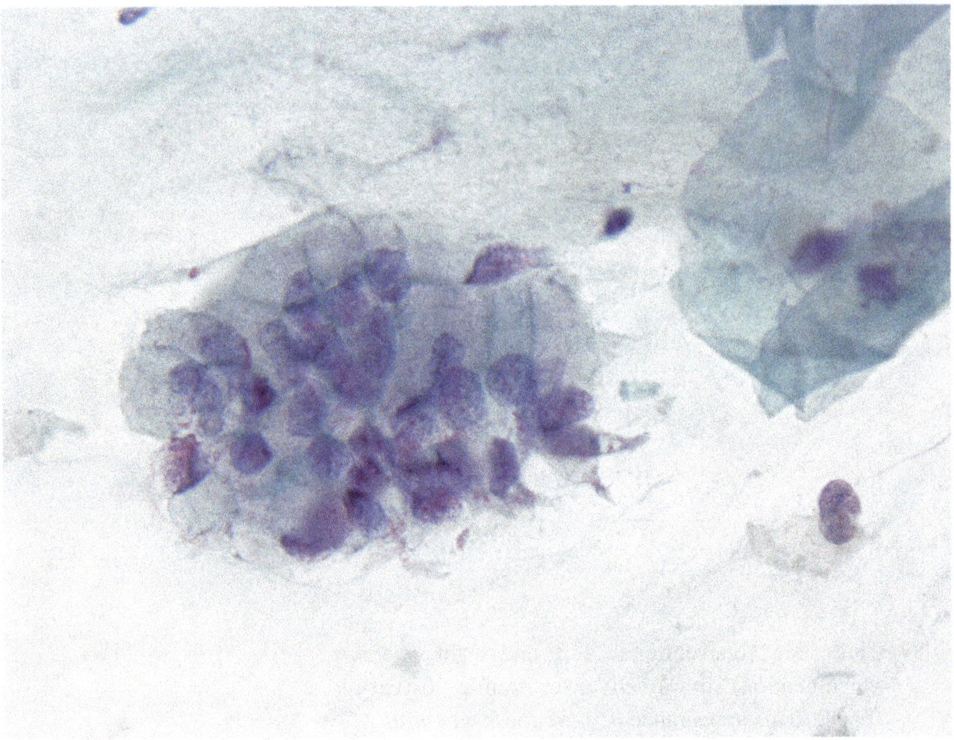

Q-88. This finding from a 29-year-old woman (ThinPrep, high magnification) is consistent with which of the following interpretations?
(a) Hemosiderin-laden macrophages
(b) LGSIL
(c) HGSIL
(d) Endocervical cells
(e) Lower uterine sampling

Fig. 3.89

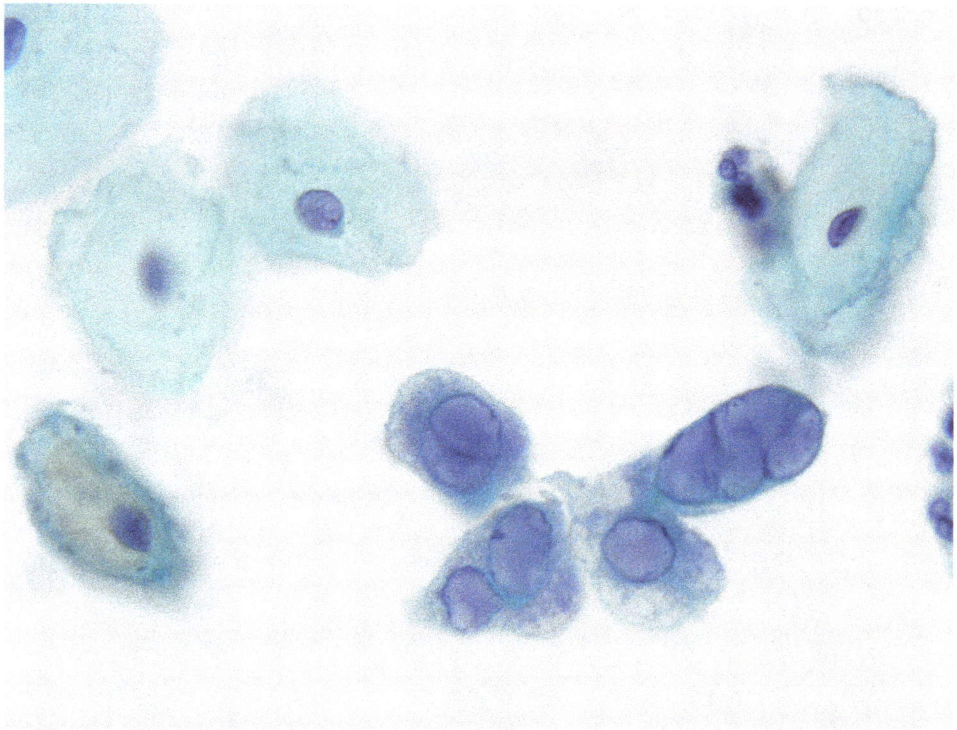

Q-89. This finding was discovered in a gynecologic sample from a 32-year-old female (ThinPrep, high magnification). It is most consistent with:

(a) CMV
(b) Herpes
(c) LGSIL
(d) HGSIL
(e) Adenovirus

Fig. 3.90

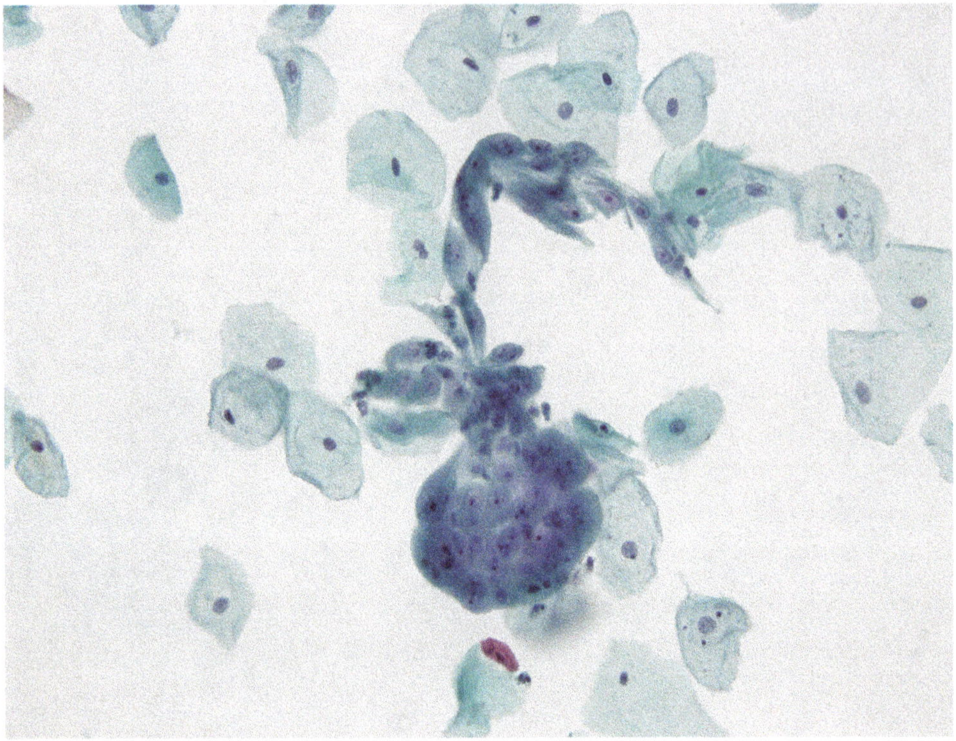

Q-90. Several groups such as this were found in the ThinPrep sample (medium magnification) from a 34-year-old woman. The most likely interpretation is that these cells represent:

(a) AGUS, endocervical origin
(b) AGUS, endometrial origin
(c) Repair
(d) LGSIL
(e) HGSIL

3.4 Answers and Discussion of Text-Based Questions 1–30

A-1. (c) **Intermediate and superficial**
In normal women of childbearing years, the usual cyclical influence of estrogen and progesterone serves to make these two cell types the most frequently found. Basal cells are seldom if ever seen in the absence of ulceration. Parabasal cells also indicate a lack of influence of estrogen and are usually only seen pre or post menopause, after delivery, and/or during lactation. Superficial and parabasal cells would seldom be seen together.

A-2. (b) **Palisading two-dimensional groups**
Endocervical cells tend to maintain either their normal side-by-side arrangement or, if viewed on end, a honeycomb arrangement. This structure may round up slightly in liquid-based preparations. Three-dimensional groups are associated with endometrial cells, ribboning is associated with repair, and syncytial groups with carcinoma in situ or invasive carcinoma.

A-3. (d) **Squamous metaplasia**
Squamous metaplasia resembles normal parabasal cells almost exactly. One can often draw a conclusion of the type of cell by examining the overall hormonal pattern of the slide. An overall low estrogenic pattern (mainly parabasal and some intermediate cells) would be present if the cells were parabasal. But occasional groups of these cells in a background of normal intermediate to superficial cells would indicate a higher estrogenic state and be more suggestive of squamous metaplasia. Hyperkeratosis is the presence of anucleated superficial squamous cells. Parakeratosis is made up of miniature superficial squamous cells. Either or both of these represent a benign protective reaction which overlies the normal epithelium to provide additional protection. Inflammatory cell changes include polychromasia, small perinuclear halos, and slight nuclear enlargement.

A-4. (b) **5–10**
Endometrial cell balls are most likely found towards the end of the menstrual cycle. These cell balls have a characteristic "double-walled" appearance.

A-5. (b) **35 μm²**
This size of the normal intermediate cell nucleus is used by the Bethesda System as a standard to gauge the degree of nuclear enlargement in abnormal conditions. Fifty square microns is the size of an average ASC-US cell nucleus, and 100 μm² is the average size of the nuclei in squamous intraepithelial lesions.

A-6. (c) **Multinucleated histiocyte**
Patients with a history of radiation therapy often have multinucleated histiocytes in their samples. They are characterized by the foamy-appearing cytoplasm and the uniform, benign appearance of the nuclei. The finely granular chromatin would not be consistent with squamous cell carcinoma. Radiation effect may have multinucleation but would not have frothy cytoplasm indicating the histiocytic nature of the cell. Herpes simplex is multinucleated but also shows molding and "ground-glass" marginated chromatin pattern.

A-7. (b) **Small orangeophilic cells with dark, pyknotic nuclei**
This pattern sometimes found in atrophy has been called pseudoparakeratosis. It consists of occasional immature parabasal cells undergoing degeneration, staining orangeophilic, and displaying a dark, degenerated nucleus. One should note the usual rounded cell shape, degenerated-looking nuclei, and occurrence in a background of atrophic cells. Vacuolization of the cytoplasm is not usually found and superficial cells would not be displayed in an atrophic slide. If the pattern were balanced between all cell types, it would not be atrophic. Finally, feathering of endocervical cells is usually a feature found in AIS of the endocervix.

A-8. (b) **Trichomonas**
The clinical findings of greenish discharge and reddened cervix (strawberry cervix) are most consistent with a diagnosis of Trichomonas. The cytologic finding of small perinuclear halos and slightly increased cytoplasmic stain is most consistent with either Trichomonas or Candida infection. Candida, however, usually produces a whitish discharge. Herpes, Aspergillus, or HPV infection would not produce this set of clinical and cytologic findings.

A-9. (a) **Leptothrix**
Leptothrix is a term often used for long filamentous bacteria, including Actinomyces or mixed lactobacilli. These long thin curving "spaghetti-like" strands are seldom found without Trichomonas, but Trichomonas may often occur by itself. Aspergillus and Entamoeba histolytica are both rare findings in Pap smears and have no relationship with Trichomonas. Candida is a common finding, but only occasionally may be found with Trichomonas.

A-10. (**d**) **Candida**
Women who are pregnant, diabetic, or on oral antibiotics may experience a change in the normal vaginal flora due to changes in the vaginal glycogen or pH. These may lead to a Candida infection which causes symptoms. Other risk factors include immunosuppression, chemotherapy, and steroids. None of the other infections is associated with this set of risk factors.

A-11. (**c**) **Staining characteristics**
Although the size and shape of Candida spores is very similar to spermatozoa, the presence of the pseudohyphae of Candida usually leads to the correct diagnosis. Occasionally, however, the hyphae may be scanty or the Candida species may be Torulopsis and not have hyphae. The classic deep blue biphasic staining of spermatozoa in which the head of the sperm has both a light area and a darker blue staining area can help differentiate in these occasional situations. The distribution on the slide would not be of assistance in differentiating between these two entities.

A-12. (**a**) **Candida**
The pseudohyphae of Candida has been shown on electron microscopy to actually pierce the epithelial cells, causing the frequent finding in which the cells are lined up along the pseudohyphae (string of pearls pattern). None of the other organisms mentioned cause this cytologic pattern.

A-13. (**c**) **IUD**
This description is consistent with Actinomyces and its presence is most closely associated with IUDs. However, it may also be noted in the presence of other foreign objects in the gyn tract, such as pessaries or tampons. Pregnancy is associated with Candida infection. Radiation does not have an association with an infectious organism. A past history of Candida infection is not associated with Actinomyces infection.

A-14. (**b**) **Herpes simplex**
Herpes simplex in the gyn tract is usually multinucleated, although some cells may only have single nuclei. However, the other changes of molding of the nuclei and margination of the chromatin are characteristic. The chromatin has a "ground-glass" appearance and there may be eosinophilic intranuclear inclusions in the nuclei. Cytomegalovirus almost always has only one nucleus and does not display molding. The intranuclear inclusion is quite large with a small halo around it giving an "owl-eye" appearance. Trichomonas does not fit the description at all, since it is a protozoon. Candida is a fungus and has pseudohyphae and small spores.

A-15. (**c**) **Cytomegalovirus**
Of the choices given, only herpes and Cytomegalovirus (CMV) have intranuclear inclusions. However, only CMV also may have cytoplasmic inclusions as well. There are no morphologic changes visible in HIV infection and HPV infection leads to large perinuclear halos and nuclear abnormalities, but has no inclusions.

A-16. (**c**) **HPV**
While infection with Candida or Trichomonas may cause an inflammatory cell change evidenced by small ill-defined perinuclear halos, these should be differentiated from the large perinuclear halos caused by HPV infection. These halos are also well defined with sharp borders and are found in conjunction with some type of nuclear abnormality such as hyperchromasia, bi- or multinucleation, enlargement of the nucleus, and smudgy chromatin. Cytomegalovirus has a very large intranuclear inclusion body with a small halo between it and the edge of the nucleus, giving an "owl-eye" appearance to the cell.

A-17. (**c**) **16**
Although HPV 16 is considered a "high-risk" subtype (and is the one most commonly found in cervical cancer), it is also the most common type found in LGSIL as well. More than 80 % of LGSIL is caused by high-risk viruses; low-risk viruses do cause warts and LGSIL, but do not go on to develop into invasive cancer. Thus, 5 and 11 are low-risk HPV subtypes but are not the most commonly found in LGSIL, and HPV 31 is a high-risk subtype, but is not as common as HPV 16.

A-18. (**b**) **Infection with HPV**
The combination of large perinuclear halos, hyperchromasia, and nuclear abnormalities is most consistent with infection with HPV. Candida or Trichomonas might cause small, ill-defined perinuclear halos, and in CMV, there is a very large intranuclear inclusion in the nucleus.

A-19. (**d**) **HPV**
HPV infection (and keratinizing dysplasias) may coexist with the findings of abnormal keratin pearls, atypical parakeratosis, and hyperkeratosis. Candida, Trichomonas, and repair do not usually elicit these keratinizing types of changes in the cells.

A-20. (**a**) **Doderlein (lactobacilli)**
Doderlein lactobacilli make up the normal flora of the vagina and help to maintain the usual slightly acidic pH by metabolizing the glycogen found in intermediate cells. The other organisms are not normally found.

A-21. (**c**) **Cytolysis**
Cytolysis occurs when the normal lactobacilli of the vagina begin to break down the intermediate cells. This results in many nuclei without their cytoplasm, cellular debris, and large numbers of the bacilli present in the smear. This occurs most often in the latter part of the menstrual cycle. Gardnerella vaginalis do not cause cytolysis, although they are associated with bacterial vaginosis. Hyperkeratosis is the presence of large numbers of anucleated squamous cells. Actinomyces is associated with IUDs and does not cause the destruction of cells.

A-22. (**b**) **Syncytial trophoblasts**
These cells derive from the placenta and may occasionally be found in one of the physiologic states associated with current or recent pregnancy. Although decidual cells are also associated with pregnancy, they are derived from cervical stroma. They do not usually have multiple nuclei and have large, reactive-looking nuclei with nucleoli. Microglandular hyperplasia is associated with oral contraceptive use and is made up of pools of small degenerated endocervical cell nuclei. Endocervical polyps would cause large groups of cells with maintained polarity and reactive-appearing nuclei. However, the cytoplasm would not be dense and the overall shape of the cluster would not be tapering.

A-23. (**a**) **Navicular cells**
Navicular cells are somewhat boat shaped (hence the name) with one end of the cell being somewhat pointed and the other rounded. They are common in the last two thirds of pregnancy. While the other choices are also associated with pregnancy, they do not fit the description given.

A-24. (**c**) **Hyperkeratosis; uterine descensus**
Prolapse of the uterus (uterine descensus) may commonly be due to failure of the round ligaments, especially after pregnancy, to suspend the uterus in its usual position. This causes irritation of the cervix and vagina where hyperkeratosis may develop as a result. While microglandular hyperplasia is associated with oral contraceptive use and Arias-Stella change is associated with pregnancy, neither of these causes white plaques that are visible on clinical exam. Candida is not associated with a history of radiation.

A-25. (**b**) **These cells may overlie a more serious lesion**
Both hyperkeratosis and parakeratosis may overlie a more serious lesion. Parakeratosis is even more significant than hyperkeratosis in this regard. Although the cells often stain orangeophilic, usually there is no confusion with a squamous cell carcinoma as the cells are small and do not have significantly enlarged nuclei. The cells are not associated with bleeding, ulceration, or the presence of an IUD.

A-26. (**c**) **Squamous metaplasia**
Hyperkeratosis contains cells without a nucleus and with transparent, thin yellow to pink cytoplasm. Parakeratosis cells are very small and polygonal and usually stain pink, yellow, or orange. Reparative cells have enlarged nuclei with nucleoli in nearly every cell and abundant streaming cytoplasm. Thus the best choice is squamous metaplasia.

A-27. (**a**) **The cells are too big for adenocarcinoma, unless there were also macronucleoli consistent with Grade 3–4 endometrial adenocarcinoma**
A is the best choice. Although an individual cell or two present in IUD effect might cause one to consider an endometrial adenocarcinoma, the surrounding cells are usually clearly benign metaplastic cells with vacuoles and occasional small nucleoli. If the slide contained endometrial adenocarcinoma, then the suspect cells are so big that the lesion would have to be high grade (3–4) which would also be accompanied by macronucleoli, a watery dirty background, and the other components of a glandular malignancy. Since those components are lacking, the suspected cells can be more confidently placed in a benign category and are assumed to be merely reactive due to the endocervical canal irritation of the placement string of the IUD. The macronucleoli and powdery chromatin description is more consistent with endometrial adenocarcinoma, as is the watery tumor diathesis. The palisading two-dimensional arrangement is most consistent with an endocervical adenocarcinoma.

A-28. (**a**) **IUD effect**
This description is consistent with "IUD cells" which, unlike neoplastic cells, occur singly and fairly rarely and are not accompanied by the usual spectrum of dysplasia. While individually these cells might mimic the cells of CIN 3, they lack the usual deeply notched

and folded hyperchromatic nuclei and they do not occur in syncytia. They are thought to be single atypical endometrial cells. CIS would have many more cells, have the usual nuclear abnormalities, and occur in syncytial groups. Repair would have large amounts of streaming cytoplasm and nucleoli. Decidual cells are associated with pregnancy (this patient delivered over a year ago) and would be much larger than the IUD cells.

A-29. (**d**) **Repair**
Microglandular hyperplasia consists of degenerated endocervical cells which are small and often occur in pools surrounded by other endocervical cells. Tubal metaplasia is frequently seen due to the widespread use of the endocervical brush which can sample higher in the endocervical canal than previously. These cells are endocervical and often ciliated and occur as crowded, hyperchromatic sheets. Nonkeratinizing squamous cell carcinoma would have hyperchromatic irregular chromatin and a syncytial or isolated arrangement. The best choice is repair.

A-30. (**c**) **Inflammatory cell changes**
These types of changes are often seen in conjunction with infection by Candida or Trichomonas but may also be found in the presence of inflammatory cells without infectious agents. Repair has nucleoli and no polychromasia. HGSIL would have hyperchromatic nuclei and no halos. HPV would have large, well-defined halos with nuclear abnormalities.

3.5 Answers and Discussion of Image-Based Questions 31–90

A-31. (**a**) **Repair**
These cells show enlarged hypochromatic nuclei with prominent nucleoli in almost every cell. Also note the cohesive nature of this sheet of cells. These are features of classic repair found in a gynecologic sample. Squamous metaplasia is not a consideration due to the prominent nucleoli in most cells. The cells are neither hyperchromatic nor a loose group nor syncytial which would be expected in squamous cell carcinoma. Hyperkeratosis is made up of anucleated squamous cells and these cells have their nuclei. These cells are squamous in origin and not endocervical.

A-32. (**c**) **Chronic follicular cervicitis**
These are groups of somewhat variably sized lymphocytes, caught up in a matrix of proteinaceous debris. The population of cells seems to be reactive rather than neoplastic and there is a tingible body macrophage (lower end of group, right). This is consistent with chronic follicular cervicitis. Acute inflammation would be made up of neutrophils, not lymphs. These cells do not have endocervical morphology. Their nuclei are smaller than those of the intermediate cells. Although they are lymphoid in origin, they are not malignant, lacking nucleoli, pleomorphism, and nuclear protrusions. Finally, these cells are not consistent with small cell carcinoma of the cervix, which would have a greater variation in size, and would be unlikely to have tingible body macrophages accompanying them.

A-33. (**b**) **Herpes**
These multinucleated cells are displaying the classic signs of herpes: molding of the nuclei, margination of the chromatin, and multinucleation. Repair does not have multinucleation as displayed here or the "ground-glass" nuclei. CMV can have "viral"-looking nuclei, but is almost always seen with only a single nucleus and a very large nuclear inclusion. These can also have cytoplasmic inclusions in a minority of cases. Although the N:C ratio might suggest a HGSIL, the nuclei are not coarsely granular but are smudgy and consistent with viral infection. Finally, adenovirus usually affects with columnar cells of the endocervix and displays perinuclear halos, which are not seen in these cells.

A-34. (**b**) **Second trimester pregnancy**
A woman who contracts herpes during her pregnancy is at risk to deliver an infant with several serious problems which can even include death from viral encephalitis or brain damage. As a precaution, these women are often advised to deliver by C-section, avoiding possible transmission to the infant during delivery. A previous history of HGSIL, postmenopausal status, day 6 of a normal menstrual cycle, or history of IUD placement would not be as clinically important as pregnancy with this diagnosis.

A-35. (**d**) **IUD wearer**
The cells on the left are vacuolated metaplastic cells, consistent with IUD effect. The image on the right is consistent with Actinomyces, which can be found in women wearing an IUD or any other foreign device, such as a forgotten diaphragm or a pessary. Although radiation may cause vacuolization, Actinomyces is not associated with it. There are no perinuclear halos consistent with adenovirus infection. The cells lack the nucleoli and the cytoplasmic streaming associated with repair. Also, they do not display the multinucleation, margination, and molding of the nuclei consistent with herpes.

A-36. (**b**) **Pregnancy**
These images are consistent with the morphology of Candida: eosinophilic pseudohyphae with oval-shaped budding. Risk factors for Candida include pregnancy, use of antibiotics, and diabetes. None of the other choices are a risk factor for Candida.

A-37. (**e**) **Days 22–28**
The last days of the menstrual cycle (days 22–28) are the most likely to reveal this pattern of cytolysis in which the normal lactobacilli digest the glycogen present in the generally intermediate cell pattern. This causes lysis of the cells, release of naked nuclei, and the presence of cellular debris in the background. These three features are seen in these images.

A-38. (**e**) **Trapping of air under the coverslip**
This brownish granular appearance on the surface of the cells is known as "cornflake artifact" and is caused by allowing the film of xylene on the surface of the slide to evaporate prior to applying the mounting media and the coverslip. This allows air to be trapped between the top surface of the cells and the coverslip, resulting in this artifact. Rapid application of the mounting media and the coverslip, and coverslipping the slides one by one as they are removed from the xylene (rather than trying to remove several slides at a time and "batch" them), will help to avoid this artifact. The other choices are all pigments rather than trapped air and would be distributed in the cytoplasm, rather than just appearing centrally in the cell.

A-39. **(d) Granuloma inguinale**

The image on the left is consistent with a granuloma, with palisading epithelioid histiocytes and chronic inflammatory cells. The presence of the small, closed safety pin organisms within histiocytes on the right is consistent with Donovan bodies. These organisms (Klebsiella granulomatis) are the causative agent of granuloma inguinale, a sexually transmitted disease that leads to ulcerative nodules. The closed safety pin appearance is best seen with air-dried or formalin-fixed material. Tuberculosis and sarcoidosis may both have granulomas; however, mycobacteria are small and very difficult to identify without special stains for TB, and there is no identifiable causative agent for sarcoidosis. Chlamydia is too difficult to reliably identify on gynecologic material without ancillary testing and it does not cause granulomas. Coccidioides immitis would have the typical "marbles in a bag" appearance of organisms within the double-walled outer structure.

A-40. **(e) Repair**

These images are most consistent with a reparative process having prominent nucleoli in most cells, a cohesive "streaming" cellular pattern, and a finely granular chromatin pattern. LGSIL would tend to have more hyperchromatic chromatin and show either an increased N:C ratio or large perinuclear halos as are found in HPV infection. HGSIL would have even more hyperchromasia and significant increase in N:C ratio. Additionally, in cases consistent with a biopsy diagnosis of CIS, a "salt and pepper" coarse chromatin pattern may be present and there may be syncytial groups in evidence in the cytology. Squamous cell carcinoma would additionally have a tumor diathesis of blood, fibrin, and cellular necrosis. Choriocarcinoma would show evidence of multinucleation, as well as other features of malignancy such as necrosis, macronucleoli, and coarse chromatin pattern.

A-41. **(d) Repeat Pap in 1 year**

These images are consistent with a diagnosis of chronic follicular cervicitis in a ThinPrep slide. Note the lymphocytes of various degrees of maturity. Often in liquid-based preparations, the lymphocytes seem to be caught up in a proteinaceous matrix. Tingible body macrophages may be seen as well but they are not a necessary component for the diagnosis. This condition may be found at any time but it often occurs in postmenopausal women, due to decreased protection of the epithelium because of the onset of atrophy. Other than being an indication of a chronic inflammatory process, this diagnosis does not require any special follow-up other than a routine Pap. Thus, the Pap should be repeated in 1 year. The other follow-up recommendations are too extensive for this diagnosis. One key to this diagnosis is in recognizing that the small dark cells are of lymphoid origin and are not HGSIL, small cell carcinoma of the cervix, or other neoplastic entities.

A-42. **(e) Herpes**

These images show the multinucleation, margination of the chromatin, and molding of adjacent nuclei that are characteristic of infection with herpes simplex. The image on the right also shows eosinophilic inclusions in the nucleus. These intranuclear inclusions are also present on the left, but are not as distinctly seen. The molding of the nuclei as well as the multinucleation and ground-glass nuclei excludes all of the other choices from consideration.

A-43. **(d) Blood**

It is important to be able to recognize the broken-down blood which often shows on liquid-based preparations as pinkish granular material. The Doderlein bacilli which are normal inhabitants of the gynecologic sample are lactobacilli and would seldom appear as granular debris. Gardnerella and coccobacilli would also display as distinct shapes, rather than granular, ill-defined material. Candida spores also would be distinct oval shapes unlike the material seen on this sample.

A-44. **(c) Trichomonas**

The small, ill-defined perinuclear halo is most consistent with infection by either Candida or Trichomonas. The Trichomonas organisms can be seen in several places in the image, including just underneath the cell with the arrow. HPV has much larger, well-defined halos. Although Candida can also cause a similar-appearing perinuclear halo, there are no Candida organisms present in the image. Nonspecific inflammatory cell changes can also produce a perinuclear halo, but there are no accompanying neutrophils. Herpes does not usually produce this change.

A-45. **(d) Degenerated parabasal cell**

Occasional eosinophilic cells may be present in atrophic slides. The cells are usually small and rounded with dense cytoplasm and they represent degenerated parabasal cells. These should be distinguished from parakeratotic cells (which have thinner cytoplasm, orangeophilia, and a polygonal shape). Hyperkeratotic cells are normal in size and orange to yellow, have thin transparent cytoplasm, and lack a nucleus.

Although dyskeratotic cells of HPV might resemble this cell, in DK the nucleus is larger and appears smudgy, and the N:C ratio is larger than is seen here. LGSIL would also have an increased N:C ratio higher than the cell seen here.

A-46. (**d**) **Candida**

These strands are uniform in size, are parallel, and have areas of fainter staining alongside areas where the stain is of a more usual uniformity. They seem to protrude out from the cell cluster. These are features consistent with a diagnosis of Candida. Actinomyces is not a fungus but a higher-order bacterium. It is associated with colonies of coccobacilli out of which a "starburst" arrangement of the organisms can be seen. It is usually associated with IUD use or the presence of other "foreign" objects such as pessaries, forgotten tampons, or diaphragms. Mucin strands can be differentiated from Candida in that they are not uniformly parallel and they vary in width as well. IUD effect is most often associated with the presence of highly vacuolated metaplastic cells in small clusters. These cells from the endocervix are reactive and thought to exhibit these characteristics due to the presence of the endocervical string which is used to verify placement of the IUD. The cells often are clustered with other more normal-looking metaplastic cells, and this can help to distinguish them from neoplastic cells. Leptothrix is almost always present only with Trichomonas vaginalis, and trichomonads are not seen. Also, Leptothrix has a tendency to have looping or curving long tendrils, whereas the pseudohyphae of Candida are straighter and they are broader in width as well.

A-47. (**e**) **64-year-old postmenopausal woman, no hormone use**

This slide is showing a typical hormonal pattern of atrophy, which would be most consistent with a 64-year-old woman who is not taking hormone replacement therapy. The group of small cells in the center is most likely endocervical in origin, due to their honeycomb pattern. The other squamous cells are consistent with mostly parabasal and lower intermediate cells, and no cells suggestive of superficial cells are seen, indicating a relative lack of estrogen. Choice "a," day 2, would likely show a bloody background, endometrial cells, and cellular debris associated with menses. Choice "b," day 13, would likely show the effects of a high estrogen level and would be composed of a much higher proportion of superficial cells, with no parabasal cells. Choice "c," day 28, would show mostly intermediate cells, and there may be evidence of cytolysis: cell debris, Doderlein bacilli, and naked nuclei. Choice "d," second trimester, normal pregnancy, would most likely be made up of almost 100 % intermediate cells, since the cell pattern during pregnancy is mainly influenced by progesterone. Only the sample of a postmenopausal woman would provide the atrophic cell pattern seen here. Other causes of atrophy during childbearing years include postpartum, death of the fetus in utero, and surgical castration without hormone replacement.

A-48. (**c**) **Radiation effect**

Many of the cells in the lower power image are greatly enlarged when compared to the normal cells in the field. Additionally, (lower power image and inset) there is a great deal of cytoplasmic vacuolization present in some of these cells as well as bizarre shapes and elongated cytoplasm. Although the nuclei are somewhat enlarged, there is not a marked increase in the N:C ratio. The background appears clean. These are all features of radiation effect. Repair would not usually display the vacuolization and cytomegaly present. Also, repair usually has macronucleoli which are not evident in this image. Squamous cell carcinoma, recurrent, is not displayed in this image. A recurrent carcinoma would have cells with hyperchromasia, coarse chromatin, nucleoli, and increased N:C ratio and would present in a background of tumor diathesis. Cytomegaly and vacuolization are not characteristic for recurrent squamous cell carcinoma. Mixed Müllerian tumor and endometrial adenocarcinoma are very unlikely in a woman who has had a hysterectomy and no history of these tumors previously. Also, features of malignancy (prominent nucleoli, tumor diathesis, etc.) are not present in this sample.

A-49. (**b**) **Endocervical cells**

These endocervical cells are displaying themselves in a typical palisading arrangement (picket fence), although they appear to be in a somewhat unusual 3-D arrangement, perhaps due to an endocervical polyp. But the cells are clearly elongated with eccentric nuclei typical for normal endocervical cells. There is no apparent nuclear or cytoplasmic pleomorphism and the background of the slide appears quite clean. This is most consistent with an interpretation of normal endocervical cells. Endometrial cells are more cuboidal than tall columnar. Additionally, they occur either as pools of single cells, as double-walled endometrial cell balls in exodus (days 4–10), or in 3-D arrangements. Although colonic adenocarcinoma may occur as tall columnar cells, these cells lack the nucleoli, the nuclear pleomorphism, and the distorted architecture that metastatic adenocarcinoma may have.

Metastatic extrauterine adenocarcinomas usually have a clean background on cytology and relatively few abnormal cells, but the exception is a direct invasion of a colonic adenocarcinoma to the vagina or cervix. In the case of direct extension, the background may be quite bloody and dirty, the carcinoma may appear as tall columnar cells, and there may be large numbers of carcinoma cells present. These factors may cause a differential diagnostic problem with endocervical adenocarcinoma. Fibroblasts would not be as cohesive as these cells. Although a granuloma is composed of epithelioid histiocytes which may show evidence of palisading around the outer edge of the group, the cells depicted in the image are too cohesive and exhibit eccentric nuclei, more typical of normal endocervical cells. Additionally, there is no evidence of chronic inflammation (multinucleated histiocytes, lymphs, etc.) seen.

A-50. (**a**) **Vaginal pessary use**

These images are consistent with an interpretation of Actinomyces, a higher-order bacterium that is often associated with IUD use. Additionally, other "foreign" devices such as a pessary, forgotten tampon, or diaphragm have also been associated with this finding. Note the radiating "starburst" appearance of the thin organisms. The background may show a number of neutrophils, as seen on the right. None of the other choices, condom use, oral contraception, coexisting HPV infection, and radiation therapy, have been associated with Actinomyces.

A-51. (**d**) **Ova of Enterobius vermicularis**

This finding is consistent with an interpretation of an ovum from the pinworm, Enterobius vermicularis. Distinguishing features of this ovum include a large oval size (about 55–25 μm), a double-walled appearance, and a flattening of one end of the ovum so that it does not resemble a perfect oval. These usually stain deep pink to red, with a darker area in the central area where the embryonic worm is located. Psammoma bodies are also reddish but are usually more round, have a concentric appearance, and will sometimes appear "cracked," as if one pushed down on a hard-shelled round candy and the outer shell cracked open. Cholesterol crystals are typically rectangular in shape. Vegetable contaminants have a variety of appearances but the flattened oval is specific for pinworm ova. Suture material can sometimes be found in gynecologic samples either postpartum or after gynecologic surgery. It appears as rectangular shapes of variable lengths but a uniform width. Pinworm ova as well as vegetable contaminants are most often found as GI contamination due to poor hygiene. However, rarely pinworm ova might be due to a true gynecologic infection.

A-52. (**c**) **Leptothrix and Trichomonas**

The image on the left represents the curving, looping forms consistent with Leptothrix, and the organisms on the right and in the inset are consistent with Trichomonas vaginalis. Leptothrix is almost always found with Trichomonas but Trichomonas can often be found without Leptothrix. If Leptothrix is identified, one should then search for the Trichomonas which does need to be treated. Candida is thicker than Leptothrix, which rules out "a" as a choice. The strands of Actinomyces are quite slender and are usually found in a "starburst" arrangement. Also, they do not curve as Leptothrix usually does. Aspergillus is much thicker than Leptothrix branches at a 45° angle. Giardia lamblia is normally found in the GI system and is caught by drinking contaminated water. Although it is a flagellated parasite, it does not coexist with Leptothrix, as does Trichomonas. Giardia also does not inhabit the gynecologic system. Thus, the best answer is c.

A-53. (**b**) **Shift in vaginal flora suggestive of bacterial vaginosis**

The Bethesda System 2001 uses the above terminology for describing the pattern previously described as "clue cells." In this condition, the normal bacterial flora of the gynecologic sample is altered from the usual Doderlein bacilli to a proliferation of coccobacilli, which often coat the squamous cells and give rise to this appearance. While this appearance was previously often associated with Gardnerella vaginalis, now the diagnostic terminology is more general and covers both cocci and bacilli. As noted the specific diagnosis of Gardnerella is no longer used in TBS, so choice a is eliminated. Choice c is also not used in TBS. The appearance of these clue cells is not consistent with Doderlein bacilli or with Actinomyces.

A-54. (**a**) **Normal endometrial cells during exodus**

These cells are showing the typical "double-walled" appearance of endometrial cells as they appear in large cell balls during days 5–10 of the menstrual cycle. This time period, termed "exodus," shows both epithelial and stromal endometrial cells commonly. Endocervical cells occur in a two-dimensional group with honeycomb or picket fence arrangements, rather than the three-dimensional arrangements seen here. These cells are in a ball; however a close inspection reveals that they are too large for neutrophils or other elements of inflammation. Finally, although HGSIL cells might be this small with a high N:C ratio, the cells are more glandular in appearance, without the dark clumpy chromatin typical of HGSIL. The typical cell ball arrangement and the young age of the patient also exclude an endometrial adenocarcinoma from serious consideration.

A-55. (**b**) **Dome-shaped nodules with umbilicated margins**
This slide displays the typical appearance of molluscum contagiosum. These cells show large eosinophilic inclusions in the cells. The dermatologic symptoms include numerous raised lesions which have raised outer edges and a central depression. This disease is highly contagious and can occur in children. Postcoital bleeding, widespread reddish rash, and draining groin lymph nodes are not symptoms of this disease.

A-56. (**b**) **Donovan bodies**
These small safety pin-shaped organisms are ingested into the macrophages. The "safety pin" appearance is more easily seen in Giemsa-stained material. These organisms, *Klebsiella granulomatis*, are the causative agent of granuloma inguinale, also known as donovanosis. The organisms are also known as Donovan bodies. Schaumann bodies are calcified bodies within multinucleated giant cells, most often associated with sarcoidosis; Histoplasma capsulatum might be confused with the Donovan bodies as they both are seen within macrophages, but Donovan bodies have the unique closed safety pin appearance. Torulopsis is larger than these organisms and is more reminiscent of the size and shape of spores of *Candida albicans*. *Coccidioides immitis* usually is found within an outer structure, giving a "bag of marbles" appearance.

A-57. (**a**) **Cytolysis**
Cytolysis is a common feature of slides obtained during the latter part of the menstrual cycle, days 25–28. Superficial cells, which are more resistant to the lysing action of the Doderlein bacilli than intermediate cells, are seldom seen this late in the cycle. The intermediate cells tend to lyse, releasing naked nuclei and cytoplasmic debris into a background of abundant Doderlein bacilli. Tumor diathesis contains cytoplasmic debris as well as old and new blood and fibrin. Additionally, of course, there will also be malignant cells present. Shift in vaginal flora will not have Doderlein bacilli, the normal bacteria present in the gynecologic tract. Degenerative changes consistent with atrophy would not show these naked nuclei, abundant Doderlein bacilli, and cytoplasmic debris.

A-58 (**d**) **Chronic follicular cervicitis**
These images show cells consistent with a diagnosis of chronic follicular cervicitis, a condition which is more common in women with long-standing inflammatory conditions, such as in atrophic, postmenopausal women. In this condition, a "pool" of lymphocytes of all ranges of maturation is seen. Sometimes, tingible body macrophages with ingested nuclear debris from lymphocytes are also seen (right image). On liquid-based slides, the lymphs are often found within a matrix of proteinaceous material (left image). Although not terribly significant in terms of patient treatment, it is important to be able to differentiate this condition from other more serious conditions. Neutrophils are not a significant feature of these images so acute inflammation is not a good choice. Although some of the lymphocytes are immature, most are more mature and do not show clefting, nucleoli, or other features of lymphoma. ALL is also not a consideration, for these same reasons. Finally, small cell carcinoma of the cervix would show cells which are molding and which display significant nuclear abnormalities in small cells of neuroendocrine or squamous origin.

A-59. (**b**) **Schistosoma haematobium**
These images display several ova consistent with Schistosoma haematobium as well as an actual miracidium. These ova are approximately 150 μm by 50 μm and have a uniformly shaped oval structure which tapers to a point on one end. These ova are from flukes which utilize freshwater snails as a vector. The free-swimming organisms may penetrate the skin after swimming or bathing in infected water. The common location for ova to be found is in the bladder, where constant inflammation due to the ova is associated with squamous cell carcinoma of the bladder. Enterobius vermicularis, the pinworm ova, is a much more frequent finding due to cross contamination from the GI tract, where these parasites usually reside. Its ova can be distinguished as they are not uniformly oval, but have one flattened end. These structures are quite uniform in size and shape and do not contain nuclei, as would vegetable cells. Lubricant artifact also might be a differential, especially if it contained plant cells which simulated the ova. However, the miracidium is conclusive for Schistosoma infection.

A-60. (**b**) **Endocervical cells**
These cells in this honeycomb-type arrangement are consistent with endocervical cells. Note the uniformity of the size and shape of the cells and the columnar appearance at the edge of the group in the upper

edge of the image. These cells are too small for squamous metaplastic cells, which are somewhat more polygonal and have more abundant cytoplasm. Endometrial cells would have less cytoplasm and would tend to occur in three-dimensional groups, such as cell balls. HGSIL cells would be much less uniform, have squamous-appearing cytoplasm, and have darker coarser chromatin. They would also tend to occur with dysplastic cells and not be found in this regular honeycomb pattern.

A-61. (**c**) **Leptothrix**
This image shows a "ball" of Trichomonas organisms. They show the eccentric nucleus and ill-defined cytoplasm of these organisms. Flagella are usually lost in processing but can occasionally be seen. Leptothrix vaginalis is a Gram-positive anaerobic bacterium that is almost always found with Trichomonas vaginalis. The finding of Leptothrix should institute a thorough search for Trichomonas. HPV changes, adenovirus, molluscum contagiosum, and Actinomyces are not associated with Trichomonas vaginalis.

A-62. (**d**) **Leptothrix**
The curving structures in the image are consistent with Leptothrix. These organisms are usually associated with Trichomonas, although Trichomonas often occurs in the absence of Leptothrix. These Gram-positive anaerobic bacteria are usually rather long and can curve without breaking, unlike Actinomyces and Doderlein bacilli which are usually much shorter and do not curve. The flagella from Trichomonas are seldom seen and, in any case, are much shorter than the organisms seen here. Aspergillus is a thicker fungus with septate hyphae which branches at a 45° angle.

A-63. (**b**) **Thick white discharge with pruritus**
This image shows Candida hyphae as pinkish staining pseudohyphae with small oval-shaped spore forms. Infection with Candida is frequent in pregnant patients, in patients on antibiotic therapy, or in diabetic patients. Symptoms due to Candida include irritation and pruritus and a thick white vaginal discharge. A watery discharge with a "fishy" odor is most commonly associated with bacterial vaginitis due to Gardnerella vaginalis. Abnormal bleeding and cramping is more often associated with miscarriage or other intrauterine abnormalities. A greenish discharge with skin irritation is associated with Trichomonas infection.

A-64. (**a**) **Actinomyces**
These images illustrate the appearance of Actinomyces in a gynecologic sample. The organisms are associated with the use of an IUD or other foreign device such as a pessary. They occur as starburst-shaped rods emerging from a colony of associated coccobacilli. The structures often appear almost "fuzzy" looking. Often there is an accompanying inflammatory exudate with this finding. Aspergillus is a fungal organism and several times wider than the thin bacteria of Actinomyces. While Actinomyces often occurs in the presence of an IUD, the finding of "IUD effect" is reserved for cases in which there is cytoplasmic vacuolization and a reactive appearance to the metaplastic cells of the endocervical canal, probably due to irritation by the IUD string. Trichomonas and Leptothrix are not identified on this sample. Cytolysis is the physiologic lysing of intermediate cell cytoplasm due to the action of Doderlein bacilli. It is recognized by cell debris, naked nuclei, and abundant short Doderlein bacilli in the background of the slide.

A-65. (**e**) **Shift in vaginal flora suggestive of bacterial vaginosis**
This image shows many coccobacilli coating the surfaces of the squamous cells. These cells are sometimes referred to as "clue cells." In the most recent Bethesda System terminology, the term "shift in vaginal flora…" indicates that the bacteria encountered on the slide are not the normal Doderlein bacilli and that this finding suggests bacterial vaginosis. Trichomonas are not identified on the slide. Doderlein bacilli do not usually coat the squamous cells and coccoid forms are not seen. Actinomyces are found in colonies with accompanying bacteria and they show a starburst appearance. Finally, Candida species are fungi, not bacteria, and are thus wider than the organisms seen here.

A-66. (**c**) **Hyperkeratosis**
The finding of a number of plaques or abundant single cells without nuclei is consistent with a diagnosis of hyperkeratosis. This finding can overlie an abnormality such as LGSIL or HGSIL, especially if the lesion is keratinized. The cells are usually pink to orange staining and often show a "ghost" nucleus, a pale area where the nucleus previously was located. Although hyperkeratosis might coexist with HPV, it is not a diagnostic feature to look for. HPV changes usually show a clear large perinuclear halo and some abnormality in the nucleus (hyperchromasia, smudginess, multinucleation, increase in N:C ratio). LGSIL also would include the diagnostic features of HPV as well

as any cells which had an N:C ratio of at least one-third the diameter of the cell. Parakeratosis is another benign proliferative change, as is hyperkeratosis. In parakeratosis the abnormal cells appear similar to superficial squamous cells, but are much smaller in overall size. PK cells are about one-tenth the size of normal squamous cells and they have a small, pyknotic nucleus.

A-67. (**c**) **Days 12–16**
The image shows almost all of the squamous cells to be superficial cells. This is most highly correlated with a very high level of estrogen in the patient. The highest level of estrogen occurs about days 12–16 in the menstrual cycle, peaking just prior to ovulation. The other days of the cycle would have a different appearance. Days 0–5 would be during or just after menstruation and the slide would be bloody, have endometrial cell balls present, and have more intermediate cells and fewer superficial ones. Days 6–11 would coincide with the proliferative phase of the cycle in which the newly shed endometrium is built back up to a proper thickness for implantation after ovulation. Days 17–21 are postovulatory as the estrogen level falls and progesterone levels increase. This is associated with a decline in the number of superficial cells and a relative increase in the number of intermediate cells. During days 22–28, the progesterone levels are high and the pattern is mostly intermediate with cytolysis often occurring in the background. Thus, an estimate of days 12–16 is the best answer. However, it should be noted that hormonal levels vary between women and various patterns may be seen as a number of factors affect these average trends.

A-68. (**d**) **Polymorphonuclear leukocytes**
These inflammatory cells are mainly polymorphonuclear leukocytes, the most common type of inflammatory cell seen in gynecologic samples. In fact, it is rare that a few of these "polys" do not appear in the slide. If they are very numerous, they may interfere with optimally viewing the slide and the diagnosis may change to "unsatisfactory for evaluation due to obscuring inflammation." Lymphocytes are small and round and have very little cytoplasm. This contrasts with the three to four lobes seen in the polys. Plasma cells usually have a round, eccentrically placed nucleus with a markedly coarse chromatin pattern. Histiocytes are larger with abundant frothy cytoplasm and bean-shaped nuclei. Eosinophils are associated with allergic responses or parasitic infections. They have two nuclei in cytoplasm with eosinophilic granules.

A-69. (**b**) **Mucin**
These cells are endocervical cells, tall columnar cells which produce mucin for the endocervix. The yellowish material seen at one end of the cell is ready to be expelled into endocervical canal. Glycogen is produced by squamous cells at certain times but not mucin. Lipofuscin is a "wear and tear" pigment that is occasionally found, but not usually in a gynecologic sample. It is not usually this color. Melanin is usually not found on normal Pap smears, but if present, it appears as golden yellow to brown pigment in the cytoplasm of the melanocytes. Hemosiderin may sometimes become ingested into the cytoplasm of histiocytes if bleeding is taking place. However, the only material that is consistent with the type of cells and the setting is mucin.

A-70. (**d**) **Hyperkeratosis**
These orangeophilic cells have lost their nucleus, and with the information that many of these were seen in the sample, an interpretation of hyperkeratosis can be made. One can note the pale central area where the nucleus was previously located. This is sometimes referred to as a "ghost" nucleus. Hyperkeratosis is a benign proliferative change and can be found in a number of situations such as coexisting LGSIL or HGSIL, uterine descensus, or post hysterectomy. Due to the lack of nuclei in a number of cells, the diagnosis of hyperkeratosis (HK) is appropriate. If, however, the cells were rare, anucleated squamous cells on a slide might represent contamination from the handling of the slide (fingertip cells). Squamous metaplasia would have denser, more immature cytoplasm and the cells would have nuclei. Inflammatory cell changes may have a faint, ill-defined halo near the nucleus, but the nucleus is maintained, unlike this case. Finally, pseudoparakeratosis (also known as microglandular hyperplasia) is made up of degenerated endocervical columnar cells which are quite small, have lost their columnar appearance, stain orange, and show small, dark degenerated nuclei. These cells in the image do not have nuclei and they are too big and polygonal to suggest pseudoparakeratosis.

A-71. (**c**) **Atrophy**
Most of the normal-appearing blue cells in this image are parabasal cells, reflective of the lack of estrogen normally present in a postmenopausal woman. The small rounded orange cells with dense cytoplasm are commonly found in atrophic slides. They are thought to be degenerated immature forms of parabasal cells. Squamous metaplasia would have

a different N:C ratio than these cells and would usually stain blue, indicative of the immaturity of its cytoplasm. Although parakeratosis (PK) is the primary differential for these cells, PK has smaller, more condensed pyknotic nuclei and a thinner more transparent polygonal cytoplasm. They have been described as miniature superficial cells and that is an apt description. A keratinizing LGSIL would show the typical perinuclear halo consistent with HPV infection and/or cells with hyperchromatic nuclei and orange staining cytoplasm and an increase in N:C ratio. These features are not present in this image.

A-72. (**d**) **Radiation effect**

The atypical cells in this image have enlarged, multiple nuclei and vacuolated cytoplasm and, despite being larger than the normal cells in the image, have a more or less normal N:C ratio. These features are characteristic of radiation effect, which can be seen in samples many years after radiation therapy is completed. Repair would have prominent nucleoli, pale chromatin, and streaming cytoplasm. It does not usually have the multinucleation and cytoplasmic vacuolization noted here. Recurrent SCCA would have hyperchromatic enlarged nuclei with an increased N:C ratio and nucleoli. The cells are much too large in comparison to the normal cells in the background and cannot be classified as normal cells. Finally, the atypical cells seem to be squamous in origin and display polygonal, sharply defined cytoplasm, rather than the columnar, vacuolated cytoplasm of endocervical cells.

A-73. (**a**) **Squamous metaplasia**

The smaller rounded cells in this image are consistent with squamous metaplasia. This is one of the most common benign proliferative changes seen in gynecologic samples. Morphologically they cannot be distinguished from parabasal cells, but using the patient's age, expected level of hormone production, and the occurrence of the cells on the slide can usually help to distinguish between them. True parabasal cells are reflective of a reduced hormonal status, and if that is the case, the cells are evenly distributed over the slide. If the cells are squamous metaplasia, however, most of the slide is normal intermediate and superficial cells and occasional areas contain squamous metaplasia, as seen in this image. Atrophy therefore is not a good choice for this patient as the age and occurrence of the cells does not fit. Inflammatory cell changes would include polychromasia, small ill-defined perinuclear halos, and inflammation in the background. LGSIL would have cells of normal size but with larger, more hyperchromatic nuclei and with an increase N:C ratio. Navicular cells are boat-shaped intermediate cells with glycogen found in pregnant patients. Thus, the best answer is a.

A-74. (**e**) **Repair**

This image shows cells with nucleoli, streaming cytoplasm, and a cohesive arrangement. Additionally, the nuclei are hypochromatic with finely granular chromatin. These are features which best describe repair. Endocervical adenocarcinoma would have larger nucleoli and coarser chromatin and would occur in glandular groupings with tall columnar cells. Endometrial adenocarcinoma is usually a three-dimensional group with enlargement of the nuclei, nucleoli, and powdery chromatin. AIS of the endocervix would have cytoplasmic feathering, elongated nuclei with coarse chromatin, but usually rare nucleoli, unlike the frequent nucleoli present here. HGSIL should display cells with hyperchromatic enlarged nuclei, coarse chromatin, and increased N:C ratio. Thus, the best choice is repair.

A-75. (**a**) **Chronic follicular cervicitis**

This image shows a variety of mature and immature lymphocytes caught up in proteinaceous debris. This appearance in liquid-based preparations is common, contrasting with the "pool" of a single population of lymphs as is seen on conventional slides. Note the slight irregularities in the nuclear size and shape, indicating the presence of both mature and immature lymphs. Trichomonas may form balls of organisms but will not stain this dark purple color and instead will stain gray to lavender with an eccentric ill-defined nucleus. Small cell carcinoma of the cervix would have larger cells with hyperchromatic nuclei and small amounts of cytoplasm. This is also true of HGSIL. Detecting the lymphocytic nature of the cells of chronic follicular cervicitis is an important first step in reaching the correct diagnosis. Careful inspection of these cells will show that although the cells are lymphocytes, they do not have the irregular chromatin, nucleoli, and nuclear clefts or protrusions common in lymphoma.

A-76. (**c**) **Herpes**

These cells show the common features found in herpes infection: multinucleation; smudgy, ground-glass chromatin pattern; and molding of the nuclei. The image on the left also shows the eosinophilic inclusion bodies which may be found in herpes. Adenovirus only occurs in endocervical cells and it is not multinucleated. CMV usually has only one nucleus and has a very large basophilic intranuclear inclusion which gives an owl-eye appearance to the slide. HGSIL would not feature the marked smudgy ground-glass chromatin and molding featured on this slide, and LGSIL would not have the intranuclear inclusions, molding, and multinucleation seen here.

A-77. **(a) Soak in glycerin for 30 min; restain**
This image is an example of "cornflake" artifact, in which a golden brown pigment-like substance seems to cover the cells. This is caused by trapping air between the cell surface and the coverslip by allowing the xylene to evaporate before the coverslip is applied. Rapid coverslipping of the slides one by one without allowing the xylene to evaporate will prevent this artifact. If it is extensive, it can interfere with interpretation of the slide and it must be remedied by removal of the coverslip and soaking the slide in glycerin for 30 min prior to restaining and prompt recoverslipping. This artifact is not involved with lengths of time in the various stains so altering those will not remove the artifact. A mixture of 50 % ETOH and xylene just prior to coverslipping would not be advisable since the water in the 50 % alcohol mixture would not be compatible with the xylene, nor would this remedy the problem.

A-78. **(b) Radiation effect**
The cells in these images are consistent with the effects of radiation therapy. We can see cytomegaly, vacuolization, bizarre shapes, and an increase in nuclear size with a corresponding increase in cytoplasmic area, leading to a mostly normal N:C ratio. Note that these changes can be seen for years or even decades after cessation of therapy. The changes seen are not consistent with inflammatory cell changes which usually have small perinuclear halos, polychromasia, and an abundance of neutrophils. Repair is also not a good choice as there are no nucleoli, streaming cytoplasm, and maintained polarity to suggest this diagnosis. This degree of cytomegaly is usually only seen in patients after radiation therapy or certain types of chemotherapy or with vitamin B12 deficiency. LGSIL would have a higher N:C ratio. Recurrent squamous cell carcinoma would generally have much smaller cells with a markedly higher N:C ratio, hyperchromasia, nucleoli, and a dirty background.

A-79. **(d) Candida**
The "moth-eaten" appearance in the cytoplasm should lead one to carefully search the slide for the appearance of Candida. The patient's history of pregnancy also suggests that Candida may be the cause of this inflammatory cell change. Although Trichomonas may also give this appearance, it was not one of the choices given. Neither CMV nor herpes will give the appearance seen here. Actinomyces would display as fuzzy-looking colonies of bacteria with a starburst configuration. Chlamydia would appear as small vacuoles with tiny organisms within the vacuoles. Thus the best answer is d.

A-80. **(a) Busy background**
A background such as this is very suggestive of an infection with either Candida or Trichomonas. This "busy" background on ThinPrep slides can be identified at low power and can instigate a search for the true cause. Common causes of a busy background are Trichomonas or Candida infection, atrophy, cytolysis, or tumor diathesis. In addition to the observation that there are too many "things" in the background (too busy), one can note a single pseudohyphae in the center of the field, which leads to a diagnosis of Candida. A tumor diathesis should have an identifiable blood and/or cellular necrosis aspect to the slide. An increase in the intensity of the stain can go along with either Candida or Trichomonas infection but this is not observed here. Endometrial cell balls are usually seen during exodus (days 7–10 of the cycle) but they are not noted here. Estrogen effect is not usually associated with a particular organism, although it might coexist with an infection. The fungal hyphae noted here is the best clue to the diagnosis of Candida.

A-81. **(b) Shift in vaginal flora suggestive of bacterial vaginosis**
The finding of coccobacilli coating the epithelial cells as seen in this image has previously been diagnosed in a variety of ways including clue cells, Gardnerella vaginalis, and coccobacilli. However, the latest version of the Bethesda System (2001) suggests using the terminology above, as these bacteria are often associated with the clinical symptoms of bacterial vaginosis. Actinomyces is not the appropriate diagnosis since the bacteria are not arrayed in a starburst arrangement as in Actinomyces.

A-82. **(d) 69-year-old patient with no exogenous hormone use**
This low-power view shows the type of hormonal pattern that would likely be seen in a postmenopausal woman not taking any exogenous hormone replacement therapy. This atrophic pattern is mainly made up of lower intermediate to parabasal type cells, reflective of the decreased estrogen status of the patient. Maturation indices for these patients usually range

from MI: 100/0/0 to MI: 50/50/0. A 17-year-old patient on day 5 would be expected to show copious blood, endometrial cell balls, other debris, and a maturation index which had more intermediate cells than superficial cells, but no parabasal cells. A 25-year-old patient in the third trimester of a normal pregnancy should normally have all intermediate cells in the smear. Small variations may occur immediate prior to delivery. A 32-year-old patient with testicular feminization would have a high estrogen level with a maturation index approaching nearly 100 % superficial cells.

A-83. (**e**) **Leptothrix and Trichomonas**

This image shows the long curving slender organisms consistent with Leptothrix. These organisms usually occur with Trichomonas; however, Trichomonas may often occur without Leptothrix. The Trichomonas organisms may be better seen in the higher power view in the lower left. We see an eccentric nucleus in a small grayish pear-shaped organism. These organisms have multiple flagella, but they are often lost in processing and are seldom identified on Pap-stained material. Doderlein are not seen in this image as the long, curving nature of the Leptothrix is not consistent with the appearance of Doderlein bacilli. Neither Actinomyces nor shift in vaginal flora is consistent with the images. Actinomyces is arranged in a starburst type of pattern in a colony of bacteria. Candida and Trichomonas seldom occur together and the Candida organisms will be several times greater in width than the Leptothrix. Entamoeba histolytica is a parasite of the GI tract and also has two distinct nuclei rather than the one seen in Trichomonas.

A-84. (**b**) **Parakeratotic cells**

Parakeratosis is a benign proliferative reaction made up of miniature superficial squamous cells. The cells are quite small and polygonal, usually stain pink to orange, and have small pyknotic nuclei. They occur on the surface of the epithelium and may occur with hyperkeratosis. Their presence has been associated with more serious lesions, especially keratinizing LGSIL. The cells are too small to be normal squamous cells. These cells do have nuclei so they are not hyperkeratosis. There is not a high enough N:C ratio to be considered for squamous cell carcinoma. These cells do not have the nucleoli and streaming cytoplasm consistent with repair. Thus, the best answer is parakeratosis.

A-85. (**c**) **LGSIL**

These cells have prominent large distinct perinuclear halos, consistent infection with HPV. This finding is classified by the 2001 Bethesda System as consistent with LGSIL. ASC-US might be considered if only a few of these cells were present or if the HPV changes were questionable. However, the changes seen here are unequivocal for HPV infection. ASC-H might be considered if only a few cells with N:C ratios suggestive of a HGSIL were seen. These cells do not have a high enough N:C ratio for an ASC-H diagnosis. Likewise, a diagnosis of HGSIL is ruled out due to the lack of a sufficiently high N:C ratio. Finally, glycogenated squamous cells would have yellowish material surrounding the nucleus and would not show the nuclear abnormalities (binucleation, hyperchromasia, smudgy chromatin) seen here.

A-86. (**c**) **HPV**

The large distinct perinuclear halos in cells which contain nuclei with some type of abnormality such as binucleation, hyperchromasia, or smudgy chromatin are consistent with infection by HPV. We now know that HPV infection is the cause of virtually all squamous cell carcinomas of the uterine cervix as well as most of the several stages of noninvasive neoplasia of squamous epithelium. Other viral infections (e.g., herpes) were at one time considered as possible precursors, but unequivocal proof has been obtained through molecular techniques that HPV infection is the cause of both LGSIL and HGSIL, as well as most squamous cancers of the cervix. Herpes has features of multinucleation, molding, and ground-glass chromatin, which are not seen in this image. CMV is characterized by large "owl-eye" nuclear inclusions in cells which generally have only one nucleus. Cytoplasmic inclusions may occasionally also occur. Neither HIV nor HBV has specific morphologic changes that can be seen with a light microscope.

A-87. (**a**) **Endometrial cells**

The left image shows the classic double-walled endometrial cell ball common during days 5–10 of the menstrual cycle. The right image also shows endometrial stromal cells which have slightly more cytoplasm than the epithelial endometrial cells. Endocervical cells occur in more two-dimensional groups such as honeycomb or picket fence. Also they will have a more columnar appearance with eccentric nuclei. Syncytiotrophoblasts are multinucleated cells from the placenta which occasionally are shed during a threatened spontaneous abortion. Multinucleated histiocytes have abundant finely vacuolated cytoplasm. Severe chronic inflammation would be indicated by the presence of abundant lymphocytes, in addition to plasma cells and/or eosinophils. The cells seen here do not correspond with inflammatory cells.

A-88. (**d**) **Endocervical cells**

These cells are displaying the typical appearance of endocervical cells: tall columnar cell shape, eccentric nuclei, and picket fence arrangement. Hemosiderin-laden macrophages would contain hemosiderin pigment and show the typical finely vacuolated cytoplasm and single lying arrangement of macrophages. These cells are clearly columnar in configuration and so both LGSIL and HGSIL which occur in squamous epithelium would be eliminated. Lower uterine sampling might be a consideration but the image does not show the high cellularity, tubular structures, and hyperchromatic nuclei typical of lower uterine segment samples.

A-89. (**b**) **Herpes**

This image displays the typical features of herpes infection, multinucleation, molding of the nuclei, and ground-glass chromatin. CMV has a single large intranuclear inclusion unlike the multinucleated cell seen here. Both LGSIL and HGSIL are not likely choices because both of these should show either prominent perinuclear halos or a hyperchromatic, enlarged nucleus with an increased N:C ratio. Adenovirus is only identified in columnar cells and is not consistent with the image seen here. Thus, the best answer is herpes.

A-90. (**c**) **Repair**

These cells are showing nucleoli in nearly every cell, streaming of the cytoplasm, and generally a fine, even chromatin pattern. Along with the clean background seen in this image, these cells are typical for repair. AGUS of endocervical origin should have much greater irregularity of the chromatin pattern and should not show the streaming of the cytoplasm seen especially in the right-hand image. AGUS of the endometrium should show enlarged endometrial cells in three-dimensional groups. Small nucleoli may also be seen in AGUS of the endometrium. Neither LGSIL nor HGSIL should have so many prominent nucleoli. Additionally, they should have increased N:C ratio, hyperchromatic nuclei, and irregular chromatin pattern.

Reading List

Bibbo M, Wilbur DC. Comprehensive cytopathology. 3rd ed. Philadelphia: Saunders/Elsevier; 2008.

Cibas ES. Chapter 1: Cervical and vaginal cytology. In: Cibas ES, Ducatman BS, editors. Cytology diagnostic principles and clinical correlates. Philadelphia: Saunders/Elsevier; 2009. p. 1–66.

DeMay RM. Chapter 1: The Pap test. In: DeMay RM, editor. The art and science of cytopathology. 2nd ed. Chicago: ASCP Press; 2012. p. 2–199.

Pantanowitz L, Austin RM, Michelow P. Chapter 5: Gynecological infections. In: Pantanowitz L, Michelow P, Khalbuss W, editors. Infectious diseases. New York: Springer/Elsevier; 2012.

Solomon D, Nayar R. The Bethesda system for reporting cervical cytology. 2nd ed. New York: Springer; 2004.

Wilbur DC, Henry MR. College of American Pathologists practical guide to gynecologic cytopathology: morphology, management, and molecular methods. Northfield: CAP Press; 2008.

Squamous Lesions in the Pap Test

4

Marilee Means and Walid E. Khalbuss

Contents

M. Means, PhD, SCT(ASCP) (✉)
School of Health Professions,
University of Kansas Medical Center,
3901 Rainbow Blvd., Mail Stop 4048,
Kansas City, KS 66160, USA
e-mail: mmeans@kumc.edu

W.E. Khalbuss, MD, PhD, FIAC
Director of Cytology and Cytopathology Fellowship Program,
University of Pittsburgh Medical Center Shadyside Hospital,
5150 Centre Avenue, 2, Suite 201,
Pittsburgh, PA 15232, USA
e-mail: khalbussw2@upmc.edu

4.1 Tables and Summary

Table 4.1 Recommendations for cervical cytology screening

The American College of Obstetricians and Gynecologists (ACOG) recommendations released in Nov. 2009 suggest the following schedule for the timing of cervical cytologic screening:
Age 21: first Pap
Age 21–30: screening every 2 years
Age 30 and above: after 3 negative consecutive tests, screening every 3 years
Age 30 and above co-screened with HPV and Pap: if negative on both screenings, every 3 years
Age 65–70 with at least 3 normal Pap tests and no abnormal Paps in the previous 10 years may discontinue with consultation from physician
Post hysterectomy patients do not need to have a Pap, unless treatment was for a neoplastic condition
More frequent screening for patients with HIV, immunosuppression, DES exposure, previous cervical neoplasia

Table 4.2 Comparisons of various processing techniques

Technique	Advantages	Disadvantages
Conventional smear 50,000–300,000 cells	Inexpensive No special equipment or disposables Easy to process in the lab Abnormal cells may occur in streaks and be easier to find	Air-drying Obscuring elements Uneven thickness Distortion of cells due to smearing May be more time-consuming and difficult to screen

(continued)

W.E. Khalbuss, M. Means (eds.), *Gynecological and Breast Cytopathology Board Review and Self-Assessment*, DOI 10.1007/978-1-4614-7270-4_4, © Springer Science+Business Media New York 2013

Table 4.2 (continued)

Technique	Advantages	Disadvantages
ThinPrep 50,000–75,000 cells Filtration system	Immediate fixation Smaller area to screen Reduction of air-drying and obscuring elements Even thickness May be easier to screen Ancillary testing can be performed on remainder of vial	Expensive equipment and disposables More time-consuming to process Random sampling may disperse abnormal cells Crushed border cell artifact High grade or glandular groups may be more difficult to interpret Rounding up – smaller appearing cells and nuclei Less hyperchromasia Small nucleoli may be present in premalignant lesions May contain fewer abnormal cells
SurePath 50,000–75,000 cells Gravity system	Immediate fixation Smaller area to screen Reduction of air-drying and obscuring elements Even thickness May be easier to screen Ancillary testing may be performed on remainder of vial Combines processing and staining steps	Expensive equipment and disposables Significantly more time-consuming to process Random sampling may disperse abnormal cells High grade or glandular groups may be more difficult to interpret Rounding up – smaller appearing cells and nuclei Less hyperchromasia Small nucleoli may be present in premalignant lesions May contain fewer abnormal cells

Table 4.4 Inflammatory and infectious organisms common in gynecologic cytology

Viruses

Human papillomavirus (HPV) – koilocytes, mild nuclear abnormalities, dyskeratocytes

Herpes simplex virus (HSV) – multinucleation, ground glass nuclei, molding, +/– nuclear inclusions

Cytomegalovirus (CMV) – large nuclear inclusion (owl's eye), no molding, occasional multinucleation, may also have cytoplasmic inclusions

Bacteria

Doderlein bacilli – normal bacterial flora, helps to maintain normal acidity of vagina

Shift in vaginal flora – clue cells, coccobacilli and/or cocci, Doderlein bacilli, and inflammation are absent, associated with bacterial vaginosis

Actinomyces – higher-order bacteria, associated with IUDs, dark-blue fuzzy masses of bacteria with starburst rays of filamentous thin bacilli

Fungi

Candida species – indeterminate to pink staining pseudohyphae with oval buds (yeast forms)

May occur in "shish kebab" formations as the hyphae pierce the epithelial cells

Protozoa

Trichomonas vaginalis – gray to lavender, 8–30 μm organism with an ill-defined, eccentric nucleus; red cytoplasmic granules may be seen, flagella may occasionally be seen in LBP, and it may coexist with the long curving bacilli (Leptothrix); however, Leptothrix does not occur without Trichomonas. Can elicit a marked inflammatory response or may have a clean background

Table 4.3 Squamous cellular components of Pap smears

Squamous epithelial cells

Basal cells – seldom seen in the absence of severe atrophy or ulceration

Size 10–12 μm diameter, round, scant cytoplasm, central nucleus

Lowest level of epithelium, rests upon basement membrane, site of regeneration of cells

Parabasal cells – commonly seen in atrophic states due to low estrogen, i.e., childhood, postmenopause, postpartum

Size 15–30 μm diameter, round to oval, more abundant denser cytoplasm than basal cells, central nucleus, nuclear diameter is 8–9 μm, N/C ratio mean of 20 %

Intermediate cells – more mature state than parabasal cells, common in pregnancy and late luteal phase of the menstrual cycle, one of the two most common cells seen in normal childbearing hormonal states

May be lysed by the action of the Doderlein bacilli (cytolysis) leaving only bare nuclei

Size 35–50 μm diameter, more oval to polygonal, more abundant thinner cytoplasm than parabasal cells, central nucleus, nuclear diameter is 7–8 μm, N/C ratio mean of 3–5 %

Superficial cells – most mature state, one of the two most common cells seen in normal childbearing hormonal states

Resistant to action of Doderlein bacilli

Size 45–50 μm diameter, most polygonal and thinnest cytoplasm, small dark central nucleus, nuclear diameter is 5–6 μm, N/C ratio is 2–3 %

Table 4.5 Nonneoplastic conditions in the female genital tract

Repair and regeneration

Repair – streaming cytoplasm, preserved polarity, prominent nucleoli in 100 % of the cells, Variably enlarged hypochromatic nuclei

Reactive cells – 1–2× enlargement over intermediate cell nuclei (ICN), fine chromatin, smooth nuclear membrane, small nucleoli, pale to slightly hyperchromatic nuclei

Inflammatory conditions

Follicular cervicitis – heterogenous population of mature and immature lymphocytes and occasionally, tingible–body macrophages

Inflammatory cell change – includes polychromasia, ill-defined perinuclear halos, <2× enlargement over intermediate cell nucleus, pale chromatin, vacuolization of cytoplasm, common with Trichomonas and Candida

Benign proliferative conditions

Squamous metaplasia – resembles parabasal cells except occurs in specific areas of slide, not associated with a generalized atrophic hormonal pattern as are parabasal cells, cytoplasm is more polygonal than parabasal cells

Hyperkeratosis – annucleated superficial and intermediate cells, may overlie a more serious lesion

Parakeratosis – miniature superficial squamous cells, may overlie a more serious lesion

Table 4.6 Premalignant squamous lesions of the female genital tract

ASCUS – atypical squamous cells
ASCUS – atypical cells of undetermined significance (lack morphology and/or quantitatively too few for a diagnosis of LGSIL)
2–3× intermediate cell nucleus (ICN)
ASC-H – atypical squamous cells, cannot rule out HGSIL (lack morphology and/or quantitatively too few for a diagnosis of HGSIL)
High N/C ratios, usually too few in number for a diagnosis of HGSIL
LGSIL – low-grade squamous intraepithelial lesion
Includes koilocytes, dyskeratocytes, and cells with an increase in the nuclear size, >3× ICN, mild hyperchromasia, finely granular chromatin
HGSIL – high-grade squamous intraepithelial lesion
Includes previous categories of moderate dysplasia, severe dysplasia, and carcinoma in situ
>3× ICN, finely to coarsely granular irregular chromatin, hyperchromasia, nuclear shapes vary from round to oval in less severe lesions to highly indented, clefted, and cerebriform shapes in the most serious lesions
Cells occur singly, in sheets, or in syncytial groups. In conventional smears, they can also be seen in small clusters, rows or linear arrangements
General comments: these premalignant lesions generally do not have prominent macronucleoli, although small nucleoli may sometimes be found in liquid-based preparations. The background of the case is clean, without the old and fresh blood, cellular debris, and necrosis found in invasive squamous cell carcinoma. The slides generally show increasing numbers of abnormal cells, a gradual increase in nuclear/cytoplasmic ratio, an increase in hyperchromasia, an increase in the coarseness and irregularity of the chromatin pattern, and an increase in disorderly architecture (from sheets to syncytia) as the severity of the lesion increases. The shapes of the nuclei range from round to oval in ASCUS slides to highly indented, clefted, and irregularly shaped in HGSIL. The overall size of the nuclei increases as the severity of the lesion increases, ranging from 2 to 3 × ICN in ASCUS to >3 × ICN in HGSIL. At the same time, the overall size of the cell tends to decrease, so that the cells display a higher nuclear/cytoplasmic ratio as the severity of the lesion increases.

Table 4.8 Rare variants of squamous cell carcinoma

Verrucous carcinoma – papillary growth pattern, very well-differentiated
Warty carcinoma – marked condylomatous changes, prominent koilocytes
Papillary squamous cell carcinoma – significant nuclear atypia with papillary growth pattern
Transitional cell carcinoma – resembles transitional cell carcinoma of bladder, urothelial cell features
Lymphoepithelioma-like squamous cell carcinoma – syncytia and single cells with lymphocyte infiltrate
Spindle squamous cell carcinoma – spindle, non-keratinized, high-grade cells resembling sarcoma, CK+

Table 4.7 Subtypes of squamous cell carcinoma of the uterine cervix

	Keratinized	Non-keratinized	Small cell
Nuclei	Opaque, hyperchromatic Coarsely granular, irregular Nucleoli may be present but difficult to see due to opaque nuclei Variable N/C ratio	Coarsely granular, irregular Hyperchromatic Prominent nucleoli High N/C ratio	Very coarse, hyperchromatic Nucleoli (may be difficult to see due to small size of cells) Very high N/C ratio
Cyto plasm	Pleomorphic, spindle, tadpole, dense Largest, variably sized	More uniform, round to polygonal Medium size	Uniform in appearance Scant, delicate Smallest sized
Staining	Orange, keratinized	Cyanophilic, no keratin pearls	Cyanophilic
Occurrence	Single more than groups	Loose clusters, single, HCGs, syncytia	Syncytia, single cells
Background	Diathesis but may be less than other types due to exophytic growth pattern	Diathesis	Most severe diathesis
Diff. dx.	**Severe K dysplasia** If >10–15 % of abnormal cells are pleomorphic, favors SCCA	**Repair** If cells have lost polarity, have hyperchromasia, are single, occur in syncytia, and + tumor diathesis, favors SCCA	**Endometrial cells, atrophy, follicular cervicitis** Use diathesis, nucleoli to exclude benign conditions **Lymphoma, small cell NE carcinoma** Use ID of lymphoid cells for lymphoma, immunos for NE
Other	Least common in the USA	Most common in the USA	Intermediate frequency

While the subclassifications of squamous cell carcinoma are not utilized in the Bethesda System for reporting, nevertheless knowledge of the variety of morphologic patterns which correlate with invasive squamous cell carcinoma can be a useful guide for the cytologist

4.2 Text-Based Questions 1–40

Q-1. Recommended cervical screening guidelines (American Cancer Society) allow for cessation of screening if the patient has no previous abnormal history and if:
(a) She is older than 55 years
(b) She is older than 70 years
(c) She has a history of DES exposure
(d) She is receiving corticosteroid therapy

Q-2. The appropriate administration of prophylactic HPV vaccines:
(a) Must take place before initiation of sexual activity
(b) Has 2 doses
(c) Will successfully treat an HPV infection
(d) Will eliminate the need for Pap testing by 2017
(e) Will eliminate the risk of clear cell adenocarcinoma in DES exposed women

Q-3. Which of the following may interfere with the optimum Pap test sampling of the uterine cervix?
(a) Use of cytobrush
(b) Application of fixative after 90 seconds
(c) Taking the sample after day 14 of the cycle
(d) Use of 95 % ethyl alcohol as a fixative

Q-4. Sampling of the lower uterine segment:
(a) Should be avoided due to diagnostic difficulties
(b) Is a requirement for adequate Pap test results
(c) May be best obtained by rotating the cytobrush three to five times
(d) Helps to avoid air-drying artifact

Q-5. Which of the following is NOT a Bethesda System criteria for "unsatisfactory for evaluation"?
(a) Lack of patient identification
(b) Insufficient squamous component
(c) Absence of endocervical or transformation zone component
(d) Obscuring elements covering over 75 % of the epithelial cells
(e) Less than 5,000 squamous cells on a liquid-based preparation

Q-6. Which of these patients is the most likely to show evidence of atrophy on the cytologic sample?
(a) Patient with history of DES exposure in utero
(b) 27-year-old patient in second trimester of a normal pregnancy
(c) 42-year-old patient, LMP day 7
(d) 6-year-old child with precocious puberty and evidence of ovarian tumor
(e) 65-year-old with no history of exogenous hormone therapy

Q-7. A patient with a history of uterine descensus is most likely to display which of the following on the Pap:
(a) Hyperkeratosis and parakeratosis
(b) Candida and leptothrix
(c) LGSIL and dyskeratocytes
(d) Repair and Trichomonas

Q-8. A stain that might detect the correct origin of a multinucleated cell found in the sample from a woman in the first trimester of pregnancy is:
(a) S-100
(b) Mucicarmine
(c) Grocott
(d) HCG
(e) TTF-1

Q-9. Normal flora of the female genital tract contains:
(a) Lactobacilli
(b) Gardnerella vaginalis
(c) Leptothrix
(d) Candida albicans
(e) Actinomyces

Q-10. A 15–30 μm lavender to gray organism with an eccentric oval nucleus is:
(a) Herpes simplex
(b) Actinomyces
(c) Calymmatobacterium granulomatis
(d) Trichomonas
(e) Chlamydia trachomatis

Q-11. A patient has a history of hysterectomy and radiation for cervical carcinoma. Cells are found in the vaginal Pap with the following characteristics: cytoplasmic streaming, variable enlargement of the nuclei, finely granular chromatin pattern, frequent nucleoli, and hypochromasia. The most likely diagnosis is:
(a) Post radiation dysplasia
(b) Radiation effect
(c) Repair
(d) Recurrent squamous cell carcinoma
(e) Microglandular hyperplasia

Q-12. The two types of cells consistent with IUD effect that might most resemble which of the following:
(a) Endometrial adenocarcinoma and HGSIL
(b) Koilocytes and repair

(c) "Tissue paper" cells and squamous cell carcinoma
(d) Multinucleated histiocytes and hyperkeratosis

Q-13. In combination with host cell genes p53 and pRB, the two most important HPV genes which lead to the development of squamous cell carcinoma of the cervix are:
(a) L1 and L2
(b) E1 and E2
(c) E4 and E5
(d) E6 and E7

Q-14. The most common HPV subtype found in squamous cell carcinoma of the cervix is:
(a) HPV 6
(b) HPV 11
(c) HPV 16
(d) HPV 18

Q-15. The Bethesda System diagnosis of HGSIL includes:
(a) CIN I
(b) Koilocytes
(c) Dyskeratocytes
(d) Moderate dysplasia

Q-16. Small ill-defined perinuclear halos can often be seen in conjunction with:
(a) Infection with Candida or Trichomonas
(b) HPV infection
(c) Chronic follicular cervicitis
(d) Microglandular hyperplasia
(e) Lower uterine segment

Q-17. A diagnosis of ASCUS is most often made in the presence of:
(a) Rare cells with high N/C ratios
(b) Rare cells with morphologic changes short of LGSIL
(c) Moderate numbers of spindled, keratinizing cells
(d) Moderate numbers of cells with nucleoli, enlarged pale nuclei, and streaming cytoplasm
(e) Very small, discohesive dark cells with high N/C ratios

Q-18. Almost one-half of LGSIL lesions:
(a) Progress on to invasive lesions
(b) Have nucleoli
(c) Will regress even without treatment
(d) Should be treated with a LEEP procedure
(e) Are high-risk HPV positive and should be tested for the presence of HPV infection

Q-19. HGSIL:
(a) Has a significant risk of progression to carcinoma
(b) Usually occurs in large, mature squamous cells
(c) Contains nucleoli
(d) Has hypochromatic nuclei
(e) Shows feathering of nuclei from the edge of cohesive groups of cells

Q-20. The most common malignant tumor (75 %) of the cervix is:
(a) Endocervical AIS
(b) Endocervical adenocarcinoma
(c) Squamous cell carcinoma
(d) Adenosquamous carcinoma

Q-21. A differential diagnosis for HGSIL includes:
(a) Squamous metaplasia
(b) Koilocytes
(c) Estrogen effect
(d) Microglandular hyperplasia
(e) ASCUS

Q-22. Tadpole and fiber cells are the most likely to be seen in which type of squamous cell carcinoma?
(a) Neuroendocrine type
(b) Non-keratinizing type
(c) Small cell type
(d) Keratinizing type
(e) Behçet disease

Q-23. The correct immediate treatment for a patient with a diagnosis of ASC-H is:
(a) Repeat Pap in 6 months
(b) Repeat Pap in 12 months
(c) Testing for high-risk HPV
(d) Colposcopically directed biopsy
(e) LEEP procedure

Q-24. For a patient with a diagnosis of ASC-H, the positive predictive value for histologic CIN 2,3 is:
(a) Higher than for ASCUS
(b) About the same as ASCUS
(c) Lower than for ASCUS
(d) Higher than for HGSIL

Q-25. In a normal nonpregnant woman of childbearing years, for the slide to be considered as containing adequate evidence of transformation zone sampling, there must be at least:
(a) 10 metaplastic cells
(b) 10 endocervical cells

(c) 10 cells of either metaplastic or endocervical cell origin
(d) 10 parabasal cells

Q-26. For a slide to be considered as unsatisfactory due to blood or inflammation, there must be at least _______% of the cells obscured.
(a) 25
(b) 50
(c) 75
(d) 100

Q-27. What would be the expected cytomorphologic effects of the administration of progesterone to a pregnant female, who has a more mature cell pattern than expected for a normal pregnancy?
(a) Increased maturation
(b) Will have no effect
(c) May induce a decrease of maturity to intermediate levels
(d) May induce a decrease of maturity to 100 % parabasal cells

Q-28. The most frequent type of dysplasia is:
(a) Non-keratinizing
(b) Metaplastic
(c) Keratinizing
(d) Mixed metaplastic and keratinizing

Q-29. The type of SIL which is most likely to progress to CIN 3 is:
(a) Non-keratinizing
(b) Metaplastic
(c) Keratinizing
(d) Mixed metaplastic and keratinizing

Q-30. The type of squamous cell carcinoma which has the worst prognosis is:
(a) Non-keratinizing
(b) Keratinizing
(c) Small cell
(d) All of these have a similar prognosis

Q-31. Which characteristic of repair is the most helpful in distinguishing it from squamous cell carcinoma?
(a) Macronucleoli
(b) Preserved nuclear polarity
(c) Syncytia
(d) Presence of free cells
(e) Clumping of chromatin

Q-32. Which of the following has the highest percentage of macronucleoli?
(a) CIS
(b) Non-keratinizing squamous cell carcinoma
(c) Keratinizing squamous cell carcinoma
(d) Squamous metaplasia

Q-33. In which of the following diagnoses would the cells have the largest nuclei?
(a) Squamous metaplasia
(b) SIL
(c) Keratinizing squamous cell carcinoma
(d) Non-keratinizing squamous cell carcinoma

Q-34. Nuclear membrane interruption and irregular chromatin are nuclear features most abundant in which lesion?
(a) ASCUS
(b) ASC-H
(c) LGSIL
(d) HGSIL

Q-35. Cells with the following characteristics are noted in a 42-year-old female: enlarged cells, hypochromasia, sheet arrangement, enlarged nuclei, macronucleoli. The most likely diagnosis is:
(a) CIS
(b) Squamous cell carcinoma
(c) Repair
(d) Endometrial adenocarcinoma
(e) Moderate dysplasia

Q-36. Which of the following diagnoses most often displays syncytial groupings?
(a) ASCUS
(b) ASC-H
(c) LGSIL
(d) HGSIL
(e) Repair

Q-37. Glycogenated lower intermediate squamous cells, often found in pregnant patients, are sometimes shaped with a pointed end on one side of the cell and a rounded end on the other. These cells are referred to as:
(a) Syncytiotrophoblasts
(b) Decidual cells
(c) Navicular cells
(d) Pickle cells
(e) Pencil cells

Q-38. In the absence of exogenous hormonal therapy, a post-menopausal woman can display an estrogen effect due to:
(a) Obesity
(b) Cytolysis
(c) Sertoli-Leydig tumor
(d) Air-drying artifact

Q-39. Radiating starburst-like golden refractile structures found in a Pap smear and associated with pregnancy are termed:
(a) Cytotrophoblasts
(b) Syncytiotrophoblasts
(c) Decidual cells
(d) Cockleburrs

Q-40. Squamous cell carcinoma in liquid-based preparations usually will demonstrate:
(a) Cytomegaly
(b) Cytoplasmic vacuoles
(c) Eccentric hyperchromatic nuclei
(d) Clinging tumor diathesis
(e) Polychromasia

4.3 Image-Based Questions 41–100

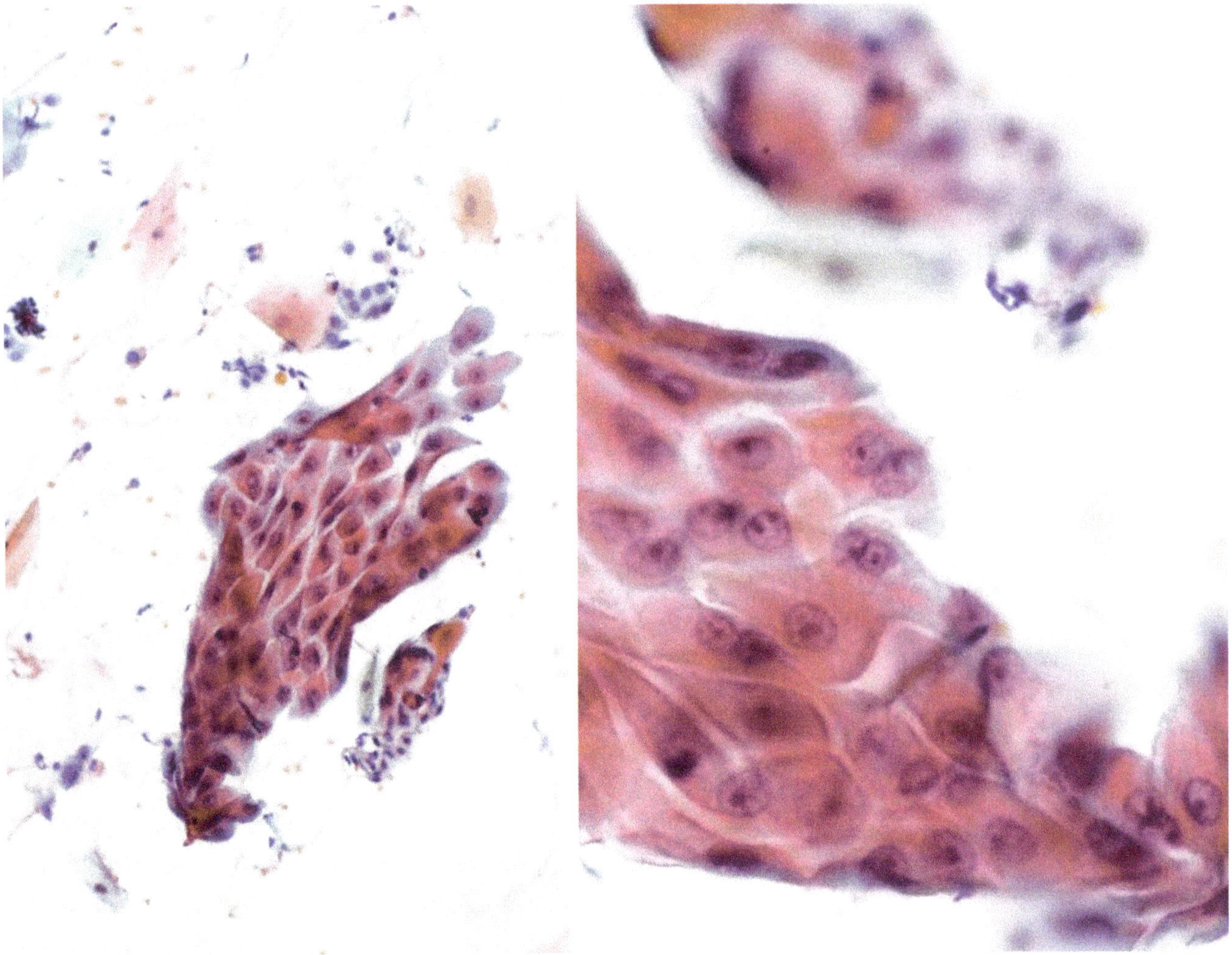

Fig. 4.41

Q-41. These images were from a cervical/vaginal smear on a 36-year-old woman (conventional, low and high magnification). The cellular material is most consistent with:
(a) Endocervical cells
(b) HGSIL
(c) Repair
(d) Squamous cell carcinoma
(e) Endocervical adenocarcinoma

Fig. 4.42

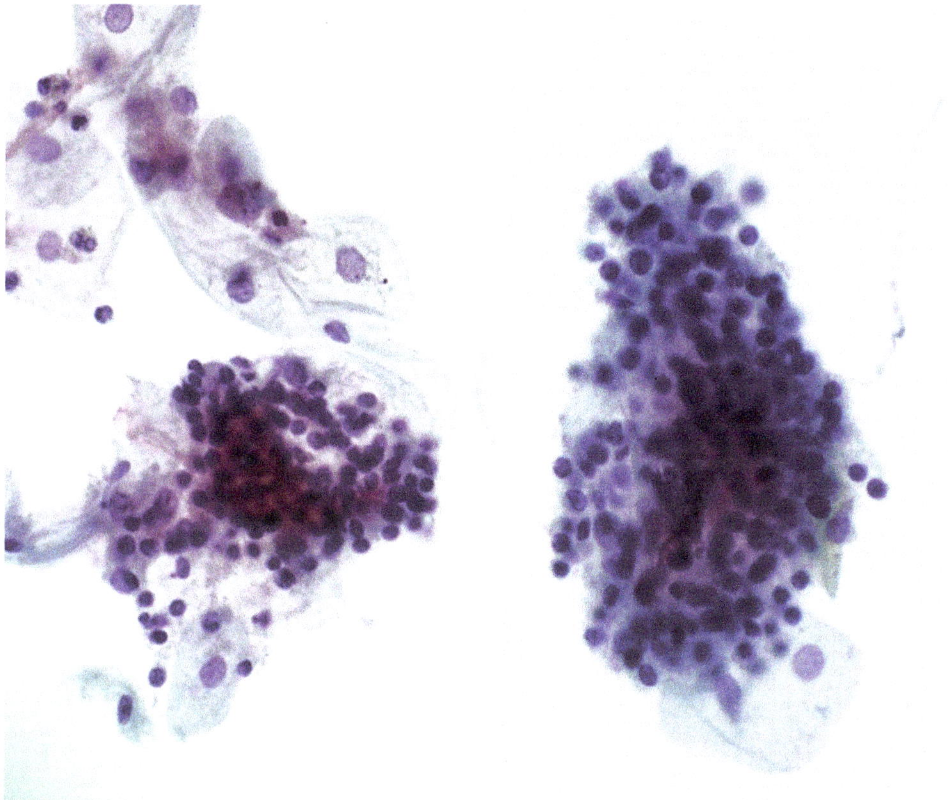

Q-42. Several clusters of cells such as these were found on the cervical/vaginal smear of a 56-year-old woman (ThinPrep, medium and high magnification). These cellular groups are most consistent with a diagnosis of:

(a) Small cell carcinoma of the cervix
(b) Endometrial adenocarcinoma
(c) Chronic follicular cervicitis
(d) HGSIL (CIS)
(e) Normal endometrial cells

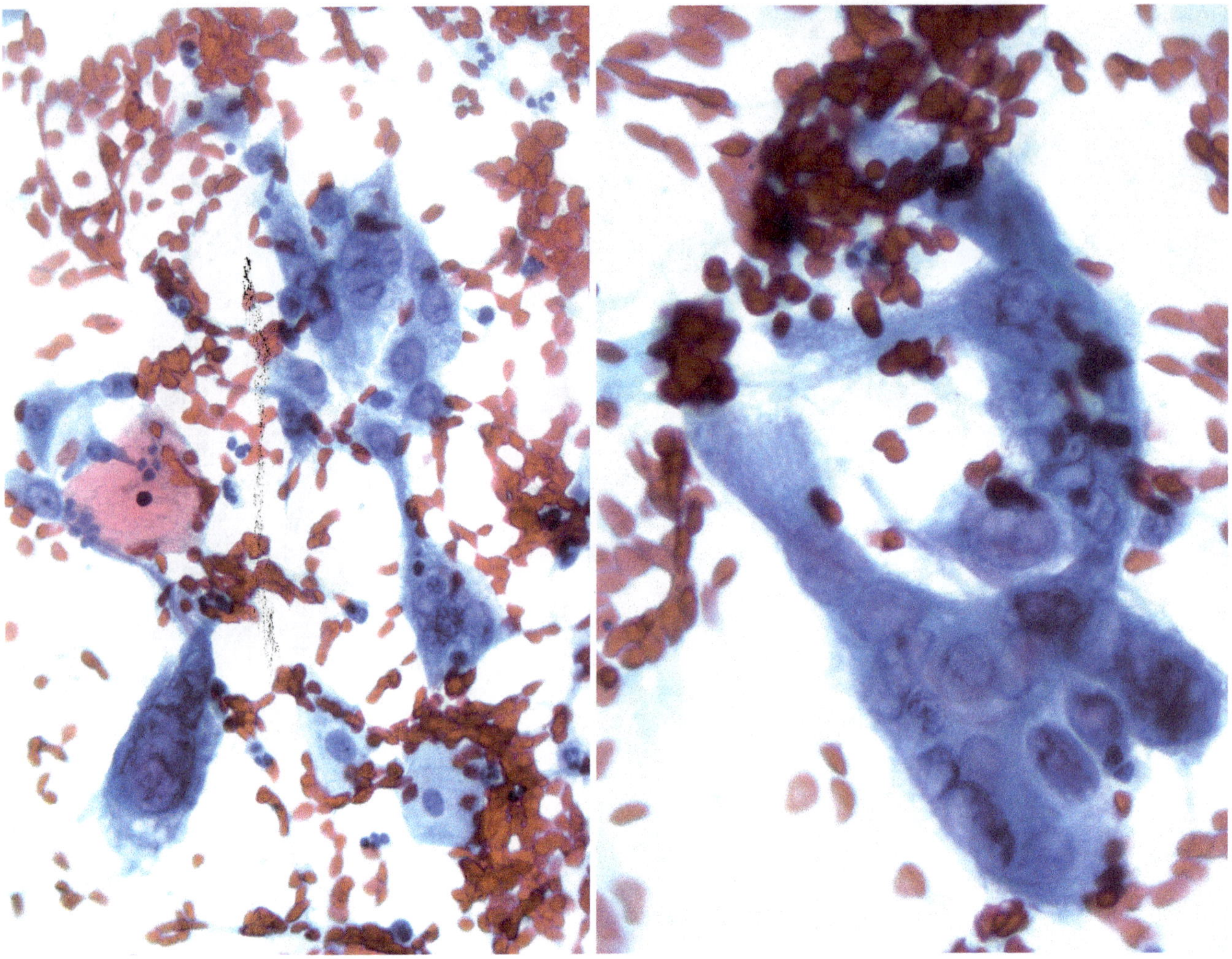

Fig. 4.43

Q-43. These cells were found in the cervical/vaginal smear of a 16-year-old female (conventional, medium and high magnification). Characteristics of the lesion include all of the following EXCEPT:
(a) Multinucleation
(b) Nucleoli
(c) Smudgy, ground glass chromatin
(d) Margination of the chromatin
(e) Eosinophilic inclusion bodies

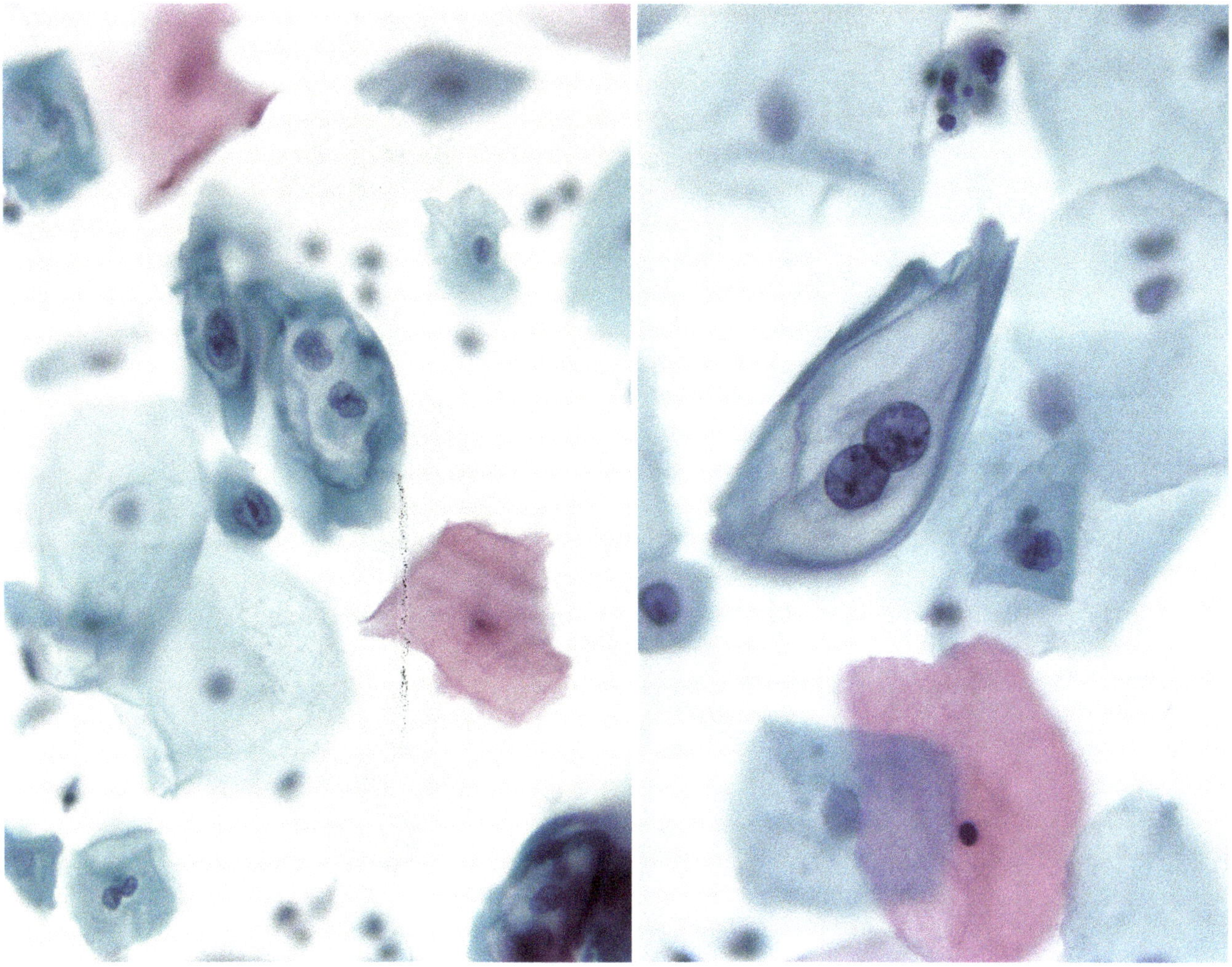

Fig. 4.44

Q-44. Cells such as these were seen in moderate numbers throughout the slide from a 26-year-old woman (Sure Path, medium and high magnification). The most likely diagnosis is:

(a) Syncytiotrophoblast
(b) Glycogen-filled cells consistent with pregnancy
(c) Multinucleated histiocytes
(d) LGSIL
(e) HGSIL

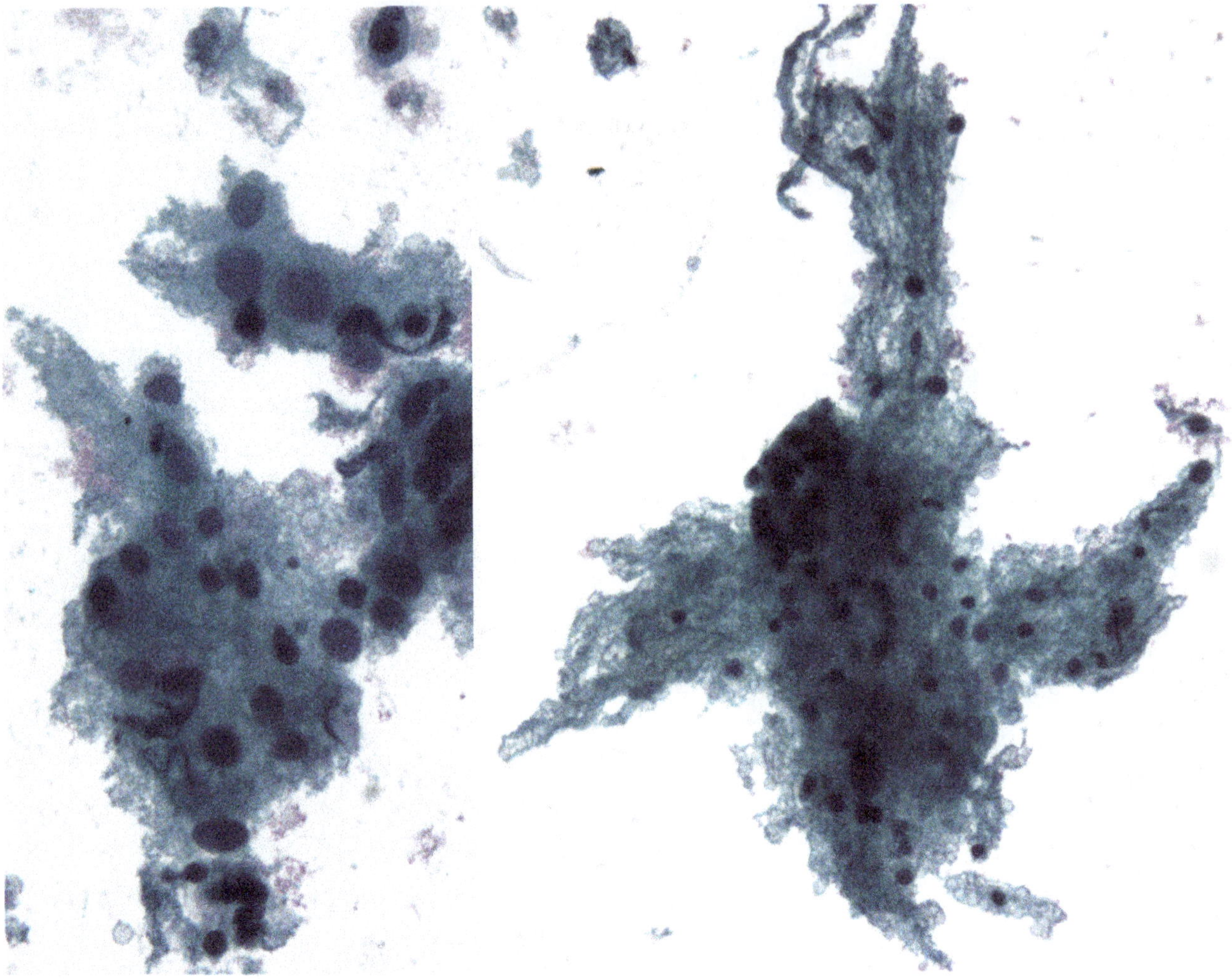

Fig. 4.45

Q-45. This 67-year-old patient had a cervical smear processed by ThinPrep, and the slide had this appearance over the entire surface (medium and low magnification). Which of the following is the most appropriate diagnosis?

(a) Unsatisfactory due to obscuring blood
(b) Quality indicator: thick, shift in vaginal flora, NILM
(c) Quality indicator: obscuring blood, HGSIL, cannot rule out invasion
(d) Shift in vaginal flora, LGSIL

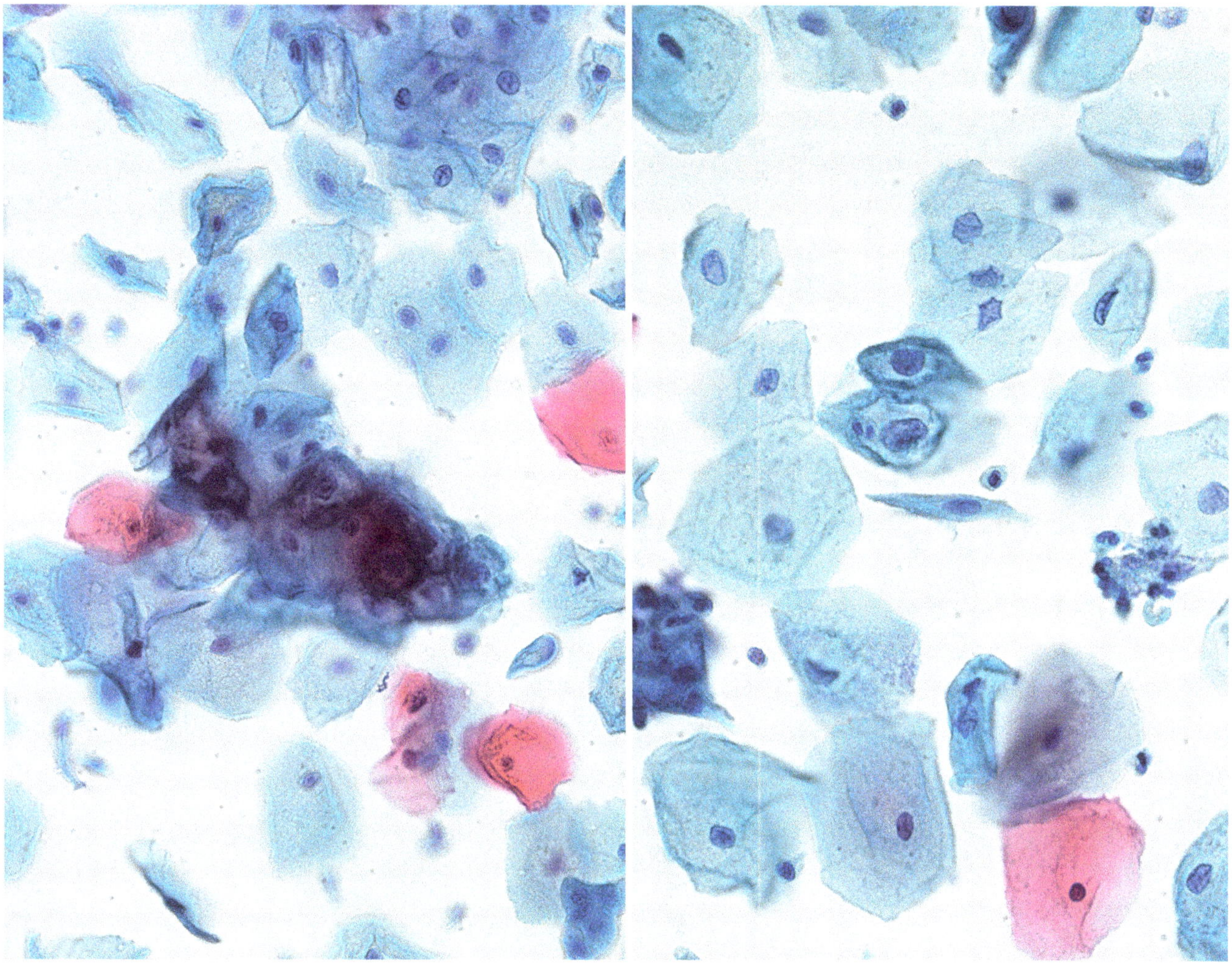

Fig. 4.46

Q-46. This slide from a 32-year-old female contained several cellular groups as seen in these two photomicrographs (SurePath, medium and high magnification). The best cytologic diagnosis of this case would be:

(a) LGSIL
(b) HR HPV 16 or 18+
(c) HGSIL
(d) Repair

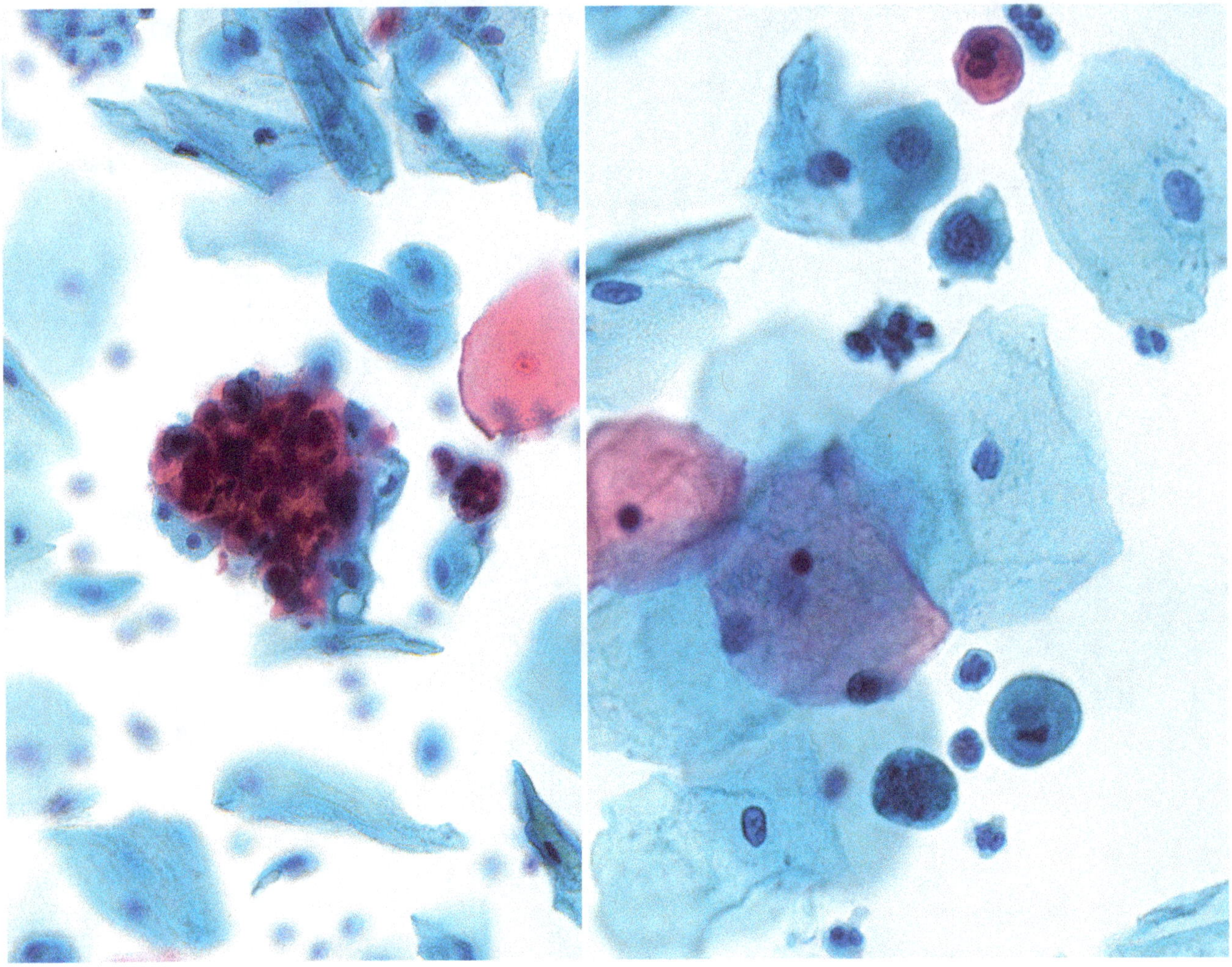

Fig. 4.47

Q-47. A 49-year-old female was found to have numerous groups of cells on her SurePath slide resembling those seen here (medium and high magnification). A clean background was noted and in other areas of the slide, some pleomorphic cells in tadpole shapes were noted. Some of the cells were noted to have deeply eosinophilic or orangeophilic cytoplasm. The most likely diagnosis is:

(a) Repair
(b) LGSIL
(c) HGSIL
(d) Endocervical AIS

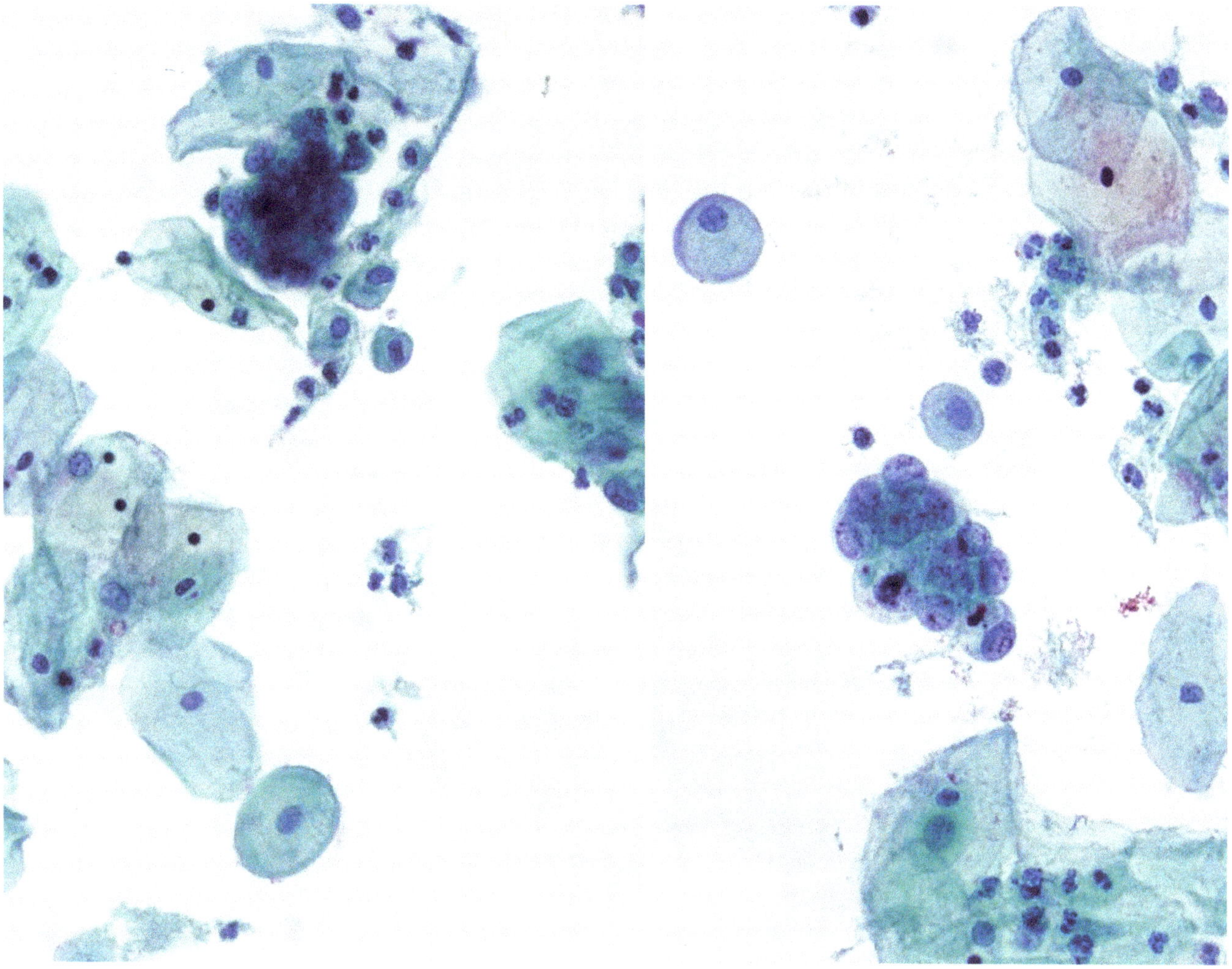

Fig. 4.48

Q-48. This patient is a 76-year-old female with a moderate number of clusters of cells such as these on her slide (ThinPrep, medium magnification). The most likely diagnosis is:
(a) Squamous cell carcinoma
(b) Endocervical adenocarcinoma
(c) Endometrial adenocarcinoma
(d) LGSIL

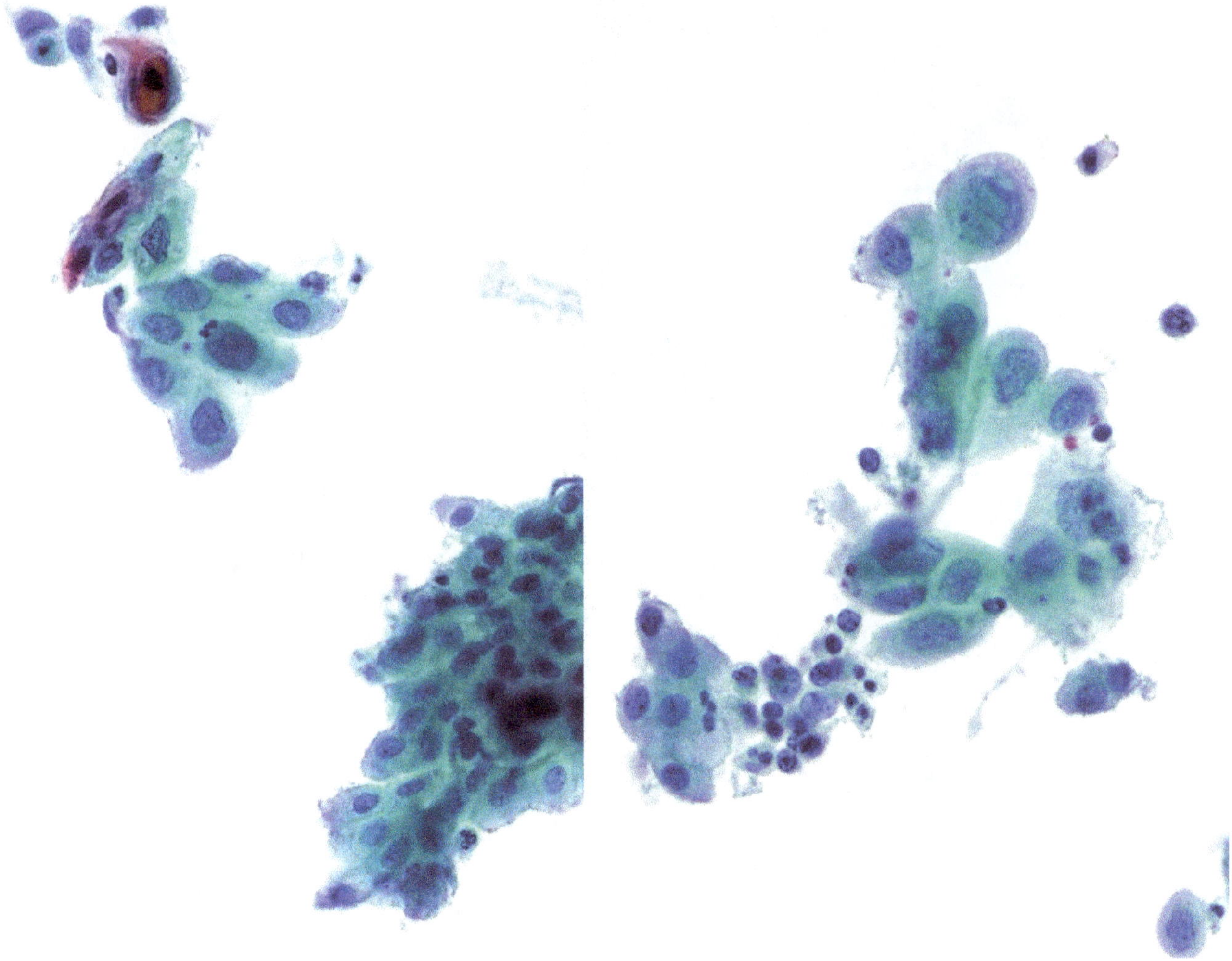

Fig. 4.49

Q-49. A 59-year-old female has numerous cells with this appearance on a Thin Prep cervical/vaginal slide (medium magnification). The most likely diagnosis is:

(a) Squamous metaplasia
(b) Endocervical AIS
(c) LGSIL
(d) HGSIL
(e) Squamous cell carcinoma

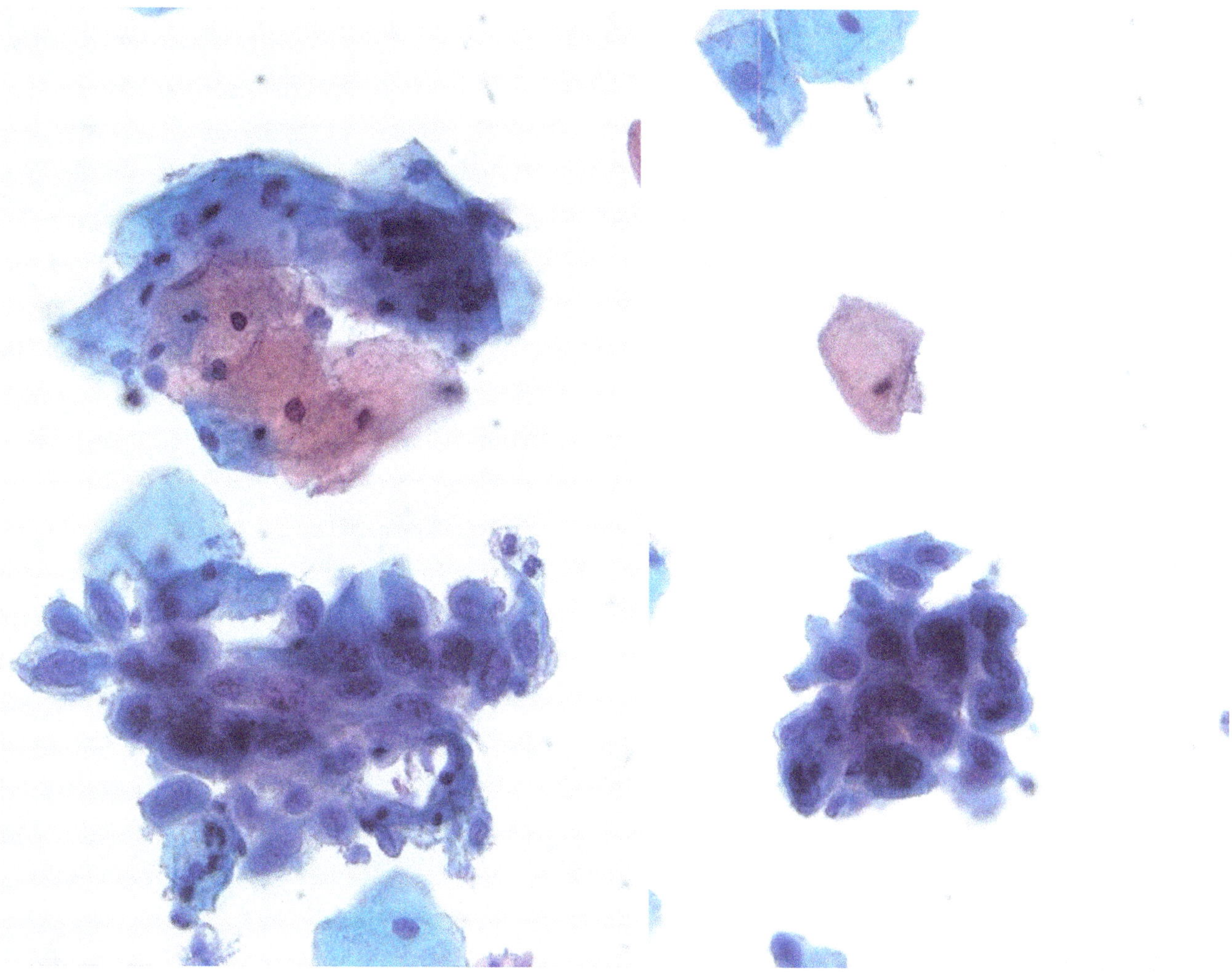

Fig. 4.50

Q-50. A 49-year-old woman had a cervical/vaginal sample processed by the ThinPrep method which showed cells such as seen in these images (medium magnification). Blood or other debris was not noted in the background. The most likely diagnosis is:

(a) Squamous metaplasia
(b) ASCUS
(c) LGSIL
(d) HGSIL
(e) Squamous cell carcinoma

Fig. 4.51

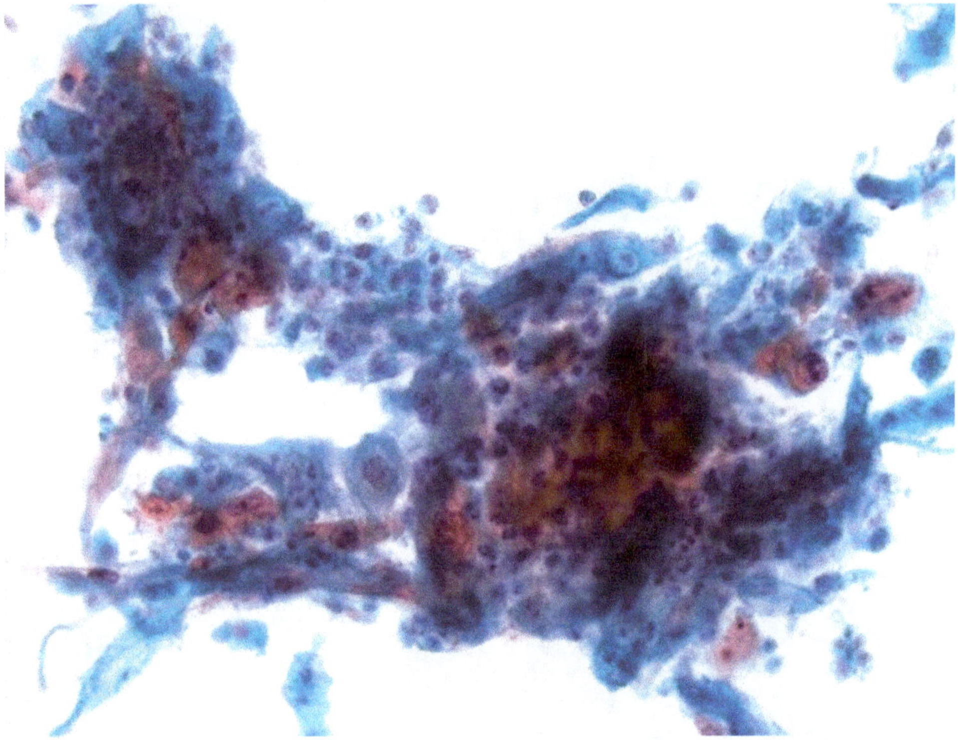

Q-51. A 64-year-old woman had a history of irregular spotting for the last 4 months. Cellular material such as seen in this image was abundant in the SurePath slide (medium magnification). The most likely diagnosis is:
(a) Repair
(b) LGSIL
(c) HGSIL
(d) Squamous cell carcinoma
(e) Adenocarcinoma, NOS

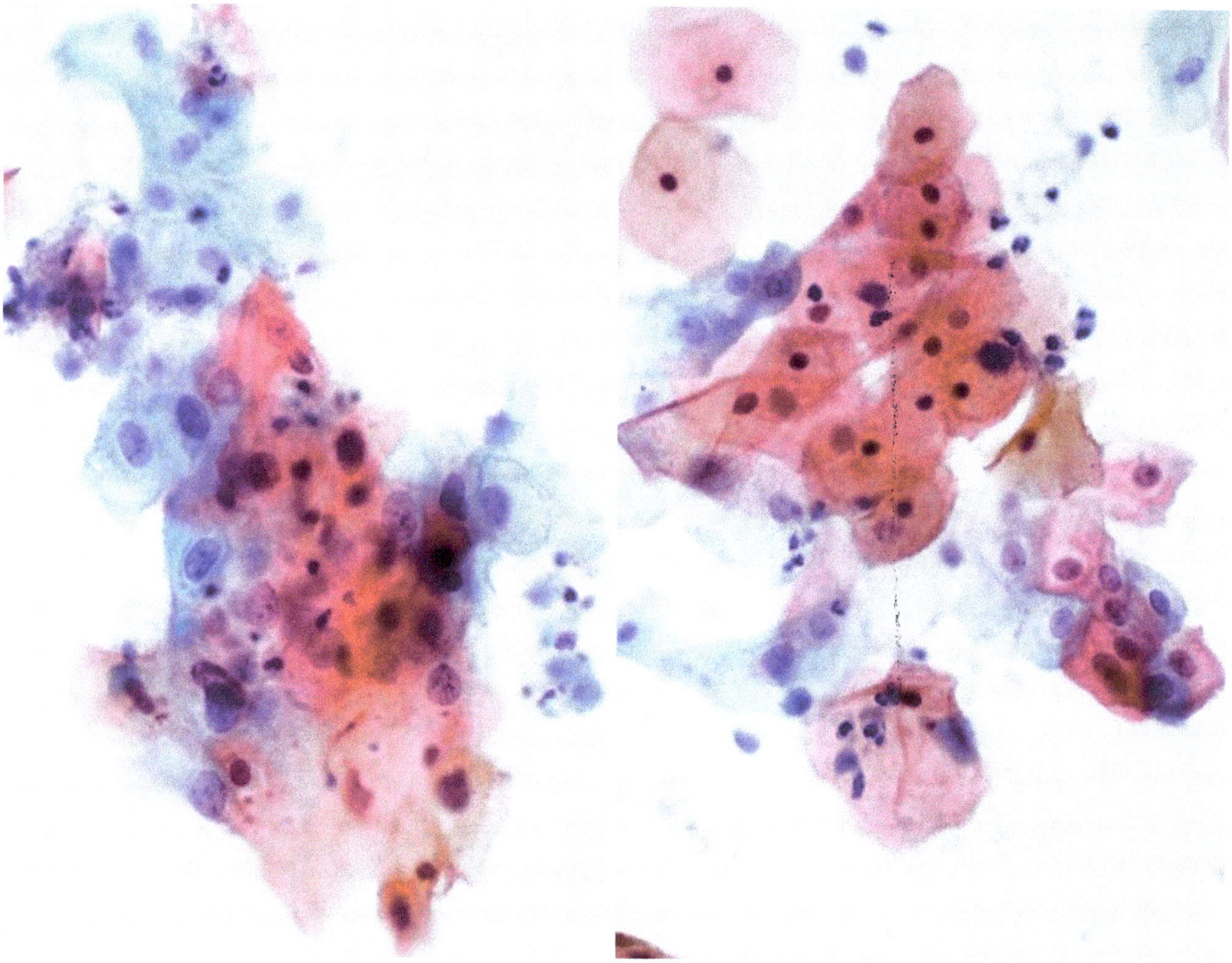

Fig. 4.52

Q-52. This woman's cervical/vaginal ThinPrep slide (medium magnification) showed many cells similar to those seen in these images. The best diagnosis is:
(a) NILM
(b) ASCUS, Trichomonas
(c) LGSIL, Trichomonas
(d) Reactive atypia, Trichomonas

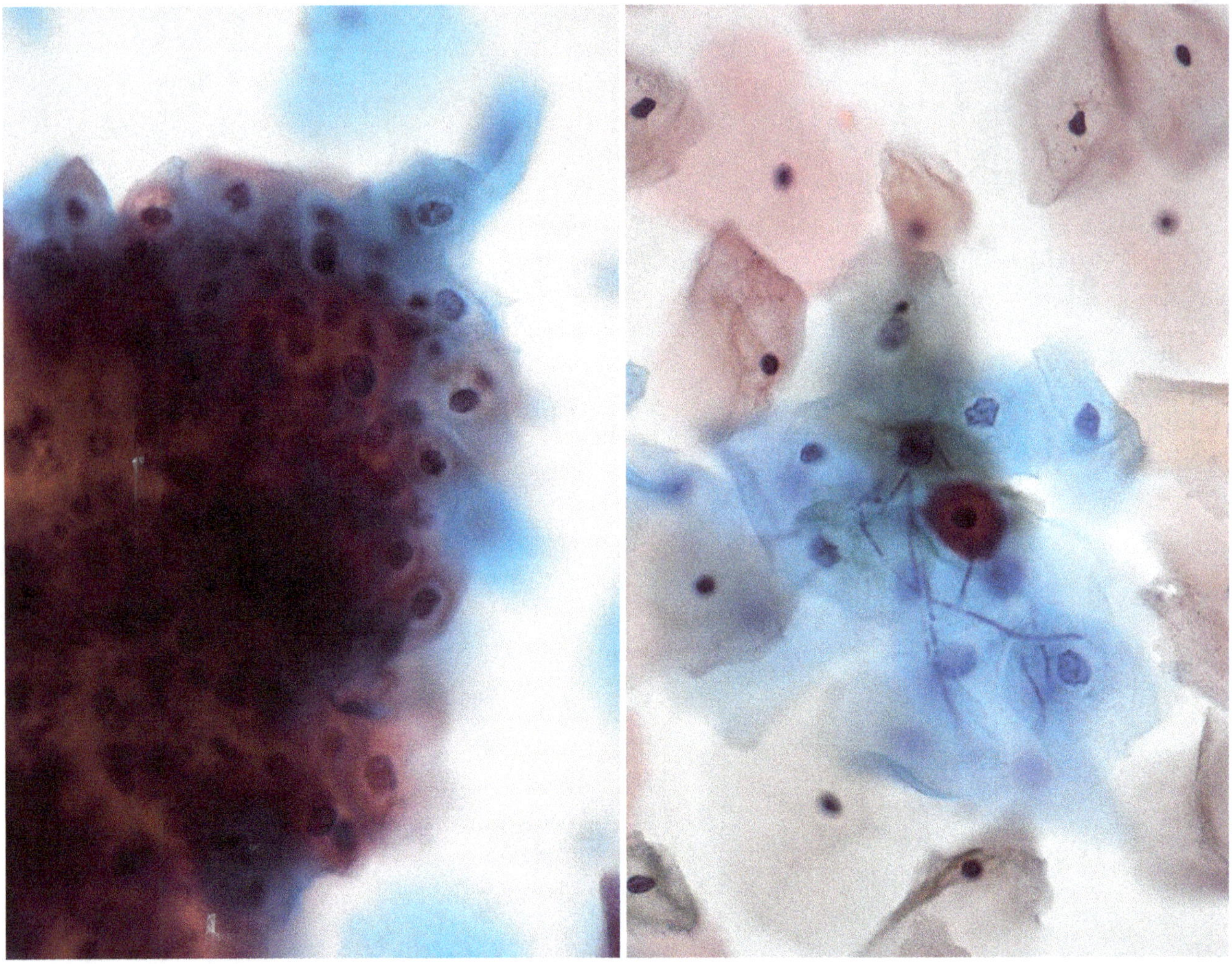

Fig. 4.53

Q-53. This slide was prepared by the SurePath methodology (medium magnification) from the cervical/vaginal material of a 26-year-old patient. The best diagnosis is:

(a) NILM
(b) ASCUS, Candida
(c) LGSIL, Candida
(d) NILM, contaminant fungi
(e) NILM, reactive atypia, Candida

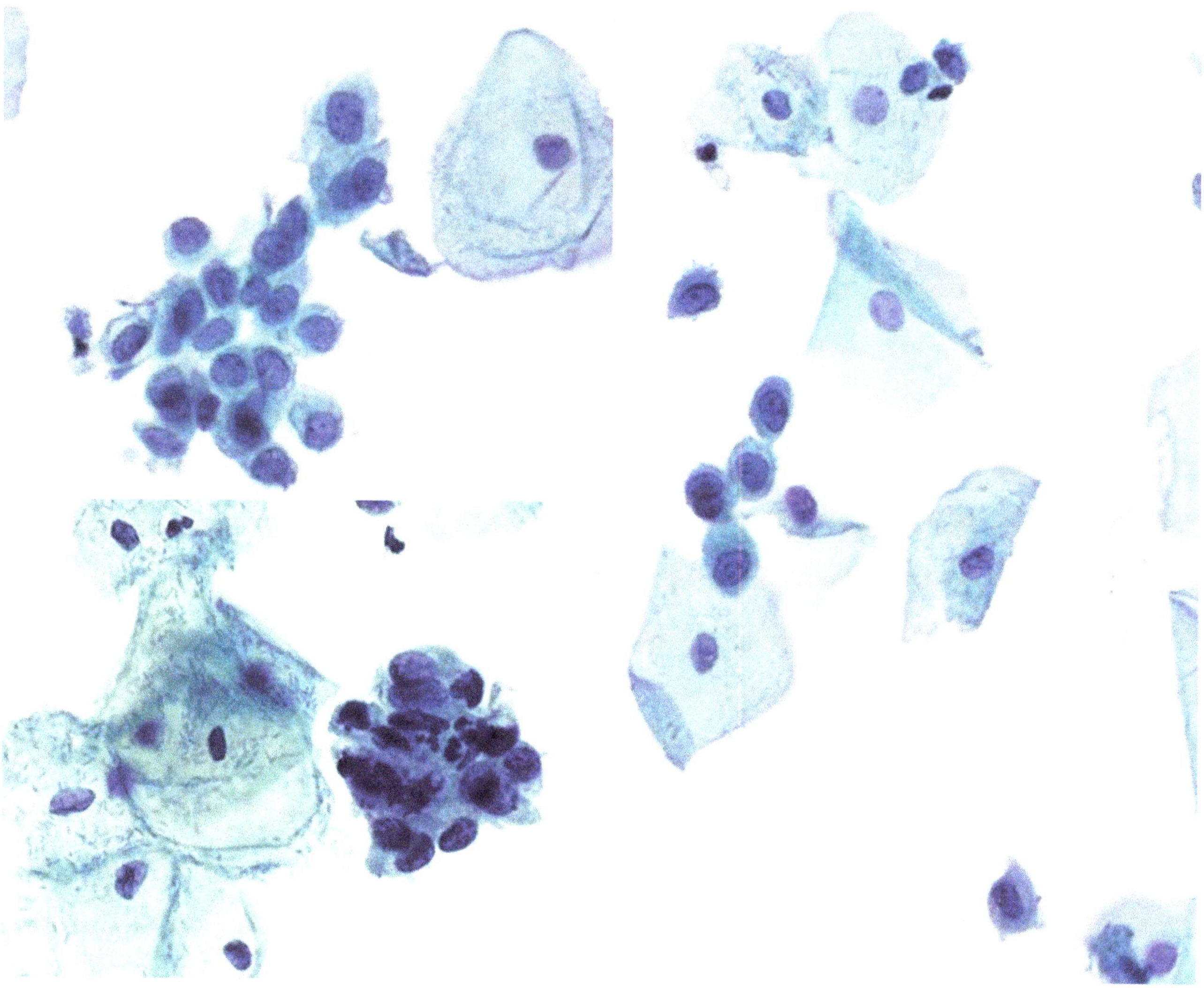

Fig. 4.54

Q-54. Several groups of cells such as these were found in the cervical/vaginal slide (ThinPrep, medium magnification) of a 38-year-old woman with no previous history. The most likely diagnosis is:

(a) Normal endometrial cells
(b) Normal endocervical cells
(c) Squamous metaplasia
(d) ASC-H
(e) HGSIL

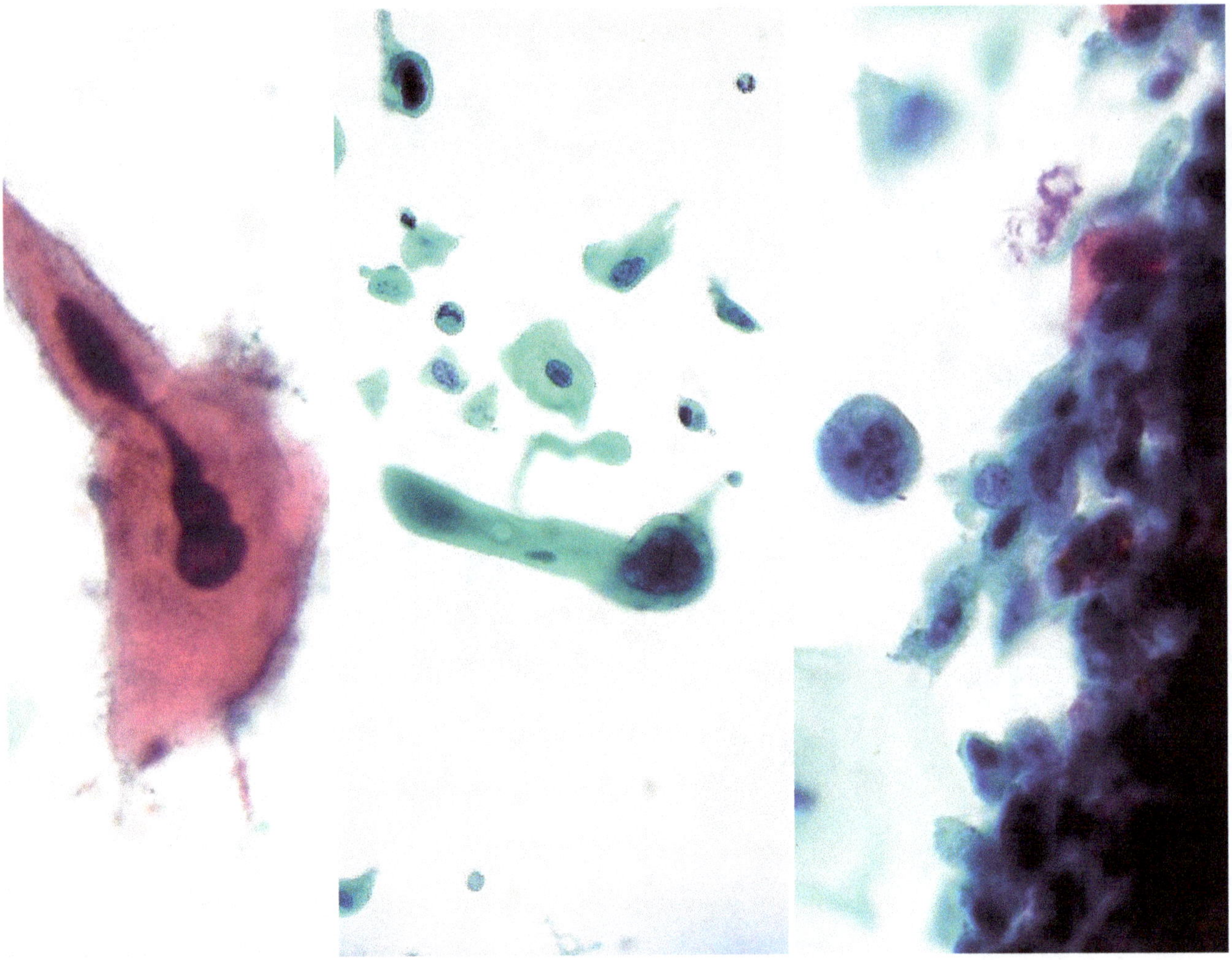

Fig. 4.55

Q-55. Numerous cells similar to those seen in these images were seen in the SurePath preparation of a 59-year-old female (high magnification). The most likely diagnosis is:

(a) Repair
(b) Endocervical adenocarcinoma
(c) Reactive atypia
(d) Tubal metaplasia
(e) Squamous cell carcinoma

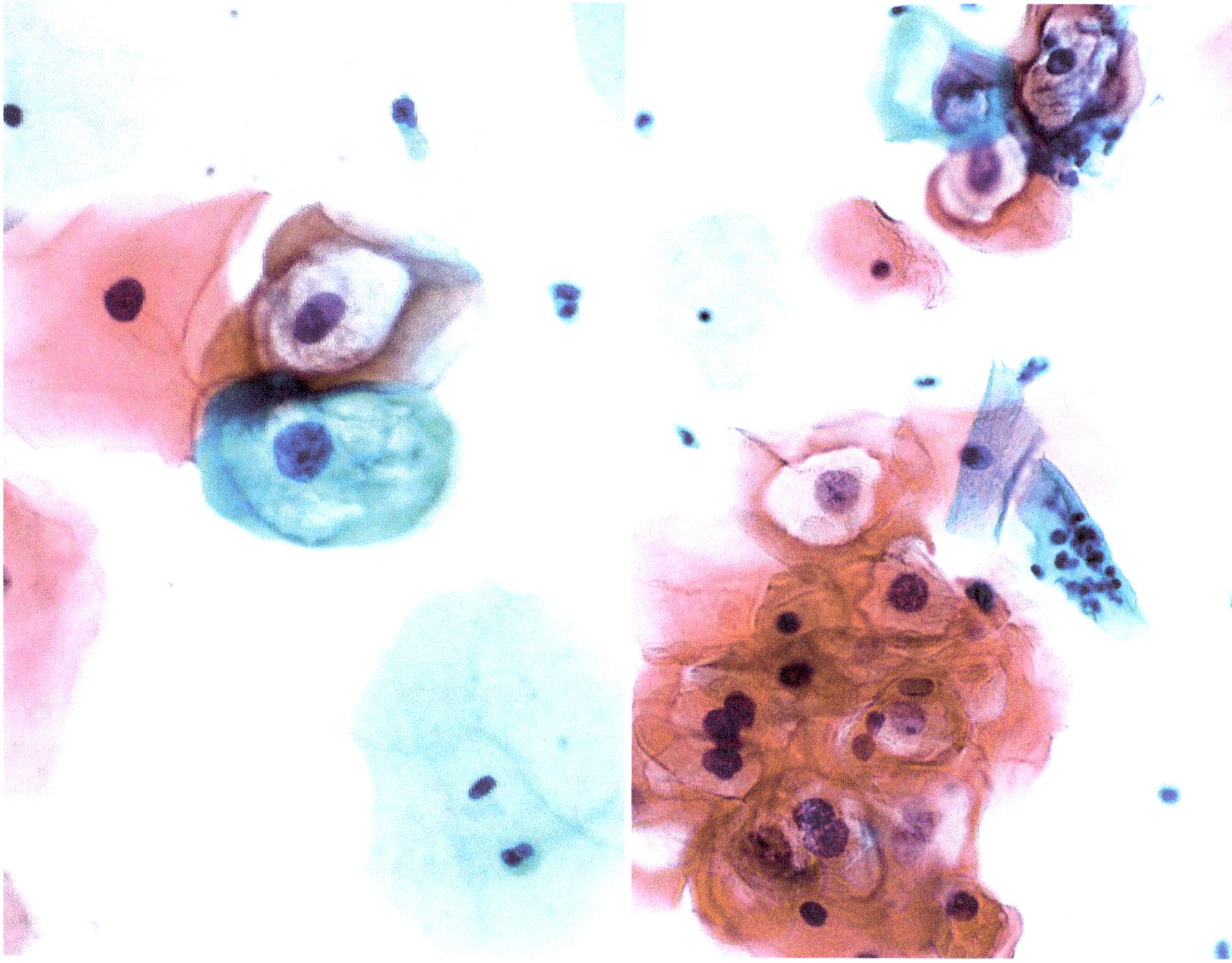

Fig. 4.56

Q-56. Cells such as these were found in the cervical sample from a 29-year-old female (ThinPrep, high and medium magnification). The most likely diagnosis is:
(a) NILM, reactive atypia
(b) ASCUS
(c) LGSIL
(d) Radiation effect

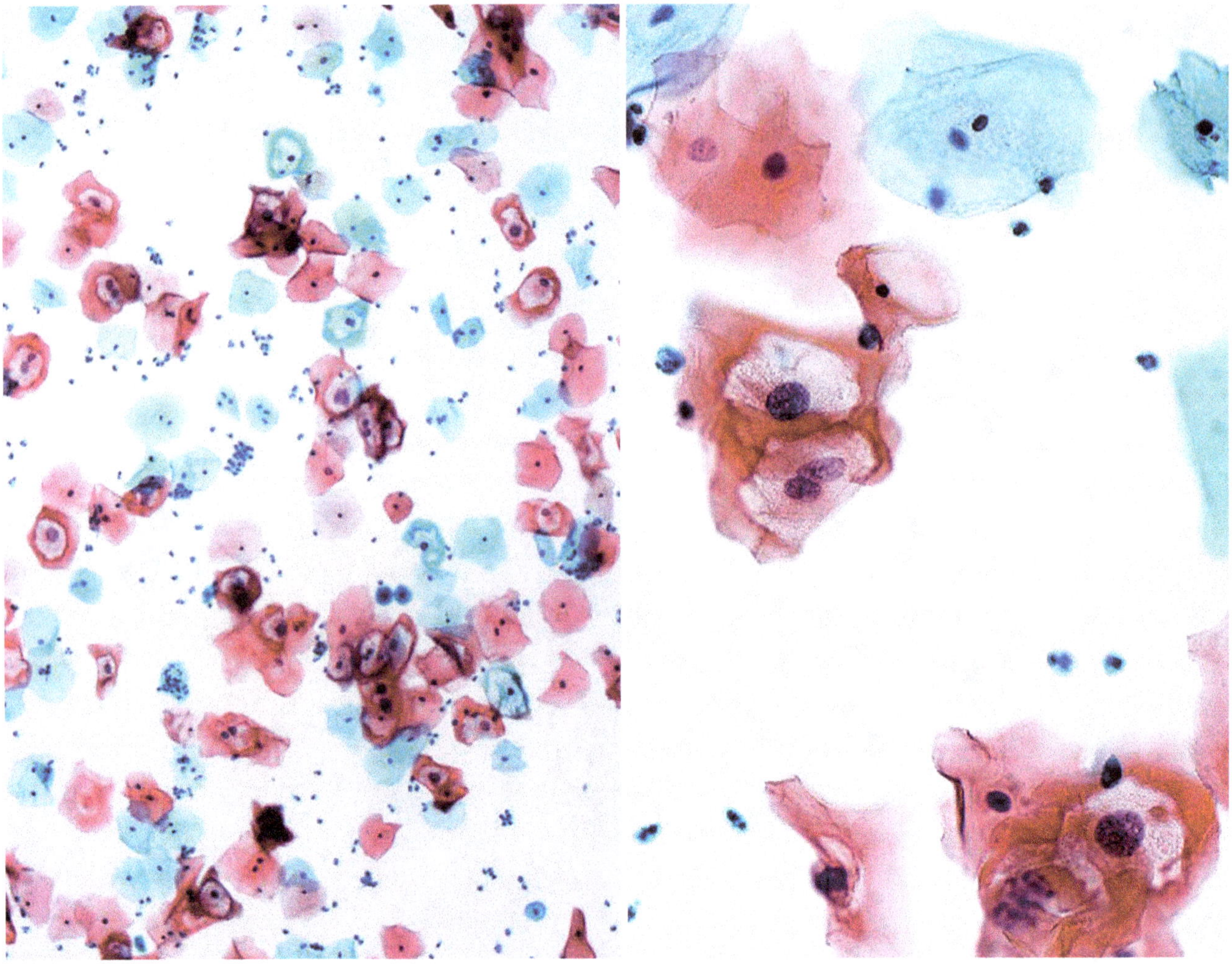

Fig. 4.57

Q-57. Many cells such as these were seen in the cervical material of a 32-year-old woman. The material was processed by ThinPrep (low and medium magnification). The best immediate next step in the follow-up of this patient would be:

(a) Send remaining material for HR HPV testing
(b) Send remaining material for LR and HR HPV testing
(c) Perform a p16 molecular test on the remaining material
(d) Send patient for colposcopically directed biopsy
(e) Repeat Pap in 12 months

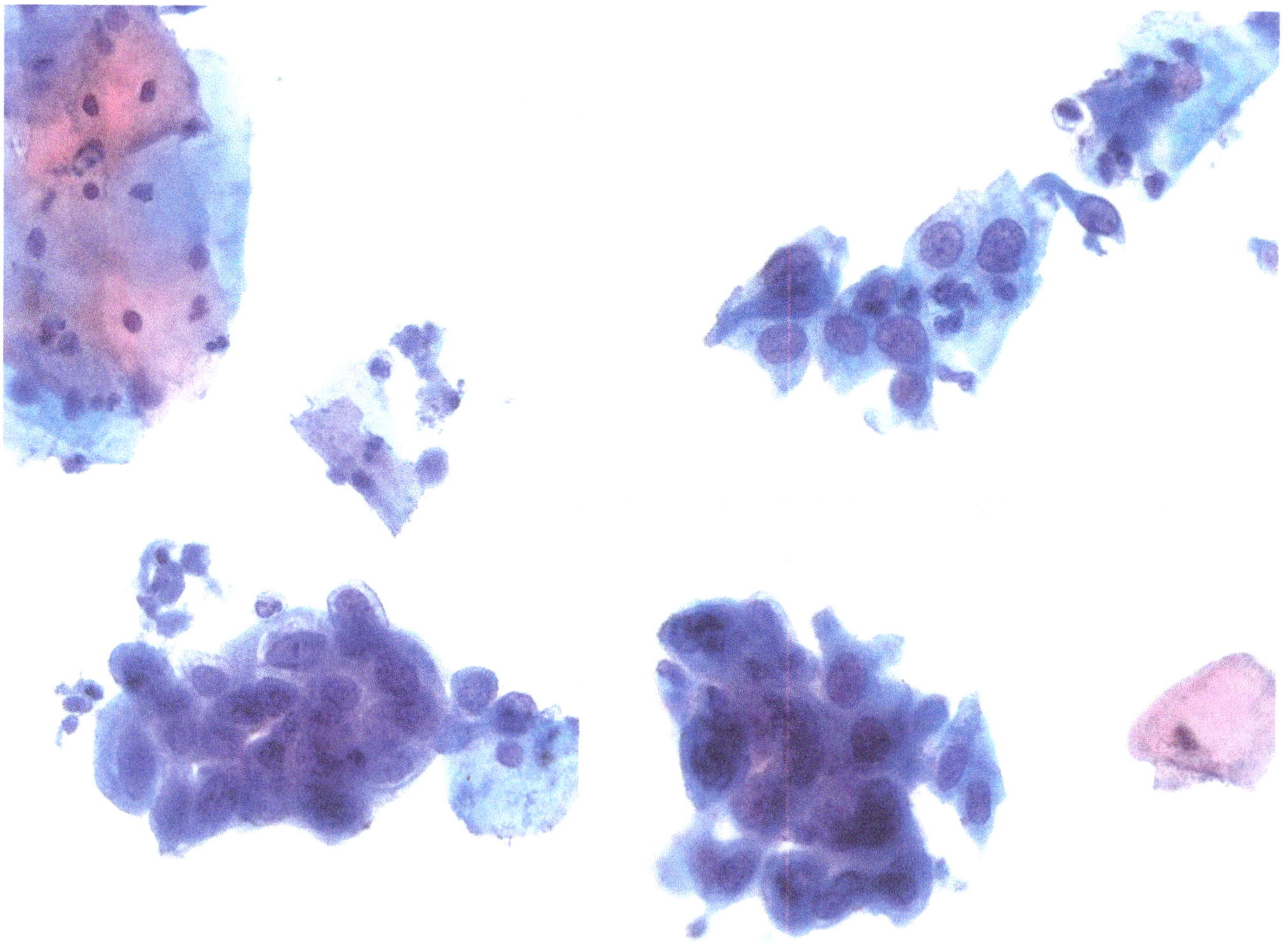

Fig. 4.58

Q-58. A number of cells such as those illustrated here were found in the gynecologic sample of a 44-year-old female (ThinPrep, medium magnification). The best diagnosis is:
(a) Endocervical AIS
(b) Normal endometrial cells
(c) LGSIL
(d) HGSIL
(e) Squamous cell carcinoma

Fig. 4.59

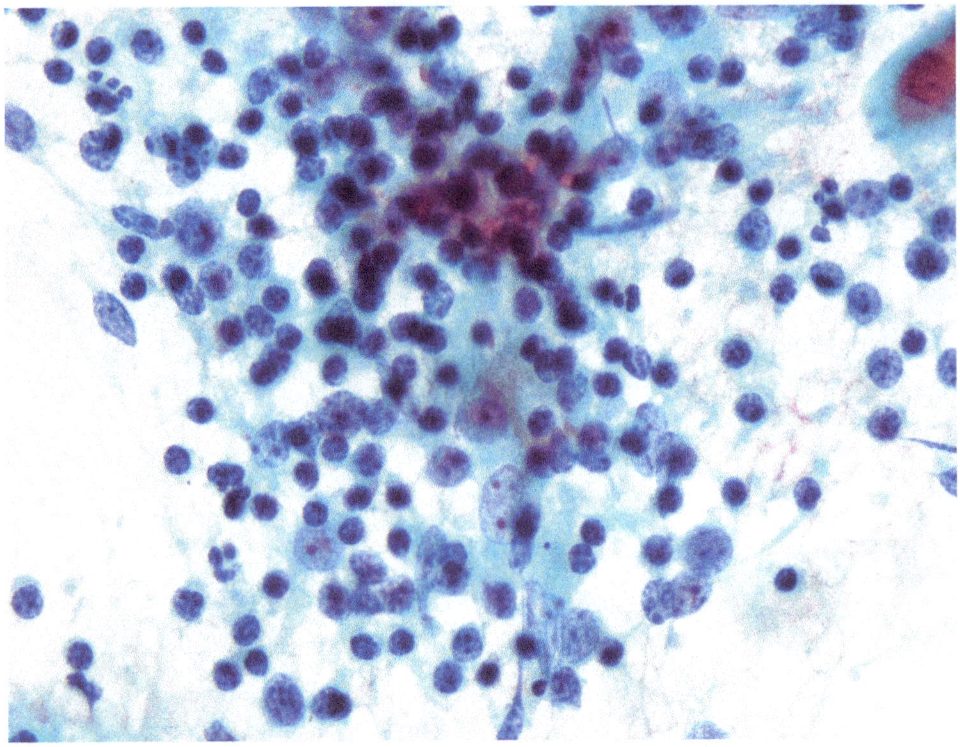

Q-59. A 52-year-old female with a past history of Chlamydia infection presents with no clinical complaints. These cells were discovered on her conventional Pap smear (high magnification). The most likely diagnosis is:
(a) Leukemia
(b) Severe acute inflammation
(c) Small cell carcinoma of the cervix
(d) Chronic follicular cervicitis

Fig. 4.60

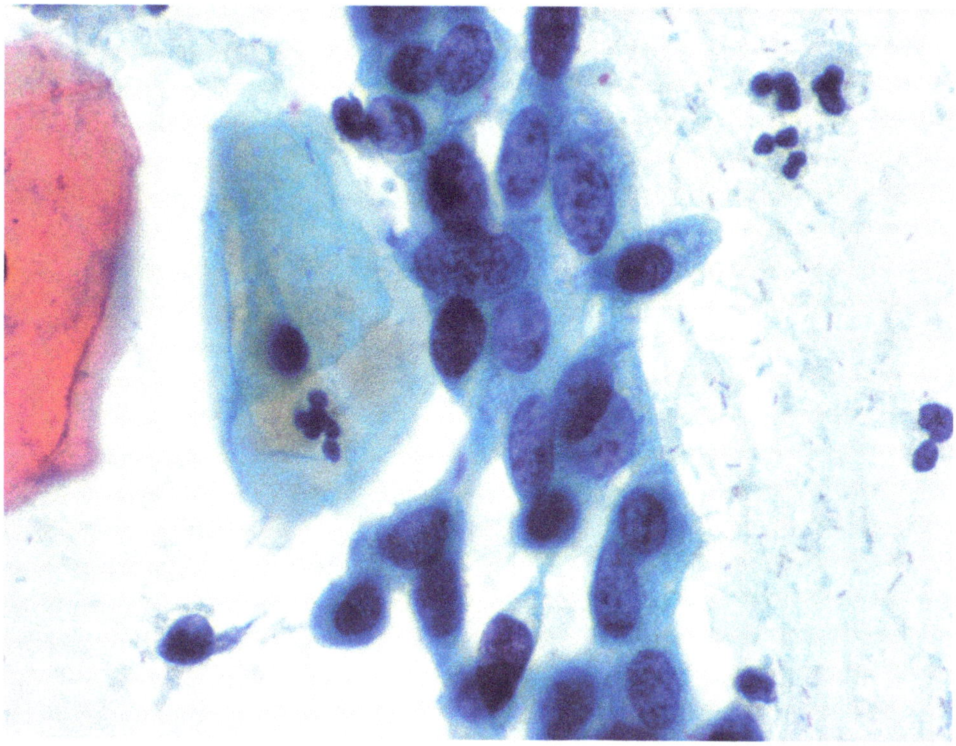

Q-60. A 36 year-old female demonstrated many cells such as these in a conventional Pap smear (high magnification). The background appeared clean. The most likely diagnosis is:

(a) LGSIL
(b) HGSIL
(c) Squamous cell carcinoma
(d) Endometrial adenocarcinoma

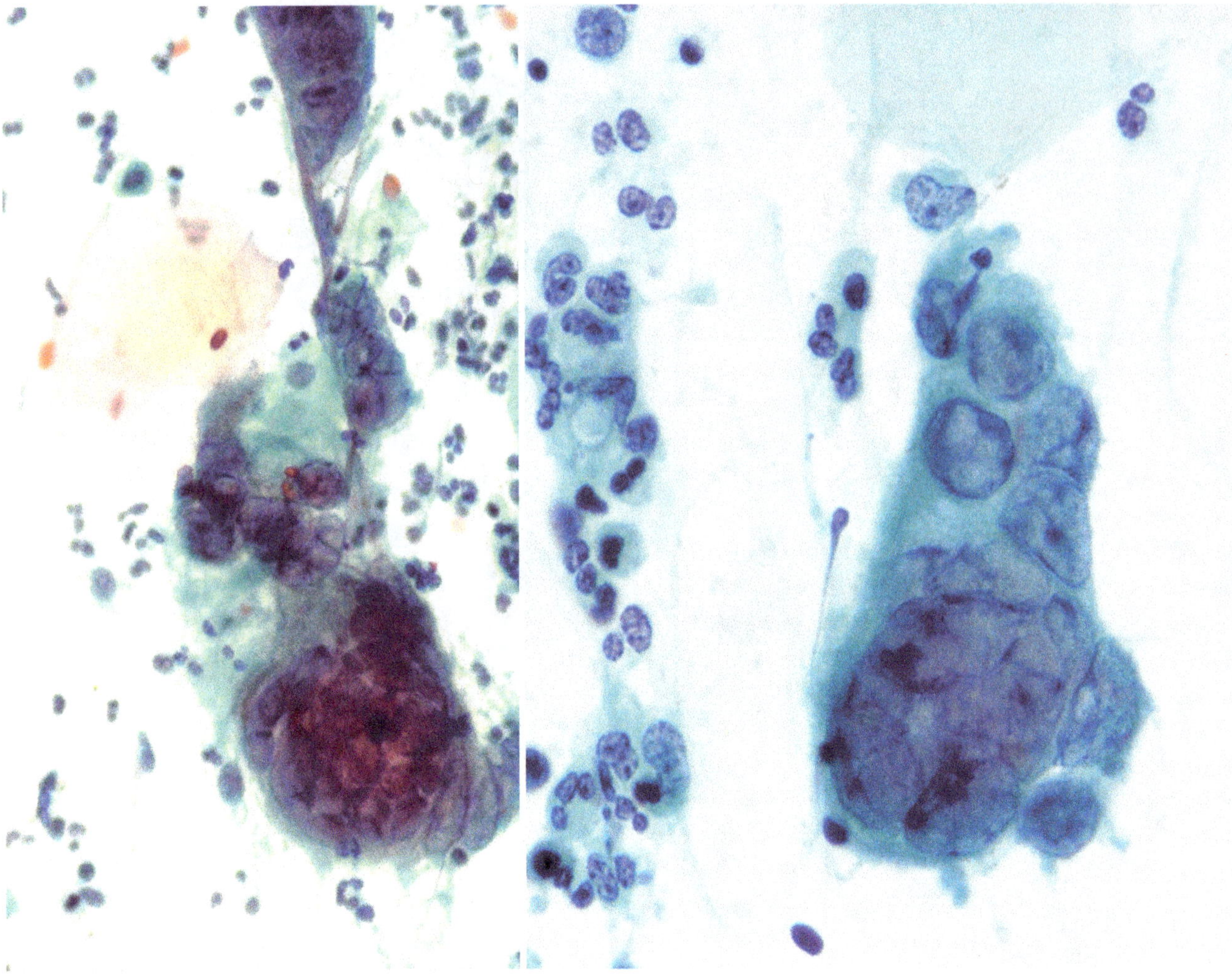

Fig. 4.61

Q-61. This 36-year-old patient is seen for her first prenatal care at 8 months gestation. Several clusters of cells such as these were seen on the conventional Pap (medium and high magnification). The most likely diagnosis and appropriate follow-up is:

(a) Syncytiotrophoblasts, schedule a D and C for incomplete miscarriage
(b) Multinucleated histiocytes, no follow-up needed
(c) Herpes simplex, plan for Cesarean section at delivery
(d) HGSIL, schedule colposcopically directed biopsy after delivery

Fig. 4.62

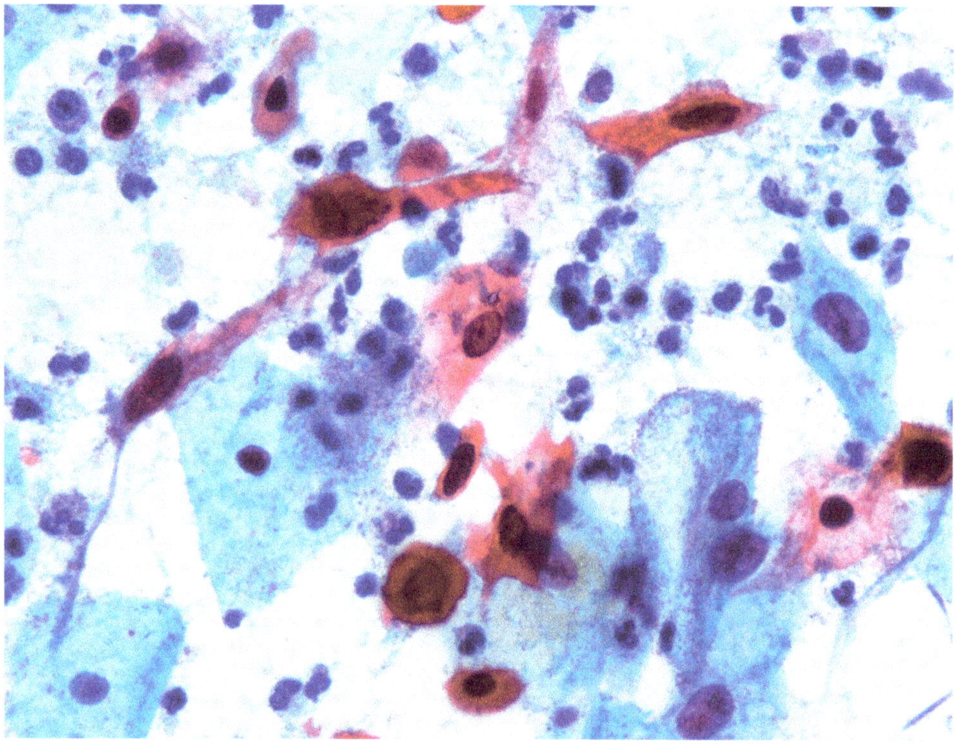

Q-62. This 58-year-old patient presented with a history of occasional spotting and back pain. She did not have a Pap in the last 8 years (conventional, high magnification). The most likely diagnosis with its accompanying risk factor is:

(a) Squamous cell carcinoma, HPV subtype 16 or 18 infection
(b) Endometrial adenocarcinoma, obesity
(c) Endocervical adenocarcinoma, HPV subtype 16 or 18
(d) Ovarian adenocarcinoma, herpes simplex infection

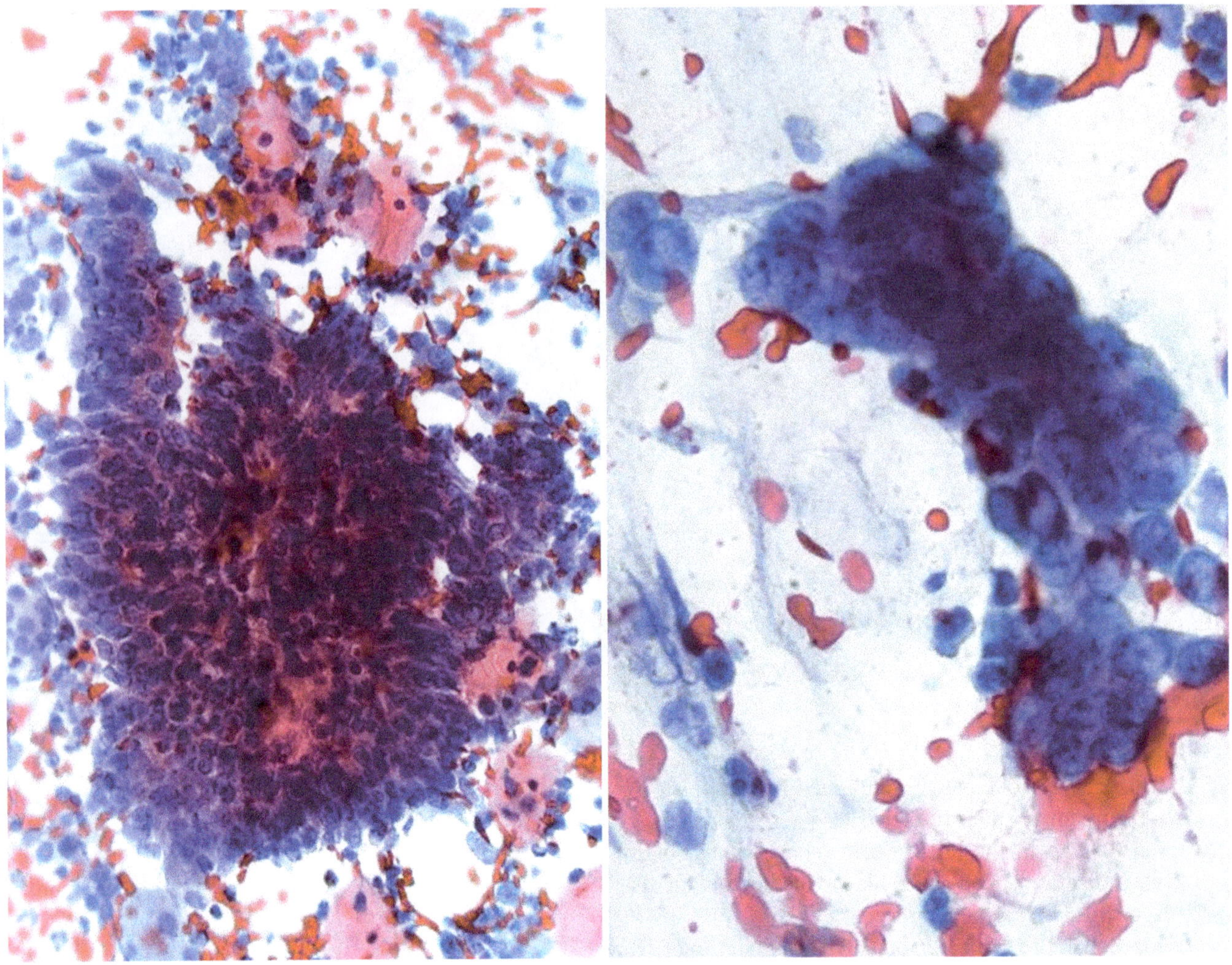

Fig. 4.63

Q-63. A 32-year-old woman has a past history of an abnormal Pap smear and current clinical history of postcoital spotting. Many groups of cells with the cellular morphology displayed are noted in the conventional slide (low and high magnification). Nucleoli are inconspicuous or absent. The most likely diagnosis is:
(a) Squamous cell carcinoma
(b) HGSIL (CIS)
(c) Endocervical adenocarcinoma
(d) Endocervical adenocarcinoma in situ

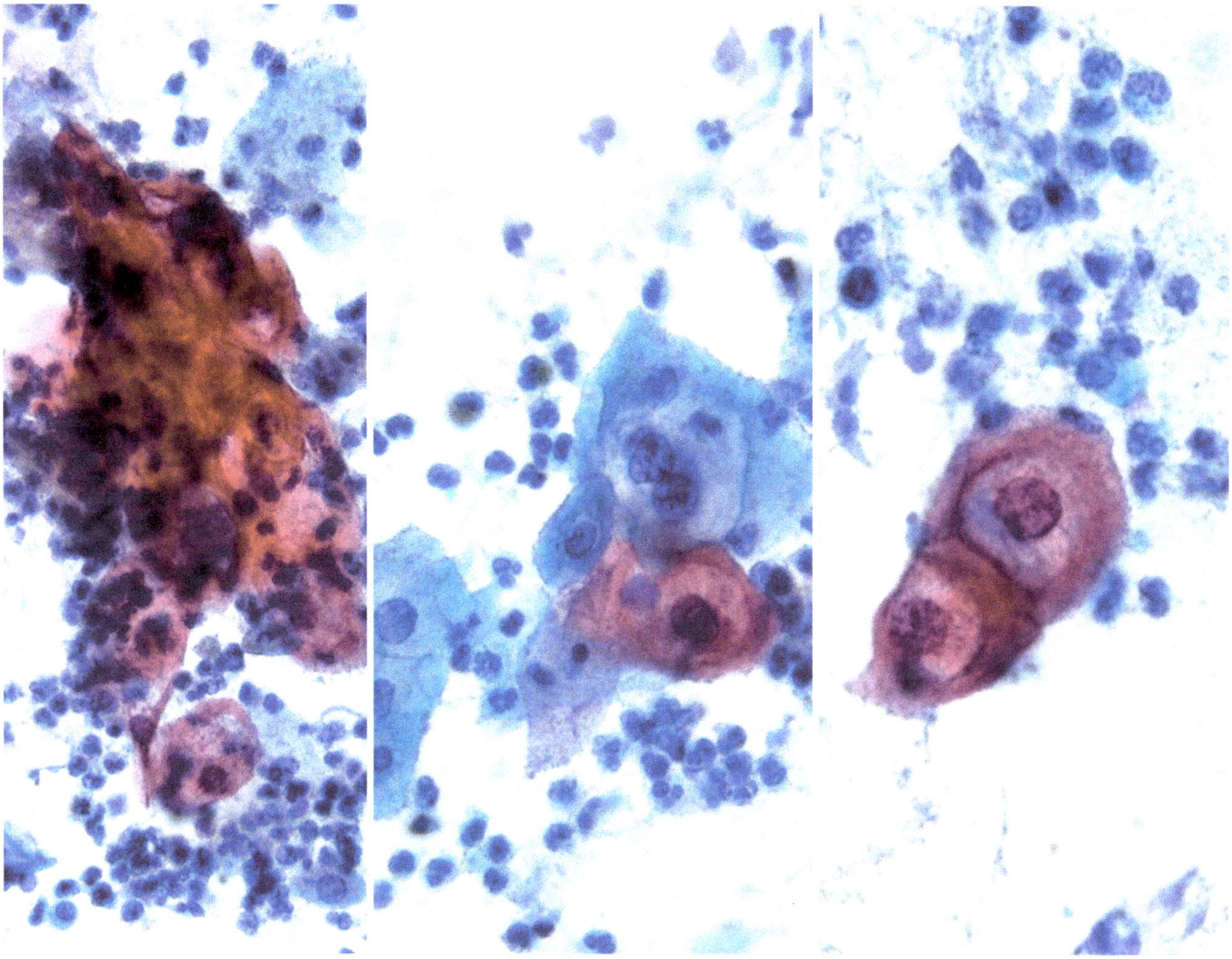

Fig. 4.64

Q-64. Cells of this type were identified within the conventional Pap smear of a 19-year-old woman (medium magnification). The most likely diagnosis is:

(a) Reactive inflammatory cell changes
(b) ASCUS
(c) LGSIL
(d) HGSIL

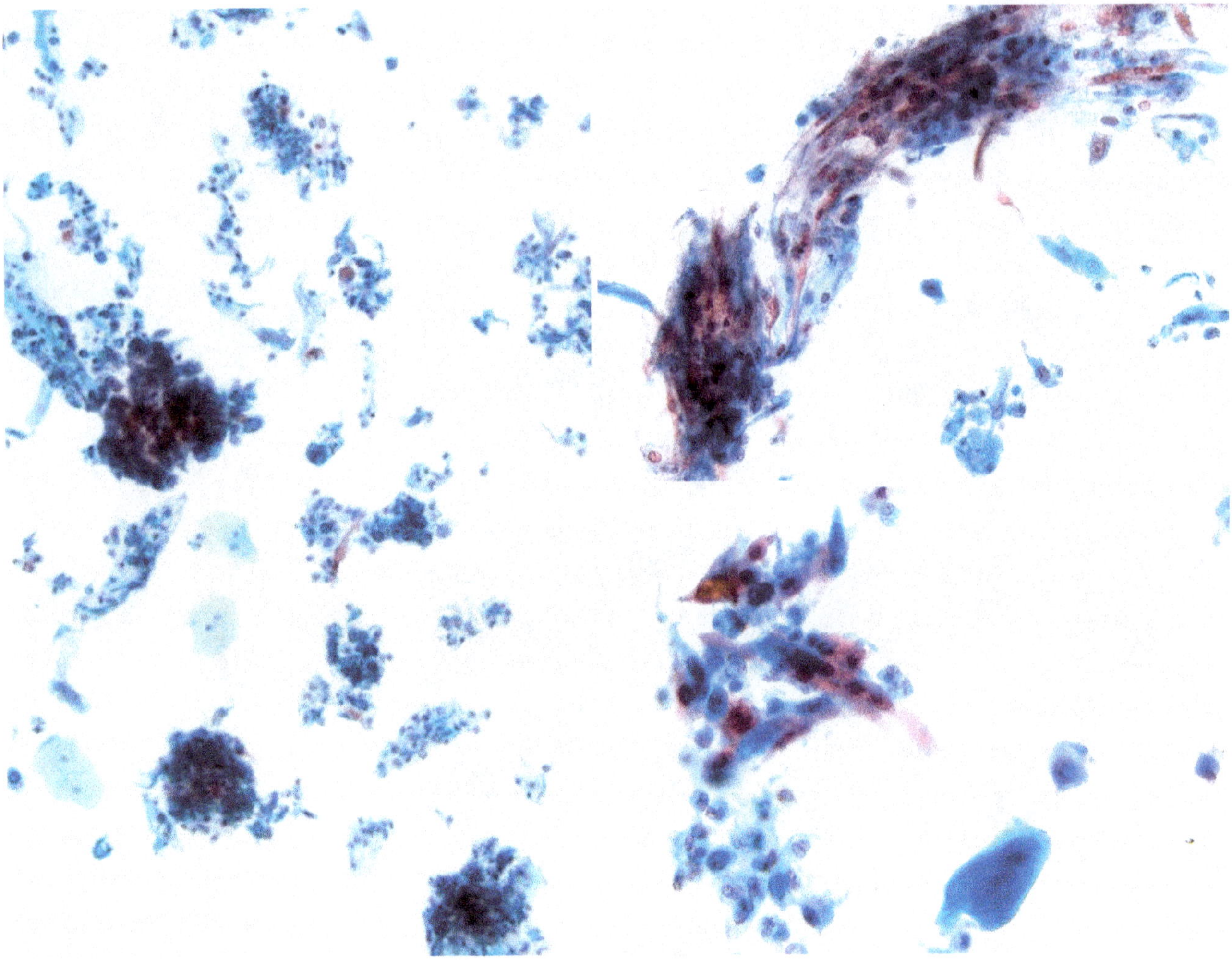

Fig. 4.65

Q-65. (SurePath, low magnification left and upper right, high magnification on the lower right). The anatomic site of origin of these cells is most likely:

(a) In the endometrium
(b) In the endocervical glands
(c) In the fallopian tubes
(d) From the squamocolumnar junction

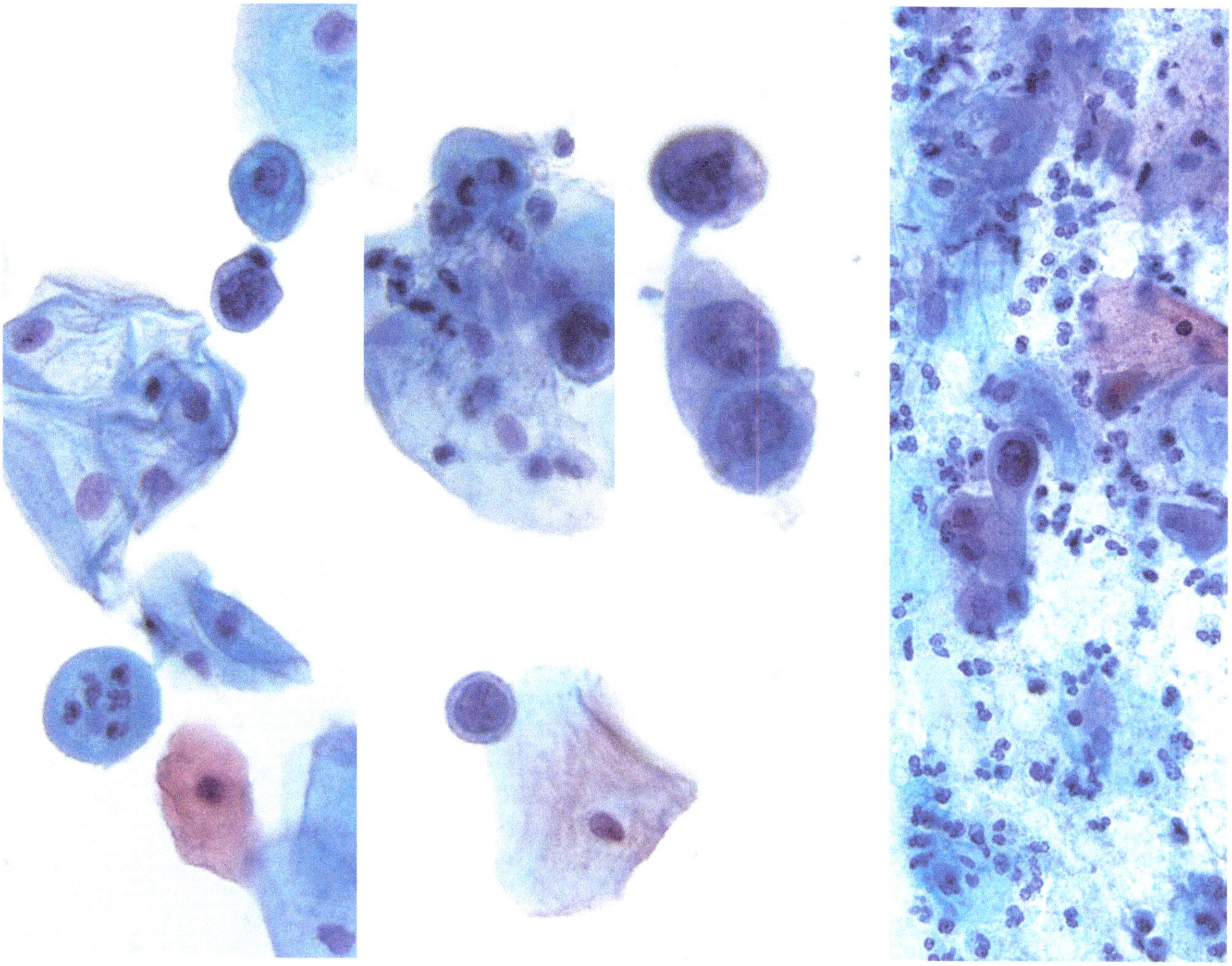

Fig. 4.66

Q-66. A relatively small number of cells such as these were found in the ThinPrep slide (medium magnification except right middle panel which is high magnification) from a 41-year-old woman. The most appropriate diagnosis and follow-up for this case is:

(a) Reactive endocervical cells, NILM, repeat Pap in 1 year
(b) ASCUS, HR HPV testing
(c) ASC-H, HR HPV testing
(d) ASC-H, immediate colposcopically directed biopsy

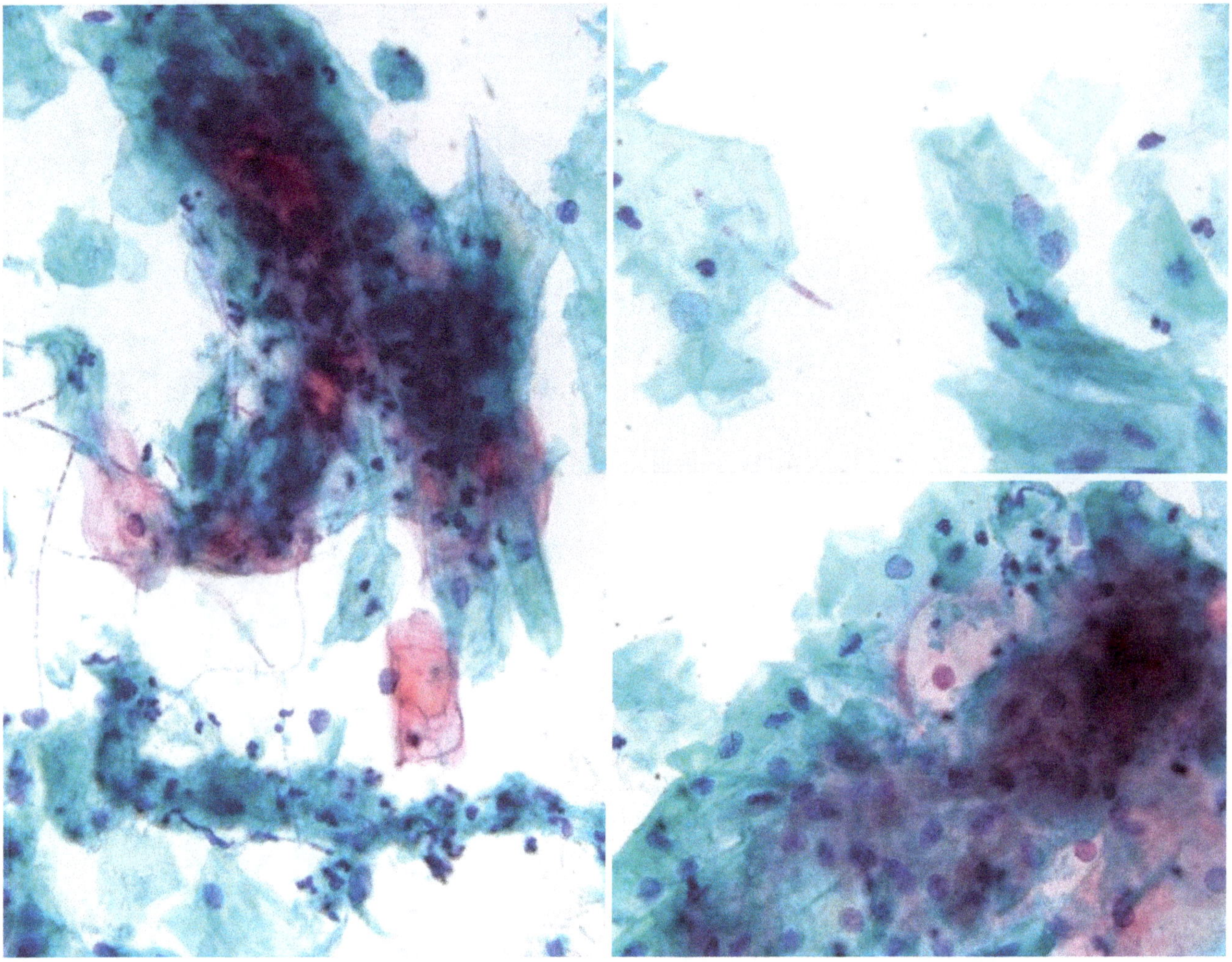

Fig. 4.67

Q-67. A 36-year-old female in the fourth month of pregnancy presents to the gynecologist with clinical symptoms of irritation and vaginal discharge. The cytologic presentation is seen in these three images (ThinPrep, medium left panel and right lower panel, high upper right panel). The most likely diagnosis is:

(a) Candida
(b) Syncytiotrophoblasts
(c) Repair
(d) CMV

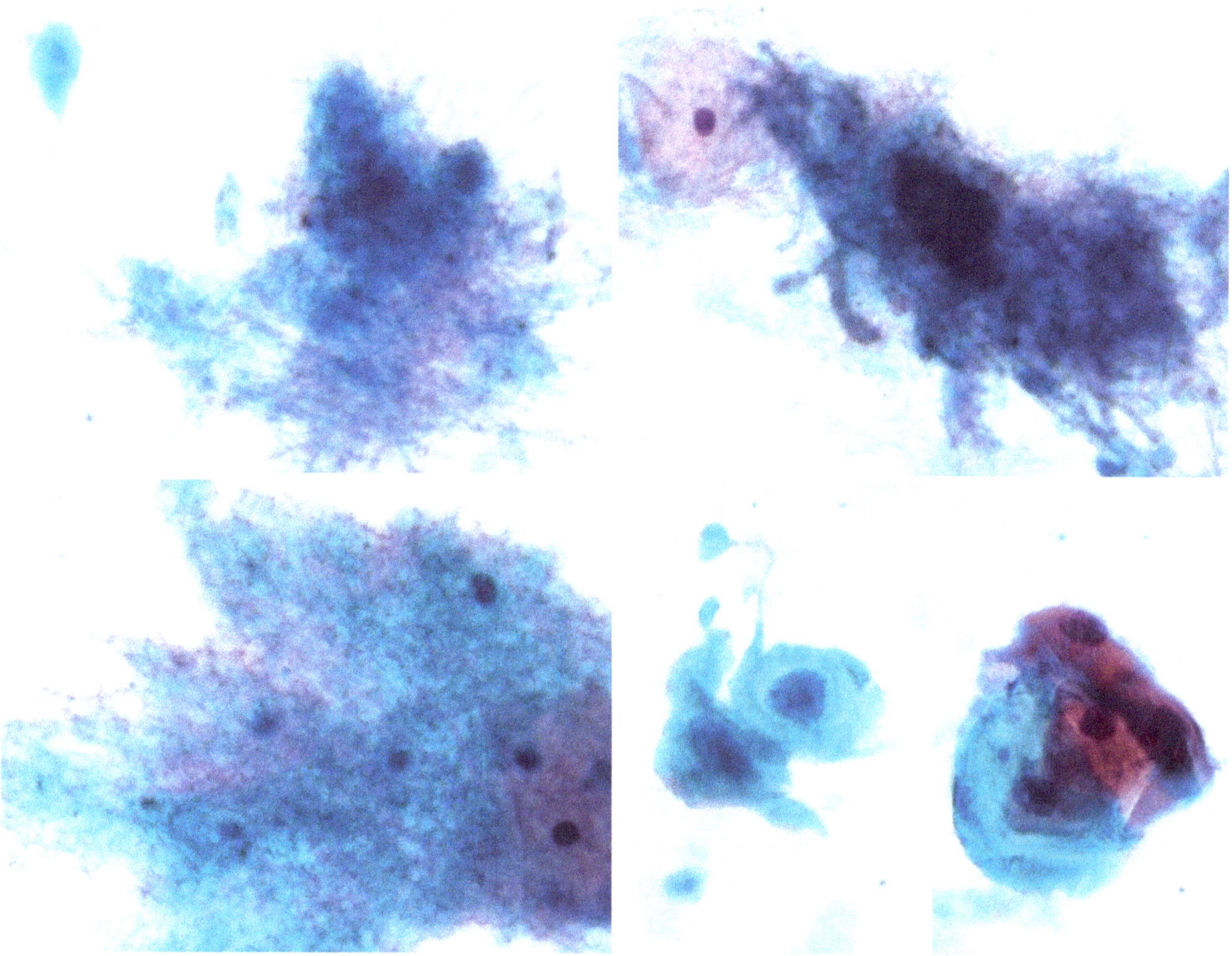

Fig. 4.68

Q-68. Identify two infectious organisms in these panels (ThinPrep, medium magnification, left two panels and right upper panel, high magnification, bottom right and center):

(a) Herpes, Candida
(b) Actinomyces, Trichomonas
(c) CMV, cytolysis
(d) Actinomyces, Candida

Fig. 4.69

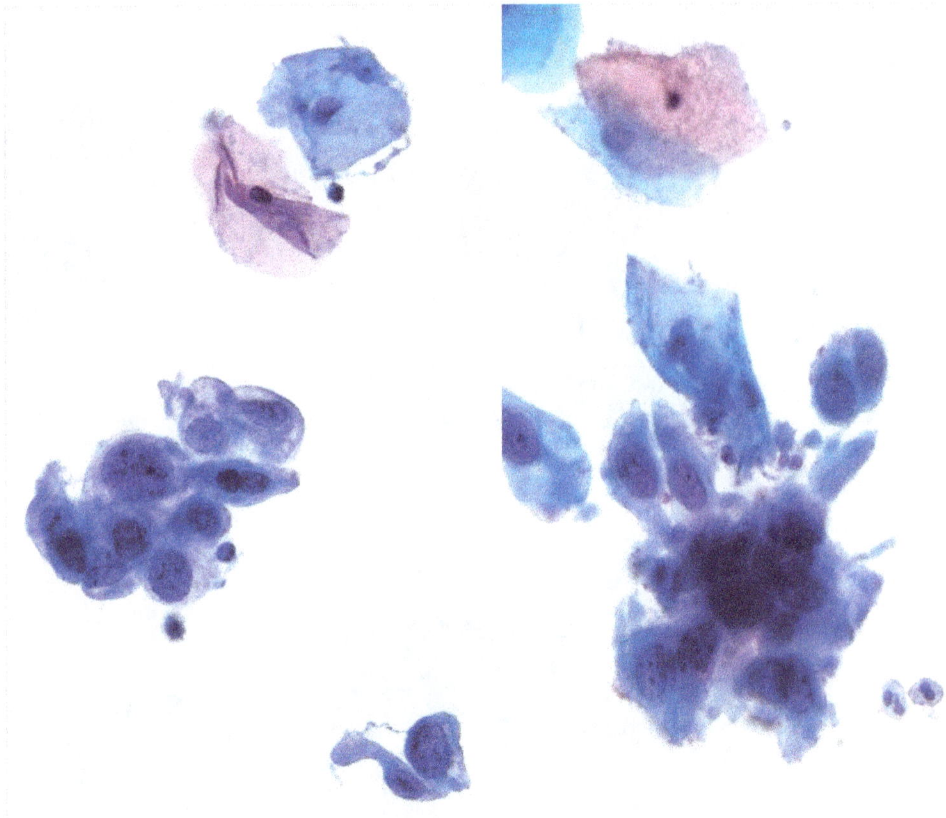

Q-69. A number of cells such as these were found on the gynecologic sample from a 48-year-old female (ThinPrep, medium magnification). High-risk HPV subtyping was also performed. The most likely results from the HPV test are:

(a) HPV subtype 6 positive
(b) HPV subtype 11 positive
(c) HPV subtype 16 positive
(d) HPV subtype 40 positive

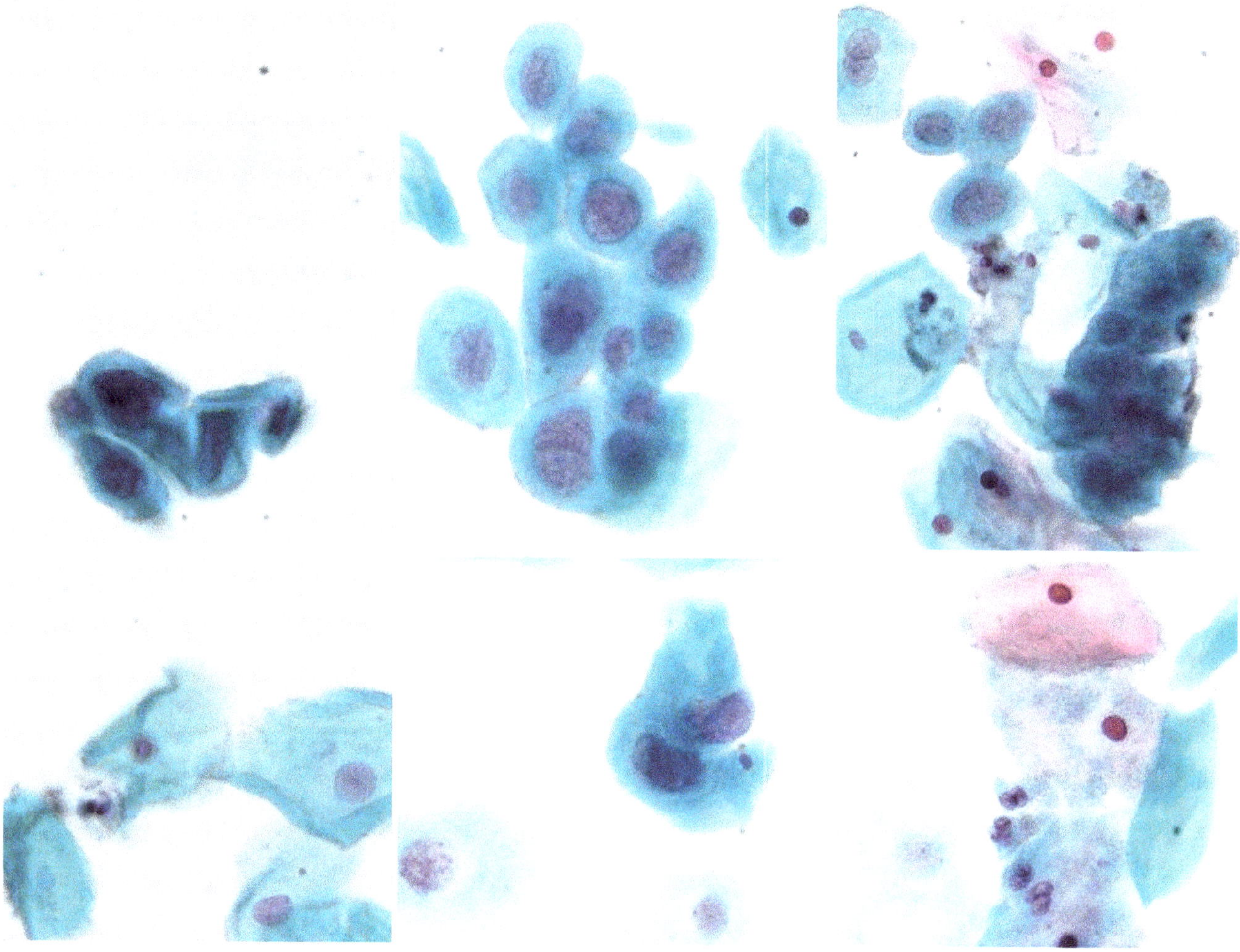

Fig. 4.70

Q-70. These cells were found in the gynecologic sample of a 28-year-old woman. The most likely diagnosis is:

(a) Folic acid deficiency, NILM
(b) Squamous metaplasia, NILM
(c) Herpes, NILM
(d) Reactive endocervical cells, NILM
(e) HGSIL

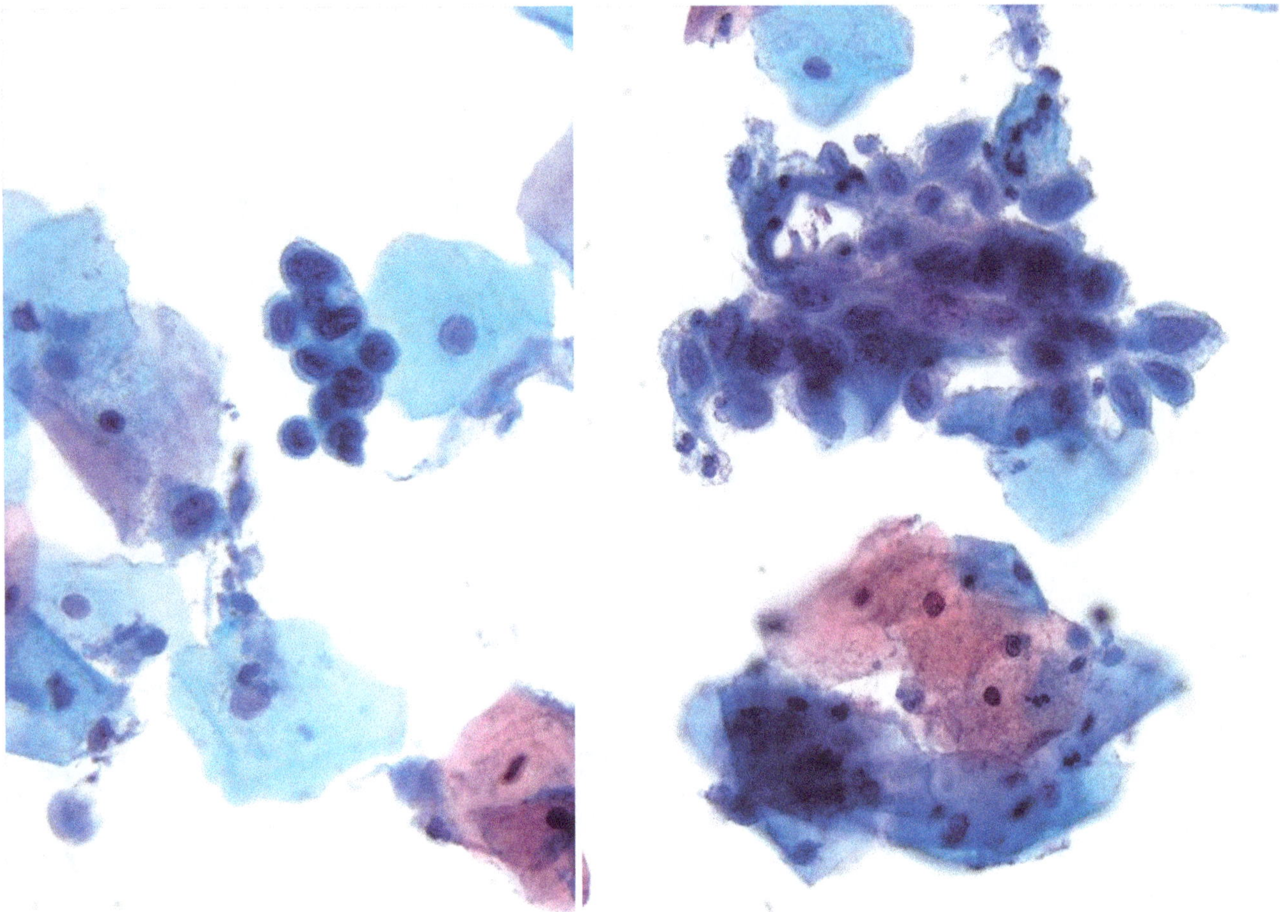

Fig. 4.71

Q-71. A 29-year-old patient displayed a number of these cells on her gynecologic sample (ThinPrep, medium magnification). The best diagnosis would be:
(a) Endometrial cells, NILM
(b) Chronic follicular cervicitis, NILM
(c) Squamous metaplasia, NILM
(d) HGSIL

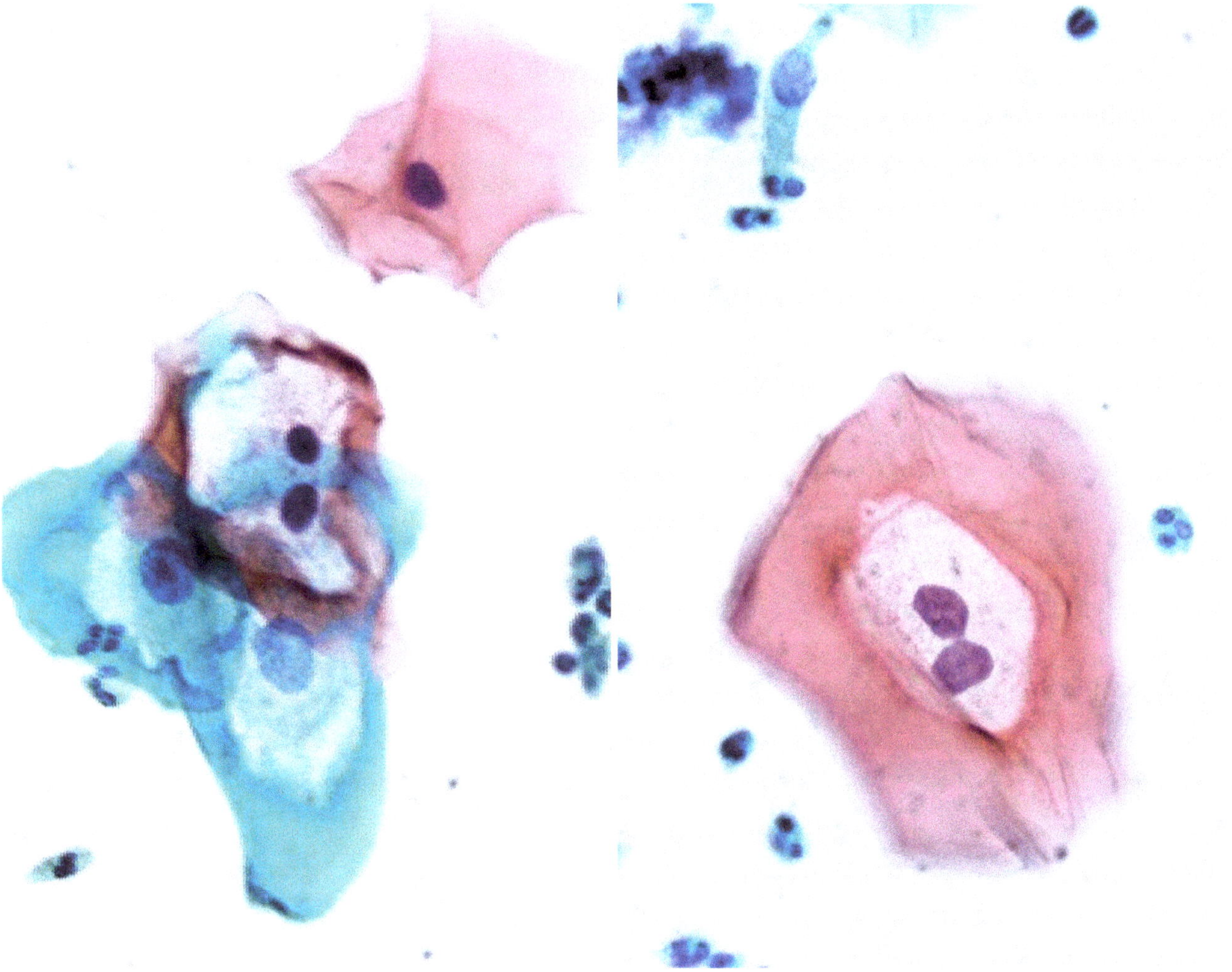

Fig. 4.72

Q-72. Which of the following statements is true about the lesion depicted here (ThinPrep, high magnification)?

(a) >80 % of LGSIL contains HR HPV subtypes
(b) Almost all CIN 3 lesions contain high-risk HPV subtypes.
(c) Pregnant patients frequently display glycogen in the perinuclear area of the cell.
(d) All patients with this lesion should receive HR HPV testing.

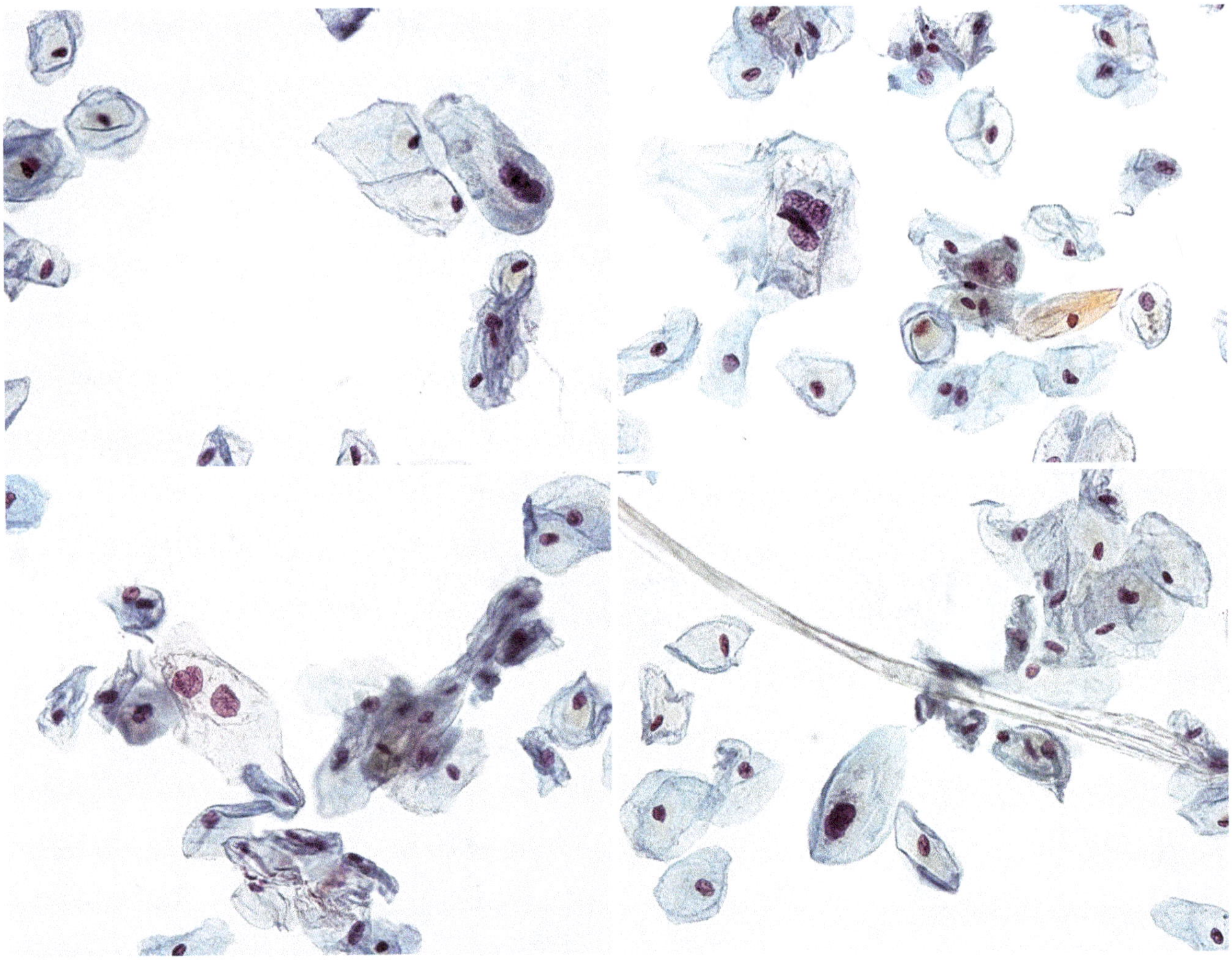

Fig. 4.73

Q-73. A 32-year-old woman with no previous abnormal history occasionally displayed the following cells in her gynecologic sample (ThinPrep, medium magnification). She was G2P1 and in the fifth month of her pregnancy. The most likely diagnosis is:

(a) LGSIL
(b) Radiation effect
(c) Folic acid deficiency
(d) IUD effect

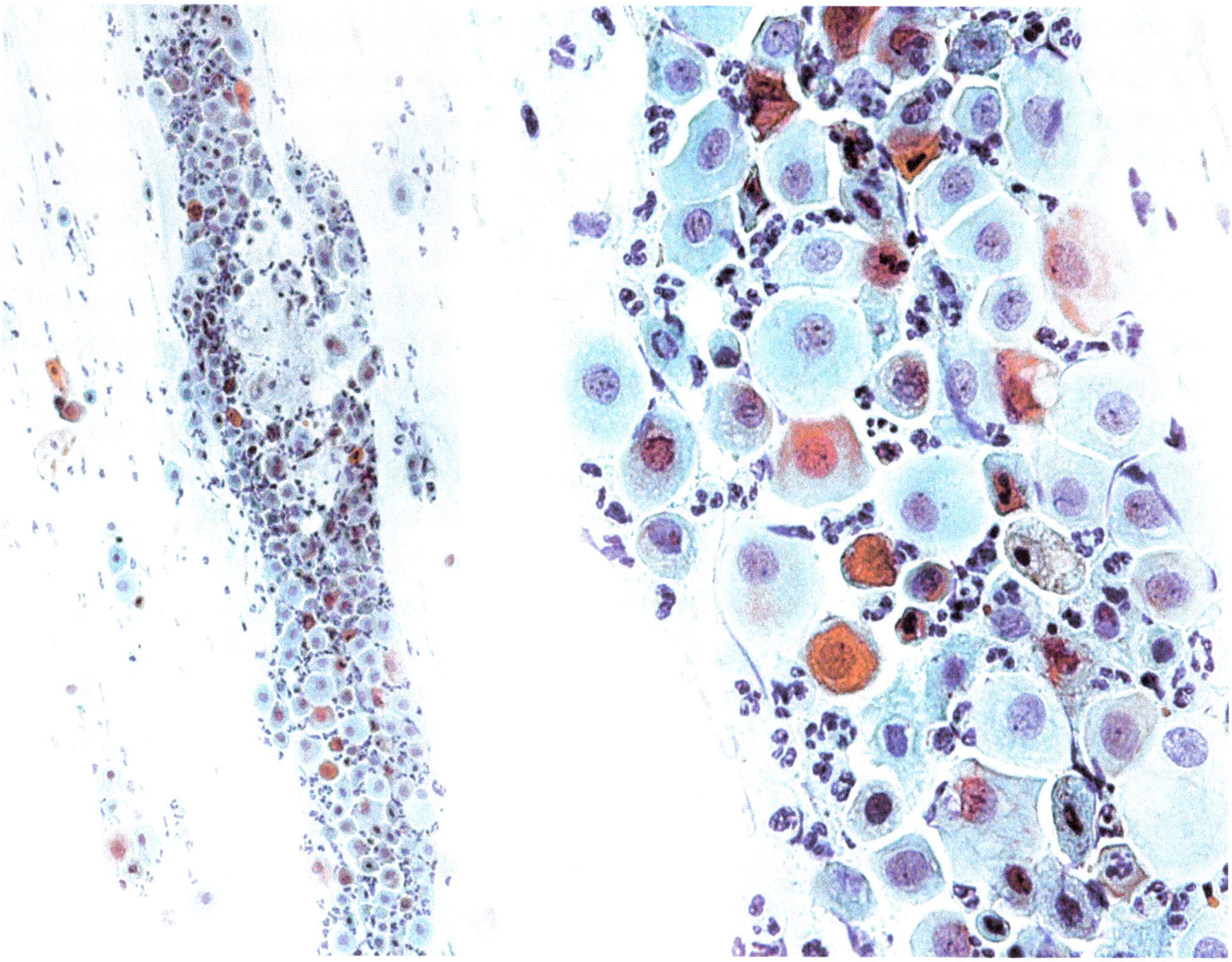

Fig. 4.74

Q-74. These cells were uniformly present in the gynecologic sample of a 65-year-old woman (conventional, low and medium magnification). The orange small cells are most likely:

(a) Degenerated parabasal cells
(b) Parakeratosis
(c) Squamous metaplasia
(d) HGSIL

Fig. 4.75

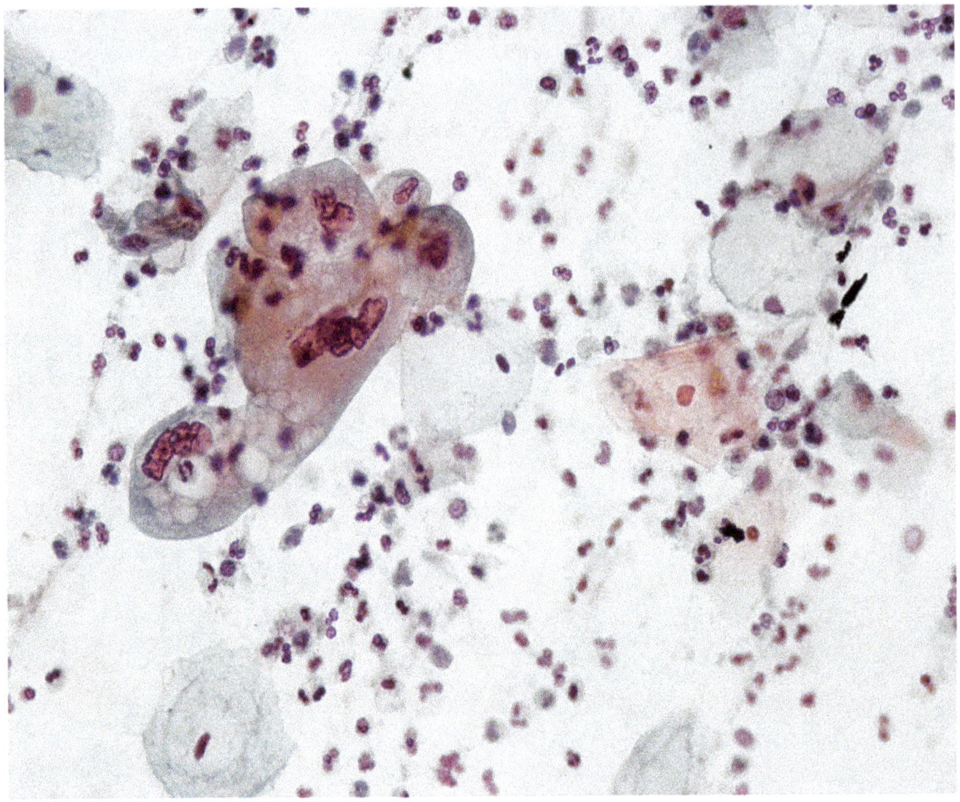

Q-75. Cells such as these were found in a 65-year-old woman with a history of squamous cell carcinoma of the cervix, hysterectomy, and radiation (conventional, medium magnification). They are most likely:
(a) Endocervical repair
(b) Radiation effect
(c) Herpes
(d) Recurrent squamous cell carcinoma

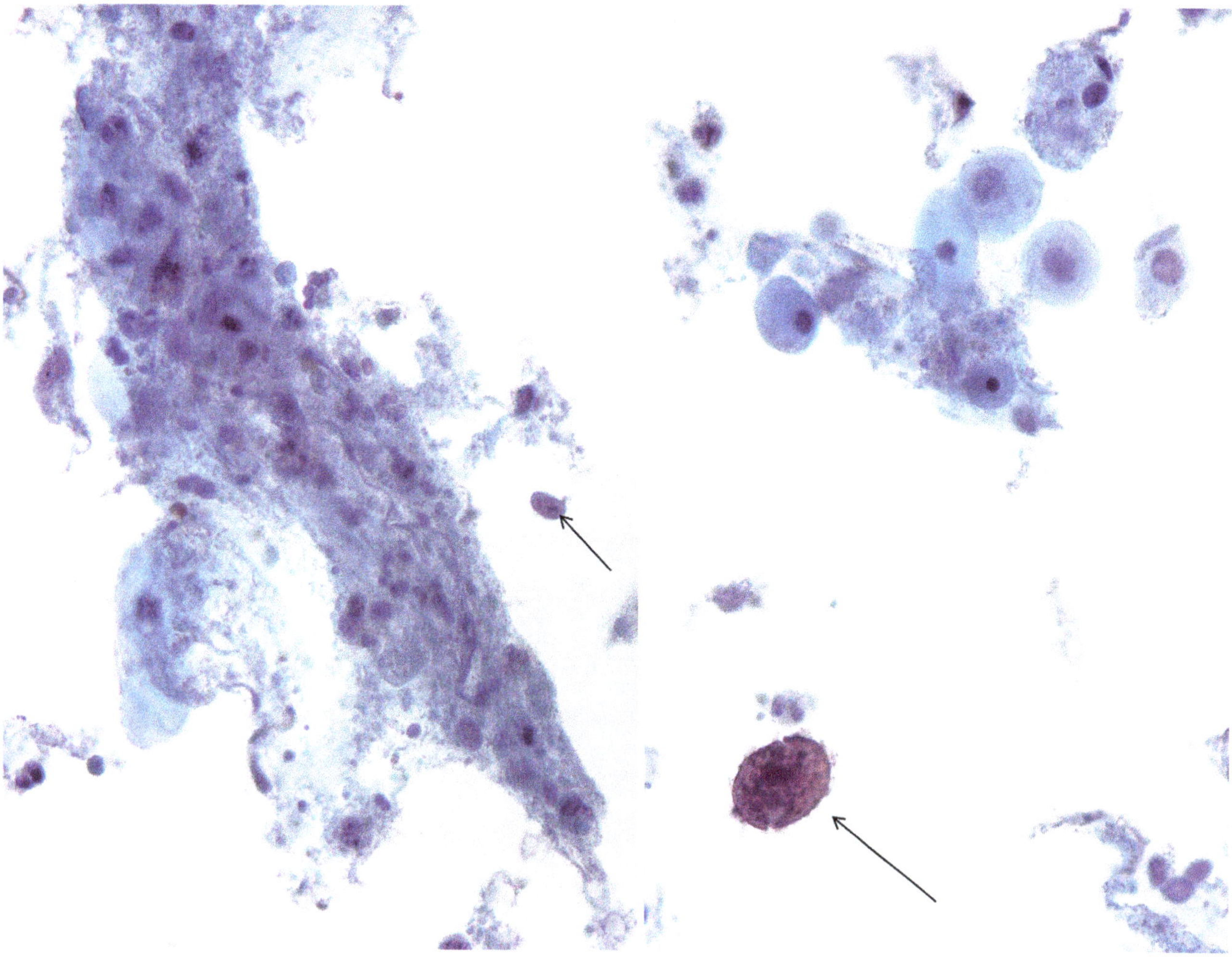

Fig. 4.76

Q-76. A 69-year-old patient with no history of previous abnormal cytology and no history of hormone replacement therapy displayed findings such as these on her Thin Prep slide (low and high magnification). The most likely cause of the blue to violet rounded structures (arrows) is:

(a) Degenerated parabasal cells
(b) AGUS – endometrial
(c) ASCUS
(d) Pollen contaminant

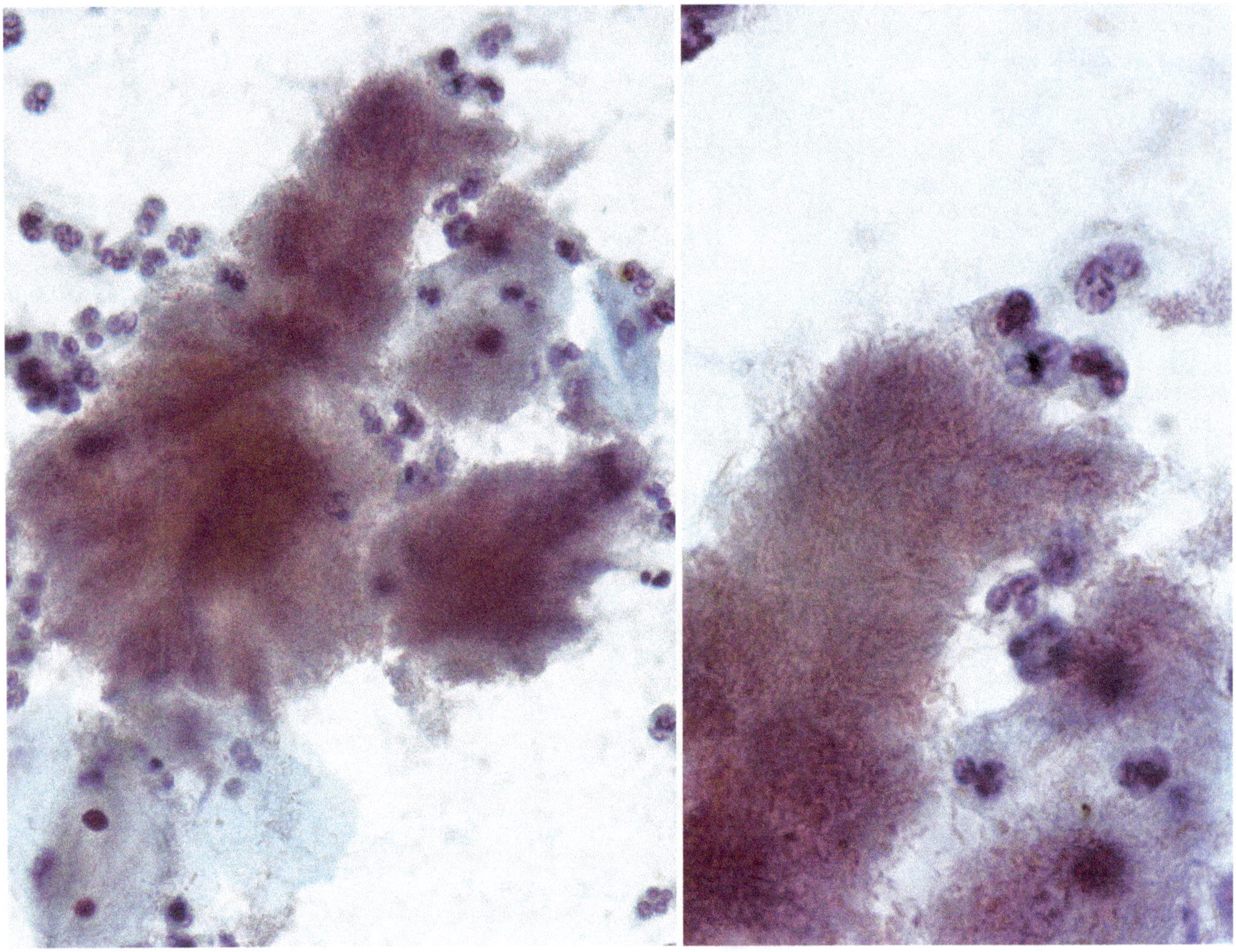

Fig. 4.77

Q-77. A 33-year-old woman presented to her physician for routine screening. These findings were observed on the slide (ThinPrep, low and high magnification). The best diagnosis is:

(a) Candida infection
(b) Actinomyces infection
(c) Leptothrix
(d) Shift in vaginal flora

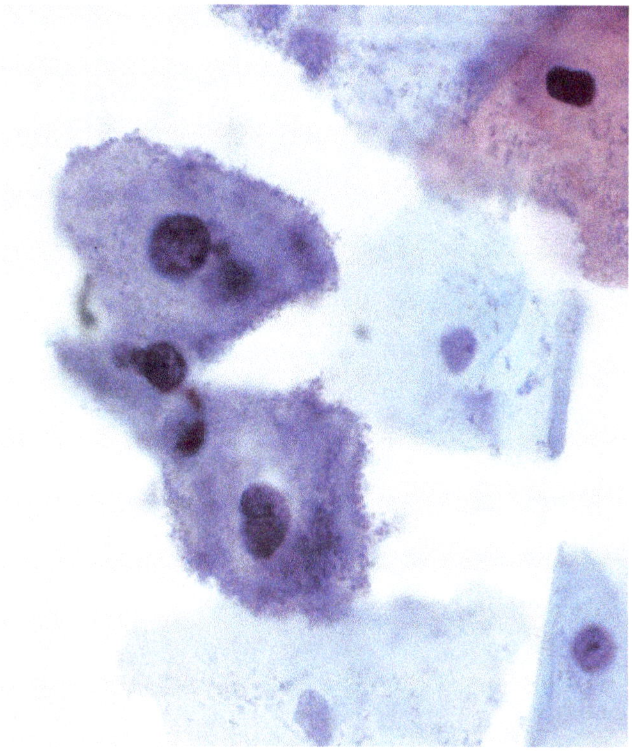

Fig. 4.78

Q-78. This 36-year-old patient had a clinical symptom of vaginal discharge, absence of lactobacilli and inflammatory cells on the rest of the slide (SurePath, high magnification) and a number of cells such as these. The best diagnosis is:

(a) Doderlein bacilli
(b) Gardnerella vaginalis
(c) Haemophilus vaginalis
(d) Clue cells
(e) Shift in vaginal flora suggestive of bacterial vaginosis

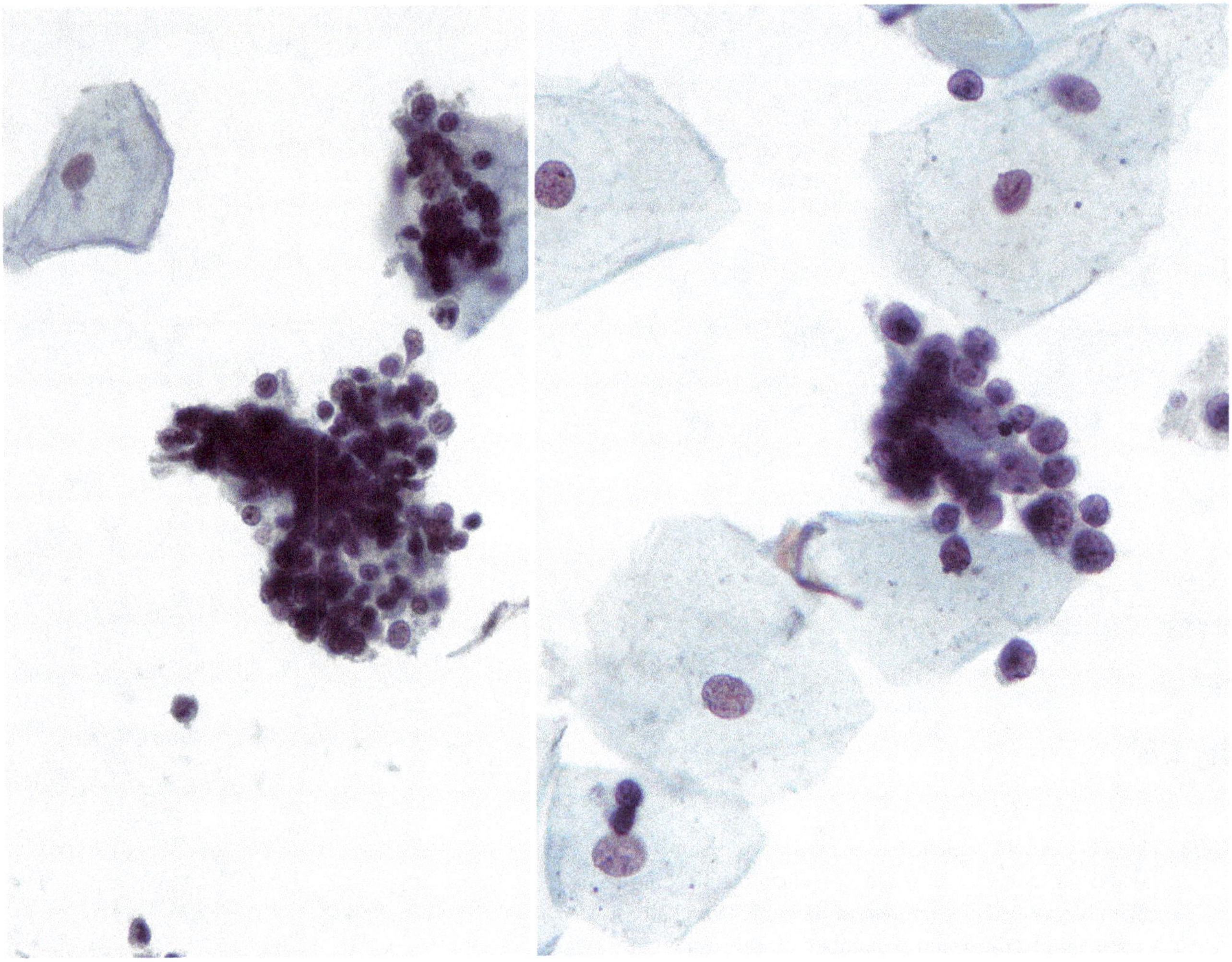

Fig. 4.79

Q-79. Cells such as these were found in several areas of a ThinPrep slide (medium and high magnification) from a 47-year-old female. The most likely diagnosis is:
(a) Acute inflammation
(b) ASC-H
(c) HGSIL
(d) Chronic follicular cervicitis
(e) Endometrial cells

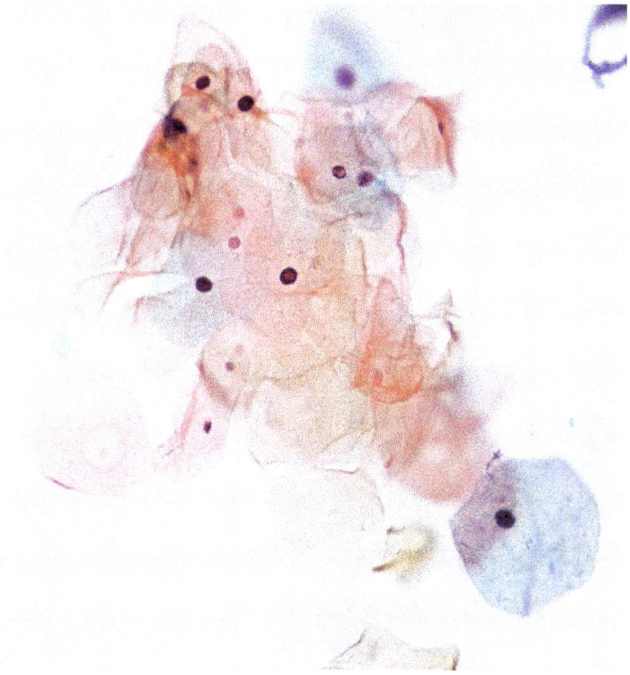

Fig. 4.80

Q-80. A 46-year-old patient had cells such as these in many areas of the slide (ThinPrep, medium magnification). The correct diagnosis is:

(a) Parakeratosis
(b) Dyskeratosis suggestive of HPV infection
(c) Hyperkeratosis
(d) Microglandular hyperplasia

Fig. 4.81

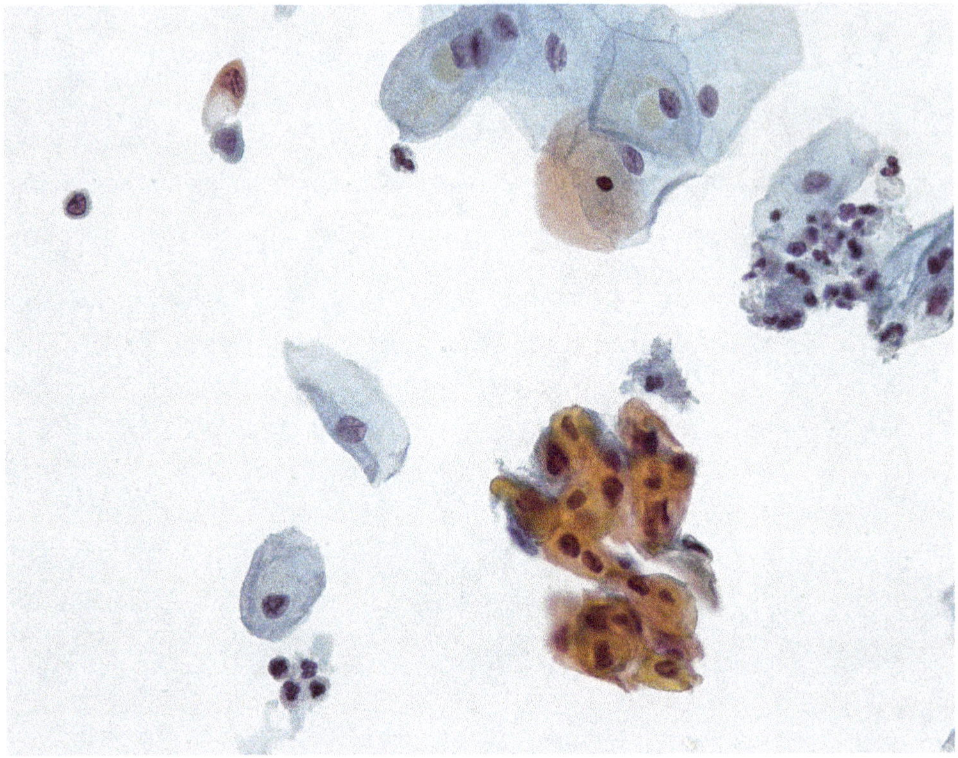

Q-81. Many cells such as these were found in the Thin Prep slide (medium magnification) of a 29-year-old woman. What other types of cells are the most likely to also be seen on this slide?

(a) Squamous cells with small, ill-defined perinuclear halos
(b) Endocervical cells with hyperdistended vacuoles
(c) Parabasal cells with autolytic atrophy
(d) Mature squamous cells with large, well-defined perinuclear halos

Fig. 4.82

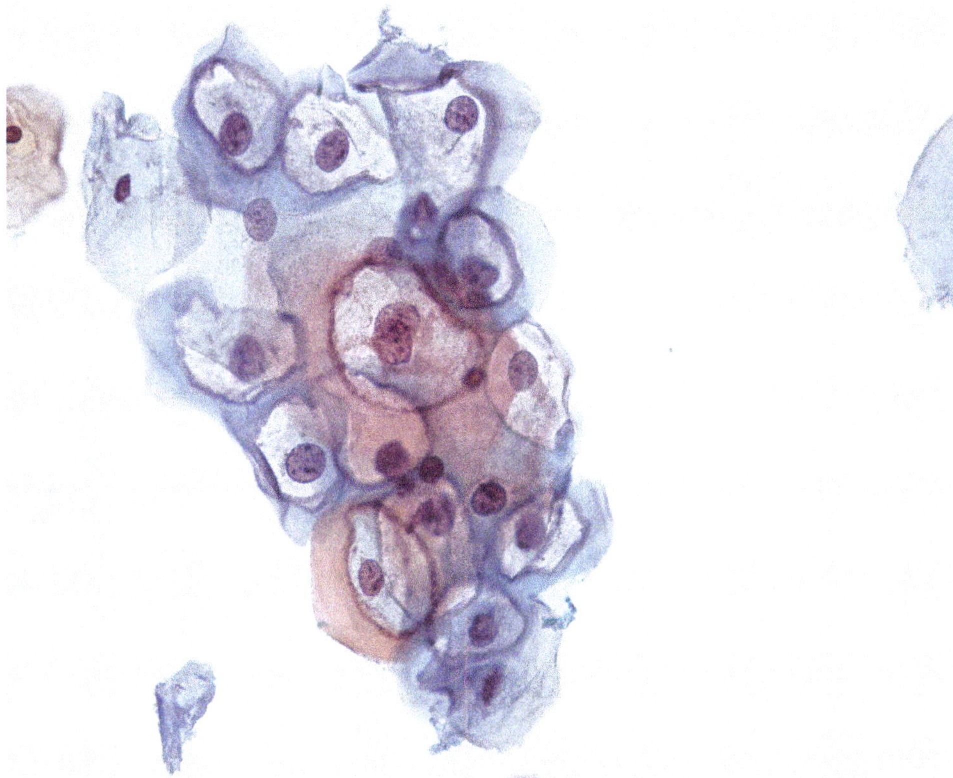

Q-82. The large clear areas in these cells are most likely due to (ThinPrep, medium magnification):
(a) Effects of chemotherapy
(b) Effects of radiation
(c) Inflammatory cell changes
(d) Effects of HPV infection
(e) Hyper-vacuolization

Fig. 4.83

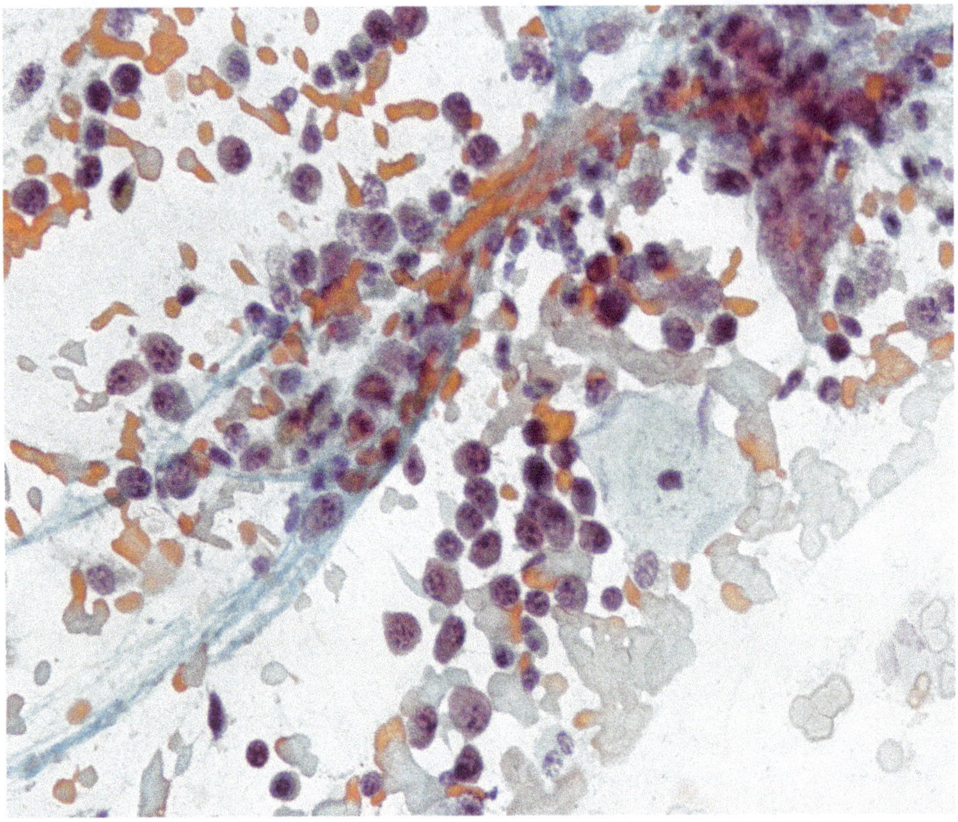

Q-83. The small cells with eccentric nuclei and scant cytoplasm are consistent with (conventional, high magnification):
(a) Lymphocytes, mature and immature
(b) Plasma cells
(c) Histiocytes
(d) Endometrial cells
(e) Small cell carcinoma of the cervix

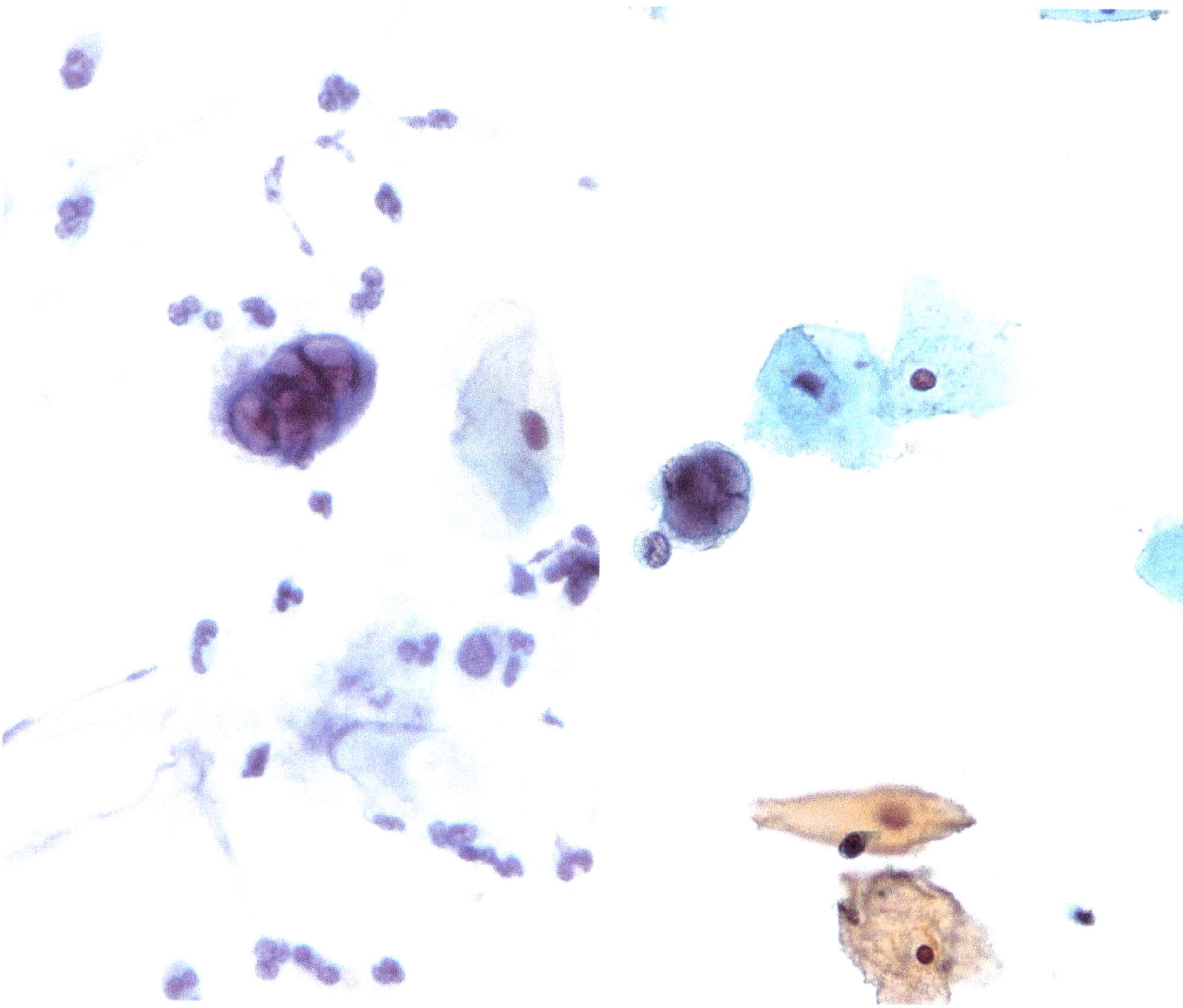

Fig. 4.84

Q-84. Several clusters of cells such as these were found in the gynecologic sample from a 32-year-old female (ThinPrep, medium). The most appropriate diagnosis is:

(a) Herpes
(b) Multinucleated histiocytes
(c) LGSIL
(d) ASC-H

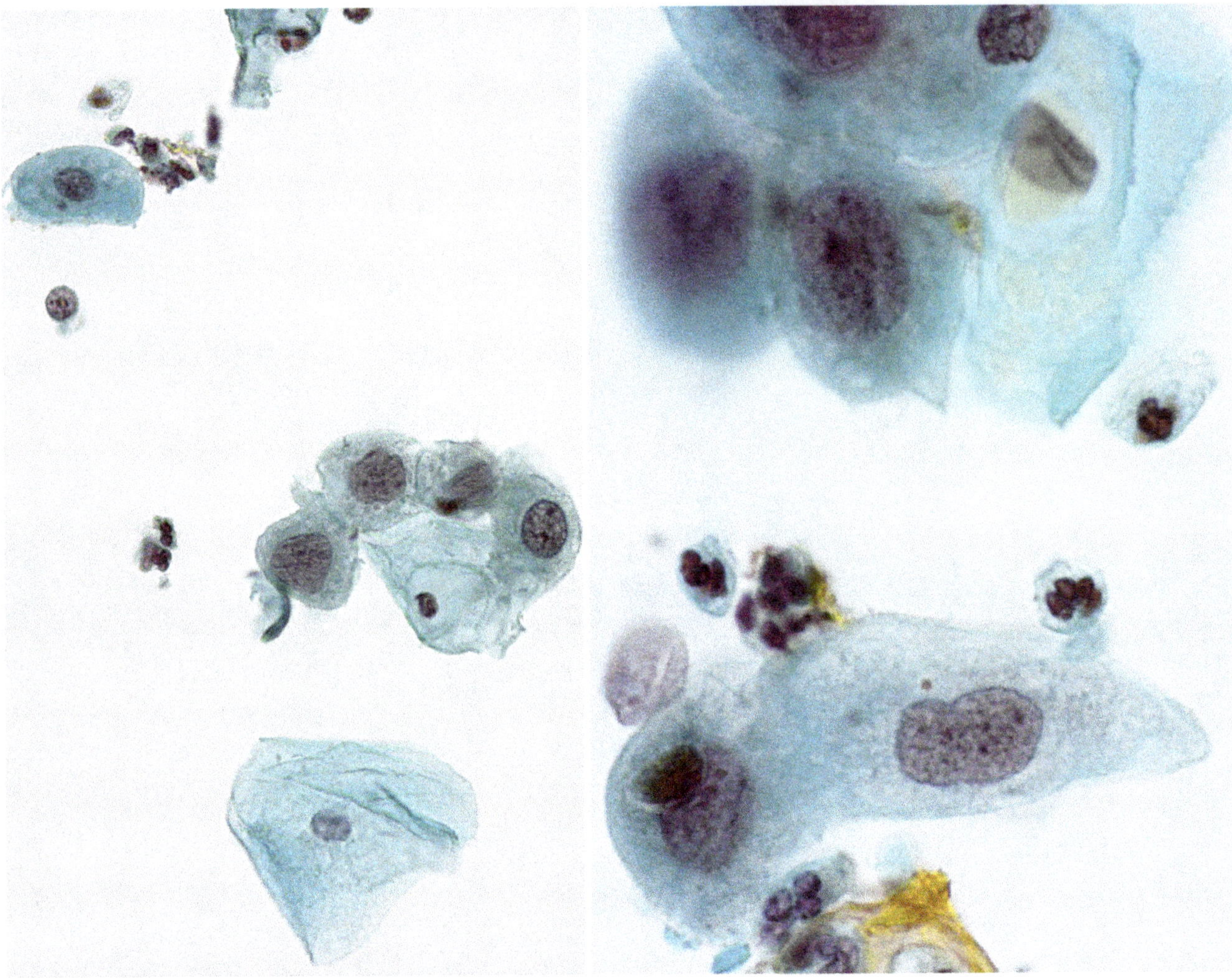

Fig. 4.85

Q-85. A 46-year-old woman had several clusters and scattered cells such as these on the slide (ThinPrep, medium and high magnification). The most appropriate diagnosis in this case would be:

(a) Squamous metaplasia
(b) LGSIL
(c) HGSIL
(d) Repair

Fig. 4.86

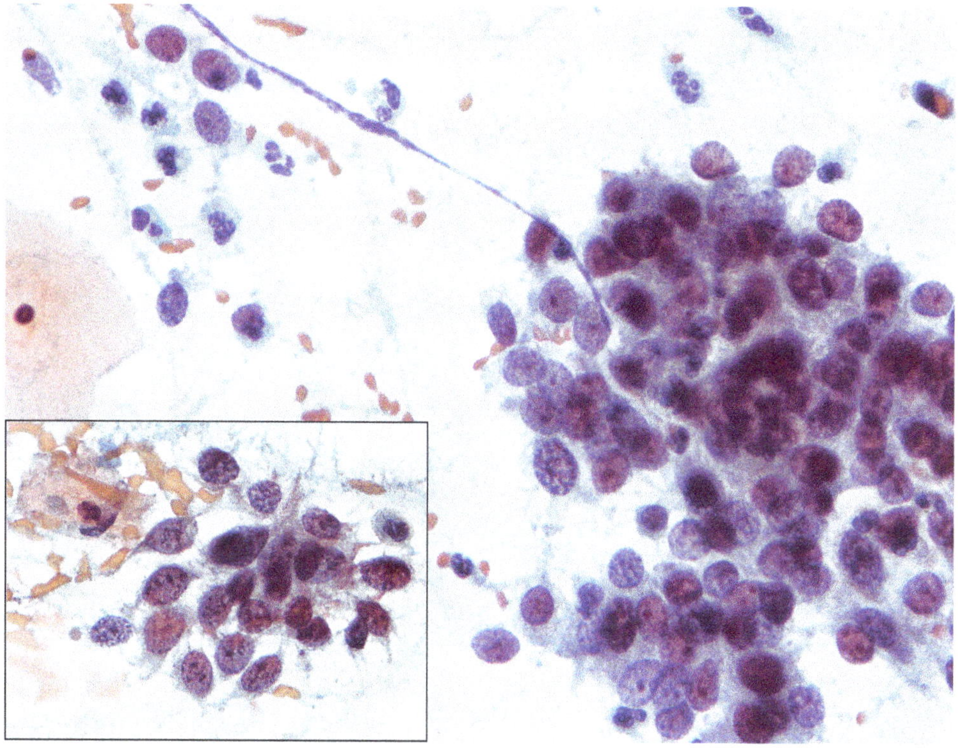

Q-86. Many cells such as these were found in the conventional slide of a 52-year-old woman (high and medium magnification in inset). The most likely diagnosis for this case is:

(a) Endometrial cells
(b) Adenocarcinoma of endometrial origin
(c) HGSIL
(d) Squamous cell carcinoma
(e) Adenocarcinoma of the endocervix

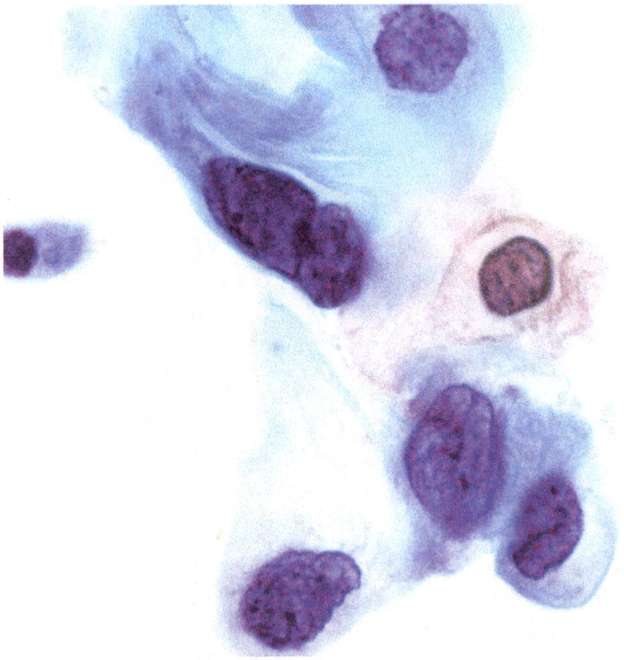

Fig. 4.87

Q-87. In order to determine the severity of the abnormality seen in these cells (ThinPrep, high magnification), one should most carefully observe which of the following?

(a) Whether there are koilocytes on the slide
(b) The irregularity of the nuclear membranes
(c) The color of the cytoplasm
(d) The appearance of the background
(e) The color of the nuclei

Fig. 4.88

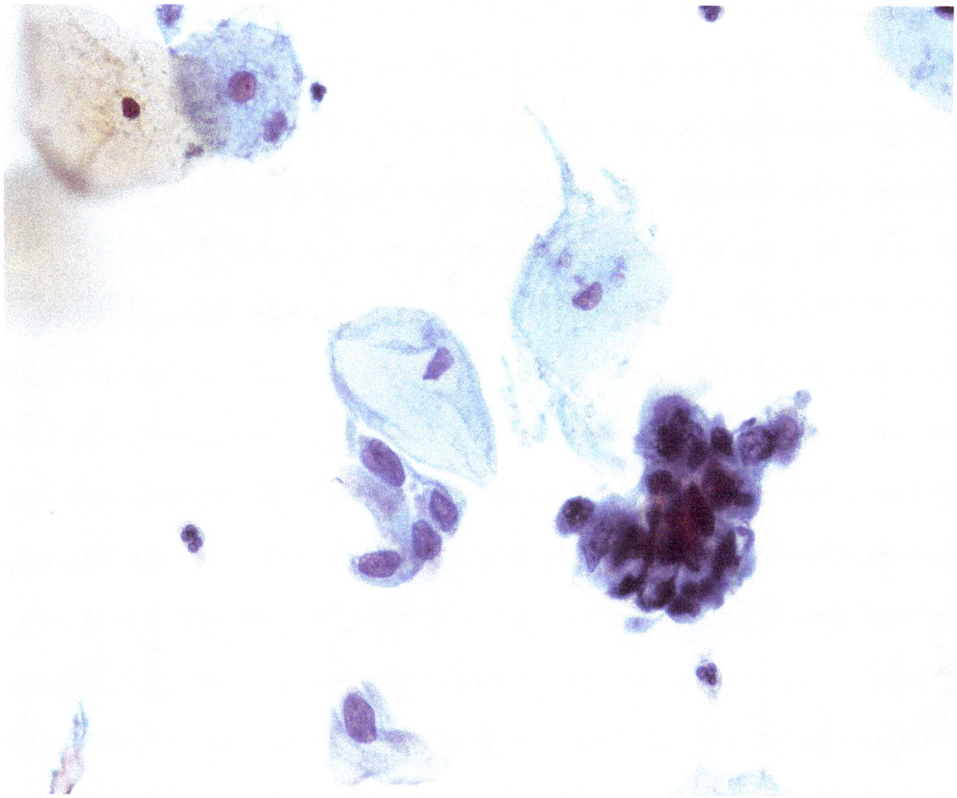

Q-88. A number of cells such as these were found in the gynecologic sample of a 47-year-old woman (ThinPrep, medium magnification). The most likely diagnosis is:
(a) ASCUS
(b) LGSIL
(c) HGSIL
(d) Squamous cell carcinoma

Fig. 4.89

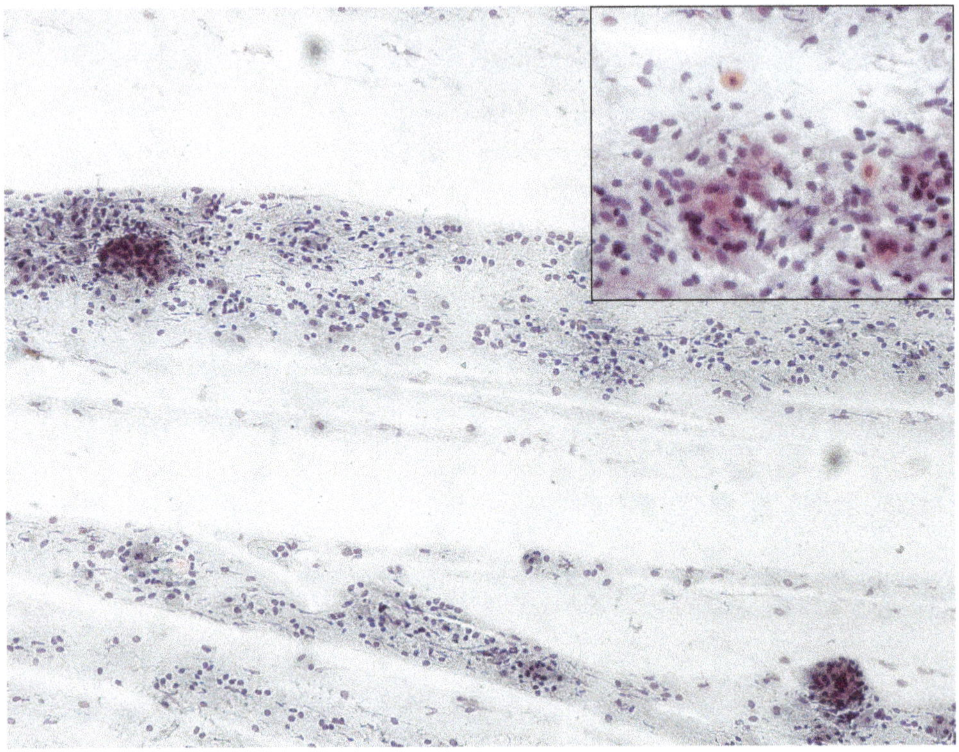

Q-89. A 65-year-old woman was seen in her gynecologist's office for a routine exam. The cells on the conventional slide resembled those illustrated here (low magnification and medium in inset). The most likely diagnosis is:

(a) Endometrial adenocarcinoma
(b) Endocervical adenocarcinoma
(c) Squamous cell carcinoma with evidence of keratinization
(d) Atrophy

Fig. 4.90

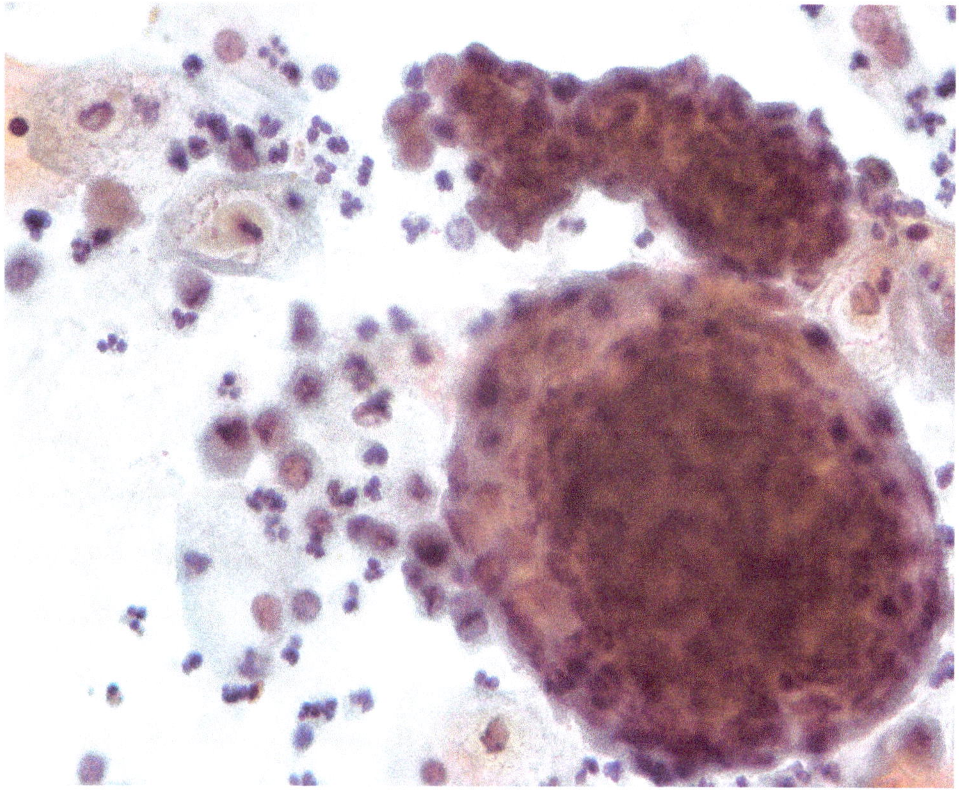

Q-90. Cells such as these were found in the gynecologic sample of a 32-year-old female (ThinPrep, high magnification). Clinical history from the patient included a previous "abnormal" Papanicolaou test result about 3 years earlier, G3P3, and LMP 7 days ago. The most likely diagnosis of these cells is:

(a) Histiocytes
(b) HGSIL (CIS)
(c) Endometrial cells
(d) Atrophy
(e) Chronic follicular cervicitis

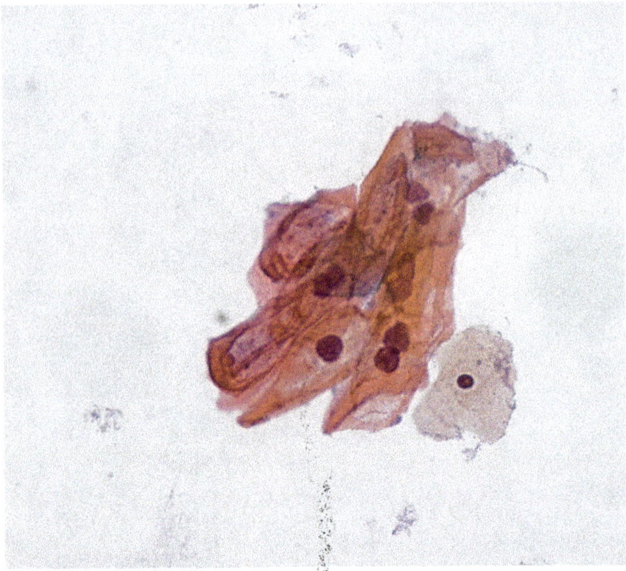

Fig. 4.91

Q-91. The best differential diagnosis for a case with a number of cells (ThinPrep, medium) such as these would be between:

(a) NILM and ASCUS
(b) ASCUS and LGSIL
(c) LGSIL and HGSIL
(d) HGSIL and SCCA

Fig. 4.92

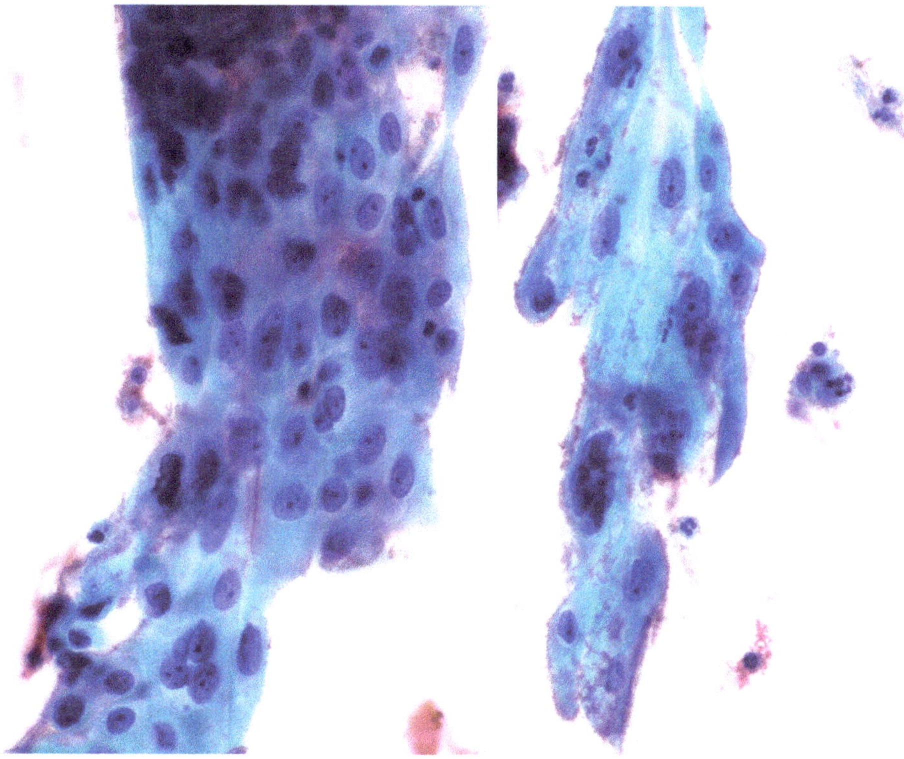

Q-92. A 56-year-old patient displayed cells such as these on her routine Pap smear (ThinPrep, medium and high magnification). The background contained small amounts of lysed blood, but no inflammation or organisms. The cells occurred in sheets such as these. The most likely diagnosis is:

(a) Atrophy
(b) Repair
(c) Squamous metaplasia
(d) LGSIL

Fig. 4.93

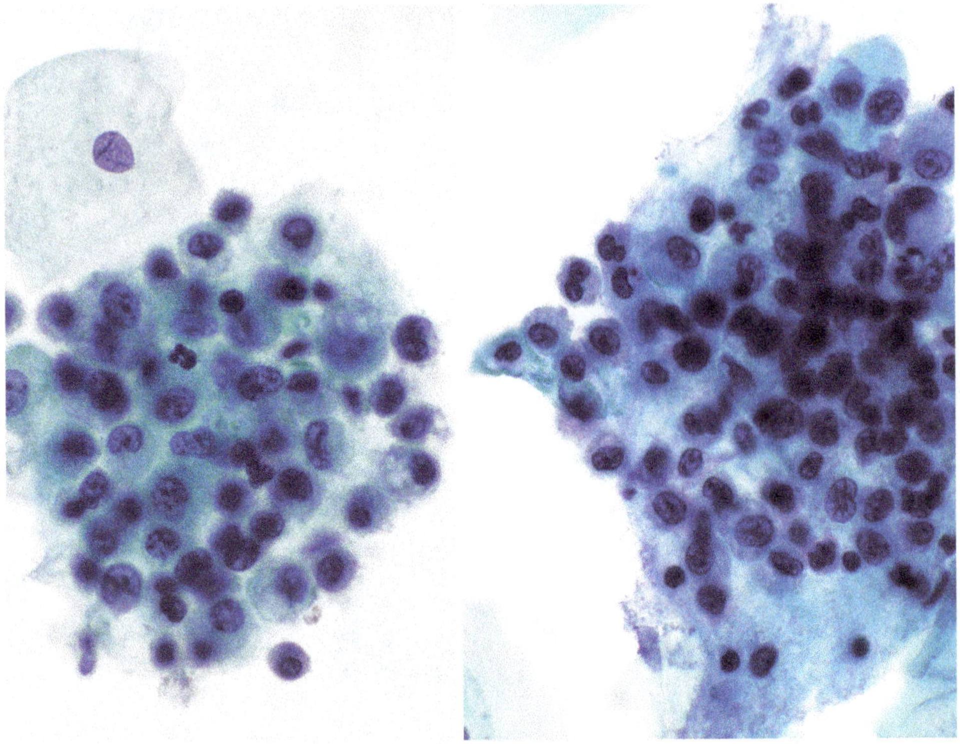

Q-93. Several clusters of cells such as these were found in the ThinPrep Pap (high magnification) of a 38-year-old female. The most likely diagnosis is:

(a) Endometrial cells
(b) Reactive endocervical cells
(c) HGSIL
(d) Carcinoma with small cell morphology of the cervix

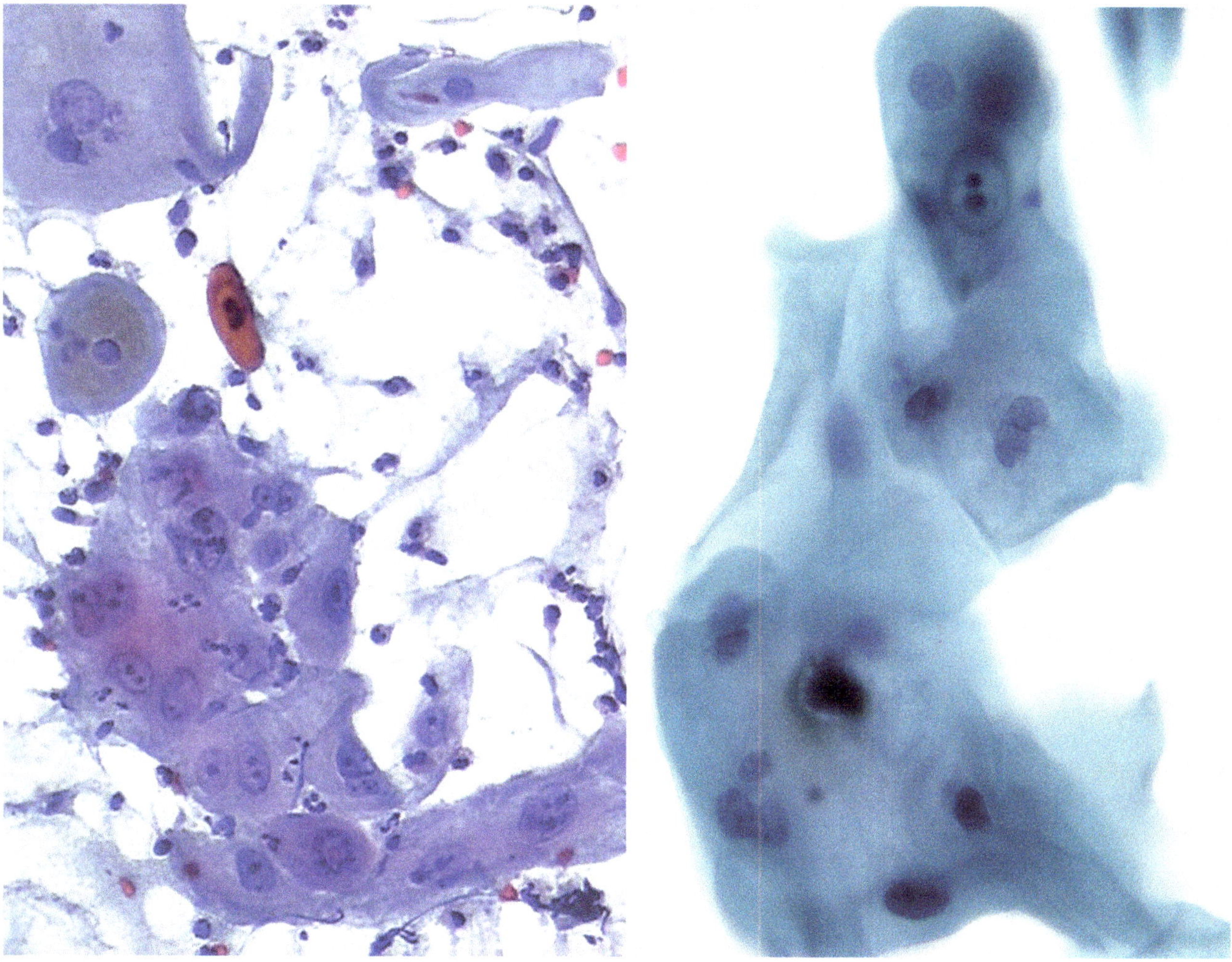

Fig. 4.94

Q-94. These cells were found in the Pap smear (SurePath, medium magnification) of a 62 year-old female with a history of squamous cell carcinoma of the cervix. She has been treated by hysterectomy and radiation completed 5 months ago. The most likely diagnosis is:
(a) Atrophy
(b) Post-radiation dysplasia
(c) Radiation effect
(d) Recurrent squamous cell carcinoma

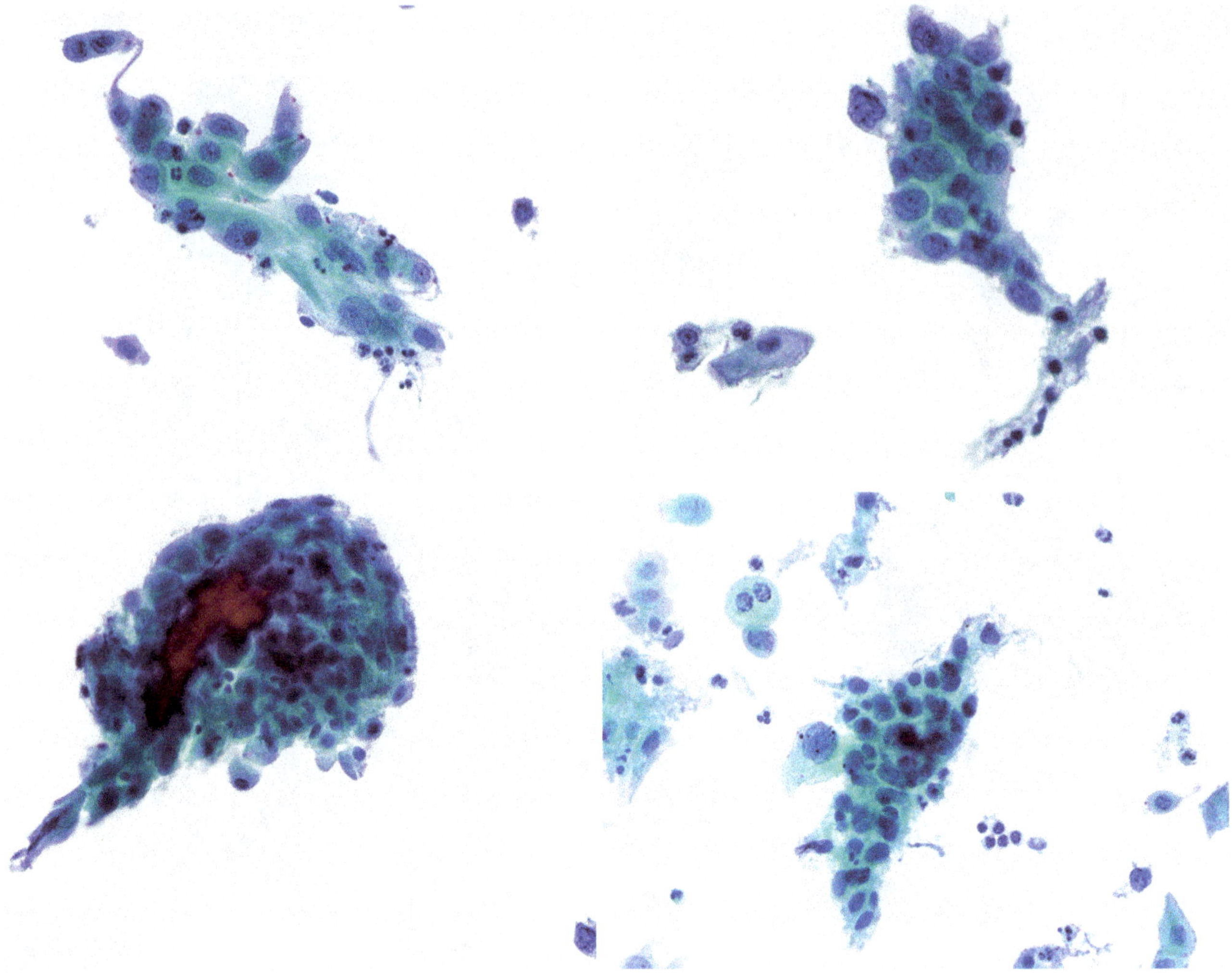

Fig. 4.95

Q-95. A number of cells such as these were found in the gynecologic sample (ThinPrep, medium magnification) of a 48-year-old woman. The most likely diagnosis is:

(a) ASCUS
(b) LGSIL
(c) HGSIL
(d) Squamous cell carcinoma
(e) Atrophy

Fig. 4.96

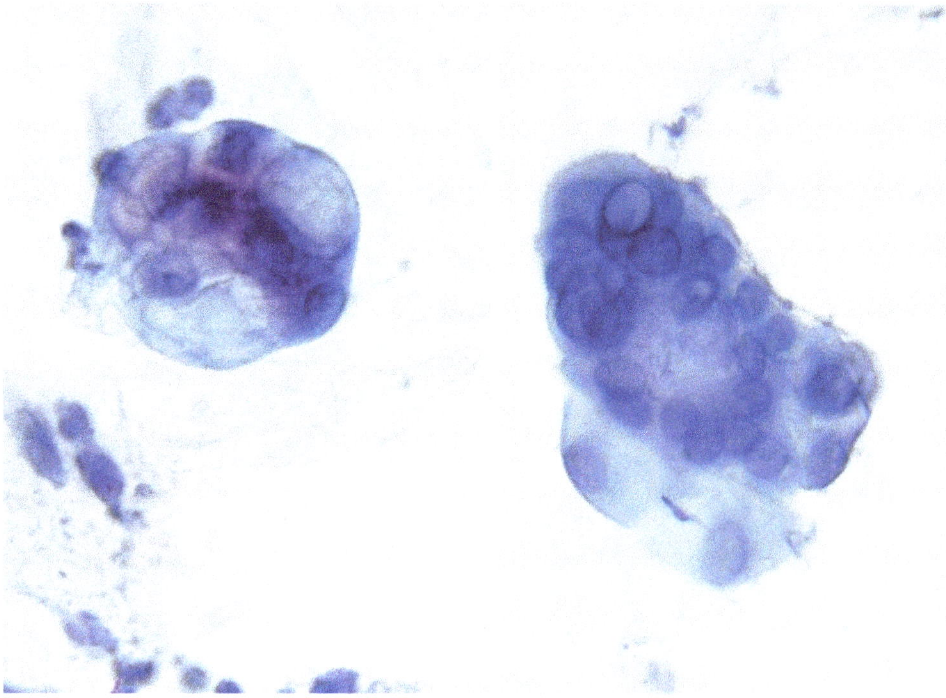

Q-96. This patient is a 24-year-old patient in for a routine checkup after placement of an intrauterine device 4 months ago. Several clusters of cells such as these were seen on the slide (ThinPrep, high magnification). The most likely diagnosis is:

(a) Clear cell adenocarcinoma associated with DES exposure in utero
(b) Multinucleated histiocytes
(c) Endocervical AIS
(d) IUD effect
(e) Squamous cell carcinoma

Fig. 4.97

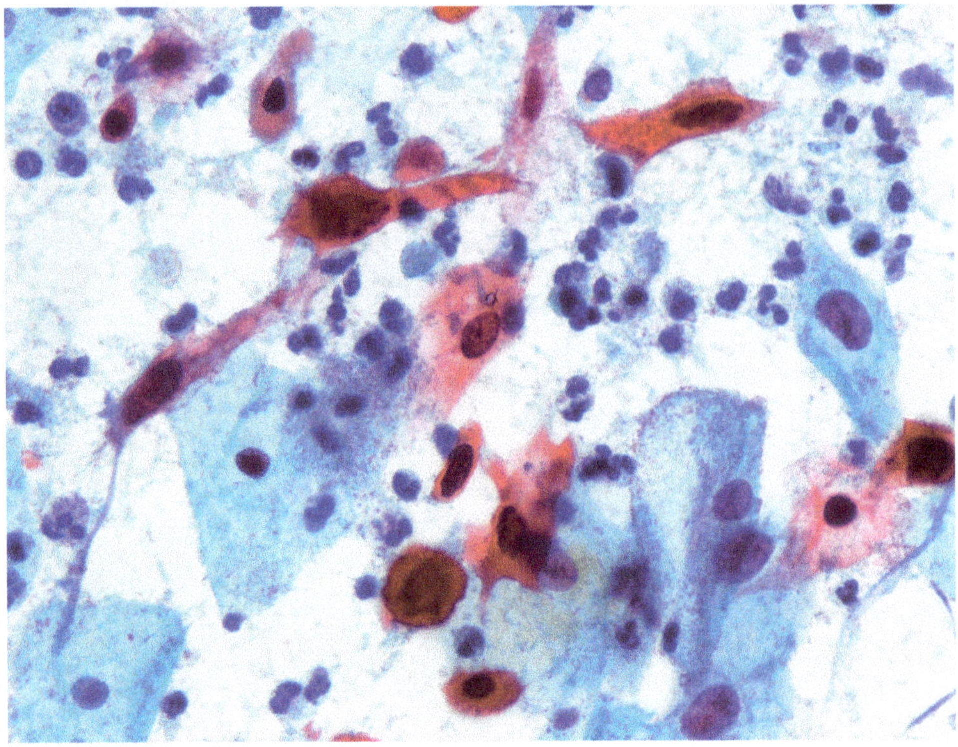

Q-97. Many cells such as these were found in the conventional slide (high magnification) from a 58-year-old woman. The most likely origin of these cells is:

(a) Internal endocervical os
(b) Endocervical glands
(c) External endocervical os
(d) Ectocervix

Fig. 4.98

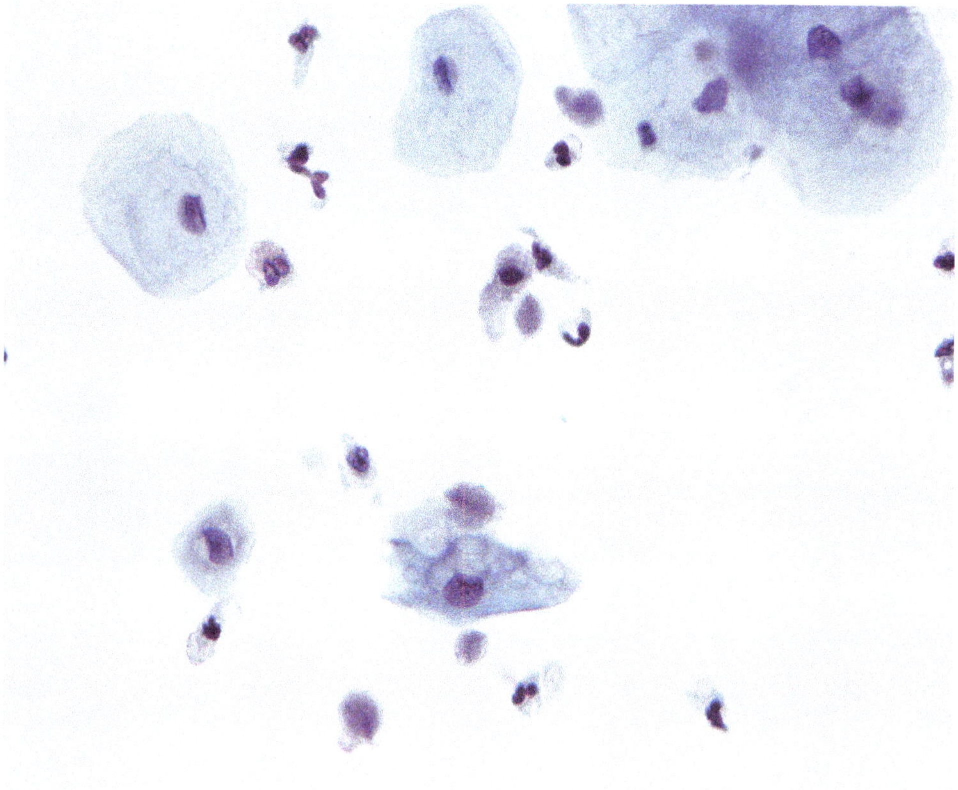

Q-98. Cytoplasmic vacuolization and perinuclear halos were seen in the ThinPrep slide (medium magnification) of a 30-year-old woman. The most likely causative agent in this case is:

(a) HPV 18
(b) HPV 11
(c) Gardnerella vaginalis
(d) Trichomonas vaginalis

Fig. 4.99

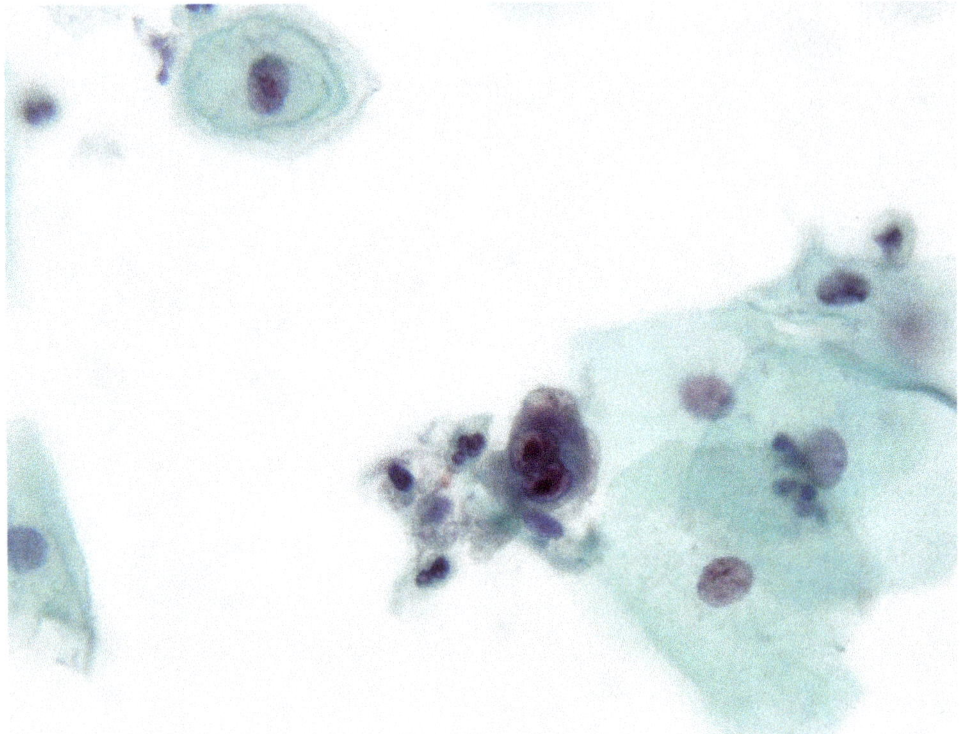

Q-99. Several cells such as these were found in the gynecologic sample from a 56-year-old patient (ThinPrep, high magnification). Most of the cells had a single nucleus and this one had two nuclei. All of the nuclei were pale and had a single large eosinophilic structure as seen in this image. The most appropriate diagnosis is:

(a) Endometrial adenocarcinoma
(b) Repair
(c) Herpes simplex
(d) Cytomegalovirus

Fig. 4.100

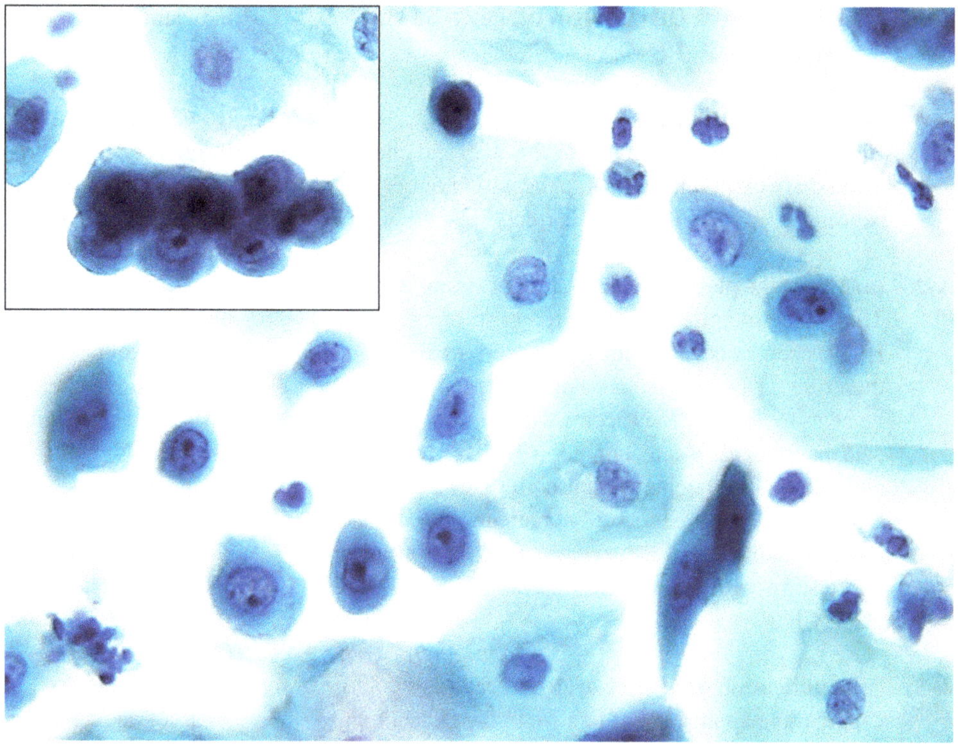

Q-100. A 38-year-old woman presented with mouth and vaginal ulcers of 14 months duration. She reported painful swallowing and a 40 lb weight loss over this period. Many cells such as these were found in groups and clusters within the gynecologic sample processed by SurePath (high magnification). Given this clinical history and the appearance of these cells, the most appropriate diagnosis is:

(a) Repair
(b) Herpes simplex
(c) CMV
(d) Pemphigus vulgaris

4.4 Answers and Discussion of Text-Based Questions 1–40

A-1. **(b) She is older than 70 years**
Choice a is not recommended by the ACS and choices c and d are contraindications for cessation of cervical cancer screening. Choice b is correct.

A-2. **(a) Must take place before initiation of sexual activity**
The protective effect of the three dose prophylactic HPV vaccines occurs prior to exposure to HPV, and therefore, girls and young women ages 9–26 are targeted as recipients. The vaccine will not treat or eradicate a current HPV infection nor is it effective against clear cell adenocarcinoma caused by DES exposure. Decades will pass before all women are able to take advantage of the vaccine, and the need for continued Pap testing will continue into the future, far beyond 2017. Choice a is correct.

A-3. **(b) Application of fixative after 90 seconds**
Delay in the application of fixative to the gynecologic slide will result in air-drying artifact and may interfere with the diagnostic accuracy of the specimen. The use of the cytobrush, restricting collection of the sample to the latter half of the cycle, and the use of 95 % ethyl alcohol as a fixative all have a beneficial effect on the accuracy of the slide. The correct answer is b.

A-4. **(a) Should be avoided due to diagnostic difficulties**
Sampling of the LUS may inadvertently occur due to the use of the cytobrush, especially in women with a shortened endocervical canal. However, the dark glands and tissue fragments with hyperchromatic nuclei and with a high nuclear/cytoplasmic ratio may be confused with either squamous or glandular lesions such as HGSIL or AIS. The finding of well-preserved glandular tubes and stromal cells should help to confirm the diagnosis of LUS. The cytobrush should only be rotated one-quarter turn and should never be inserted so that the lowest bristles are not visible. Air-drying artifact should be avoided by rapid fixation, either by the use of liquid-based preparation methods or by immediate fixation with 95 % ethyl alcohol.

A-5. **(c) Absence of endocervical or transformation zone component**
The addition of a determination of adequacy in the Bethesda System beginning in 1988 was an important advancement in Pap test reporting. In 2001, the lack of transformation zone component was changed from being "unsatisfactory" to a comment under "quality indicator." The other choices are all appropriate choices to designate a case as "unsatisfactory."

A-6. **(e) 65-year-old with no history of exogenous hormone therapy**
The most common reason for an atrophic pattern to be detected on a gynecologic sample is the normal physiologic postmenopausal state in which the production of estrogen has declined. Patients exposed to DES in utero do not show an atrophic pattern, second trimester pregnant patients should show an intermediate pattern, a cyclic female also will not be atrophic, and a 6-year-old child with precocious puberty may have an estrogen producing ovarian tumor and the pattern will be indicative of the presence of estrogen. Other low estrogen states include premenarche, postpartum, Turner syndrome, and post bilateral oophorectomy. The correct choice is e.

A-7. **(a) Hyperkeratosis and parakeratosis**
Uterine prolapse (or "descensus") can be the cause of areas of leukoplakia seen on the cervix or vaginal wall. However, hyperkeratosis and especially parakeratosis may also overlie a more serious lesion such as HGSIL and large white plaques should be removed gently by the clinician using gauze prior to taking the sample. Choice "b" would be of an infectious nature and descensus does not cause this, choice "c" would indicate HPV infection, and choice "d" would also not be associated with prolapse of the uterus. Choice a is correct.

A-8. **(d) HCG**
Multinucleated cells found during or immediately after pregnancy may be derived from placental origin (syncytiotrophoblasts) and may be infrequently but not reliably associated with impending loss of the pregnancy. Helpful confirming stains include immunostaining for human chorionic gonadotrophin (HCG) and human placental lactogen. Other differentials would include multinucleated histiocytes or herpes infection. The nuclei of syncytiotrophoblasts are usually more coarse and hyperchromatic than those of multinucleated histiocytes. The nuclei of herpes should have the classic "ground glass" and molded appearance. Of the stains listed, only HCG would detect placental origin. The correct answer is d.

A-9. **(a) Lactobacilli**
Lactobacilli are the normal bacterial inhabitants of the gynecologic tract. They are gram-positive rods and the maintenance of the slightly acidic pH of the vagina

seems to be related to the production of lactic acid as the bacilli metabolize glycogen from the squamous cells. As normal flora, their presence is expected and is not reported. However, absence of lactobacilli and replacement by mixed bacteria, cocci, or coccobacilli is reported as "shift in vaginal flora suggestive of bacterial vaginosis." The correct answer is a.

A-10. (**d**) **Trichomonas**

Trichomonas is a relatively frequent finding in gynecologic samples. It is a protozoa with an eccentric nucleus and flagella. However, the flagella are usually lost in the processing of the specimen and are not often identified. Two usual patterns are seen in the background of the slide: abundant polymorphonuclear leukocytes with wreath and ball formations or a very clean background with few polys, often with a slightly intensified staining reaction. Either of these patterns may be accompanied by other inflammatory changes such as small ill-defined perinuclear halos, polychromasia, or a "moth-eaten" appearance of the cytoplasm. Herpes is a virus and the changes seen are found in epithelial cells. Actinomyces is a higher-order bacteria and shows a starburst type of arrangement arising in a colony of bacteria. Calymmatobacterium is the causative organism of granuloma inguinale, and Chlamydia infection often displays small cytoplasmic vacuoles within the epithelial cells. Chlamydia infection is too difficult to accurately diagnose on cytology and cytology labs have discontinued reporting it. The correct answer is d.

A-11. (**c**) **Repair**

One of the most common causes of repair is radiation. The criteria for repair are listed and these must be distinguished from the changes seen in invasive carcinoma. One change caused by radiation is the finding of cytomegalic cells which do not have a significant increase in nuclear/cytoplasmic ratio. The cells, often polychromatic and sometimes having bizarre shapes, may continue for decades after the cessation of radiation therapy. A post radiation dysplasia should be differentiated from repair or radiation effect by the increase in nuclear/cytoplasmic ratio. This finding puts the patient at increased risk for recurrent carcinoma within 3 years of treatment. Recurrent squamous cell carcinoma should have a markedly increased N/C ratio, hyperchromasia, and may have nucleoli. A dirty background should be present as well as irregular chromatin patterns. The uniform, streaming cytoplasm and the hypochromatic, finely granular nuclei of repair can also assist with this differential. Finally, microglandular hyperplasia is made up of small, dark degenerated endocervical cells and is often seen in patients taking oral contraceptives.

A-12. (**a**) **Endometrial adenocarcinoma and HGSIL**

The intrauterine contraceptive device has been noted to cause abnormalities in the cells seen in the gynecologic sample. One of the cell types is glandular and might resemble an endometrial adenocarcinoma due to the presence of occasional nucleoli, cytoplasmic vacuolization, and ingested polys. However, the size of the abnormal appearing cells usually leads one to a correct diagnosis, particularly if the patient history (childbearing years, history of IUD use) is consistent with that finding. Although the size of the nucleus of a cell of high grade endometrial adenocarcinoma (grade III or IV) might look similar, usually the nucleoli of high-grade adenocarcinoma are quite prominent. The other clue is that a high-grade lesion would have many abnormal cells in the same group, while IUD effect often has only one or two suspicious cells with small nucleoli within a small cluster of otherwise normal appearing metaplastic cells. This also leads to a benign diagnosis. The other worrisome cell seen in IUD effect resembles HGSIL. It has a very high N/C ratio and a dark, hyperchromatic nucleus. However, HGSIL usually does not have nucleoli, such as IUD effect cells have, and the number and surrounding companions of these cells are too few and too benign appearing to lead to that diagnosis. A is the best answer.

A-13. (**d**) **E6 and E7**

E6 binds to the p53 gene and transforms it from a proto-oncogene into an oncogene blocking the normal process of apoptosis (cell death). E7 binds to the pRB gene and halts its usual tumor suppressor function of regulation of the cell cycle which leads to unregulated cellular proliferation. The loss of the two normal gene functions thus leads to an unregulated proliferation of cells which do not die. These two HPV genetic factors seem to be the most important in the multiple changes that lead to squamous cell carcinoma. D is the correct answer.

A-14. (**c**) **HPV 16**

HPV 16 is the most common HPV subtype found both in squamous carcinoma as well as in the precursor lesions of LGSIL and HGSIL.

A-15. (**d**) **Moderate dysplasia**

The first three choices would all be diagnosed as LGSIL with adequate numbers of abnormal cells present on the slide. Only "d" should be included in the diagnosis of HGSIL.

A-16. **(a) Infection with Candida or Trichomonas**
One of the changes often seen with infectious organisms such as Candida or Trichomonas is the presence of a small, ill-defined perinuclear halo. This halo should be differentiated from the much larger, sharp-bordered, perinuclear halo seen in koilocytes. HPV infection results in a distinct, often thick-edged halo, as well as some type of nuclear abnormality such as hyperchromasia, bi-nucleation, slight enlargement, smudginess, etc. Chronic follicular cervicitis, although it may be found in the presence of long-standing cervical infections, does not cause the perinuclear halos itself. Microglandular hyperplasia and the sampling of lower uterine segment also do not lead to the formation of perinuclear halos. The correct answer is a.

A-17. **(b) Rare cells with morphologic changes short of LGSIL**
Although ASCUS is one of the most common abnormalities seen on gynecologic samples, its description, criteria, and reproducibility have all been areas of study and diagnostic controversy. The newest 2001 Bethesda system subdivided the category of "atypical cells" into ASCUS, "atypical cells of undetermined significance" or ASC-H, "atypical cells, cannot exclude HSIL." The quantity, degree of morphologic change, clinical history, and maturity of the cytoplasm all should be evaluated in reaching this decision. However, most cytologists agree that a diagnosis of ASCUS generally means the finding of cells which do not quite meet either the morphologic degree of change or the number of abnormal cells found in a LGSIL, or both. However, they also do not meet guidelines for normal cells. This is a significant lesion, however, and 10–20 % of ASCUS cytology samples are found to contain HGSIL on biopsy. About 30–40 % of cases contain high-risk HPV when tested with molecular diagnostic tests. Thus, these patients should be properly followed up, tested for high-risk HPV, and further followed with colposcopy if high-risk HPV positive. The criteria of rare cells with high N/C ratios better describes a diagnosis of ASC-H. Moderate numbers of spindled keratinized cells would more likely lead to a diagnosis of at least LGSIL, if not HGSIL. Cells with streaming cytoplasm and nucleoli with pale chromatin are most consistent with repair, and very small, dark, high N/C ratio cells would be unlikely to be diagnosed as ASCUS. The correct answer is b.

A-18. **(c) Will regress even without treatment**
Based on a meta-analysis of the natural history of SIL, 47 % of LGSIL lesions regress and only 21 % were found to progress to HGSIL. Nucleoli are not a feature of LGSIL and a LEEP procedure is reserved for biopsy-proven HGSIL lesions. A large majority of LGSIL lesions were found to be positive by high-risk HPV molecular testing and it would not be cost-effective to do this testing for that reason. Therefore, the best answer is c.

A-19. **(a) Has a significant risk of progression to carcinoma**
The cells of HGSIL do have a significant risk (1.4 % in meta-analysis) of progressing to invasive carcinoma. The cells are usually immature with either syncytial arrangements, sheets, or an isolated occurrence. The nuclear atypia is usually marked with hyperchromasia, irregular coarse chromatin patterns, and a very high nuclear/cytoplasmic ratio. Nucleoli and hypochromatic nuclei are more characteristic of repair and are not a characteristic feature of HGSIL. The nuclei are usually hyperchromatic, although it is somewhat less prominent in liquid-based preparations than in conventional slides. Feathering of the bordering nuclei is a feature seen in endocervical neoplasia. Prominent increased N/C ratio, chromatin irregularities, single cell, sheet, or syncytial arrangements, and the numbers of abnormal cells help to diagnose HGSIL. The best answer is a.

A-20. **(c) Squamous cell carcinoma**
By far the most common malignancy of the cervix is squamous cell carcinoma. HPV 16 accounts for 50–60 % of all squamous cell carcinomas worldwide. The incidence of AIS is only 2 % of that from CIN3. Endocervical adenocarcinoma makes up about 15 % of female genital tract tumors and adenosquamous carcinoma is rarer but increasing in incidence. The best answer is c.

A-21. **(a) Squamous metaplasia**
One difficulty that beginning cytologists often encounter in discriminating squamous metaplasia from HGSIL comes from the fact that squamous metaplasia often occurs in immature cells with dense, cyanophilic cytoplasm, just as many HGSIL cells do. However, the irregular chromatin pattern, anisonucleosis, and hyperchromasia of the HGSIL cells should contrast with the more finely granular, evenly distributed, uniform nuclear chromatin pattern of squamous metaplasia. Additionally, the overall size of the HGSIL cells will often be larger than those of immature squamous metaplasia. Occasionally, however, the HGSIL cells may be single or in small groups of 2–3, quite small, and therefore more difficult to detect. The key to their detection is the presence of hyperchromatic nuclei

which are seldom seen in squamous metaplasia. Cases such as this require diligent screening to detect. Koilocytes are more associated with cases of LGSIL, not HGSIL. Estrogen effect would be reflected in the increase in the number of superficial cells above those expected for the physiologic state of that patient. Microglandular hyperplasia is diagnosed by the presence of pools of small, degenerated glandular cell nuclei, most often much smaller than the cells associated with HGSIL. Also, the cytoplasm seen is usually finely vacuolated in microglandular hyperplasia. The cells of ASCUS have only mildly enlarged nuclei which do not even meet the criteria for LGSIL and thus, should not usually be confused with HGSIL. The correct answer is a.

A-22. (**d**) **Keratinizing type**

Tadpole and fiber cells refer to the sometimes bizarre cell shapes that are most often associated with keratinizing types of squamous cell carcinoma. Keratinizing squamous cell carcinoma often also has orangeophilic cytoplasm, very hyperchromatic, opaque nuclei, unusual nuclear shapes, a lack of prominent nucleoli, and a somewhat less prominent tumor diathesis than the other types of squamous cell carcinoma. Additionally, it is often associated with hyperkeratosis and/or parakeratosis. Neuroendocrine and small cell types of squamous cell carcinoma usually have rather small round to oval cells which are fairly uniform in their size and shape. Non-keratinizing squamous cell carcinoma usually contains larger cells, with more abundant cytoplasm. They may occur in syncytial arrangements as well as in clusters, but the usual shape is more round to polygonal and bizarre shapes such as are seen in tadpole or fiber cells do not often occur. Behçet disease is a rare benign chronic dermatologic disease presenting with ulcers in the oral cavity and vulva. The smears may show dark pleomorphic nuclei and keratinized cytoplasm with large prominent nucleoli. Since it is not a type of squamous cell carcinoma but is a benign differential with squamous cell carcinoma, e is not the correct answer. Clinical history and close follow-up may be needed to help make this distinction. D is the correct answer.

A-23. (**d**) **Colposcopically directed biopsy**

ASC-H is a significant diagnosis with a high rate of biopsy-proven HGSIL (50 %). Therefore, according to the suggested follow-up protocol of the ASCCP (2007), the appropriate follow-up for these patients is an immediate colposcopically directed biopsy (Choice D). These patients, of course, should not have HPV testing as their first therapeutic choice, as it would not be cost-effective (84 % positivity), nor repeat Pap test. A LEEP procedure is not recommended without first obtaining biopsy confirmed evidence of HGSIL or worse disease.

A-24. (**a**) **Higher than for ASCUS**

The positive predictive value for histologic CIN 2,3 for a cytologic diagnosis of ASC-H is 50 %. This is markedly higher than ASCUS (17 %) and somewhat lower than HGSIL cytologic diagnoses (63 %). The correct answer is a.

A-25. (**c**) **10 cells of either metaplastic or endocervical cell origin**

As defined by the 2001 Bethesda System for the evaluation of the presence of an endocervical sample, either 10 endocervical and/or squamous metaplastic cells should be present. The absence of such endocervical components does not make the sample "unsatisfactory," but is mentioned as a "quality indicator." The correct answer is c.

A-26. (**c**) **75**

The 2001 Bethesda System defines an obscuring component making the slide unsatisfactory as covering more than 75 % of the epithelial cells. The correct answer is c.

A-27. (**c**) **May induce a decrease of maturity to intermediate levels**

The normal pattern in pregnancy changes to an almost entirely intermediate cell pattern by the second trimester. If the pattern is more mature than expected (a higher number of superficial cells), then the administration of progesterone will decrease the maturation to the normal intermediate cell pattern. If a pregnancy is normal, the administration of estrogen will have no effect and will not increase the number of superficial cells seen. A pattern of nearly 100 % parabasal cells is ominous for the continuation of the pregnancy and may be seen in cases of intrauterine fetal demise. The correct answer is c.

A-28. (**a**) **Non-keratinizing**

The most common type of dysplasia is the non-keratinizing type. In a series of 2,453 cases, it occurred about 7 times more frequently than metaplastic type and 25 times more often than the keratinizing type. Mixed metaplastic and keratinizing types seldom occur together; the most common mixture is the non-keratinizing and metaplastic types. The correct answer is a.

A-29. **(b) Metaplastic**
Early studies found that the most significant subtype of squamous intraepithelial lesion in terms of progression to CIN 3 was the metaplastic type. The other subtypes listed were less likely to progress.

A-30. **(c) Small cell**
Five-year survival rates for small cell carcinomas were found to be only 20 %, versus 79 % in non-keratinizing types and 48 % in keratinizing types. Small cell tumors were found to be more biologically aggressive and are considered the most poorly differentiated of these three types of tumors. The correct answer is c.

A-31. **(b) Preserved nuclear polarity**
Macronucleoli are not a useful characteristic to distinguish between repair and carcinoma since both lesions have nucleoli. Repair usually does have the characteristic of having virtually 100 % of the cells contain nucleoli; carcinoma may approach this level but may also have a much smaller percentage of cells that contain nucleoli. Syncytial groupings, free cells, and clumpy chromatin are all features of carcinoma. Thus b, preserved nuclear polarity, is a feature of repair which distinguishes it from squamous carcinoma in which the polarity of the cells is not preserved.

A-32. **(b) Non-keratinizing squamous cell carcinoma**
CIS and squamous metaplasia do not usually display prominent macronucleoli. Non-keratinizing squamous cell carcinoma has traditionally been described as having the most macronucleoli. Keratinizing squamous cell carcinoma may show nucleoli in occasional syncytial groupings but the opaque, dark nuclei usually seen in the orange, pleomorphic cells does not allow for visualization of nucleoli. The typical features of non-keratinizing carcinoma also include sheets, syncytial arrangements, and single cells, a tumor diathesis, hyperchromatic irregular chromatin, and a high nuclear/cytoplasmic ratio. The correct answer is b.

A-33. **(b) SIL**
Dysplasias on average have larger nuclei than most carcinomas. In fact, some dysplastic cells (LGSIL) may have the largest neoplastic nuclei found in squamous lesions. This may occur with a concomitant increase in the overall cell size, so that the cells show an appropriate N/C ratio for a LGSIL diagnosis. Usually the very high N/C ratios found in carcinomas are due to the enlargement of the nuclei along with a marked decrease in the amount of cytoplasm. The correct answer is b.

A-34. **(d) HGSIL**
The nuclei of ASCUS and LGSIL are generally finely granular, with evenly distributed chromatin. The nuclear borders are smooth. HGSIL more often has raisinoid nuclear shapes, with nuclear membrane interruption, especially in the severe dysplasia to CIS range. Although ASC-H may have some changes in this range, usually the changes are inadequate or the abnormal cells are too few in number for an outright diagnosis of HGSIL. Therefore, d is the correct answer.

A-35. **(c) Repair**
The combination of features of enlarged cells and nuclei, sheet or ribbon-like arrangement, hypochromasia, and macronucleoli are most consistent with a diagnosis of repair. CIS and squamous cell carcinoma usually do not have macronucleoli or hypochromasia. Also the arrangement of CIS and squamous cell carcinoma is usually syncytial groups. Endometrial adenocarcinoma also would usually occur as small three-dimensional clusters of cells with small nucleoli. A moderate dysplasia usually has hyperchromasia and does not have nucleoli. C is the correct answer.

A-36. **(d) HGSIL**
Syncytial groupings are most often found in carcinoma in situ, now included in the HGSIL category. The cells of ASCUS and LGSIL are more commonly single or in sheets. Repair displays as cohesive ribbons with streaming cytoplasm. Although a rare case of ASC-H might display a syncytial group, generally they are more often found in HGSIL. D is the correct answer.

A-37. **(c) Navicular cells**
These cells, shaped somewhat like a boat (hence the name navicular), are often found filled with glycogen in the Pap of a pregnant woman. Syncytiotrophoblasts are a very uncommon finding, as are decidual cells. Both of these cells do not contain glycogen. "Pencil cells" is the name given to extremely elongated endocervical cells. Pickle cells are from the lower layer of the epidermis and are not glycogenated.

A-38. **(a) Obesity**
Excess weight can contribute to an estrogen effect in a postmenopausal woman due to the production of estrogen by adipose tissue. In fact, in women who are morbidly obese, premalignant and even malignant endometrial cancers have been found in women who are premenopausal and are much younger than the

usual postmenopausal age group. Cytolysis usually displays an intermediate cell pattern, as superficial cells are more resistant to the lytic effects of the Doderlein bacilli. Sertoli-Leydig tumors produce progesterone and would not create an estrogen effect. Air-drying artifact may create an artificially pink staining smear but does not truly affect the maturation of the cells. A is the correct answer.

A-39. **(d) Cockleburrs**
The only crystalline, starburst-like appearance of any of these choices is the so-called cockleburr. While all of these may be associated with pregnancy, the cockleburr is a structure of about 50–100 μm in diameter and composed of thick, spoke-like rays, often with accompanying histiocytes. While most commonly associated with pregnancy, less than 5 % of pregnant women have them. Their presence has no effect on the prognosis of mother or fetus. Choices "a" and "b" are cells derived from placental tissue. Choice "c" derives from altered stromal cells and indicates decidualization of the cervical stroma. D is the correct answer.

A-40. **(d) Clinging tumor diathesis**
The appearance of invasive squamous cell carcinoma in liquid-based preparations perhaps varies most from its usual presentation in conventional slides due to the more subtle appearance of the tumor diathesis in the preparation. Instead of a grossly bloody, prominent tumor diathesis as is common in conventional slides, the spaces between the abnormal cell clusters appear deceivingly "clean" and free from the classic tumor background. However, if one observes carefully around the edges of the abnormal cells in LBP, one can detect old and fresh blood, cellular debris, necrosis, and fibrin. This "clinging tumor diathesis" is a subtle but important clue in coming to a malignant diagnosis. The other choices are more common in radiation effect (a and b), in glandular cervical lesions (c), or in infectious conditions (e). The correct answer is d.

4.5 Answers and Discussion of Image-Based Questions 41–100

A-41. (**c**) **Repair**

These cells are most consistent with repair. They have preserved polarity, streaming cytoplasm, nucleoli in nearly 100 % of the cells, hypochromatic finely granular chromatin pattern, and a clean background. Although there are some red blood cells visible in the background, a true tumor diathesis is made up of old and fresh blood, necrotic cellular debris, and often fibrin strands. In liquid-based preparations (LBP) the tumor diathesis is often found clinging to the groups of malignant cells. Endocervical cells would occur in a more honeycomb architectural arrangement and have less polygonal cytoplasm. HGSIL is not a consideration due to the presence of prominent nucleoli, lack of hyperchromasia, and lack of irregular chromatin pattern. Also the nuclear/cytoplasmic ratio (N/C ratio) is not as markedly uniformly increased as in HGSIL. Endocervical adenocarcinoma is not a consideration because these cells appear as flat, ribbon-like sheets, and not in syncytial-like arrangements or loose strips. These cells are also polygonal, indicating squamous origin, rather than endocervical columnar cells with eccentric nuclei. Also, endocervical adenocarcinoma usually has a pronounced tumor diathesis.

A-42. (**c**) **Chronic follicular cervicitis**

These cells are fairly hyperchromatic and seem to be occurring in a "pool" which contains both very small round cells as well as slightly larger cells. Nucleoli are inconspicuous to absent, and there seems to be a proteinaceous matrix in which these cells reside. The clue to this diagnosis is the presence of the very small, perfectly round cells which are mature lymphocytes. These cells are too small to represent small cell carcinoma of the cervix, endometrial adenocarcinoma, or HGSIL (even if CIS) (Compare their size with the squamous cell nuclei in the image.). Although some of the larger, more immature lymphocytes might overlap these categories in their size range, the smaller ones do not. Also note that these cells are non-cohesive. Although tingible body macrophages can often be seen with chronic follicular cervicitis, they are not a requirement to make this diagnosis. This condition commonly occurs with *Chlamydia* infection and is more often seen in postmenopausal women, although it can occur at any age. Normal endometrial cells also are slightly larger than these cells. The perfect roundness of the mature lymphocytes precludes consideration of normal endometrial cells.

A-43. (**b**) **Nucleoli**

This is an example of herpes and shows many of the characteristic elements: multinucleation, margination (thickening) of the nuclear membrane, molding of the nuclei, and "ground glass" chromatin. Eosinophilic inclusion bodies are not well seen in this example but may be present in herpes. The chromatin pattern usually lacks distinct particles and appears pale and smudgy. Nucleoli are not a feature of herpes. The eosinophilic inclusion which may be seen in herpetic cells is well-defined and is an intranuclear inclusion. However, this feature may or may not be present in the infected cells.

A-44. (**d**) **LGSIL**

These cells are characteristic of those with HPV infection. Note the large, perinuclear halos with sharply defined edges. Additionally, HPV infected cells have nuclear abnormalities of some type. These may include enlargement, hyperchromasia, smudgy chromatin, and bi- or multinucleation. Syncytiotrophoblasts usually have many more nuclei and have a more vacuolated appearance to the cytoplasm, since they arise from placental tissue. Additionally, the nuclei are often bland and similar in their staining, size, and shape. Glycogen-filled cells have yellow granular material in the cytoplasm and do not have the nuclear irregularities seen in HPV. Multinucleated histiocytes also have bland, uniform appearing nuclei without hyperchromasia, smudginess, or enlargement. Additionally, they often contain frothy finely vacuolated cytoplasm, unlike these cells which have hard, sharp-edged cytoplasm of squamous origin. HGSIL cells would be expected to have a much higher nuclear/cytoplasmic ratio than is seen here. Thus, these cells are consistent with HPV infection and the best diagnosis is LGSIL.

A-45. (**c**) **Quality indicator**: **obscuring blood**, **HGSIL**, **cannot rule out invasion**

A diagnosis of "unsatisfactory" is unacceptable as there are clearly abnormal cells in the slide. Any abnormality, even if accompanied by a qualifying adequacy factor, must be diagnosed and not read out as "unsatisfactory." Although the blood appears granular in the background, it should be recognized as such and not diagnosed as bacteria. Additionally, the abnormal N/C ratio of the cells precludes a NILM diagnosis. The high nuclear/cytoplasmic ratios are inconsistent with a diagnosis of LGSIL. Of these choices, "HGSIL, cannot rule out invasion" is the best choice. The groups seem to include "clinging tumor diathesis" as well as abnormal cells. Tumor diathesis on liquid-based preparations will often appear as seen on this slide and will contain fresh and old blood, as well as necrotic debris from degenerating and dying cells. Before an "unsatisfactory" diagnosis is rendered, the slide should be carefully screened even when there are obscuring factors such as blood to rule out the presence of abnormal cells.

A-46. (**a**) **LGSIL**

These cells are consistent with infection by HPV. They show large, clear halos, and some type of nuclear irregularity (enlargement, wrinkling of the nuclear membrane, and hyperchromasia). Although infection with HR HPV 16 or 18 might be present, it is impossible to diagnose on cytology what specific type of HPV is causing the cellular abnormality. A molecular diagnostic test would be required. The cells depicted do not show the increased N/C ratio consistent with HGSIL. Also, they do not have the cytoplasmic ribboning, prominent nucleoli, and hypochromasia typical of repair.

A-47. (**c**) **HGSIL**

This slide most likely represents HGSIL, probably of keratinizing type. The slide shows cells with a high N/C ratio and deeply eosinophilic cytoplasm (suggestive of abnormal keratinization). Additional history given indicates a clean background, numerous abnormal cells, and occasional pleomorphism. These features are characteristic of HGSIL, keratinizing type. In cases in which the pleomorphic cells make up greater than 10 % of the abnormal cells, a keratinizing squamous cell carcinoma should be considered. The differential diagnosis should not include LGSIL, due to the very high N/C ratio present. Also, indications of pleomorphism are most often seen in higher grade lesions rather than LGSIL. The lack of nucleoli and ribboning excludes repair. Endocervical AIS might be considered due to the clean background and cytoplasmic eosinophilia; however, the pleomorphism, abnormal keratinization, and polygonal appearance of these cells should exclude this from consideration.

A-48. (**c**) **Endometrial adenocarcinoma**

The most likely diagnosis of this case is endometrial adenocarcinoma. The cells are seen in clusters rather than sheets or syncytial groups. They have a distinctly three-dimensional appearance. The background seems to contain delicate wisps of tumor diathesis. Conventional slides often will have a watery, bluish, granular tumor diathesis. Liquid-based slides often have a "stringy" diathesis and some "clinging" tumor diathesis. However, the blatantly bloody tumor diathesis of endocervical adenocarcinoma or squamous cell carcinoma is not present. Additionally the cells are not markedly hyperchromatic, as would be expected with a squamous cell carcinoma and to a somewhat lesser degree, endocervical adenocarcinoma. The cytoplasm is finely vacuolated, frothy, and the nuclei are considerably enlarged from the standard size of a normal intermediate cell nucleus. Nucleoli can be observed in the right hand panel. LGSIL is not a consideration since these cells have a glandular configuration and cytoplasmic appearance rather than the sharply defined cytoplasm of cells of squamous origin.

A-49. (**d**) **HGSIL**

These images show cells in sheet arrangements with high nuclear/cytoplasmic ratios. The nuclei are hyperchromatic and some of them are very angular or irregularly shaped. Note for example in the left panel, in the upper left corner, the nucleus which is crescent-shaped, the one a little lower which is shaped almost like a triangle, and the several which are spindle-shaped. Normal nuclei should be round to oval and this degree of angularity is quite abnormal. Also note the anisonucleosis present in the groups, as well as the indication of abnormal keratinization in the left panel. The background appears clean. While there are some normal squamous metaplastic cells present, the abnormal cells are larger, with higher N/C ratios and more hyperchromasia. Endocervical AIS is not a consideration as these cells are not glandular or columnar in shape and do not have the palisading common in AIS. The N/C ratio is too high for LGSIL. There are no classic features for squamous cell carcinoma such as nucleoli, dirty background, highly pleomorphic cells, and extremely high N/C ratio or syncytial groups.

A-50. (**d**) **HGSIL**

These cells have a high N/C ratio, irregular nuclear shapes, hyperchromasia, and some nuclear grooves and wrinkling. Their arrangement seems to be sheet-like with some cells approaching a syncytial arrangement. This is most consistent with HGSIL. The cells are too large with too high an N/C ratio to be squamous metaplasia. Compare the abnormal cells with the normal squamous cells present in the image. The N/C ratio is too high for the consideration of ASCUS or LGSIL as a diagnosis. The cells also lack nucleoli and do not appear to have any clinging tumor diathesis in the background. Thus, squamous cell carcinoma is not a consideration.

A-51. **(d) Squamous cell carcinoma**

These cells show hyperchromasia, irregular chromatin patterns, anisonucleosis, clinging tumor diathesis, and indications of abnormal keratinization. The chaotic, haphazard arrangement of the cells is also an indication of malignancy. Repair would have much less hyperchromasia and a more finely granular, uniform chromatin pattern. Also, this case lacks the ribbon-like arrangements frequent in repair. The consideration of LGSIL or HGSIL is highly unlikely due to the very high N/C ratio present in these cells and the dirty background. Nucleoli are also present in this image and would be highly unlikely in premalignant lesions. While an adenocarcinoma might be considered due to the patient's age and history, the cells themselves have sharp-edged distinct cytoplasm and polygonal shapes, indicating their squamous origin. The cells also lack a two dimensional picket fence arrangement (as would be seen in endocervical adenocarcinoma) or a three-dimensional cluster or papillary grouping (as would be seen in endometrial adenocarcinoma).

A-52. **(d) Reactive atypia, Trichomonas**

There are at least four trichomonads in the left panel, right lower edge, as well as several that can be observed in the right panel. These flagellated amoeba are probably among the most commonly seen infectious agents in Pap smears. The flagella are seldom observed, although since the advent of liquid-based preparations, they can more often occasionally be seen. There are several common patterns of staining and morphology observed with a Trichomonas infection. One commonly seen pattern is an extreme inflammatory reaction with many polymorphonuclear leukocytes, sometimes in wreaths and ball formations in the background. Another common pattern is as seen here, in which, paradoxically, there is virtually no background of polys at all. These slides also often display an unusually bright, intense staining reaction, as seen here. Also, the presence of the Trichomonas causes a slight edema of the nuclei, which is seen as very slight nuclear enlargement in the slide. Also, some cytoplasmic irregularities may be seen, including a "moth-eaten" appearance, or some small indistinctly edged perinuclear halos (seen on the right). One should be careful not to overcall these as evidence of LGSIL. Additionally, the very slight nuclear enlargement is insufficient for a diagnosis of either ASCUS or LGSIL. The Trichomonas should be reported so that the clinician can properly treat the patient for the infection.

A-53. **(e) NILM, reactive atypia, Candida**

The right panel shows the typical appearance of Candida in a cervical/vaginal sample. Note the pseudohyphae and somewhat irregular staining showing the septate growth pattern of the fungal organisms. Candida is associated with pregnancy, diabetes, and immunosuppression. Note also the small, ill-defined perinuclear halos in the cell group on the left. These are reactive changes caused by the Candida infection. While slight nuclear enlargement can be seen, it is most consistent with one and one-half to two times the size of a normal intermediate cell nucleus. The nuclei that are visible have maintained a normal N/C ratio and do not appear to have nuclear irregularities. This excludes both ASCUS and LGSIL as diagnostic possibilities. Thus, since the right panel shows typical features of Candida species, the best answer is e.

A-54. **(e) HGSIL**

These cells are quite small with very high N/C ratios. Careful examination may be required to arrive at the correct interpretation. These cells seem to contain sharp-edged, crisp cytoplasmic borders, and the largest of these cells (top section of the left panel) clearly shows their squamous origin. They have a somewhat polygonal shape with a central nucleus. This eliminates normal endocervical cells which have eccentric nuclei. The cytoplasm in normal endometrial cells would be less well-defined, finely vacuolated, and the cells tend to occur in 3D groups or loose clusters. Also, endometrial cell nuclei are less uniformly round to oval and often show reniform or irregularly shaped nuclei. The N/C ratio is too high and they are too hyperchromatic for squamous metaplastic cells. While ASC-H is a morphologic consideration, the history given and the several images would indicate that these abnormal cells are sufficiently abundant in number to qualify for a diagnosis of HGSIL. When the abnormal cells are quite few in number, care must be taken to locate and properly diagnose cells with this morphology as ASC-H, as these cases were found to have CIN2 or worse in 30–40 % of patients in the ALTS trial.

A-55. **(e) Squamous cell carcinoma**

These cells have the characteristic appearance of squamous cell carcinoma. Pleomorphism, abnormal keratinization, and extremely hyperchromatic, irregular nuclei are noted. Note also the dense, very sharp-edged cytoplasm. Nucleoli are not well observed in this sample, probably due to the extreme hyperchromasia often present in cells originating from a keratinizing type of squamous cell carcinoma. These types of carcinoma may have a relatively cleaner background than either non-keratinizing or small cell squamous cell carcinoma due to their often exophytic growth pattern. However, some evidence of clinging tumor diathesis may be seen, especially in the panel on the left. Differentiating between a HGSIL lesion and an invasive keratinizing squamous cell carcinoma may thus present difficulties. The best procedure is to determine the approximate percentage of abnormal cells which display pleomorphism. If it is greater than 10 %, an invasive keratinizing squamous cell carcinoma should be considered.

A-56. **(c) LGSIL**

These cells have the characteristic features of cells derived from HPV infection. These koilocytes have large, clear, distinctly defined perinuclear halos, along with nuclear abnormalities. Nuclear abnormalities may include enlargement (from slight up to one-third the diameter of the cell), smudginess, bi- and multinucleation, and hyperchromasia. Even in cells without appreciable nuclear enlargement, if one of the other nuclear abnormalities is present along with the clear, large halo, they can be designated as koilocytes and a diagnosis of LGSIL is appropriate. Small, ill-defined perinuclear halos accompany reactive atypia, such as is seen in Trichomonas or Candida infections. These HPV halos are much bigger, take up more of the cytoplasm of the cell, and some of them have thickened dense cytoplasm at the edge of the halo. If the halos were not characteristic for HPV and/or the nuclear abnormalities were absent, ASCUS might be a consideration. However, that is not the case in this image. Radiation does not produce these typical koilocytotic changes, although it may produce some vacuolization in the cytoplasm. Usually this is accompanied by an enlargement of both the nucleus and the cytoplasm so that very large cells, with multiple or enlarged nuclei may be found. The key is that the N/C ratio is usually maintained within the normal range. Polychromasia, finely granular chromatin, and bizarre cell shapes may also occur in post radiation therapy.

A-57. **(d) Send patient for colposcopically directed biopsy**

These cells are koilocytes and are pathognomic of HPV infection. The clear, large perinuclear halos, abnormalities in the nuclei, and thickening of the cytoplasmic rim around the halo are classic for a diagnosis of LGSIL. The best follow-up for LGSIL patients was evaluated in the ALTS trial which determined that high-risk HPV testing (HR HPV) was positive so often (87 %) in LGSIL patients that it was not cost-effective to perform. Low-risk HPV (LR HPV) is never indicated for any reason in the cytology laboratory. A p16 molecular test would also not be cost-effective in the follow-up of this patient. The prescribed follow-up would be colposcopically directed biopsy. It must be remembered that even LGSIL has a biopsy correlation of CIN2 or above in 15–25 % of patients. Therefore, a repeat Pap in 1 year may allow up to a quarter of patients with cytologically diagnosed LGSIL to progress to even more serious lesions without proper timely care. Thus, an immediate colposcopically biopsy is the best follow-up.

A-58. **(d) HGSIL**

These images show cells that have high N/C ratios, hyperchromatic irregular chromatin, moderate anisonucleosis, an absence of nucleoli, and a clean background. Compare their size with the normal appearing cells in the left panel. The nuclei are darker, have irregular areas of clearing and clumping in the chromatin, and some cells have nuclear rim thickening. They appear to have squamous type cytoplasm, rather than glandular cytoplasm such as AIS or normal endometrial cells might have. The cytoplasm appears polygonal, and the nuclei are central. The edges of the cytoplasm seem sharp and distinctly bordered. Also, the N/C ratio is quite marked, excluding a LGSIL from consideration. On the other hand, the background appears clean and no nucleoli are noted. The absence of these features helps to rule out a diagnosis of squamous cell carcinoma.

A-59. **(d) Chronic follicular cervicitis**

The key to this diagnosis is in noticing the very small, round lymphocytes within this "pool" of lymphs of a range of maturation. Some of the more immature lymphs have much larger, hypochromatic nuclei and nucleoli, consistent with the histologic appearance of follicular groups of lymphs below the epithelium. Note how there is no molding of the nuclei, consistent with the non-cohesive nature of lymphocytes. Also, this group of lymphocytes is relatively "pure" without many other types of inflammatory cells. The only exception to this is the occasional presence of tingible body macrophages (TBM), histiocytes with lymphocytic nuclear material ingested in the cytoplasm. Although finding a TBM is not required for this diagnosis, it can help to confirm an initial suspicion. Patients with Chlamydia and postmenopausal patients are often found to have chronic follicular cervicitis. Although these are lymphocytes and a few of them are immature, the patient has a diverse population with all levels of maturation included. Leukemia would generally have only one immature type of lymph present. Acute inflammatory cells are not noted. The final possibility, small cell carcinoma of the cervix, is ruled out due to the presence of the very small, perfectly round mature lymphs. These are smaller than even the nuclei of small cell carcinoma. Also, small cell carcinoma and leukemia/lymphoma would have a more uniform appearance than the variety of lymphoid maturation apparent here.

A-60. **(b) HGSIL**
These cells have hyperchromatic chromatin, very high N/C ratios, irregular chromatin pattern, anisonucleosis, and squamous appearing, hard-edged cytoplasm. These features are consistent with a HGSIL. LGSIL can be excluded because these cells have too high N/C ratio for LGSIL. Squamous cell carcinoma is not a consideration due to the lack of nucleoli, absence of syncytial groupings, and clean background. Finally, endometrial adenocarcinoma is more likely to have delicate, frothy scant cytoplasm, prominent nucleoli, and three-dimensional groupings.

A-61. **(c) Herpes simplex, plan for Cesarean section at delivery**
These cells have the typical configuration of herpes, multinucleation, molding of the nuclei, and "ground glass" chromatin. As seen here, the nuclei may be somewhat pale and powdery due to the viral infection. Sometimes, eosinophilic intranuclear inclusions can also be seen. Margination of the chromatin resulting in a thickened nuclear rim may be present. Herpes is a very significant finding in a woman towards the end of her pregnancy. If the woman is having a recurrent infection, she may already have developed antibodies and passed them on to the fetus, in which case the fetus is more likely to be protected. However, if the status is unknown and the infection occurs after week 36, the infant has a 33 % chance of developing an infection with quite serious sequelae including demise. Therefore, in this case, a Cesarean section is recommended to prevent the delivery through the infected birth canal. Syncytiotrophoblasts are occasionally seen in threatened or post abortion. However, trophoblastic cells, although multinucleated, have bland, regular nuclei without the characteristic molding and ground glass appearance of herpes. Multinucleated histiocytes may also be seen in pregnant women, but they have foamy cytoplasm and uniform bland finely granulated chromatin in the nuclei. HGSIL is not a consideration as these nuclei are not hyperchromatic and HGSIL would have distinct, irregular chromatin, unlike the powdery, ground glass pattern seen here.

A-62. **(a) Squamous cell carcinoma, HPV subtype 16 or 18 infection**
These cells are most consistent with squamous cell carcinoma. They display very hyperchromatic nuclei, with some that are even opaque. Pleomorphism is noted. There is evidence of abnormal keratinization with the cytoplasm of some cells staining deeply pink to orange. The arrangement of cells is single or in syncytial groups. The N/C ratio is extremely high and the nuclear shapes are spindle, triangular, or round to oval. Nucleoli may be seen if the hyperchromasia of the nuclei allows for it. Endometrial adenocarcinoma might be a consideration due to the patient's age, but the distinct squamous-like edges of the cytoplasm would not be consistent with this diagnosis. Endocervical adenocarcinoma might be considered due to the deep eosinophilia of the cytoplasm; however in this case, the cytoplasm lacks the granularity and glandular appearance of endocervical adenocarcinoma. Ovarian adenocarcinoma is not a consideration due to the lack of clustering, glandular cytoplasmic appearance, or prominent nucleoli.

A-63. **(d) Endocervical adenocarcinoma in situ**
The key to this diagnosis lies in the ability to distinguish a syncytial group from a glandular 2D endocervical type of architecture. Note in the left panel, how the nuclei are parallel to one another on the left side of the group. Also note the crowded parallel, pseudopalisading of the nuclei at the top of the group in the right panel. This is typical feathering of the endocervical nuclei in which the nuclei are so crowded within the cluster that the nuclei protrude outward, like the feathers of a bird's wing. Hyperchromatic crowded groups such as these should always be examined carefully to detect the architectural characteristics of the cells. Squamous cell carcinoma is excluded since this is not a syncytial grouping of cells and since nucleoli are not conspicuous. Likewise, the organized arrangement of pseudopalisading nuclei with feathering visible at the edges helps to rule out CIS. Endocervical adenocarcinoma is a consideration due to the 2D arrangement of the cells; however, these usually have very conspicuous macronucleoli or multiple nucleoli present.

A-64. **(c) LGSIL**
These cells have large, distinct perinuclear halos and have coexisting nuclear abnormalities consistent with a diagnosis of LGSIL. These changes are caused by HPV infection and morphologic evidence of this

infection is indicated by the sharp thickened cytoplasmic edge of the halo, the increase in nuclear size or bi-nucleation, and the increase in hyperchromasia of some of the nuclei. Although not clearly seen here, the nuclei are sometimes also seen as smudgy, without crisp chromatin particles. Reactive cellular changes may also sometimes show perinuclear halos in cases with Trichomonas or Candida. However, those halos are smaller, have ill-defined edges, and should not be confused with the clear, large halos seen here. The abnormal cells seen here are also clearly caused by HPV infection, so a diagnosis of ASCUS is less precise than is possible with these cells. If cells have questionable cavitations suggestive of HPV, and no clear koilocytes can be found, then ASCUS may be an acceptable diagnosis. Finally, HGSIL is not an appropriate diagnosis for these cells as the nuclear/cytoplasmic ratio is not high enough.

A-65. (**d**) **From the squamocolumnar junction**
These cells are quite abnormal and indications of a tumor diathesis are seen in the background. The "stringy" appearance of the old blood and cellular debris is common on liquid-based preparations. Clinging tumor diathesis can also be found in these types of preparations. Note the evidence of keratinization in the upper right hand panel. Combined with the elongated spindle-like appearance of the cytoplasm and the nuclei, this case is most consistent with a squamous carcinoma. Thus, the endometrium, the glands of the endocervix, and the fallopian tube are unlikely anatomic sites for this type of cancer. The squamocolumnar junction is the most common site of origin for squamous cell carcinoma of the cervix.

A-66. (**d**) **ASC-H, immediate colposcopically directed biopsy**
These cells have a very high N/C ratio, irregular nuclear outlines, hyperchromasia, and the information that relatively few of these cells were found in the ThinPrep sample. This presentation is most consistent with a diagnosis of ASC-H. The most recent guidelines for treatment from the ASCCP (2009) indicate that immediate colposcopically directed biopsy is the most cost-effective treatment for these patients. HR HPV testing for these patients is not cost-effective since they have at least a 70 % positivity rate. Additionally, this is a very significant diagnosis since at least 50 % of these cases are found to have CIN 2 or worse on biopsy. This compares to the 60–70 % CIN 2 or higher biopsy rate found with HGSIL. Thus, these lesions are quite significant on follow-up. The hyperchromasia and N/C ratio is much higher than would be found in reactive cells. The N/C ratio is also too high for a diagnosis of ASCUS. ASC-H is the correct cytologic diagnosis and, as stated above, the correct follow-up should be immediate colposcopically directed biopsy.

A-67. (**a**) **Candida**
These panels show Candida organisms with pinkish hyphae which have light and dark staining. These organisms often pierce the squamous cells and create a "string of pearls" effect with the fungus being the "string" and the squamous cells being the "pearls." Pregnancy, diabetes, and antibiotic use are common risk factors for Candida. Syncytiotrophoblasts are a very uncommon finding and are seen as multinucleated cells, often in "tadpole" like shapes. They represent placental tissue and may accompany a threatened spontaneous abortion. Reparative cells usually have streaming cytoplasm, prominent nucleoli in nearly 100 % of the cells, and pale, bland chromatin. The panel in the lower right is probably inflammatory cell changes that may accompany Candida infection. CMV should have a prominent "owl's eye" large inclusion body within the nucleus. CMV may also have cytoplasmic inclusions as well.

A-68. (**b**) **Actinomyces, Trichomonas**
The organism present in the upper left hand corner shows the typical characteristics of Trichomonas: pear-shaped, indistinct vacuolated cytoplasm, and an eccentric nucleus. Under extremely favorable conditions, the flagella of these organisms are sometimes preserved, but this is rare. The lower middle panel shows these organisms alongside some squamous cells. Actinomyces is a higher-order bacteria that forms colonies with starburst-like filaments protruding from a background of small coccoid-like bacteria. It is often found in women wearing IUDs. Herpes must have "ground glass" chromatin appearance and these images do not show this; Candida does not show the starburst arrangement seen here. CMV is not represented on the slide as owl-eye inclusions are not seen. Cytolysis is also not an organism and the bacteria represented should not be interpreted as such.

A-69. (**c**) **HPV subtype 16 positive**
The cells have the morphologic configuration of HGSIL with high N/C ratios, hyperchromatic nuclei, and squamous appearing cytoplasm. Although HR HPV typing should not be performed on HGSIL cases as it is not cost-effective, the results from subtype specific testing can be predicted in this case because the only high-risk subtype in the choices

given is subtype 16. The other choices (6, 11, and 40) are low-risk subtypes and would not have been detected in a high-risk HPV molecular test. 6, 11, and 40 might coexist with 16 but are rarely found in cancer. HPV 16 is the most common viral subtype to infect the cervix and may be associated with a range of lesions from koilocytotic atypia, LGSIL, HGSIL, and on to squamous cell carcinoma. HPV types 16, 18, 45, and 31 (in that order) make up about 80 % of the high-risk HPV types found in cervical squamous cell carcinoma.

A-70. (**e**) **HGSIL**

These cells have a very high N/C ratio as well as hyperchromasia. Note also the angularity of some of the nuclei. This is rare in the absence of neoplasia. These cells are most consistent with a high-grade lesion. Folic acid deficiency has cytomegaly without an increase in N/C ratio. The N/C ratio is also too high for normal squamous metaplasia. Herpes would have multinucleation, hypochromasia, and "ground glass" nuclei. Reactive endocervical cells would have a more elongated cytoplasm with small nucleoli present. Also, the characteristic endocervical pattern of picket fence or honeycomb arrangement is not seen.

A-71. (**d**) **HGSIL**

Although these nuclei are rather small (2–2½× a normal intermediate cell nucleus), the N/C ratio is markedly increased. They are hyperchromatic and show some nuclei with abnormal shapes (arrowhead, tadpole). They are arranged in a sheet or syncytial arrangement. Compare the sizes carefully with the surrounding normal cells. Endometrial cells would be smaller (same size as an intermediate cell nucleus) with an even higher N/C ratio in the case of epithelial or deep endometrial cells. Chronic follicular cervicitis would have a more varied size range from the perfectly round normal lymphocytes to the larger, more immature lymphs making up the lymphocytic infiltrate.

A-72. (**a**) **>80 % of LGSIL contains HR HPV subtypes**

These cellular changes are pathognomonic of HPV infection, (LGSIL). Note the large, clear, sharp-edged perinuclear halos, as well as some nuclear abnormality such as bi-nucleation, increase in nuclear size, or hyperchromatic, smudgy nuclei. Interestingly, although "low-risk" HPV subtypes are commonly associated with lower-grade lesions such as genital warts and LGSIL, more than 80 % of LGSILs contain "high-risk" HPV subtypes. This contrasts with CIN 3 lesions in which virtually all of the cases contain HR HPV. So although the statement is true, the lesion depicted is not HGSIL. Perinuclear glycogen in the cells of pregnant patients might briefly resemble the findings here, but a more thorough examination will rule this out, mainly due to the absence of the typical yellow glycogen deposits. Finally, as was determined in the ALTS trial, the majority of these cases are HR HPV positive, so performing molecular diagnostics on them is not cost-effective and they should go to immediate colposcopically directed biopsy. However, all of these would be smaller than the cells seen here. Also, the centrally placed nucleus and the squamous appearance of the small amounts of cytoplasm are more consistent with HGSIL than follicular cervicitis. These cells have too high an N/C ratio for squamous metaplasia, as well as too much hyperchromasia for a benign protective process.

A-73. (**c**) **Folic acid deficiency**

The cytomegaly seen here in these multinucleated cells is most likely due to a deficiency in one of the B vitamins, folic acid. This vitamin is utilized in DNA synthesis and a deficiency in this vitamin can mimic changes seen in radiation therapy. This change is reversible with folic acid therapy. Low levels of folic acid during early pregnancy have been associated with increased fetal risk of spina bifida, a neural tube defect. This patient's lack of previous abnormal history and relatively young age makes radiation effect unlikely. LGSIL is unlikely since the N/C ratio is not significantly increased, the cells are few, and they are quite large in comparison to normal cells. Also, due to the patient's pregnant status, IUD effect is not a tenable diagnosis. IUD effect is seen as vacuolization of metaplastic or endocervical cells.

A-74. (**a**) **Degenerated parabasal cells**

Small, pink to orange-staining cells may frequently be seen in samples from postmenopausal women who have an atrophic pattern. Note that there are also very small cells with bluish cytoplasm present as well. These changes are due to the failure of the cells to fully mature due to lack of estrogen. A key to this diagnosis is the age of the patient as well as the background pattern of marked atrophy. Although the cells are staining pink to orange, this does not indicate abnormal keratinization as might be seen with parakeratosis. The overall hormonal pattern of the slide also indicates atrophy rather than squamous metaplasia, which also usually does not stain orange. The N/C ratio in these cells and their lack of an abnormal chromatin pattern rules out a HGSIL, although atrophic slides should be screened carefully for any evidence of neoplasia.

A-75. (**b**) **Radiation effect**

These cells are showing marked enlargement, multinucleation, vacuolization of the cytoplasm, small nucleoli, and an N/C ratio that is not markedly increased. The bizarre shapes of the cytoplasm are also characteristic of radiation effect. Poly engulfment and polychromasia may also be seen occasionally. These are not endocervical repair because the cells are not streaming, with pale chromatin and prominent nucleoli in every cell, nor do they appear to have derived from endocervical epithelium, which in this case would not be present due to the hysterectomy. Although multinucleated, the nuclei are not ground glass nor molding as in herpes. Finally, the cells do not show the high N/C ratio, the abnormal chromatin pattern, and the loose syncytial arrangement that would be present in recurrent squamous cell carcinoma.

A-76. (**a**) **Degenerated parabasal cells**

These structures are relatively commonly found in postmenopausal patients with severely atrophic patterns, such as this patient. These "blue blobs" are thought to be very degenerated parabasal cells and remnants of the nuclei can sometimes be seen. The background in these patients often appears "busy" on liquid-based preparations and granularity of the background debris may give a false impression of tumor diathesis. However, the crisp chromatin pattern of neoplasia is not seen and the structures are not naked enlarged nuclei but are parabasal cells which have degenerated. Compare their overall size and shape with the other parabasal cells in the panels. The structure is too large to be of endometrial origin and lacks identifiable glandular cytoplasm. ASCUS is also a poor choice again due to the lack of identifiable cytoplasm. Pollen is usually better preserved, stains deep red to yellow, and varies in size and shape depending on the plant from which it is derived. It is important to recognize this common artifact to avoid overcalling.

A-77. (**b**) **Actinomyces infection**

"Fuzzy" appearing colonies of bluish or violet coccoid bacteria with the actinomyces organisms seen as filamentous "sunburst" rays extending outward from the colony are typical for this organism. Rarely a discharge or abdominal pain may be present. These organisms may be seen in association with IUDs or with other foreign objects such as pessaries or tampons. When seen in association with an IUD, there may be an inflammatory background. Therapy may include IUD removal, antibiotics, or both. Candida is not seen in association with colonies of symbiotic bacteria, as is actinomyces. Also, Candida is a fungus, not a higher-order bacteria, and its diameter is larger than the actinomyces filaments. Leptothrix is also a filamentous bacteria which almost always occurs with Trichomonas. It appears as a long, curving lavender lactobacilli structure with a diameter much thinner than Candida. Its long curving nature distinguishes it from the actinomyces which occurs within the bacterial colonies. "Shift in vaginal flora" is the term adopted by the Bethesda System to indicate "bacterial vaginalis." "Shift" should be used to indicate coccoid bacteria or coccobacilli which are seen coating epithelial cells ("clue" cells) or in the background.

A-78. (**e**) **Shift in vaginal flora suggestive of bacterial vaginosis**

These small coccoid bacteria usually stain bluish and may be coating the cells, as here, or in the background of the slide. Rod-shaped lactobacilli of the normal type (Doderlein) are not present. There is often a milky vaginal discharge, and inflammation is usually absent. Normal floras, i.e., Doderlein lactobacilli, are rod-shaped bacteria and are normally found in the background of the slide and not coating the epithelial cells as seen here. The other terms (Haemophilus vaginalis, Gardnerella vaginalis, and "clue cells") have been replaced in the newest Bethesda System terminology by the broader "shift in vaginal flora suggestive of bacterial vaginosis." While "shift" includes the finding of clue cells, and the other bacteria are often found in bacterial vaginosis, the newest terminology is considered a better choice as bacterial vaginosis is not caused by a single organism. The new term is not definitive for bacterial vaginosis, and clinical correlation is required to arrive at a diagnosis.

A-79. (**d**) **Chronic follicular cervicitis**

These cells are mature and immature lymphocytes. An important clue to this diagnosis is finding the smallest, perfectly round mature lymphs in the group. When these have been identified as mature lymphs, then the slightly larger, more immature lymphocytes can be identified. Often in liquid-based preparations, these lymphs seem to be caught up in a faintly visible matrix, as seen here. In conventional slides the lymphs occur in a "pool" which may extend over a large area. Tingible body macrophages may also sometimes be found but are not required for this diagnosis. This condition often occurs with Chlamydia infection. Acute inflammation would be represented by polymorphonuclear leukocytes. These cells are too small to represent a squamous lesion such as ASC-H or HGSIL. Molding is not identified as it would be in HGSIL due to the lack of cohesion of the lymphatic cells. Again, the very small round lymphs can help to rule out these options. Endometrial cells do not have such round, very small cells and their nuclei may be spindle, or bean-shaped, and may have a wrinkled raisin-like appearance. Also the size of an endometrial cell nucleus should be equal to the size of an intermediate cell nucleus; these lymphs are smaller.

A-80. (**c**) **Hyperkeratosis**

These cells are annucleated squamous cells which represent hyperkeratosis. This is a benign proliferative reaction which has pink to yellow mature cells without nuclei. One may see "ghost" nuclei, empty clear spaces where the nuclei had once occupied the cells. Some of these are faintly visible in the lower edge of the group. Parakeratosis (PK) is made of much smaller cells and has been described as "miniature superficial squamous cells." This is also a benign protective reaction and may occur with hyperkeratosis. PK is often only about 20 % or less the size of normal squamous cells. Dyskeratotic cells are also small, like parakeratotic cells but have more rounded, dense, orangeophilic cytoplasm with a slightly larger, smudgy, hyperchromatic nucleus. Microglandular hyperplasia is frequent in patients taking oral contraceptives. It is made up of degenerated glandular cells which are pink to orange, very small, rounded, and it superficially resembles parakeratosis. However, the rounded cytoplasm is finely vacuolated and glandular in appearance.

A-81. (**d**) **Mature squamous cells with large, well-defined perinuclear halos**

These small cells show the dense, rounded, orange cytoplasm typical for dyskeratocytes. Note also the enlarged, smudgy, hyperchromatic nuclei consistent with HPV infection. Thus, these cells would most likely be accompanied by koilocytes with large, well-defined perinuclear halos. Small ill-defined perinuclear halos are consistent with inflammatory changes caused by Trichomonas or Candida and they are not associated with dyskeratocytes. Endocervical cells with hyperdistended vacuoles are also not associated with dyskeratocytes. The slide seems to show a normal hormonal pattern and thus these cells are not the small orange parabasal cells sometimes seen in a background of extreme atrophy. Additionally, these cells have denser cytoplasm and have larger, darker nuclei than those found in atrophic slides.

A-82. (**d**) **Effects of HPV infection**

The large clear halos in these cells are evidence of infection by human papillomavirus (HPV). These cells, koilocytes, should have both the large clear halos seen here but also often have some abnormality of the nucleus: smudginess, hyperchromasia, increased N/C ratio, irregular chromatin, etc. Chemotherapy or radiation both lead to cytomegaly without increased N/C ratio and that is not seen here. Inflammation (Trichomonas or Candida) may cause perinuclear halos, but the halos are much smaller, more ill-defined on the inner edges, and there is not a significant increase in the N/C ratio. Also inflammatory perinuclear halos are not associated with a nuclear abnormality such as those listed above. These cells are clearly squamous cells with sharp-edged cytoplasm, and in the absence of radiation or other causes, squamous cells seldom show any vacuolization in the cytoplasm.

A-83. (**b**) **Plasma cells**

These small cells display an eccentric nucleus which has a characteristic "clock-face" or "soccer ball" appearance due to large clumps of chromatin and surrounding areas of paler chromatin. These cells are seen in cases of chronic inflammation and may be occasionally found in a pool as seen here. It is important to note their single, non-cohesive arrangement. Mature lymphs would be slightly smaller and rounder, while immature lymphs would be larger than these cells and would not have the eccentric, soccer ball appearance of the nucleus. Histiocytes would have more abundant cytoplasm and would be larger. Endometrial cells would be more cohesive and would have some bean-shaped nuclei. The normal size of an endometrial cell nucleus is the same as an intermediate cell nucleus. Endometrial cells also do not have this chromatin pattern. Small cell carcinoma of the cervix might be a consideration initially, but these cells do not show the subtle variation in size, chromatin pattern, or degree of hyperchromasia consistent with small cell carcinoma of the cervix.

A-84. (**a**) **Herpes**

These cells have the characteristic features of herpes: multinucleation, molding of the nuclei against one another, and "ground glass" chromatin. Herpes cells may also have eosinophilic intranuclear inclusion bodies. Multinucleated histiocytes do not display the molding of the nuclei or ground glass chromatin pattern as seen here. Also they will have more abundant lacy cytoplasm. LGSIL will display enlarged nuclei with an increased N/C ratio of about one-third the diameter of the cell. The chromatin pattern will be crisp and well-defined or may be dark and smudgy in koilocytes. It will not be ground glass as seen here. Some cells of LGSIL may be binucleated, particularly in koilocytes, but the nuclei will not display molding. A diagnosis of ASC-H should be reserved for cells which morphologically meet the criteria for HGSIL but are too few in number to warrant the diagnosis of HGSIL. HGSIL cells would never display the ground glass chromatin seen here and are seldom multinucleated. They should show hyperchromasia and irregular crisp chromatin patterns with high N/C ratios.

A-85. (**c**) **HGSIL**

These cells show rounded, dense, immature cytoplasm with enlarged nuclei. These nuclei show a generally finely granular, evenly distributed chromatin pattern and a high N/C ratio. Hyperchromasia is also noted. Hyperchromasia may be less pronounced in liquid-based preparations than in conventional slides. Compare the overall cell size and nuclear size with the normal squamous metaplastic cell in the upper left panel. A LGSIL would likely have a lower N/C ratio and be less likely to show the nuclear abnormalities seen here. Especially note the irregular nuclear outlines and signs of clefting and grooving of the nuclei. These nuclear abnormalities are less likely to be seen in LGSIL than in HGSIL. Repair is not a consideration due to the lack of nucleoli and streaming cytoplasm.

A-86. (**d**) **Squamous cell carcinoma**

This slide shows extensive blood, cellular debris, and necrosis in the background. The cells are small, but larger than the intermediate cell nuclei in the background. Additionally the nuclei have marked clearing and clumping of the chromatin, extremely high N/C ratios, hyperchromasia, and nucleoli can be identified. The cells appear to occur singly, in loose clusters or syncytial groups. These are all criteria for cervical carcinoma with small cell morphology. Benign endometrial cells are excluded by the presence of nucleoli and the dirty background. Also, benign endometrial cells should not be larger than the intermediate cell nuclei. Adenocarcinoma of the endometrium, although a consideration, is excluded by the marked irregularity of the chromatin, and the squamous appearance of the cytoplasm as seen in the lower right hand corner of the slide. Usually, endometrial adenocarcinoma has a more powdery, paler chromatin than the "salt and pepper" clearing and clumping observed in this slide. Also, one would expect somewhat more prominent nucleoli. The dirty background and presence of nucleoli exclude a HGSIL from consideration. Finally, adenocarcinoma of the endocervix would generally display multiple, prominent macronucleoli and architecture loosely resembling the picket fence or honeycomb arrangements seen in normal endocervical cells. Also, one would expect more abundant cytoplasm and eccentrically placed nuclei for endocervical adenocarcinoma.

A-87. (**b**) **The irregularity of the nuclear membranes**

At first glance, these cells might lead one towards a diagnosis of LGSIL, based solely on the N/C ratio. However, the nuclear membrane irregularities, as well as nuclear clefting, grooves, and hyperchromasia are markedly abnormal. One should carefully search the remainder of the slide for other evidence of HGSIL, including cells with markedly increased N/C ratios, such as is observed in the lower right hand corner of the slide. Usually LGSIL will have smooth nuclear borders, without clefting or nuclear grooves. Numbers of abnormal cells will also be a consideration, as well as the morphology. Usually HGSIL will show higher numbers of abnormal cells than LGSIL. In the case of rare cells with HGSIL morphology, ASC-H may be a consideration. The color of the nuclei or the cytoplasm generally is not a significant consideration in determining the severity of the lesion. The appearance of the background is usually only a criteria to assist when deciding between an invasive carcinoma and a CIS-type HGSIL. Since these cells do not show morphologic changes severe enough to consider that differential, the background is not an important consideration in this case.

A-88. (**c**) **HGSIL**

The most likely diagnosis is HGSIL. These cells show hyperchromasia, high N/C ratios, angular nuclear shapes, and evidence of clefting of the nuclei. Usually LGSIL cells have smooth nuclear borders and less irregularity of the sizes and shapes of the nuclei, as well as a lower N/C ratio than seen here. The finding of arrowhead, spindle, or non-isodiametric angular nuclei is an important feature, along with high N/C ratios, to diagnosis HGSIL. The N/C ratio here is much higher than would be expected in a case of ASCUS. The absence of a dirty background and nucleoli excludes squamous cell carcinoma from consideration.

A-89. **(d) Atrophy**

This slide shows the typical pattern of atrophy consistent with loss of cyclic estrogen. These cells are mainly of parabasal type with some lower intermediate cells as well. The background is not consistent with tumor diathesis, as might be seen in endometrial, endocervical, or squamous malignancies. Tumor diathesis usually contains old and fresh blood, cellular debris, necrotic material, and other evidence of the tissue destruction of normal cells by the invading cancer. However, the background illustrated here is often seen in atrophy and does not contain blood or cellular necrosis. It does contain some "streak" nuclei, evidence of the fragile nature of these atrophic cells. Also, there is a bluish background such as seen in conventional slides with atrophy. This must be differentiated from a true tumor diathesis. Additionally, the nuclei of these cells are uniform in size, shape, staining, and bland chromatin pattern. This uniformity helps to exclude any neoplastic process. Additionally, nucleoli are not seen. The patient's age is also a helpful piece of clinical history which makes the pattern seen here consistent with the expected hormonal status of the patient. The occasional finding of small orange-staining parabasal cells is often seen in atrophic slides and should not be interpreted as abnormal keratinization.

A-90. **(c) Endometrial cells**

These cells are displaying the typical pattern seen in normal endometrial cells during days 6–10 of the menstrual cycle. The cells may appear in a double walled structure called an endometrial cell ball (lower right hand corner). This is made up of endometrial epithelial cells and endometrial stromal cells. The cluster of cells in the upper right hand corner is typical for epithelial endometrial cells. A few single stromal cells are noted to the left of the cell ball, showing more abundant foamy cytoplasm than is usually seen in the epithelial cells. While a single small histiocyte is nearly identical in appearance to a single stromal endometrial cell, the three-dimensional clusters of cells seen indicate their epithelial origins. HGSIL is not a consideration since the displayed nuclei are uniform in size and staining, having bland, finely granular chromatin, and no hyperchromasia. Although the N/C ratio is high, these nuclei are the same size as an intermediate cell nucleus. HGSIL nuclei would be larger, more hyperchromatic, and have more irregular chromatin. Atrophy would be unusual in this age group, unless induced by surgical castration or immediate postpartum. Also, there is evidence of estrogen effect in the superficial and intermediate cells present. Chronic follicular cervicitis is ruled out by the cohesive nature of these cells, compared to mature and immature lymphs seen in follicular cervicitis. Follicular cervicitis lymphs are non-cohesive in appearance.

A-91. **(b) ASCUS and LGSIL**

A is most likely incorrect since these cells do have some type of morphologic abnormality as seen by the bi-nucleation, Thus, ASCUS vs. NILM is not a good choice. B is a better answer, since there is some nuclear atypia with a slight increase in the N/C ratio. There is also some indication of large perinuclear halos, although perhaps not classic for koilocytes in this field. A search of the remainder of the slide should be made to see if unequivocal koilocytes might be found. If they are not, and if the N/C ratio does not increase more than is seen here, a diagnosis of ASCUS might be appropriate. LGSIL vs. HGSIL is not an appropriate choice because the N/C ratio is not significantly enlarged, as it would be in either of those lesions. The same holds true for HGSIL vs. SCCA. The morphology is not supportive of either of those diagnoses.

A-92. **(b) Repair**

These cells have enlarged nuclei, streaming cytoplasm, nucleoli in most of the cells, and a bloody but not dirty background. The cells seem to maintain their polarity and the chromatin pattern is bland and not remarkable. Note the distinct cell borders and the cohesive sheet-like arrangement. The cells seem to have too much cytoplasm to be atrophy and atrophy does not usually contain nucleoli. Although some of the cells resemble squamous metaplasia, streaming cytoplasm and nucleoli are not found in squamous metaplasia. Also the nuclei are too variable for the usual appearance of squamous metaplasia. LGSIL does not have nucleoli and should have a more uniformly increased N/C ratio than is seen here.

A-93. **(a) Endometrial cells**

These cells are in a three-dimensional loose cluster. The nuclei are the same size as the nearby intermediate cell nucleus. Also note the bean-shaped nuclei visible within the cluster. These are indicative of endometrial origin. Additionally, the cytoplasm is fluffy or lacy appearing, indicating the glandular nature of these cells. Reactive endocervical cells are glandular but are larger in overall size, have an eccentric nucleus, and often show reactive, small nucleoli. None of these characteristics are seen in the group seen here. HGSIL would have larger cells with clearly squamous type cytoplasm. Also, the N/C ratio would be much increased over these cells, and hyperchromasia and irregular or clumpy chromatin could be observed in HGSIL. Carcinoma with small cell morphology of the cervix may have clearly squamous type cytoplasm, hyperchromasia, clumpy chromatin, and a markedly dirty background consistent with the biologic aggressiveness of the tumor. The bean-shaped nuclei of endometrial cells are not found in small cell carcinoma cells.

A-94. (**c**) **Radiation effect**
The key to this diagnosis is the presence of a couple of normal cells within the field. These two cells (one parabasal and one intermediate) are much smaller than the other cells displaying cytomegaly, nuclear and cytoplasmic vacuoles, ingested polys, and no significant increase in the N/C ratio. These cells are much too large and have too much cytoplasm to qualify for a diagnosis of atrophy. Post radiation dysplasia should display cytomegaly and other changes of radiation effect with a significant increase in the N/C ratio. A diagnosis of post radiation dysplasia within 3 years of treatment gives the patient a higher risk of having recurrent carcinoma. These cells do not have high N/C ratios, hyperchromasia, nucleoli, dirty background, or other signs of recurrent squamous cell carcinoma. Usually the persistent or recurrent tumor cells do not show effects of radiation therapy and they may be rather small.

A-95. (**c**) **HGSIL**
These cells are hyperchromatic with high N/C ratios. They appear in sheets or clusters of cells with syncytial arrangement. ASCUS is not the best choice since these cells have a much higher N/C ratio than the relatively lower N/C ratio prevalent in ASCUS. Also the N/C ratio is higher than it would be in LGSIL. HGSIL would have this scanty amount of cytoplasm and a large, hyperchromatic nuclei which take up over 80–90 % of the cell. The background is clean and the nuclei do not show nucleoli as it would if it represented cancer. Therefore, the best diagnosis for this case would be HGSIL.

A-96. (**d**) **IUD effect**
The key to this diagnosis is the presence of highly vacuolated cells of probable metaplastic and/or endocervical origin. These cells become irritated by the presence of the endocervical string on the IUD and react by becoming vacuolated. Clear cell adenocarcinoma of the vagina was associated with intrauterine exposure to DES during the mother's pregnancy. This resulted in vaginal adenosis and occasional clear cell adenocarcinoma of the vagina in women in their teens and early adulthood. The cells of clear cell adenocarcinoma, however, are obviously malignant, with abundant cytoplasm, macronucleoli, and a dirty background. DES was prescribed from 1945 to 1971 and the risk of clear cell adenocarcinoma was about 1/2,000 women. Since the youngest of these women are now approaching 40, this diagnosis is becoming more and more unlikely. The cytoplasm of these cells is too dense for histiocytes and these are multiple cells, rather than two multinucleated cells. Endocervical AIS is composed of crowded, tall columnar cells with feathering and elongated nuclei and clumpy chromatin. The cells here have excessively glandular appearing cytoplasm to consider a squamous malignancy. Also a squamous cancer would have nucleoli, clumpy chromatin, hyperchromasia and a dirty background.

A-97. (**d**) **Ectocervix**
These cells show evidence of abnormal keratinization, shown by the intensely orange staining of the cytoplasm of the squamous cells. Note also the pleomorphic shapes, the dark, opaque nuclei, and the overall squamous appearance of the cytoplasm. Keratinizing squamous cell carcinoma is most likely to originate on the ectocervix of the patient and is often associated with hyperkeratosis or parakeratosis. Nucleoli may be difficult to discern due to the intensely dark nuclei. Also, as these keratinizing lesions are often exophytic in their growth pattern, the background may not have as much tumor diathesis as non-keratinizing or small cell types of cervical carcinoma. The internal endocervical os would not be a good choice for the location of the origin of this squamous cell carcinoma. Endocervical glands would also not be a likely source for these cells. External endocervical os might have some involvement with a tumor such as this, but the most likely anatomic location is the ectocervix.

A-98. (**d**) **Trichomonas vaginalis**
There are about four to five trichomonas organisms in this field. These are protozoa which are pear- to oval-shaped with a faint elongated eccentrically located nucleus. Infection with Trichomonas and Candida may cause the small ill-defined perinuclear halos and the so-called "tissue paper" cells with cytoplasmic vacuolization. The organisms range in size from about 8–30 μm. These cells may have a somewhat "moth-eaten" appearance on ThinPrep. The halos produced by either HPV 18 or HPV 11 would be larger and the nuclei would be enlarged, smudgy, or have other abnormalities. The changes seen with Gardnerella vaginalis are the appearance of "clue cells" and background bacteria in the slide.

A-99. **(d) Cytomegalovirus**

Cytomegalovirus (CMV) is often described as having an "owl's eye" appearance due to the relatively large intranuclear inclusion body found within a pale appearing nucleus. CMV is distinguished from herpes simplex infection in that the cells of herpes are usually more abundant in the slide, are usually multinucleated, show evidence of nuclear molding, and have "ground glass" chromatin. Although CMV has similar chromatin, it is most usually found as cells with one single nucleus, and it has a quite large eosinophilic or basophilic inclusion body. CMV may also have blue cytoplasmic inclusions (25 %) unlike herpes. Note also that in this unusual case with two nuclei, they overlap one another and do not display the nuclear molding seen in herpes. Repair will also have pale nuclei but crisp chromatin particles will be visible, unlike the "ground glass" chromatin seen in virally infected cells. Also, repair should have streaming cytoplasm and occur in cohesive ribbons, rather than single cells. Finally, these cells do not display the delicate foamy cytoplasm and powdery, irregular chromatin characteristic of endometrial adenocarcinoma.

A-100. **(d) Pemphigus vulgaris**

This rare autoimmune disease was often fatal before the advent of corticosteroid treatment. Clinically the patient suffers from blistering, ulceration, and loss of mucosal and skin tissues, due to a loss of the desmosomes which anchor the cells to one another. The cytologic presentation shows groups and single cells with a prominent, eosinophilic bar-shaped nucleolus. The nuclei are round with pale chromatin. The cells do not show the cohesive streaming characteristics of repair. The nuclei are not "ground glass" as in herpes and the cells are not multinucleated. Also, the nuclei are not smudgy and pale, as they appear in CMV. Additionally, the nucleolus is not as large in relation to the size of the nucleus as the inclusion body is in CMV. This very painful disease may also cause blistering on the epidermis and both the loss of fluids and difficulties in swallowing may lead to significant weight loss, as in this patient. Thus, this clinical history and the appearance of the cells lead to the diagnosis of pemphigus.

Reading List

Cibas ES. Cervical and vaginal cytology. In: Cibas ES, Ducatman BS, editors. Cytology diagnostic principles and clinical correlates. Philadelphia: Saunders/Elsevier; 2009.

Cox JT, Solomon D, Schiffman M. Prospective follow-up suggests similar risk of subsequent CIN 2 or 3 among women with CIN 1 or negative colposcopy and directed biopsy. Am J Obstet Gynecol. 2003;188:1406–12.

DeMay RM. The Pap test. In: DeMay RM, editor. The art and science of cytopathology. 2nd ed. Chicago: ASCP Press; 2012.

Melnikow J, Nuovo J, Willan AR, et al. Natural history of cervical squamous intraepithelial lesions: a meta-analysis. Obstet Gynecol. 1998;92(4 Pt 2):727–35.

Money D, Steben M, et al. Guidelines for the management of Herpes Simplex virus in pregnancy. J Obstet Gynaecol Can. 2008;208:514–9.

Patten SF. Morphologic subclassification of preinvasive cervical neoplasia. In: Weid GL, Keebler CM, Koss LG, et al., editors. Compendium on diagnostic cytology. 6th ed. Chicago: Tutorials of Cytology; 1988.

Salazar-Martínez E, Lazcano-Ponce EC, Lira-Lira GG, et al. Case–control study of diabetes, obesity, physical activity and risk of endometrial cancer among Mexican women. Cancer Causes Control. 2000;11(8):707–11.

Sherman ME, Solomon D, Schiffman M, (for the ALTS group). Qualification of ASCUS. A comparison of equivocal LSIL and equivocal HSIL cervical cytology in the ASCUS LGSIL Triage Study. Am J Clin Pathol. 2001;116:386–94.

Sherman ME, Castle PE, Soloman D. Cervical cytology of atypical squamous cells-cannot exclude high-grade squamous intraepithelial lesion (ASC-H): characteristics and histologic outcomes. Cancer. 2006;108(5):298–305.

Shoff SM, Newcomb PA. Diabetes, body size, and risk of endometrial cancer. Am J Epidemiol. 1998;148(3):234–40.

Smith RA, Cokkinides V, Eyre HJ. American Cancer Society guidelines for the early detection of cancer, 2006. CA Cancer J Clin. 2006;56(1):11–25; quiz 49–50.

Vooijs GP, van Aspert-van Erp AJM, Bulten J. Benign proliferative reactions, intraepithelial neoplasia, and invasive cancer of the uterine cervix. In: Bibbo M, Wilbur DC, editors. Comprehensive cytopathology. 3rd ed. Philadelphia: Saunders/Elsevier; 2008.

Wied GL. Hormonal cytology. In: Keebler CM, Somrak TM, editors. The manual of cytotechnology. 7th ed. Chicago: ASCP Press; 1993.

Wied GL, Bibbo M. Hormonal cytology. In: Bibbo M, editor. Comprehensive cytopathology. 2nd ed. Philadelphia: Saunders; 1997.

Wilbur DC, Maurer S, Smith NI. Beçhet's disease in a vaginal smear: report of a case with cytologic features and their distinction from squamous cell carcinoma. Acta Cytol. 1993;37:525–30.

5 Glandular Lesions in the Pap Test

Walid E. Khalbuss and Marilee Means

Contents

W.E. Khalbuss, MD, PhD, FIAC (✉)
Director of Cytology and Cytopathology Fellowship Program,
University of Pittsburgh Medical Center Shadyside Hospital,
5150 Centre Avenue, 2, Suite 201,
Pittsburgh, PA 15232, USA
e-mail: khalbussw2@upmc.edu

M. Means, PhD, SCT(ASCP)
School of Health Professions,
University of Kansas Medical Center,
3901 Rainbow Blvd., Mail Stop 4048,
Kansas City, KS 66160, USA
e-mail: mmeans@kumc.edu

5.1 Tables and Summary

Table 5.1 Cytomorphology of repair in the Pap test

Two-dimensional cohesive sheets with "streaming effect"
Well-defined cell borders
Mild nuclear enlargement
Round or oval nuclei with smooth nuclear contour and fine chromatin
Prominent nucleoli or multiple nucleoli
Abundance of cytoplasm, may be cyanophilic or vacuolated
Mitotic activities may be present
Neutrophils often present
No nuclear overlapping
No single cells
No high N/C ratio

Table 5.2 Differential diagnosis of cells with prominent nucleoli in Pap test

Repair
Treatment effect
Decidual changes
Pemphigus vulgaris
Adenocarcinoma
Nonkeratinizing squamous carcinoma
Metastatic tumor (melanoma, lymphoma, etc.)

Table 5.3 Differential diagnosis of "naked" nuclei in the Pap test

Autolysis of cytoplasm in menopause
Cytolysis
Degenerative changes in endocervical cells
Arias-Stella reaction
HSIL
Squamous cell carcinoma
Metastatic malignancies

W.E. Khalbuss, M. Means (eds.), *Gynecological and Breast Cytopathology Board Review and Self-Assessment*,
DOI 10.1007/978-1-4614-7270-4_5, © Springer Science+Business Media New York 2013

Table 5.4 Pap test with post hysterectomy glandular cells, possible etiology

Wrong history
Columnar cell metaplasia in atrophic vagina
Mesonephric duct remnants
Bartholin glands
Rectovaginal fistula
Supracervical hysterectomy
Endometriosis
Vaginal adenosis
Prolapsed fallopian tubes
Glandular metaplasia following radiation or chemotherapy

Table 5.5 Differential diagnosis of hyperchromatic crowded groups in Pap test

Reactive endocervical cells
Tubal, squamous, or transitional metaplasia
Benign endometrial cells
Lower uterine segment
Endometriosis
Follicular cervicitis
Atrophy
Polyp
Herpes infection
AGC
HSIL
AIS
Adenocarcinoma
Squamous cell carcinoma
Other primary malignancies
Metastatic malignancies

Table 5.6 Hyperchromatic crowded groups (HCG): benign vs. neoplastic

Benign
Polarity maintained (architecture and nuclear)
Cilia in benign glandular cells (tubal metaplasia)
Biphasic glandular and stromal cells (endometrial clusters)
Minimal cellular and nuclear overlap and crowding
Minimal nuclear pleomorphism (uniform and round nuclei)
Low N/C ratio
Smooth nuclear contours
Evenly dispersed chromatin
Smudgy chromatin
Neoplastic
Disordered (chaotic) polarity (cellular arrangement)
Loss of nuclear polarity within cell groups
Associated single atypical and/or malignant cells
Feathering, rosettes, or acini typical of AIS
Background tumor diathesis concerning for malignancy
Pleomorphic crowded cells with nuclear overlap
High N/C ratio and irregular pleomorphic nuclei
Hyperchromasia with coarse chromatin
Macronucleoli suggest an invasive process
Numerous mitoses

Table 5.7 Tubal metaplasia vs. adenocarcinoma in situ (AIS)

Tubal metaplasia
Few cell groups
Less crowded groups without stratification
Round to oval nuclei
Hyperchromatic and finely granular nuclei
Inconspicuous nucleoli
Absent of mitosis
Ciliated
Adenocarcinoma in situ (AIS)
Risk factors: HPV16 and HPV 18 (seen in 50–90 % of cases)
Average age, 35–40 years at presentation; range, 27–74 years
Precursor to most cases of cervical invasive adenocarcinoma
Hyperchromatic crowded groups (HCG) of glandular cells with large nuclei (at least 2× the size of a normal endocervical cell)
The N/C ratio is increased
The chromatin is coarsely granular but evenly distributed
Mitoses and apoptotic bodies (small nuclear breakdown fragments)
Nucleoli are variably present but are usually small
Architecturally, the HCG show distinctive features including pseudostratified strips of columnar cells, feathered edges (nuclei and cytoplasmic protrusions from the group margins), and the presence of epithelial rosettes (gland formations)
No tumor diathesis (as diathesis is caused by the tissue destruction that occurs with invasive growth) but can be associated with an increased number of inflammatory cells in the background
Immunostain: CEA+, p16+, Ki 67+, vimentin−, ER−, PR−

Table 5.8 Atypical endocervical cells vs. atypical endometrial cells vs. adenocarcinoma in situ (AIS)

Atypical endocervical cells
Cells in sheets and strips (quantity low)
Crowding and nuclear overlap (mild)
Rare feathering or rosetting
Ill-defined cell borders
Nuclear enlargement (two to three times normal endocervical cells)
Increased N/C ratio
Diminished cytoplasm
Mild hyperchromasia
Nucleoli may be present
Mitoses are rare
Atypical endometrial cells
Small and few groups of 5–10 cells per group
Nuclear enlargement
Scant to moderate cytoplasm ± vacuoles
Ill-defined cell borders
Hyperchromasia
Nucleoli may be present
Adenocarcinoma in situ (AIS)
Hyperchromatic crowded groups (HCG) of glandular cells with large nuclei (at least 2× the size of a normal endocervical cell)
The N/C is increased
The chromatin is coarsely granular but evenly distributed
Mitoses and apoptotic bodies (small nuclear breakdown fragments)
Nucleoli are variably present but are usually small

Table 5.8 (continued)

Architecturally, the HCG show distinctive features including pseudostratified strips of columnar cells, feathered edges (nuclei and cytoplasmic protrusions from the group margins), and the presence of epithelial rosettes (gland formations)
No tumor diathesis (as diathesis is caused by the tissue destruction that occurs with invasive growth) but can be associated with an increased number of inflammatory cells in the background

Table 5.9 AIS vs. endocervical adenocarcinoma vs. endometrial adenocarcinoma

Adenocarcinoma in situ (AIS)
Hyperchromatic crowded groups (HCG) of glandular cells with large nuclei (at least 2× the size of a normal endocervical cell)
The N/C is increased
The chromatin is coarsely granular but evenly distributed
Mitoses and apoptotic bodies (small nuclear breakdown fragments)
Nucleoli are variably present but are usually small
Pseudostratified strips of columnar cells, feathered edges (nuclei and cytoplasmic protrusions from the group margins), and epithelial rosettes (gland formations)
No tumor diathesis (as diathesis is caused by the tissue destruction that occurs with invasive growth) but can be associated with inflammatory cells in the background
Immunostain: CEA+, HPV+, p16+, vimentin–
Endocervical adenocarcinoma
Highly cellular with numerous atypical cells
Tends to show "in situ" 2-D configuration, due to their lack of opportunity to "round up"
The nuclei are large (two to three times normal endocervical cells)
Cells have irregular hyperchromatic chromatin and irregular nuclear envelopes
Prominent nucleoli
Scant to abundant cytoplasm
Columnar morphology of the cells in well-differentiated variants
Many of the architectural features of AIS are present: honeycombed group configuration, presence of pseudostratified strips of cells, and rosette formation
A tumor diathesis (clumped and clinging granular material) in LBC
A diffuse granular breakdown material (tumor necrosis) in conventional slides
Immunostain: vimentin+, LMW cytokeratin + (CK7, CK8/18 and CK19), ER+ and PR+, CEA–, p16–
Endometrial adenocarcinoma
Few cells/clusters in low-grade carcinoma, larger number in high-grade carcinoma, but fewer than in endocervical carcinoma
The cells and cell groupings will round up and form 3-dimensional clusters due to mucus acts like a liquid suspension
Nuclear enlargement, irregular nuclei
Prominent nucleoli and abnormal chromatin patterns
Watery or granular diathesis pattern in the background
Distinctive diathesis (no necrotic gritty breakdown material seen)
May show foamy histiocytes and with epithelial cells with large vacuoles containing neutrophils (so-called oxyphil cells)
Immunostain: CEA+, p16+, EMA+, keratin+, ER and PR+ (25 %), p53+, vimentin–, CD10–, p63–

Table 5.10 Adenocarcinoma vs. squamous cell carcinoma in Pap test

Adenocarcinoma	Squamous cell carcinoma
More in aggregates, less single cells	More single cells, less in aggregates
Cuboidal/columnar cells	Polygonal cells/tadpole cells
Pleomorphism ++	Pleomorphism ++++
Vacuolated cytoplasm	Dense cytoplasm
No keratinization	Keratinization +/–
Vesicular nuclei	Opaque nuclei
Nucleoli ++	Nucleoli +/–
Drunken honeycombing	
Gland architecture/papillae	Back-to-back arrangement
3-D aggregates/nuclear overlapping	No nuclear overlapping/crowding
Less well-defined borders	Well-defined borders
Necrotic background ++	Necrotic background ++++

Table 5.11 Differential diagnosis of AIS and adenocarcinoma

Differential diagnosis of AIS
Exfoliated endometrial cells
Abraded endometrial cells and LUS
Reactive endocervical cells
Reparative changes
HSIL
Invasive adenocarcinoma
Differential diagnosis of adenocarcinoma
AGC
AIS
Metastatic tumor
Endometritis
Histiocytes
IUCD
Squamous metaplasia
Repair
Pemphigus vulgaris
Viral infections

5.2 Text-Based Questions 1–30

Q-1. Which statement best describes the glandular lesions in Pap test?
(a) The frequency of endocervical adenocarcinoma has been increasing.
(b) The differential diagnoses of glandular lesions in liquid-based cytology include reactive conditions, high-grade squamous intraepithelial lesion (HSIL) with glandular involvement, follicular cervicitis, and low-grade intraepithelial lesions.
(c) The majority of adenocarcinoma contains HPV DNA including mucinous adenocarcinoma, but not adenosquamous carcinomas.
(d) Features of AIS include two-dimensional clustering, hyperchromatic crowded nuclei, pleomorphism, altered nuclear polarity, increased N/C ratio, feathering, apoptosis, and presence of numerous single atypical cells.

Q-2. Which is a true statement regarding the histology of the endocervical cells?
(a) The endocervix is the glandular component of the cervix that forms glands with secretory cells and ductal cells.
(b) The endocervix is a series of deep infoldings of mucosa that tunnel into endocervical stroma forming crypts that secrete mucus.
(c) The endocervical mucosa consists of multiple layers of endocervical columnar cells.
(d) Endocervical cells are morphologically similar to endometrial cells.
(e) Endocervical cells are always present in groups (strips and sheet) forming acini, papillae, and cell balls.

Q-3. Which statement best describes endocervical adenocarcinoma in situ (AIS)?
(a) The average age of AIS and adenocarcinoma is similar (52 years old).
(b) HPV 16 and 18 have been identified in AIS and adenocarcinomas in similar proportions.
(c) AIS and adenocarcinoma are morphologically not similar.
(d) AIS has not been seen in the originally negative biopsies from women that later develop invasive adenocarcinomas.

Q-4. Which statement best describes the difference between AIS and invasive endocervical adenocarcinoma in the Pap test?
(a) Three-dimensional clustering (with continuous depth of focus), pleomorphism, feathering, hyperchromatic crowded nuclei, irregular nuclear membranes, uniform stippled chromatin, increased N/C ratio, apoptosis, and presence of single atypical cells are seen in AIS but not in invasive endocervical adenocarcinoma.
(b) Invasive adenocarcinoma has different cytological features of AIS.
(c) Invasive adenocarcinoma shows more inflammation, lysed blood, irregular nuclear membranes, nucleoli, and numerous single cells.
(d) Invasive adenocarcinoma shows more inflammation, lysed blood, and irregular nuclear membranes.

Q-5. Which statement best describes clinging diathesis in Pap test?
(a) A pattern of necrosis where diathesis material adheres or surrounds clusters of malignant cells
(b) A diathesis that contains blood with lysed RBCs, inflammation, proteinaceous debris, and degenerated malignant cells
(c) A patchy pattern displaying discreet aggregates of debris and seen in liquid-based preparation
(d) A dirty background of blood, lysed RBCs, inflammation, nuclear debris, and cellular debris

Q-6. Which description is the least applicable to the architecture atypia of adenocarcinoma in situ that can be readily seen at low-magnification scanning objectives?
(a) Tightly crowded hyperchromatic groups
(b) The two-dimensionality of the groups is often apparent
(c) A group of palisaded strips, complex branched fragments, acinar or rosette architecture, and feathering
(d) Numerous small sheets, short strips, or large microbiopsy fragments

Q-7. Which of the following is true regarding the atypical glandular cell (AGC) category?
(a) In AGC of endometrial cell or of endocervical cells, nuclear atypia is the most important feature for diagnosis.
(b) In AGC of endocervical cell origin, nuclear atypia is the most important feature for diagnosis.
(c) In AGC of endocervical cell origin, architectural atypia is the most important feature for diagnosis.
(d) In AGC of endometrial cell origin, nuclear atypia is the most important feature for diagnosis.

Q-8. Which statement describes the most characteristic features of endocervical or vaginal clear cell carcinoma in Pap test?
(a) Many atypical cells retain columnar shape in well-differentiated cases.
(b) The nuclei are large (2–3× than normal endocervical cells) with irregular hyperchromatic chromatin, prominent nucleoli, irregular nuclear envelopes, and abundant to scant cytoplasm.
(c) Tumor diathesis (clumped and clinging granular material in LBC) and diffuse granular breakdown material in conventional slides.
(d) The cells have apical "hobnail" nuclei; prominent nucleoli; clear, abundant vacuolated cytoplasm; and large, pale, round to irregular nuclei, and naked nuclei are common due the delicate nature of the cytoplasm.

Q-9. Which is true regarding serous adenocarcinoma?
(a) Serous adenocarcinoma is a low-grade malignancy.
(b) It consists of well-differentiated architectural features (glands or papillae).
(c) Serous adenocarcinoma in Pap test typically shows numerous papillary clusters; coarse to smudgy, dark chromatin; prominent nucleoli; and dense, bulky cytoplasm.
(d) Bizarre tumor giant cells are rare, and psammoma bodies are not common.

Q-10. Which is true regarding endometrial adenocarcinoma in Pap test?
(a) The malignant cells are numerous than in cervical carcinoma.
(b) The nuclei are enlarged, irregular, with nucleoli and abnormal chromatin patterns.
(c) The background is typically clean with no watery or granular/watery diathesis seen.
(d) Foamy histiocytes and epithelial cells with large vacuoles containing neutrophils (so-called oxyphil cells) are rarely seen.

Q-11. Which is true regarding cellular changes associated with intrauterine device (IUD)?
(a) The cellular abnormalities induced by IUD may mimic only glandular abnormalities.
(b) The cellular abnormalities induced by IUD may mimic squamous abnormalities only.
(c) The cellular abnormalities induced by IUD may mimic glandular or squamous abnormalities.
(d) The cellular abnormalities induced by IUD are specific and cannot be seen in the absence of history of IUD.

Q-12. Which is the least likely in the differential diagnosis of follicular cervicitis?
(a) HSIL
(b) Small cell carcinoma or lymphoma
(c) AIS or adenocarcinoma
(d) AS-US or LSIL

Q-13. Which of the following is an inaccurate statement regarding cytoplasm of immature squamous metaplastic cells in Pap test?
(a) It is often dense and homogeneous with distinct borders. However, they occasionally become vacuolated and cyanophilic.
(b) Cytoplasmic vacuolation is frequently observed in the presence of inflammation.
(c) Cytoplasmic vacuolation is frequently observed in the presence or as a consequence of degeneration.
(d) Presence of atypia in immature squamous metaplastic cells (nuclear enlargement and variation in nuclear size) is indicative of dysplasia.

Q-14. Which of the following is the most accurate statement about squamous metaplastic cells in Pap test?
(a) Nuclei are round with irregular nuclear envelope and with fine chromatin and small nucleoli.
(b) Cytoplasm is dense and not vacuolated.
(c) They may show cytoplasmic projections with "spider legs" morphology due to their stromal origin.
(d) The presence of squamous metaplastic cells indicates that the transformation zone (TZ) has been sampled.

Q-15. Which of the following statements is true regarding cellular changes associated with intrauterine device (IUD)?
(a) It occurs as single cells of endometrial origin showing dark smudged nuclei with irregular nuclear contour that mimics HSIL.
(b) It may show small clusters of rounded cells of glandular origin showing individual cells with large vacuoles that push the pleomorphic enlarged nuclei toward the edge of the cluster (bubblegum vacuoles).
(c) The presence of single cells with smudged nuclei or small clusters with "bubblegum vacuoles" is specific for IUD effect.
(d) It occurs as single cells of endometrial or high endocervical origin showing dark smudged nuclei with smooth nuclear contour that mimics HSIL.

Q-16. Which statement is true about glandular cells seen in Pap test from women status post-hysterectomy?
(a) They are seen in approximately 10 % of vaginal Pap tests from women who have had a total hysterectomy.
(b) They are seen more in women who have undergone postoperative radiotherapy.
(c) They resemble normal endometrial cells.
(d) They are seen in approximately 10 % of vaginal Pap tests from women who have had a total hysterectomy.

Q-17. Tumor diathesis in Pap test is least seen in:
(a) Endocervical adenocarcinoma
(b) Endometrial adenocarcinoma
(c) Squamous cell carcinoma
(d) Extrauterine carcinoma

Q-18. Which statement is true about feathering seen in adenocarcinoma in situ (AIS)?
(a) Feathering is a distinctive and specific feature of AIS.
(b) Feathering refers to cigar-shaped enlarged nuclei at the periphery protruding beyond the confines of the cell borders. The nuclei protrude into the free space surrounding the cell group.
(c) The feathering is due to extreme nuclear crowding and discohesion to the basement membrane.
(d) It is created when the extremely crowded nuclei bounded by basement membrane are released from the confines of cell group upon rupture of the cytoplasmic membrane's attachment point.

Q-19. Adenoma malignum is a well-differentiated endocervical adenocarcinoma. Which of the following is not true about adenoma malignum?
(a) It is an abnormal glandular lesion with atypical cells in single, sheets, and clusters displaying a drunken honeycombing morphology (disorganization).
(b) The nuclei are enlarged, pleomorphic, and crowded with visible nucleoli, and the majority of the cases are negative for HPV.
(c) The cells may show intracytoplasmic "golden yellow" mucin that is positive for PAS-Alcian blue 2.5 and NHIK-1083 stains.
(d) It is a well-differentiated adenocarcinoma, and it has a better prognosis compared to other variants of endocervical adenocarcinoma.

Q-20. Which is true about repair in Pap test?
(a) Severe reactive or reparative changes may mimic SIL, AIS, or carcinoma.
(b) Reparative changes show loose cohesion, three-dimensional clusters with loss of polarity.
(c) Reparative changes show chromatin clumping and hyperchromatic nuclei.
(d) Reparative changes show prominent nucleoli and tumor diathesis.

Q-21. Which is true about decidual cells in Pap test?
(a) Decidual cells and Arias-Stella changes occur in the same cell types, and both are usually associated with pregnancy.
(b) Decidual changes are seen in endocervical or endometrial glandular epithelium, while Arias-Stella changes occur in stromal cells.
(c) Decidual changes are seen in stromal cells while Arias-Stella changes occur in endocervical or endometrial glandular epithelium.
(d) Decidual changes may mimic adenocarcinomas especially clear cell adenocarcinoma, while Arias-Stella changes may be mistaken for LSIL.

Q-22. Which of the following statements best describes atypical endometrial cells/atypical glandular cells in Pap tests?
(a) Single or clusters of small glandular cells with round to oval, darkly staining nuclei and nuclear molding
(b) Single or clusters of glandular cells with anisocytosis and apoptotic bodies (single cell necrosis)
(c) Single and clusters of glandular cells with enlarged nuclei, nuclear membrane irregularity, and prominence of nucleoli
(d) Single or clusters of glandular cells with scant cytoplasm, small vacuoles, and engulfed neutrophils

Q-23. Which of the following best describes presence of benign-appearing endometrial cells out of the cycle in women 40 years or older in Pap tests?
(a) The Bethesda System for Reporting Cervical Cytology in 2001 (TBS 2001) recommended that benign-appearing endometrial cells in postmenopausal women be reported as an "epithelial cell abnormality" based on the increased risk for endometrial adenocarcinoma (6 %).
(b) The TBS 1991 recommended that benign-appearing endometrial cells in postmenopausal women be reported as category "Other," and this was applicable only to exfoliative endometrial cells.
(c) Directly sampled lower uterine segment or abraded stromal cells/histiocytes, when present alone, should be reported under the category of "Other" according to the TBS 2001.
(d) The TBS 2001 recommended that benign-appearing endometrial cells in postmenopausal women be reported as category "Other," and this was applicable only to exfoliative endometrial cells.

Q-24. The most important feature that distinguishes atypical endometrial cells from benign endometrial cells is:
(a) The frothy, delicate cytoplasm and round cellular shape
(b) Increased nuclear size
(c) Three-dimensional configurations
(d) Prominent nucleoli

Q-25. Which is true regarding the category of atypical glandular cells (AGC) in Pap tests?
(a) This category was present in the Bethesda System (TBS) for Reporting Cervical Cytology in both 1991 and 2001.
(b) This category includes atypical glandular cells of reactive nature.
(c) This category may include cases with AIS.
(d) In this category, there is no need to further qualify the atypia into endocervical or endometrial origin.

Q-26. Which is true about endocervical or vaginal clear cell carcinoma?
(a) Clear cell carcinoma of the cervix or vagina is a rare malignancy of Müllerian origin.
(b) It always occurs in daughters of women who took diethylstilbestrol (DES) during pregnancy.
(c) It affects older women, and it has slightly worse prognosis than classical endocervical adenocarcinoma.
(d) The majority (>60 %) of clear cell carcinomas are HPV DNA positive.

Q-27. A Pap test shows numerous glandular-like cells with marked reparative changes in sheet and single cell arrangement and a clean background. Some cells show fine, evenly distributed chromatin and bullet-shaped nucleoli. The most likely diagnosis in this case is:
(a) Endocervical adenocarcinoma
(b) Adenoma malignum
(c) Pemphigus vulgaris
(d) AIS

Q-28. A Pap test shows few glandular cell clusters with papillary-like and three-dimensional configurations. Occasional concentric ringed calcified material is seen within the fibrovascular cores of papillae. The cells have hyperchromatic nuclei with finely granular chromatin and irregular nuclear contour. The background is clean. The most likely diagnosis of this Pap test is:
(a) Endocervical adenocarcinoma
(b) Cervical squamous cell carcinoma with necrosis
(c) AIS
(d) Metastatic serous carcinoma of ovarian origin

Q-29. Immunostains may be helpful in differentiating metastatic disease in Pap tests and can be performed on cell block material prepared from liquid-based samples. Which immunoprofile would best confirm a breast primary?
(a) ER+, PR+, mammaglobin+, CK7+
(b) ER+, PR+, CEA+, vimentin−
(c) ER+, PR+, CK7+, vimentin+
(d) CK7−, CK20−, CEA+, CDX2+

Q-30. Which is true regarding menstrual endometrial cells in the Pap test?
(a) They may resemble AIS, adenocarcinoma, or HSIL.
(b) They demonstrate well-preserved small, molded hypochromatic nuclei.
(c) Ball formation or histiocytes are not common.
(d) Feathering, rosettes, and strips of columnar cells may be seen.

5.3 Image-Based Questions 31–57

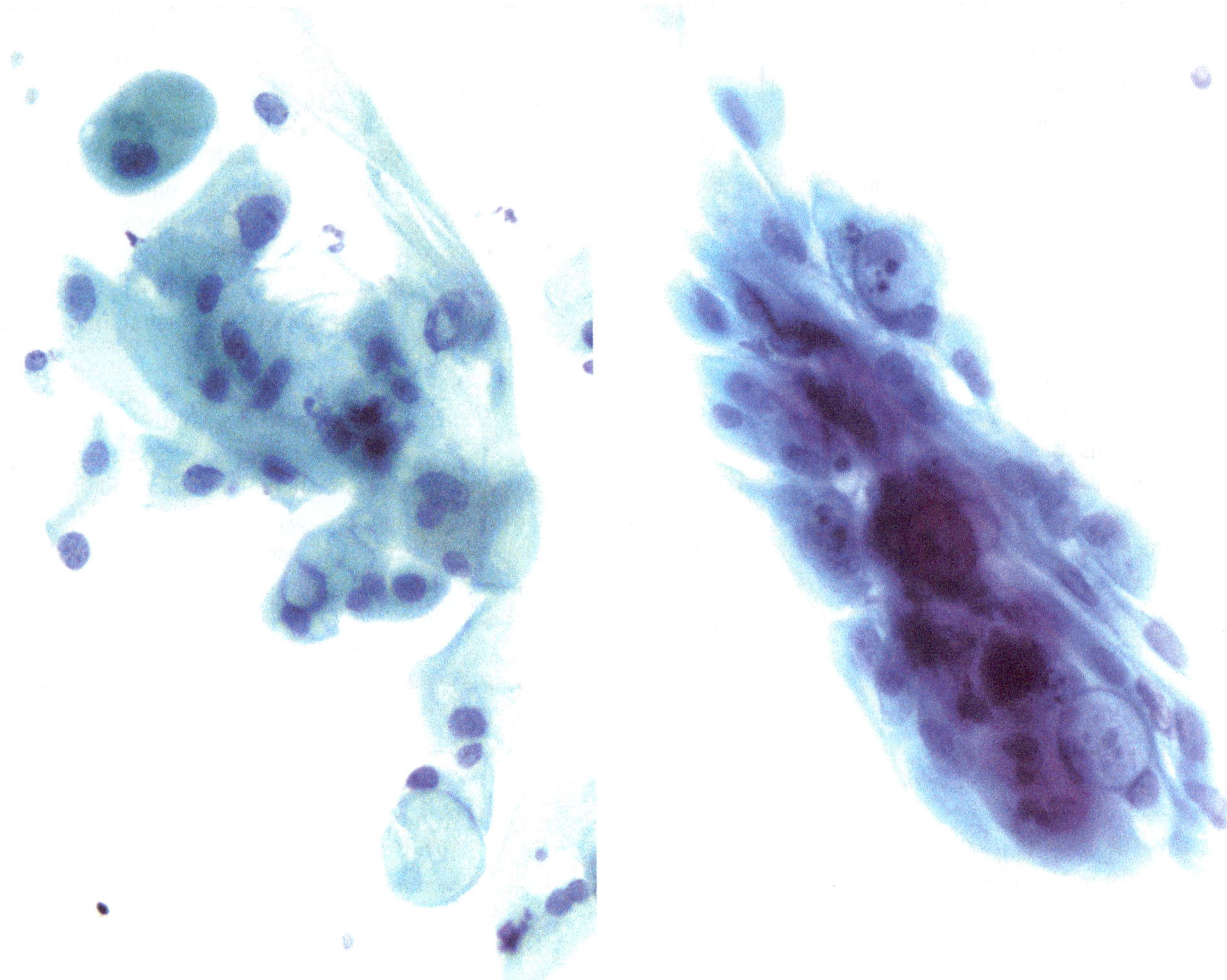

Fig. 5.31

Q-31. This image is from a Pap smear of a 41-year-old female with a history of squamous cell carcinoma. What is the most likely diagnosis?

(a) Neoplastic, recurrence of squamous cell carcinoma
(b) Neoplastic, glandular
(c) Infectious
(d) Reactive

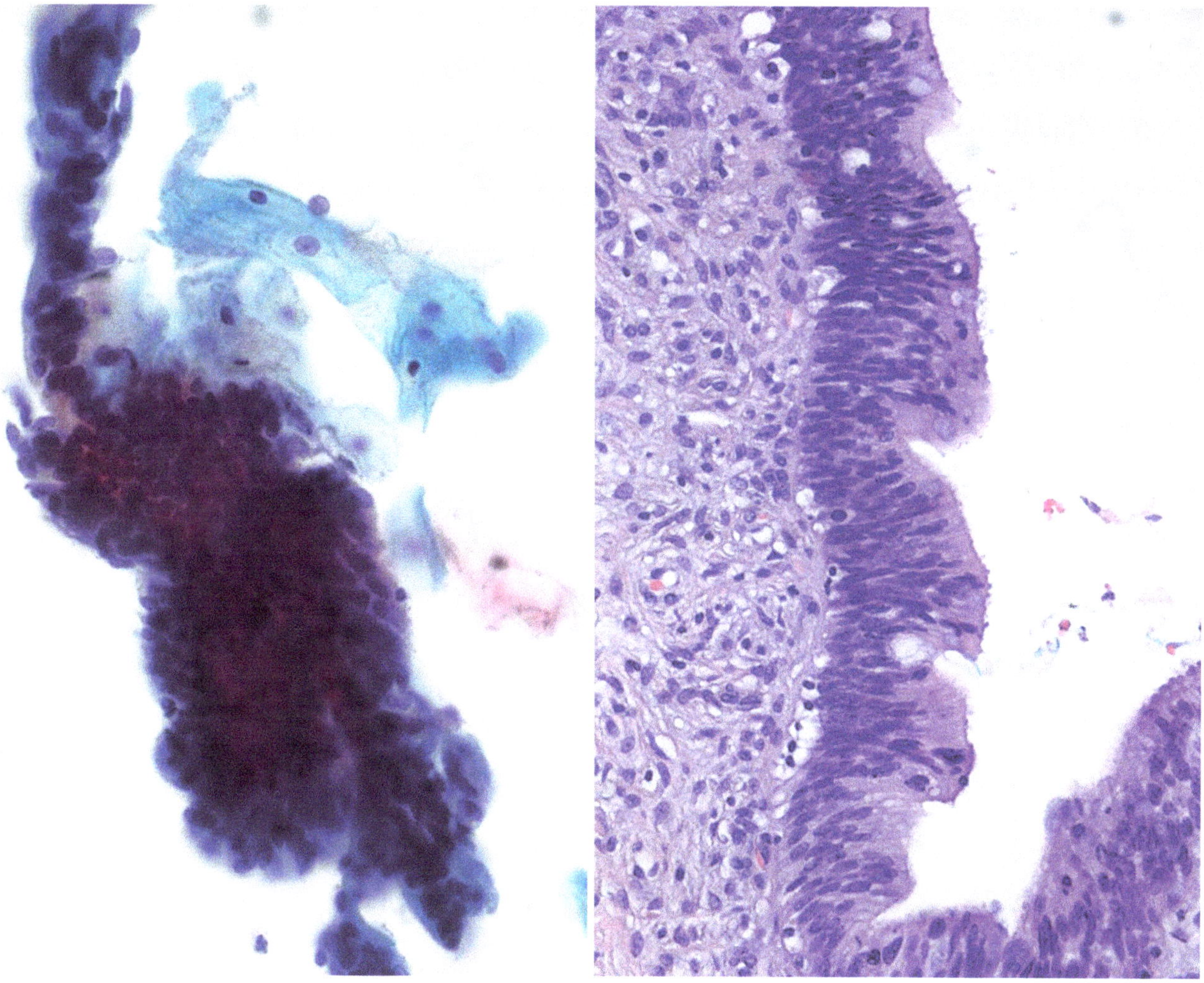

Fig. 5.32

Q-32. Which of the epithelial cell abnormality categories is most applicable to this case?
(a) Squamous cell carcinoma
(b) Adenocarcinoma
(c) Adenocarcinoma in situ (AIS)
(d) High-grade squamous intraepithelial lesion (HSIL)

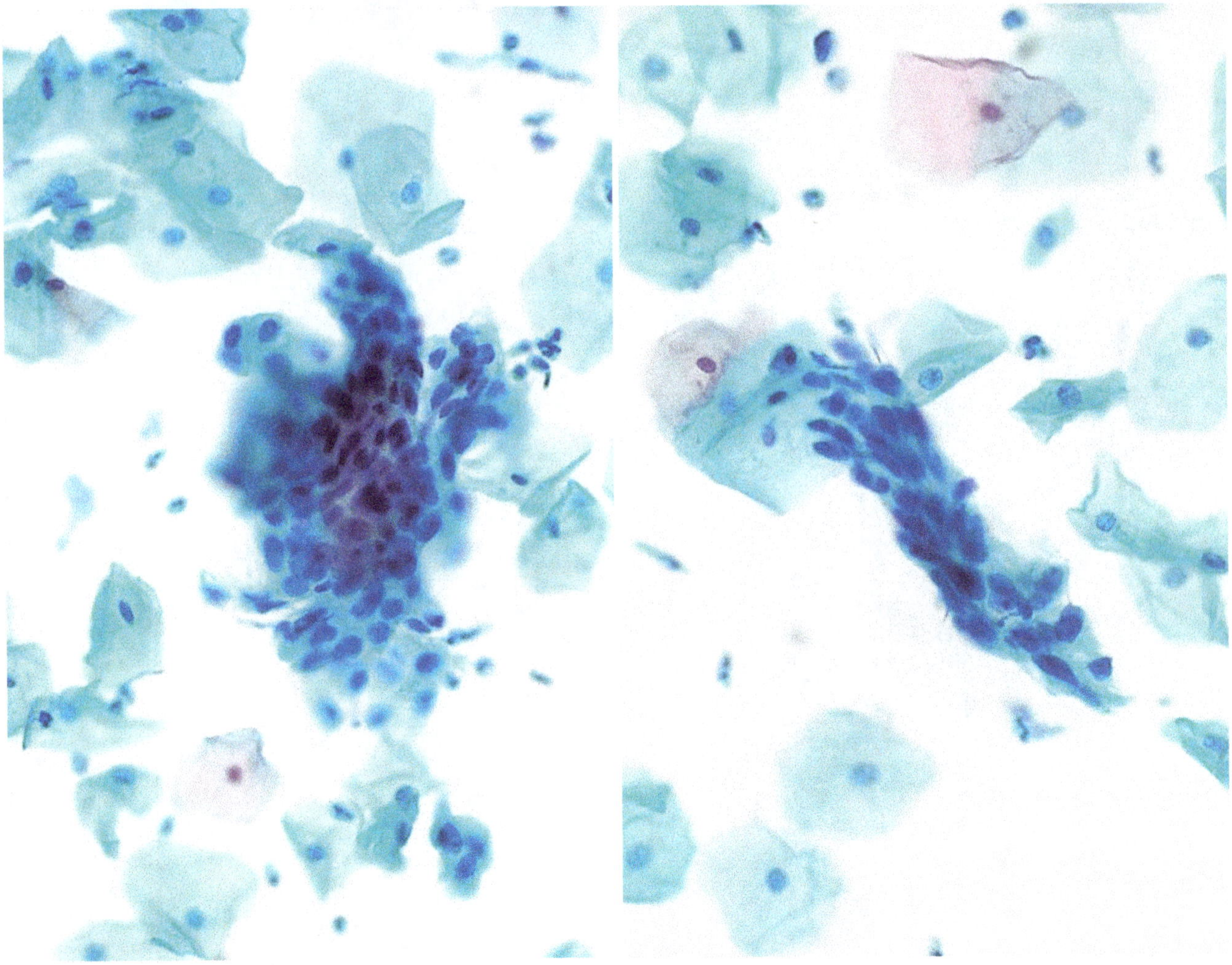

Fig. 5.33

Q-33. Which of the epithelial cell abnormality categories is most applicable to this case?

(a) Squamous cell carcinoma
(b) Adenocarcinoma
(c) Adenocarcinoma in situ (AIS)
(d) High-grade squamous intraepithelial lesion (HSIL)

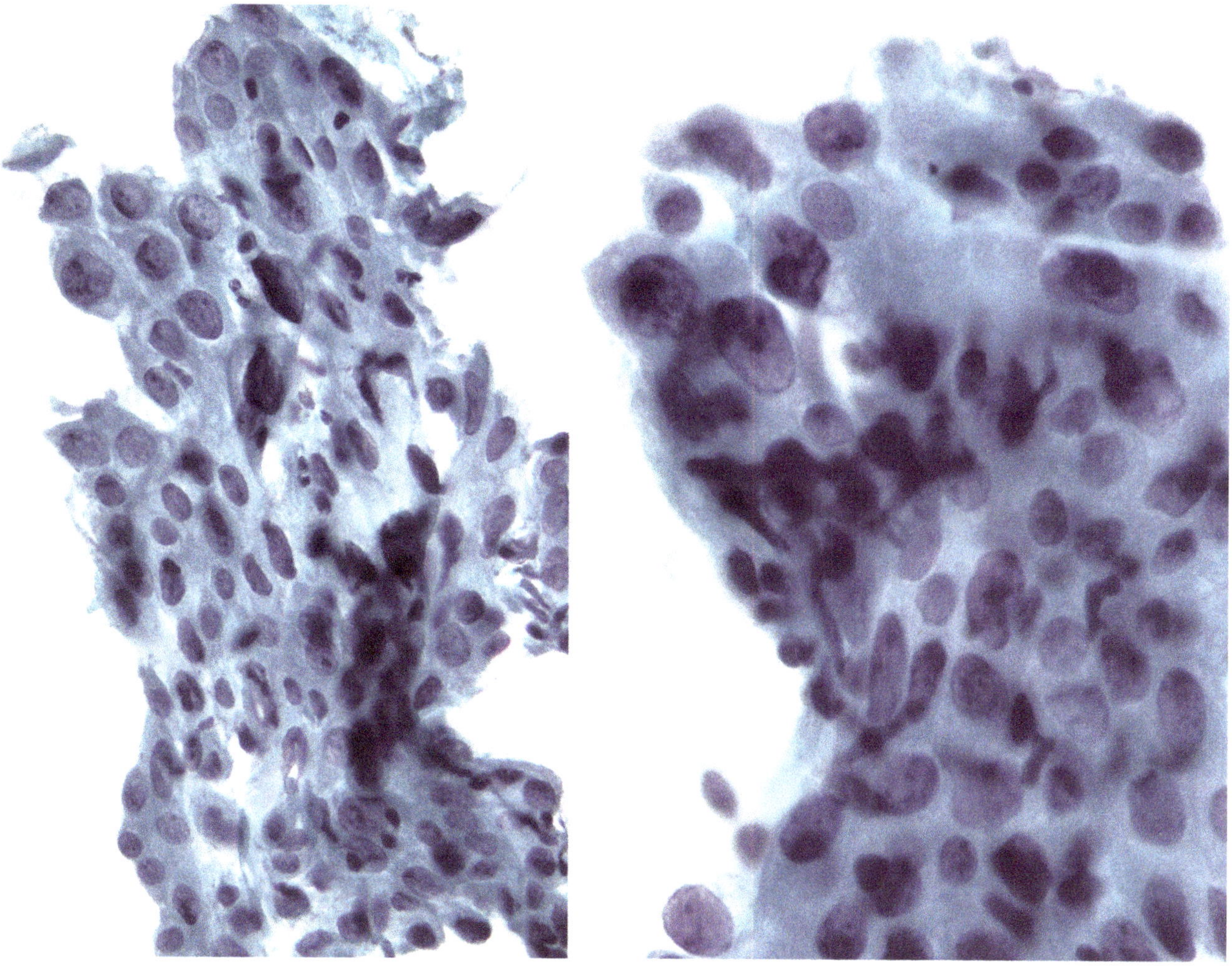

Fig. 5.34

Q-34. This liquid-based Pap test is from a 32-year-old postpartum woman who had abnormal Pap test during her pregnancy (epithelial cell abnormality—ASC). Which of the categories is most applicable to this case?

(a) Squamous cell carcinoma
(b) Adenocarcinoma
(c) High-grade squamous intraepithelial lesion (HSIL)
(d) Negative for intraepithelial lesion or malignancy (NILM)

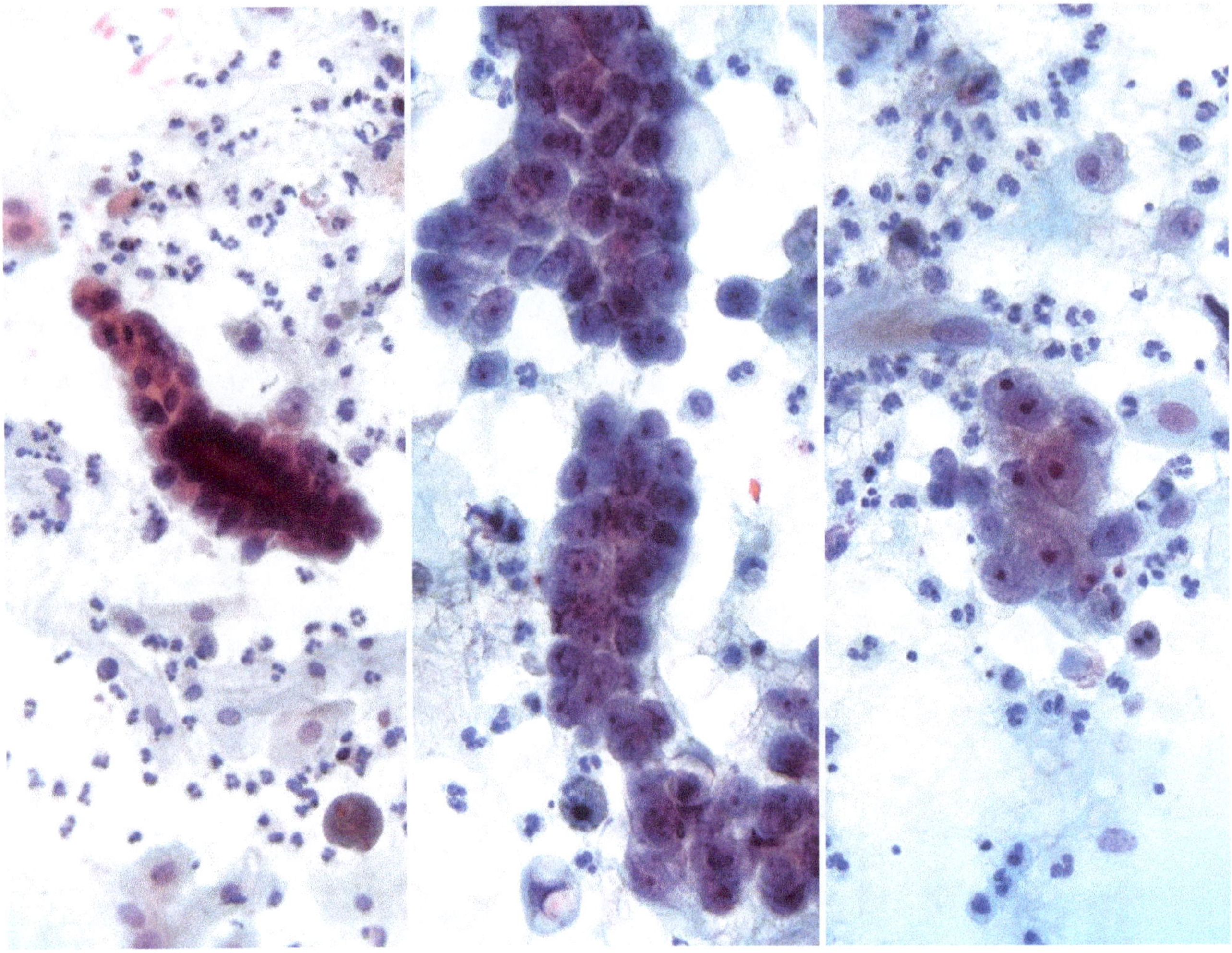

Fig. 5.35

Q-35. This Pap test is from a 62-year-old woman. Which of the categories is most applicable to this case?

(a) Squamous cell carcinoma
(b) Adenocarcinoma
(c) High-grade squamous intraepithelial lesion (HSIL)
(d) Negative for intraepithelial lesion or malignancy (NILM)

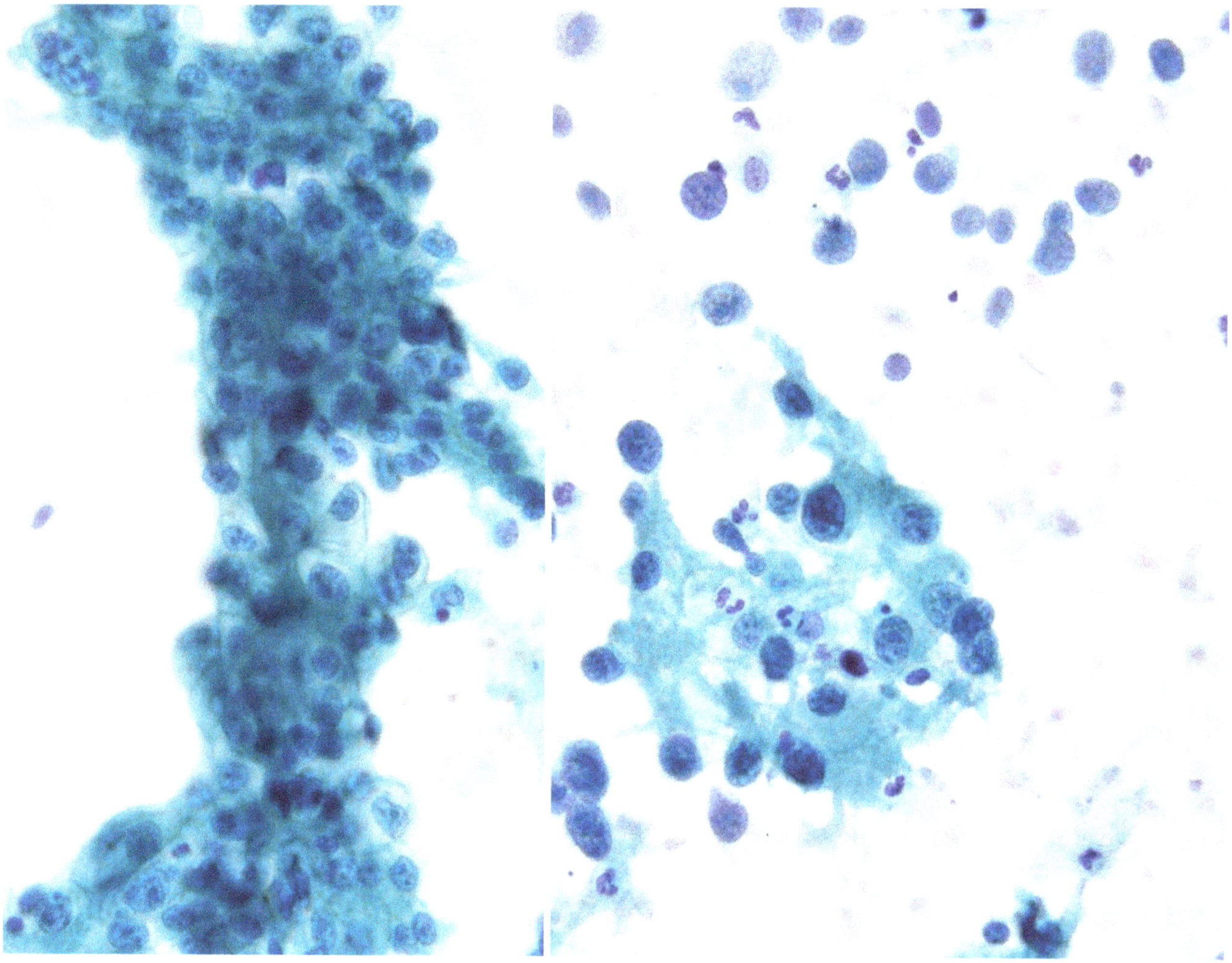

Fig. 5.36

Q-36. This image is from ThinPrep Pap Test from a 42-year-old female. What is the most likely diagnosis?
(a) Squamous cell carcinoma
(b) Adenocarcinoma in situ
(c) Adenocarcinoma with clear cell morphology
(d) Repair

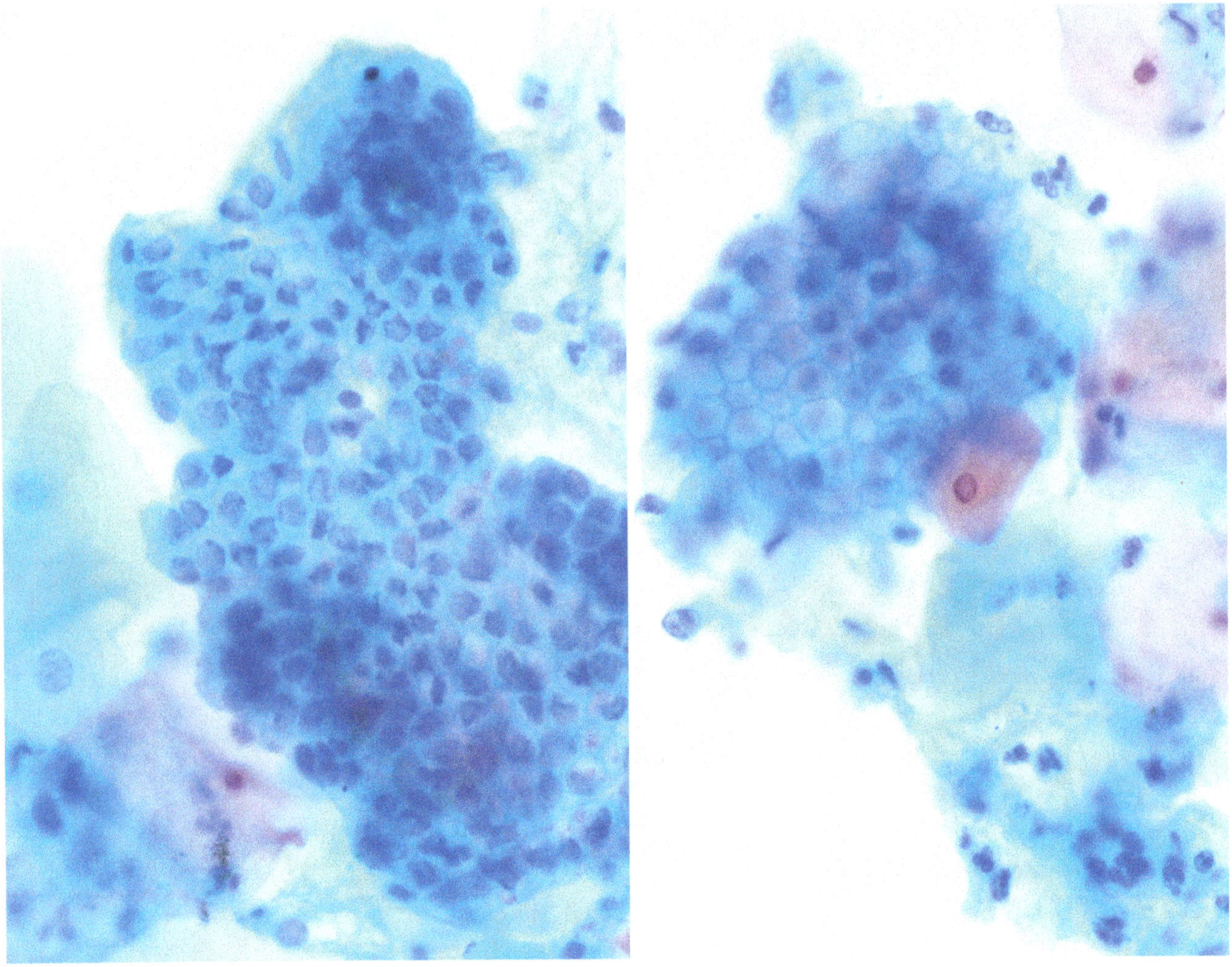

Fig. 5.37

Q-37. The predominant cells shown here represent which of the following:
(a) Intermediate cells
(b) Superficial cells
(c) Endometrial cells
(d) Endocervical cells

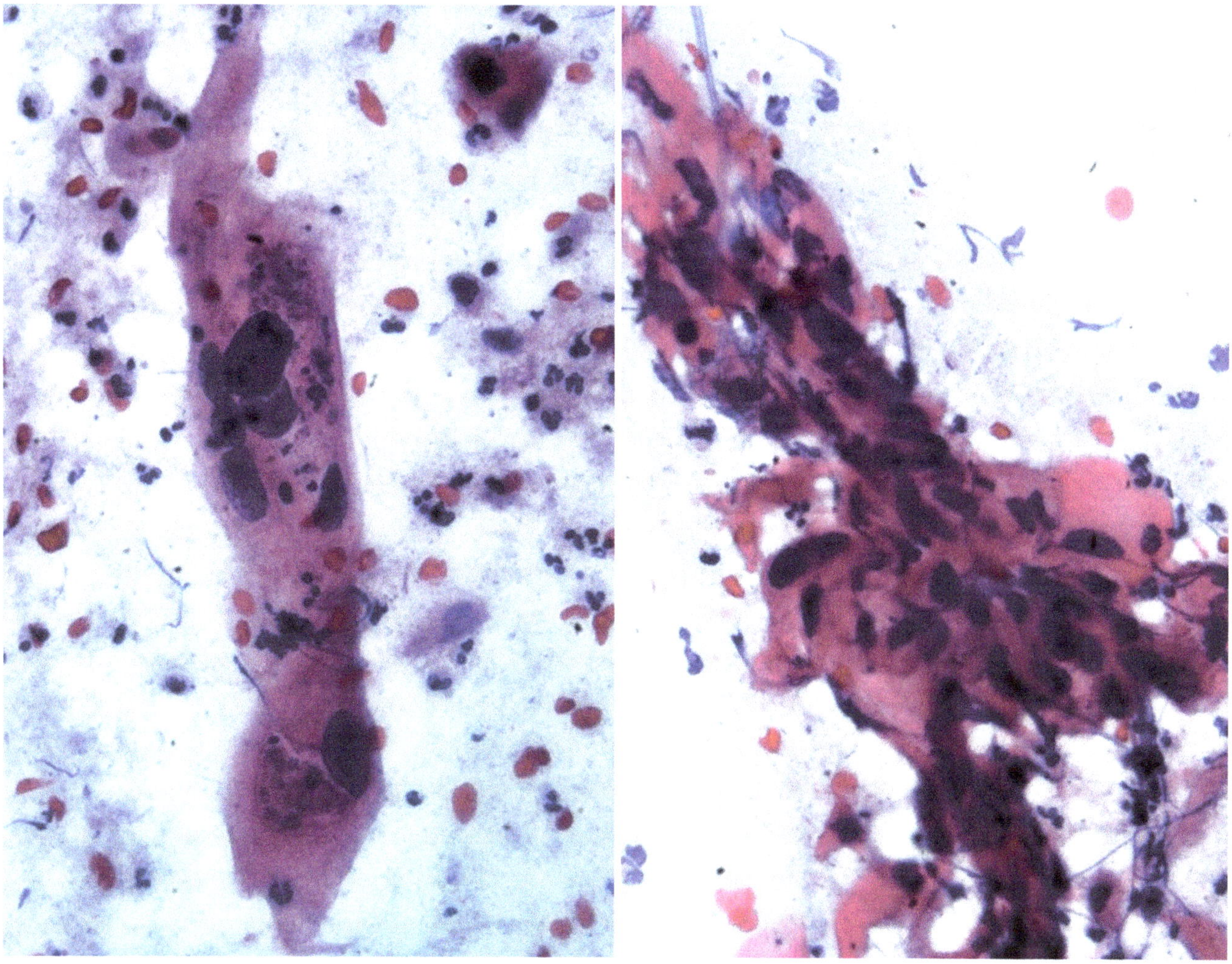

Fig. 5.38

Q-38. This image is from a conventional Pap smear from a 72-year-old female with a history of cervical squamous cell carcinoma that treated with radiation. What is the most likely diagnosis?

(a) Endocervical adenocarcinoma
(b) Endocervical adenocarcinoma in situ
(c) Recurrence of keratinizing squamous carcinoma
(d) Radiation effects

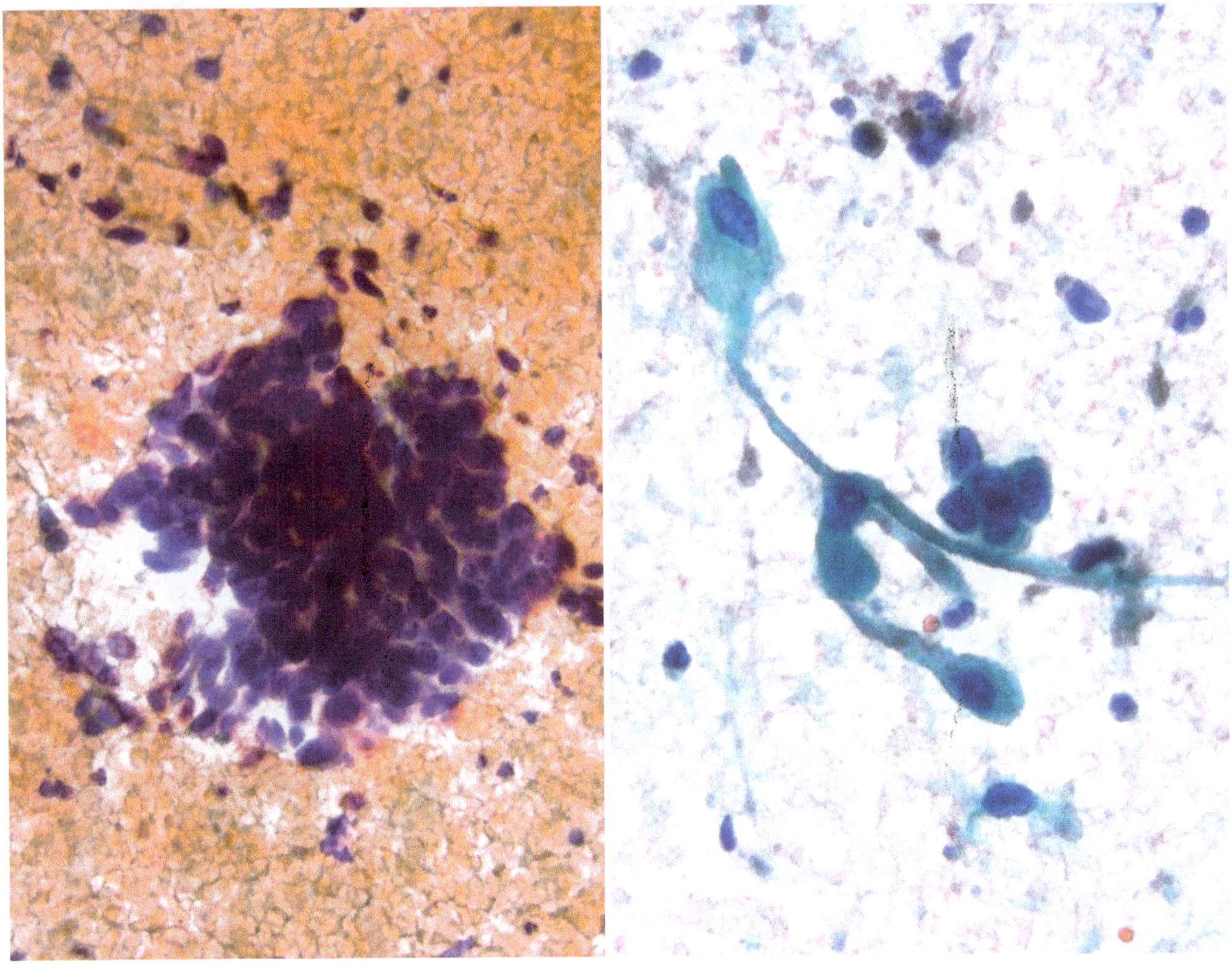

Fig. 5.39

Q-39. This image is from a conventional Pap smear. What is the most likely diagnosis?
(a) Endocervical adenocarcinoma in situ
(b) Carcinoma
(c) Follicular cervicitis
(d) Repair

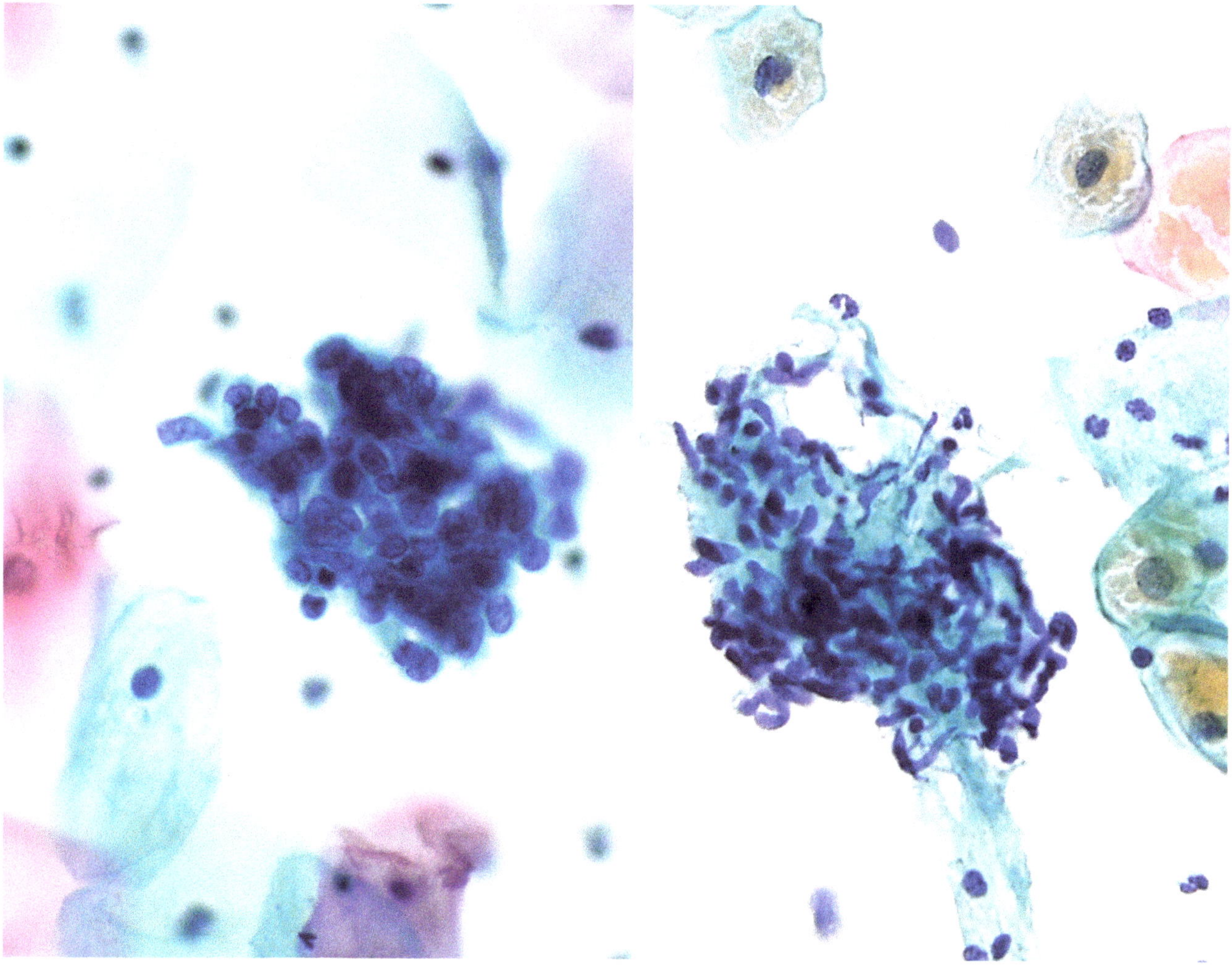

Fig. 5.40

Q-40. The origin of these cells is most likely:
  (a) Endocervical
  (b) Endometrial
  (c) Internal cervical os
  (d) Vagina

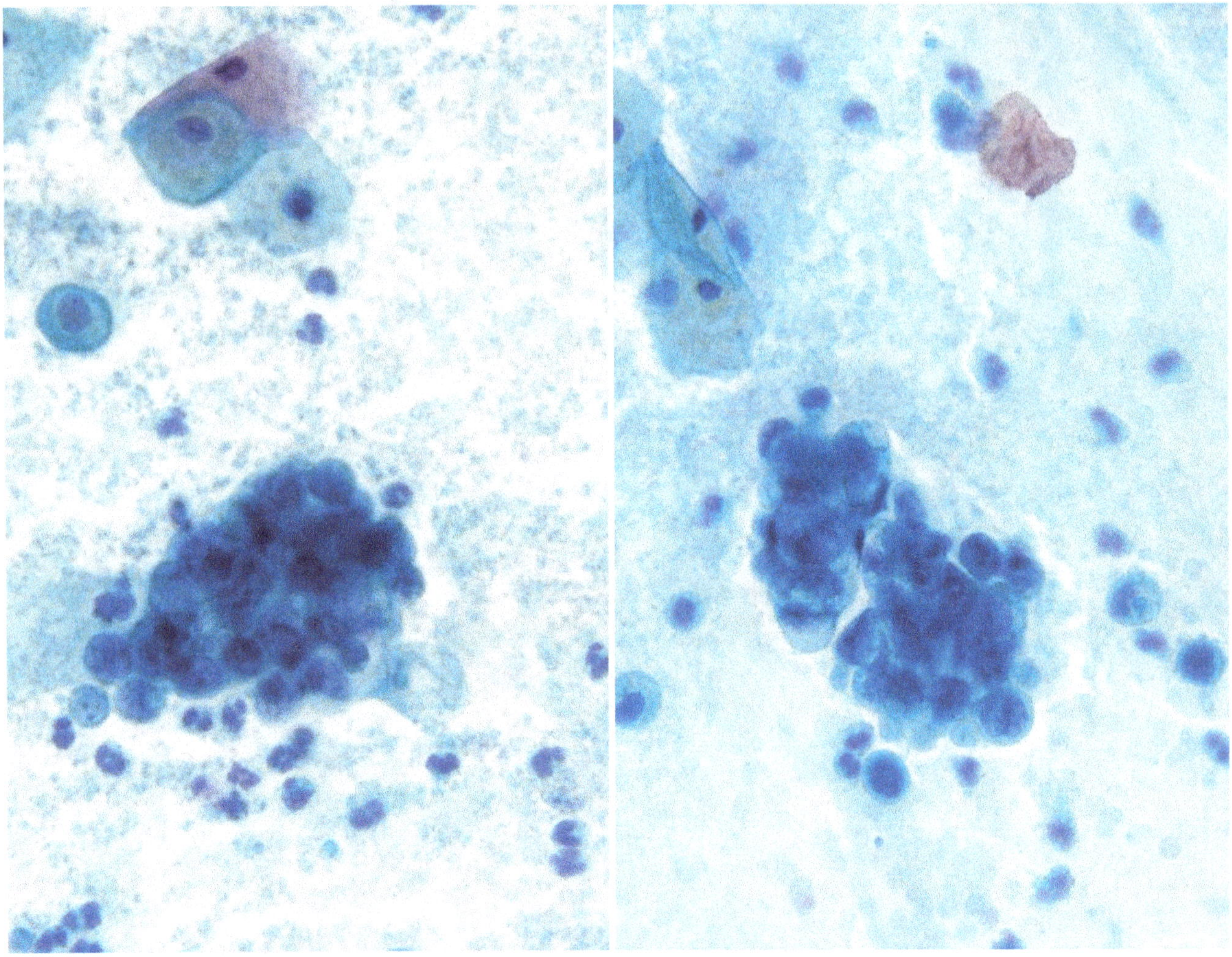

Fig. 5.41

Q-41. This image is from a conventional Pap smear from a 61-year-old female with a history of vaginal bleeding and previous diagnosis of AS-H. What is the most likely diagnosis?

(a) Adenocarcinoma
(b) Squamous cell carcinoma
(c) Small cell carcinoma
(d) Persistent of AS-H

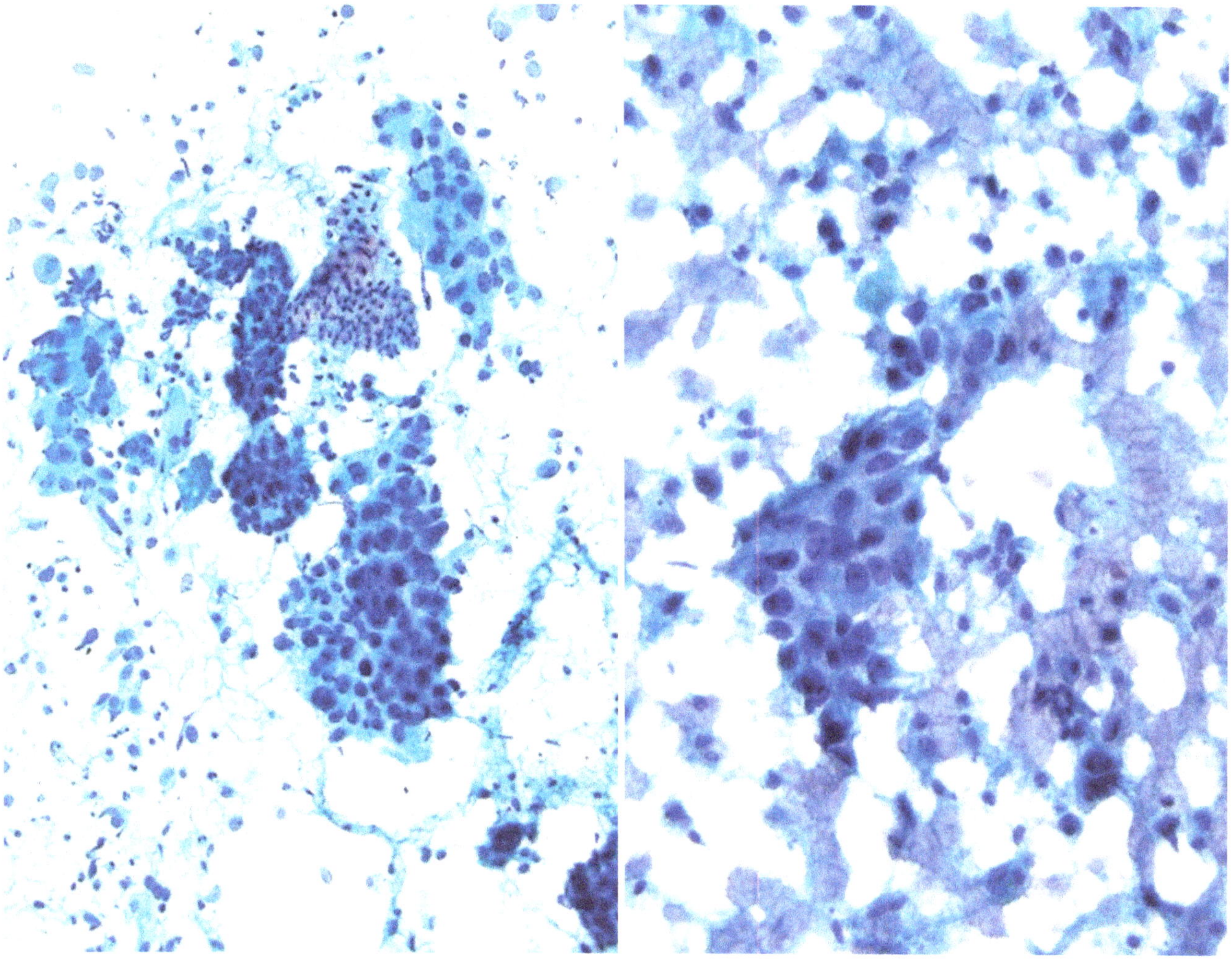

Fig. 5.42

Q-42. This image is from a repeated Pap smear of a 39-year-old female with a history of previous diagnosis of AS-US and positive HP testing. What is the most likely diagnosis?

(a) Endocervical adenocarcinoma
(b) Endocervical adenocarcinoma in situ
(c) Endometrial adenocarcinoma
(d) Squamous cell carcinoma

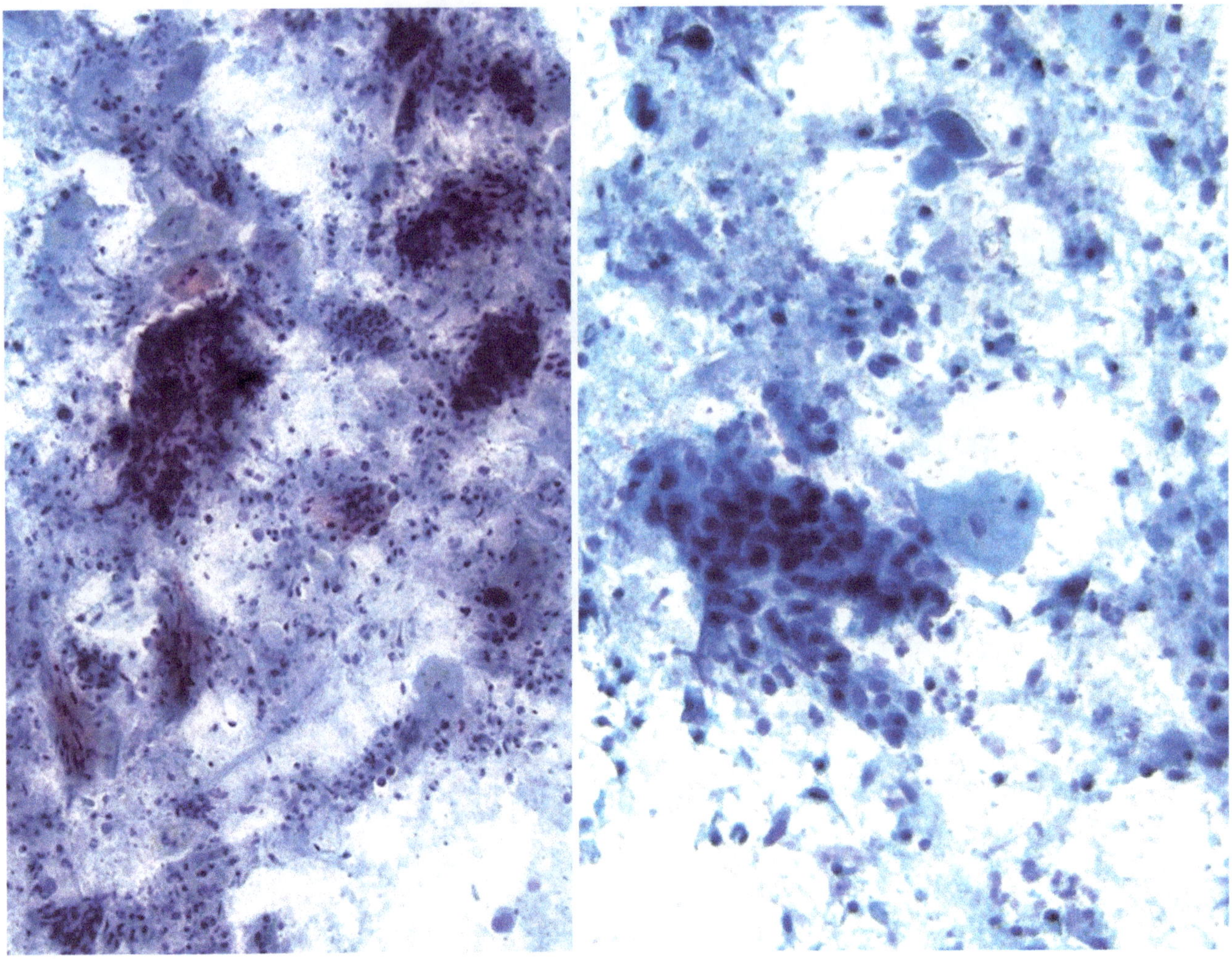

Fig. 5.43

Q-43. This image is from a Pap smear from a 51-year-old female with no previous Pap history and unknown HPV status. What is the most likely diagnosis?

(a) Endocervical adenocarcinoma
(b) Endocervical adenocarcinoma in situ
(c) Squamous cell carcinoma
(d) AS-US

Fig. 5.44

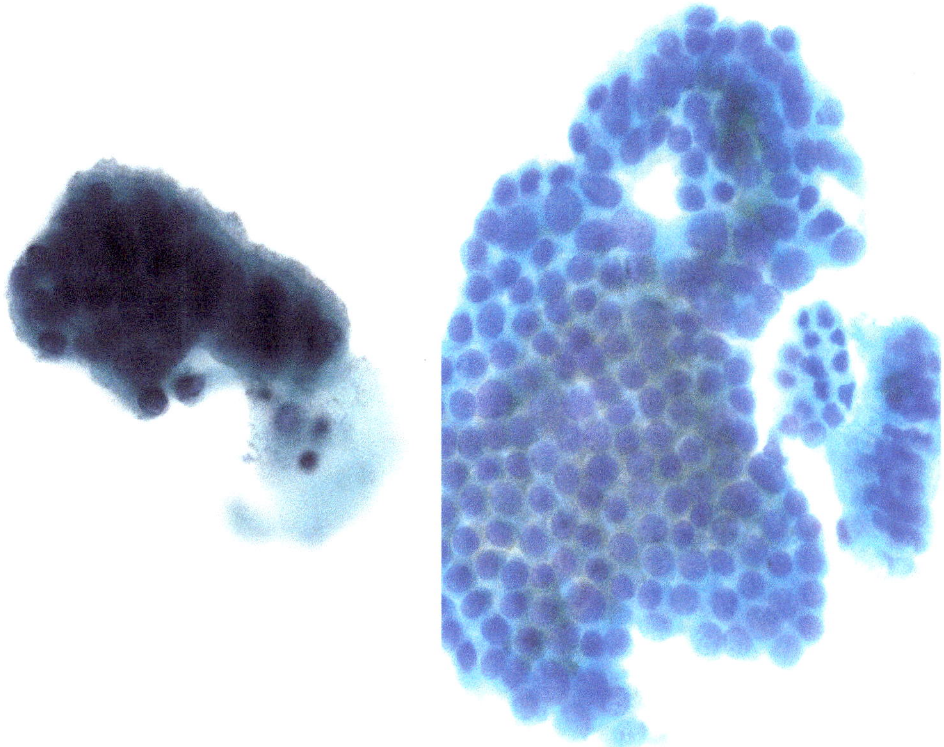

Q-44. This image is from a Pap smear of a 30-year-old female. What is the most likely diagnosis?
(a) Neoplastic, squamous origin
(b) Neoplastic, glandular
(c) Benign, reactive, infectious
(d) Dysplastic

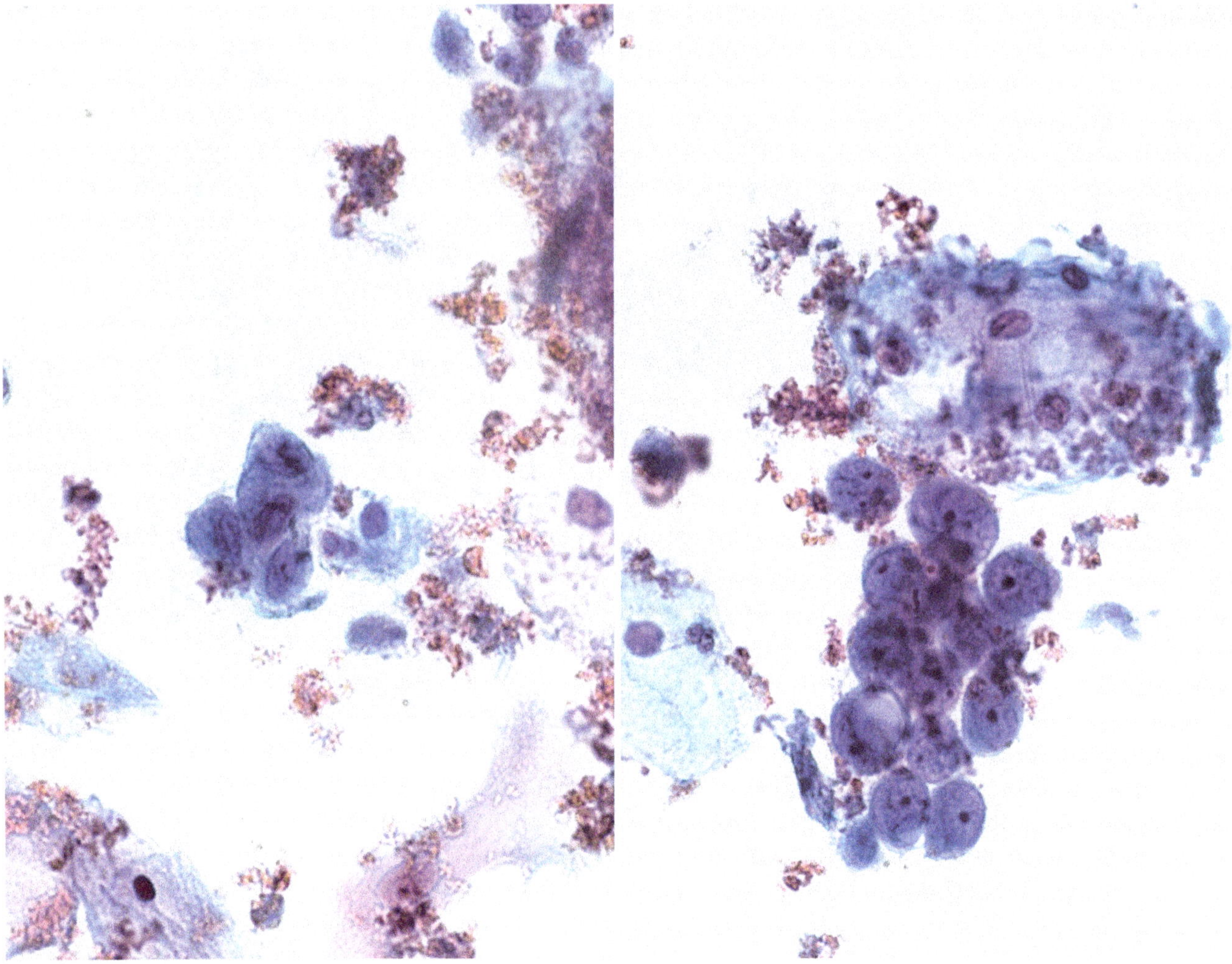

Fig. 5.45

Q-45. This image is from a repeated Pap smear of a 42-year- old female with a history of breast carcinoma. What is the most likely diagnosis?
(a) Endocervical adenocarcinoma
(b) Endocervical adenocarcinoma in situ
(c) Metastatic adenocarcinoma
(d) Benign endometrial cells in woman >40 years old

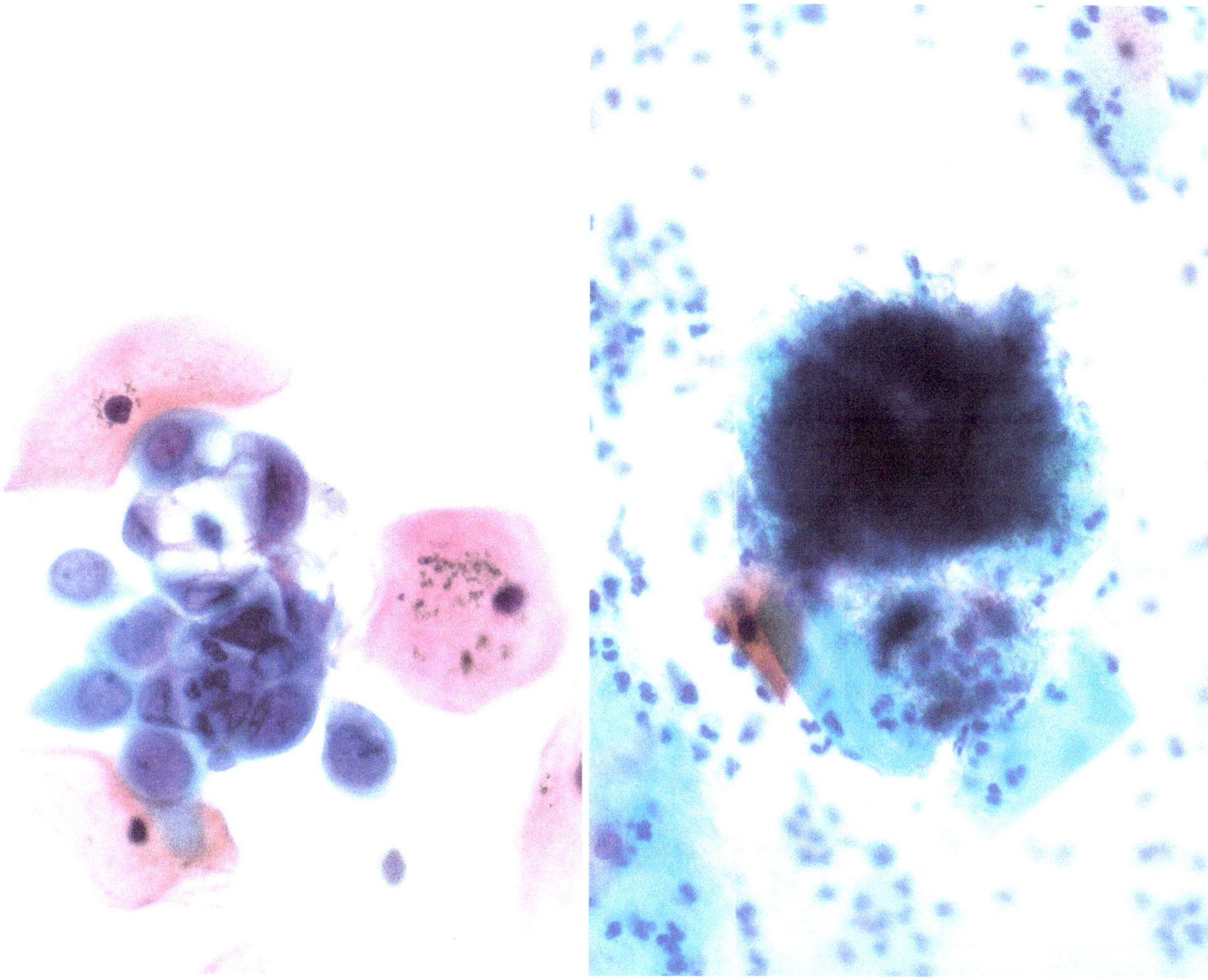

Fig. 5.46

Q-46. This image is from a Pap smear of a 24-year-old female. What is the most likely diagnosis?
(a) Neoplastic, squamous origin
(b) Neoplastic, glandular
(c) Benign, reactive, infectious
(d) Dysplasic

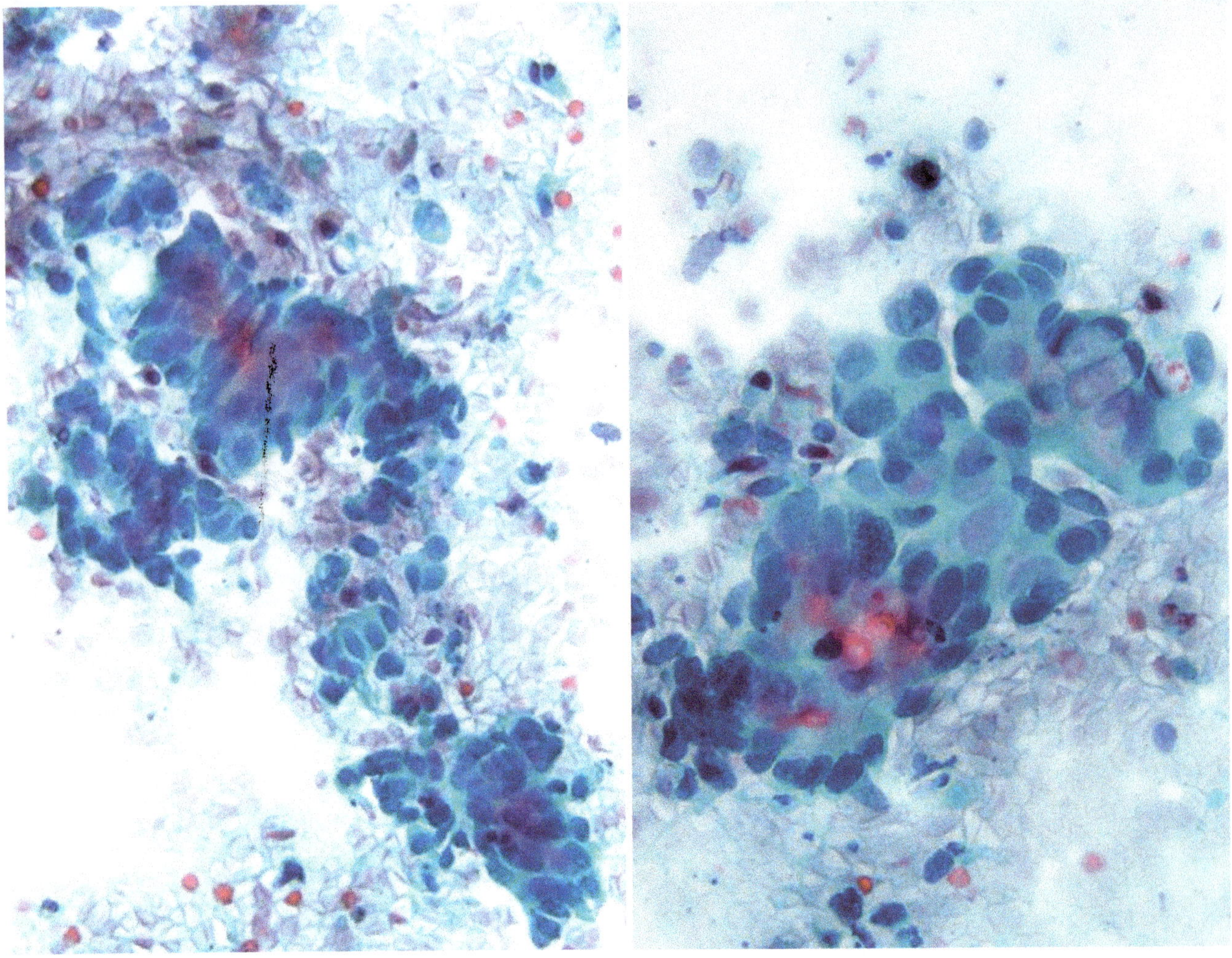

Fig. 5.47

Q-47. This image is from a Pap smear of a 47-year-old female with a history of colonic carcinoma. What is the most likely diagnosis?

(a) Endocervical adenocarcinoma
(b) Endocervical adenocarcinoma in situ
(c) Squamous cell carcinoma
(d) Metastatic colonic adenocarcinoma

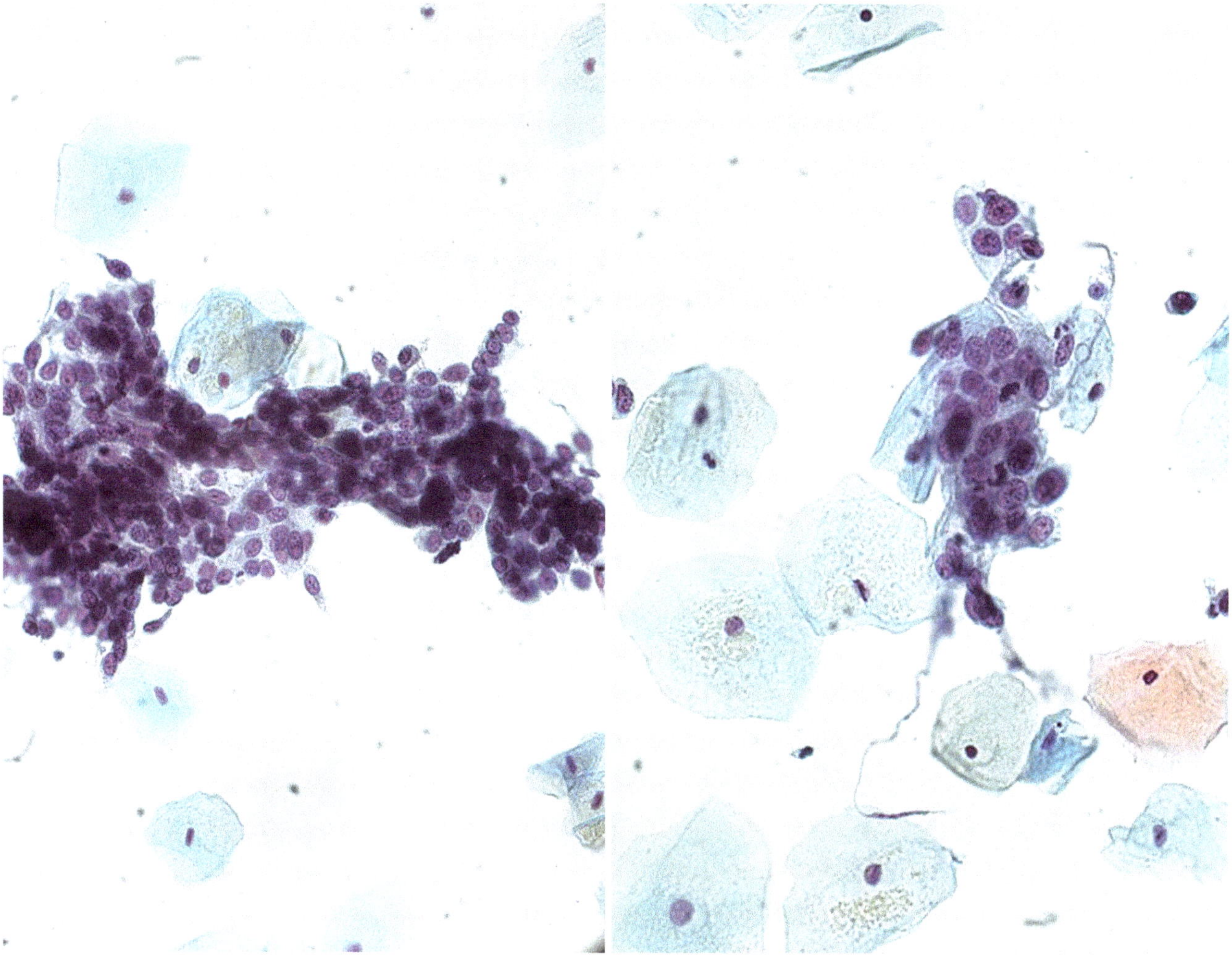

Fig. 5.48

Q-48. This image is from a Pap smear of a 27-year-old female. What is the most likely diagnosis?
- (a) Squamous cell carcinoma
- (b) Small cell carcinoma
- (c) High-grade squamous intraepithelial lesion (HSIL)
- (d) Follicular cervicitis

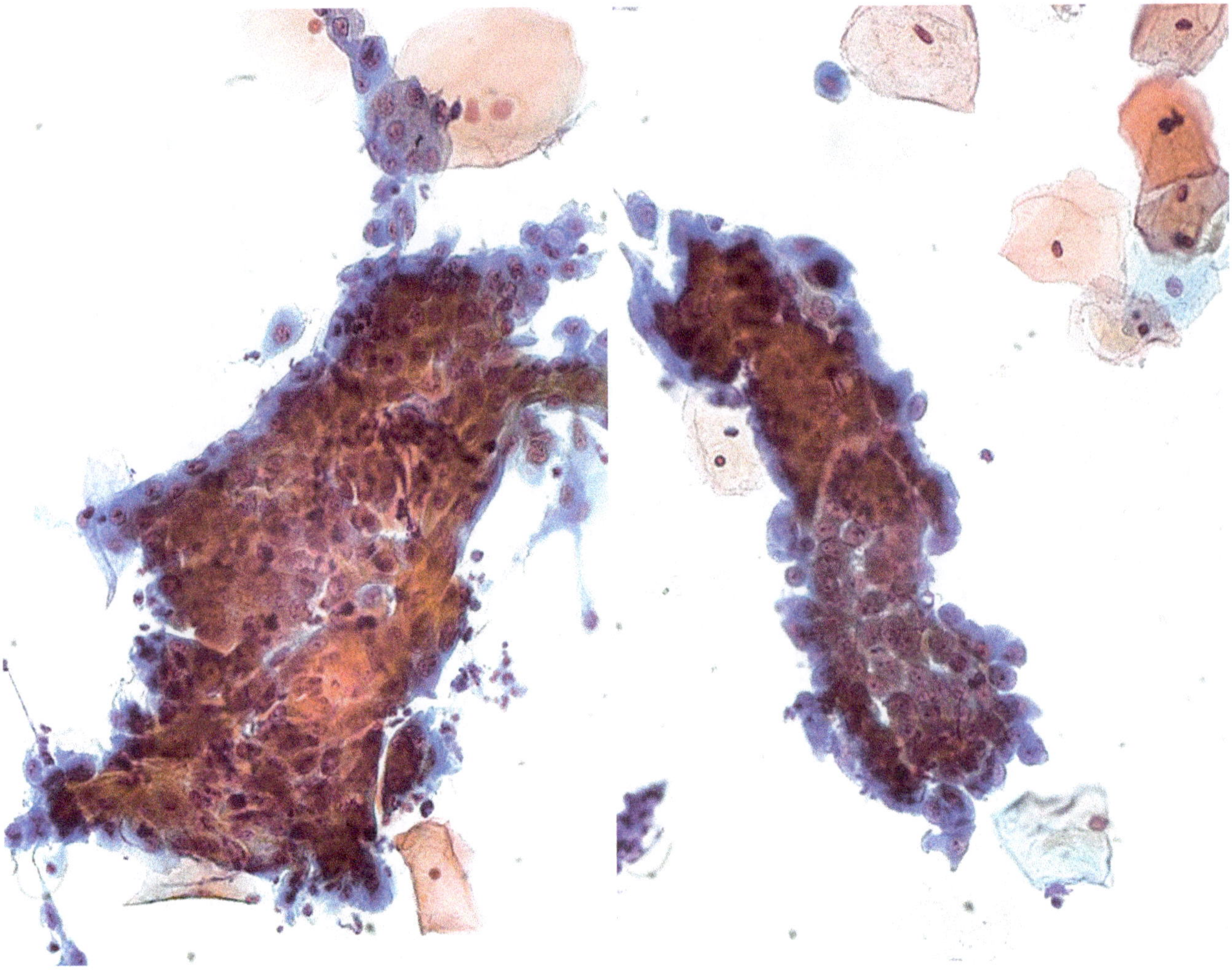

Fig. 5.49

Q-49. This image is from a Pap smear of a 35-year-old female. What is the most likely diagnosis?
(a) Neoplastic, squamous origin
(b) Neoplastic, glandular
(c) Infectious
(d) Reactive

Fig. 5.50

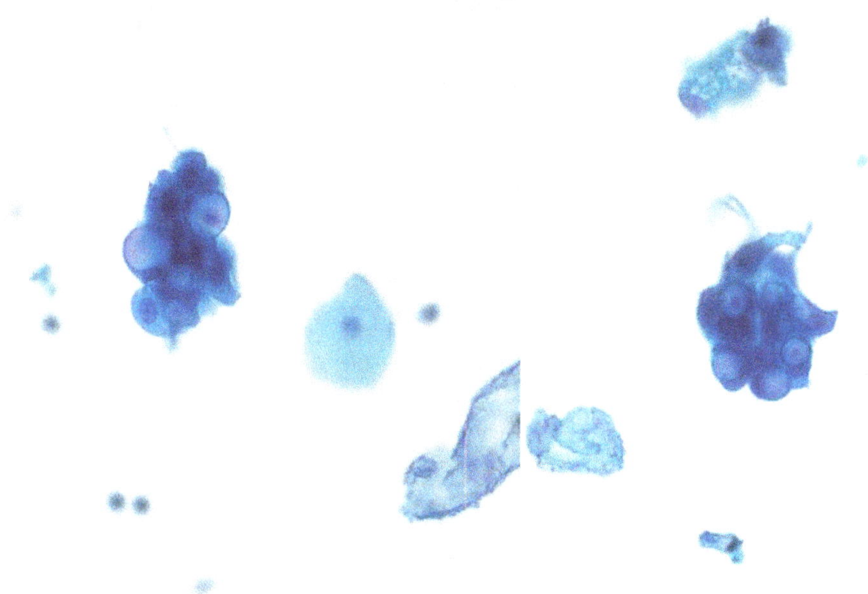

Q-50. This image is from a Pap smear of a 28-year-old female. What is the most likely diagnosis?

(a) Neoplastic, squamous origin
(b) Neoplastic, glandular
(c) Infectious
(d) Benign/reactive

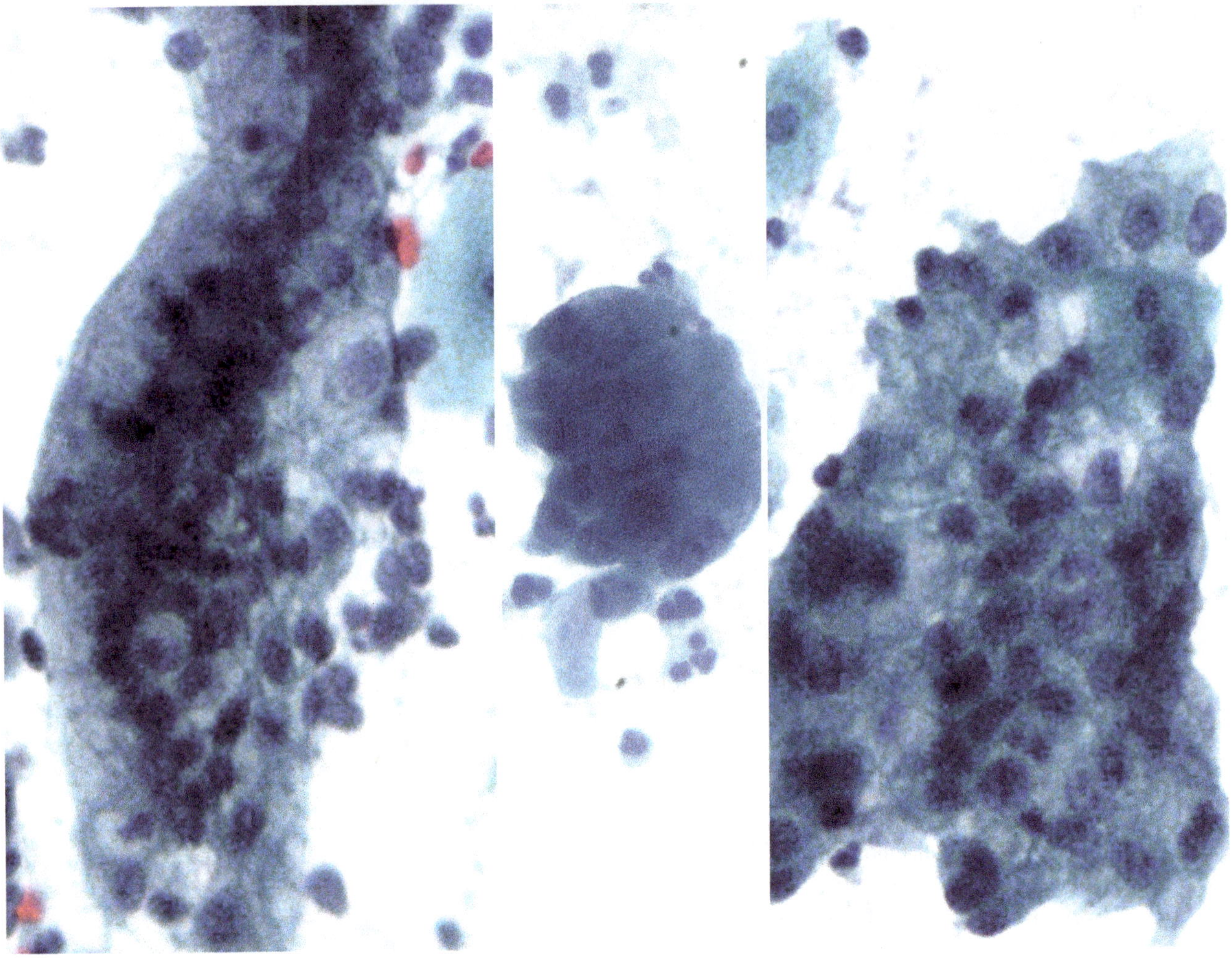

Fig. 5.51

Q-51. Which of the following is the best diagnosis of this Pap test which was obtained from a 39-year-old female with previous Pap test of atypical glandular cells (AGC)?

(a) Endocervical adenocarcinoma in situ (AIS) vs. invasive endocervical carcinoma
(b) Endometrial adenocarcinoma in situ
(c) Endometrial adenocarcinoma
(d) Metastatic breast carcinoma

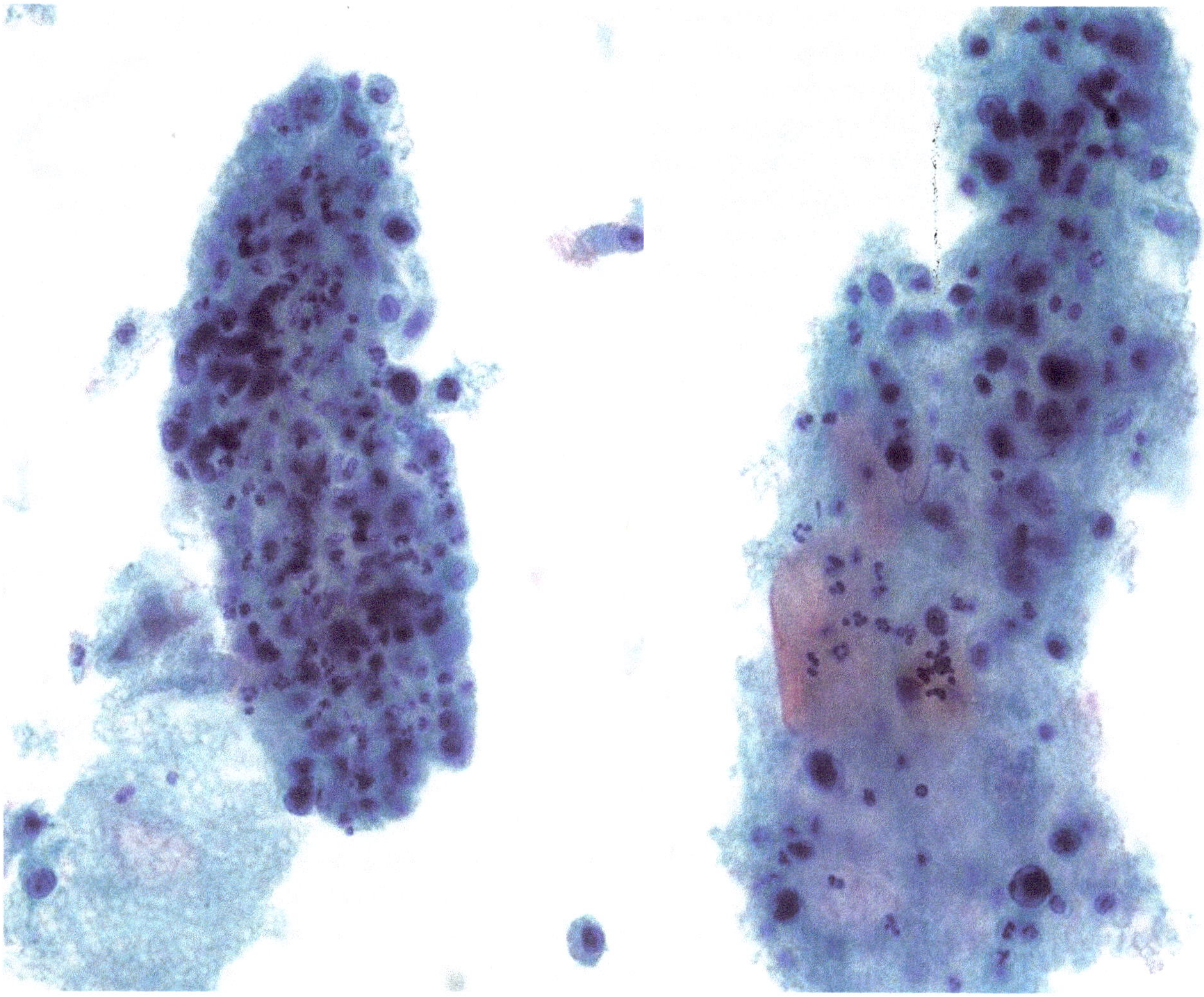

Fig. 5.52

Q-52. This image is from a ThinPrep Pap Test from a 34-year- old female. What is the most likely diagnosis?

(a) Endocervical adenocarcinoma
(b) Endocervical adenocarcinoma in situ
(c) Squamous carcinoma
(d) Repair

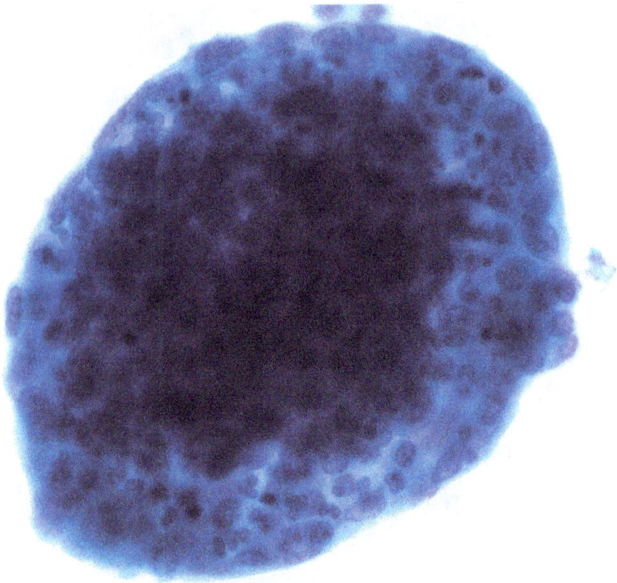

Fig. 5.53

Q-53. This image is from a Pap smear of a 28-year-old female. What is the most likely diagnosis?
(a) Neoplastic, squamous origin
(b) Neoplastic, glandular
(c) Dysplastic
(d) Benign

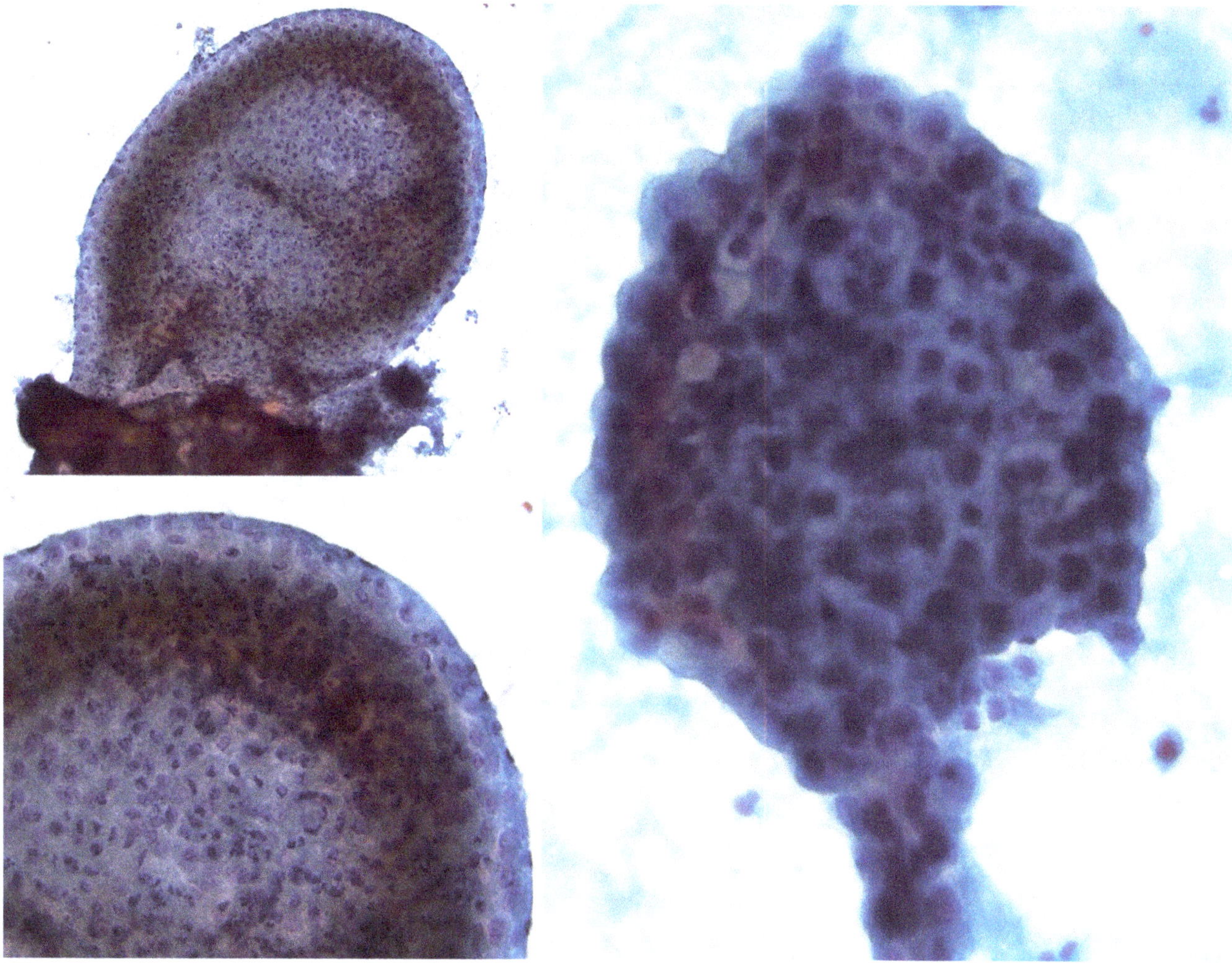

Fig. 5.54

Q-54. What is the most likely diagnosis for this Pap test from a 58-year-old woman?
(a) Adenocarcinoma
(b) Squamous cell carcinoma
(c) Endometrial cell, benign
(d) Repair

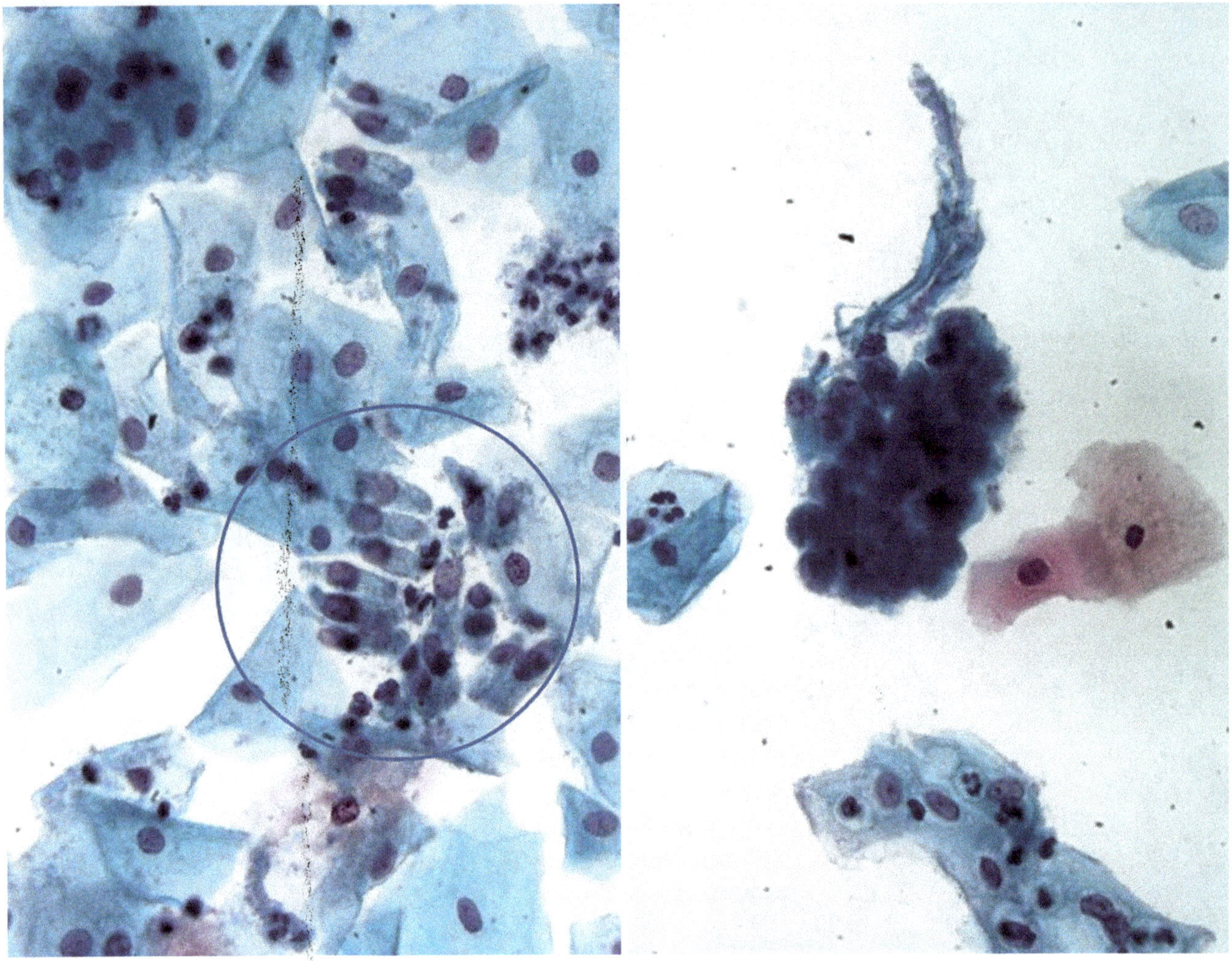

Fig. 5.55

Q-55. The cells shown within the circles represent which of the following:

(a) AIS
(b) Tubal metaplasia
(c) Benign endocervical cells
(d) Endometrial cells

Fig. 5.56

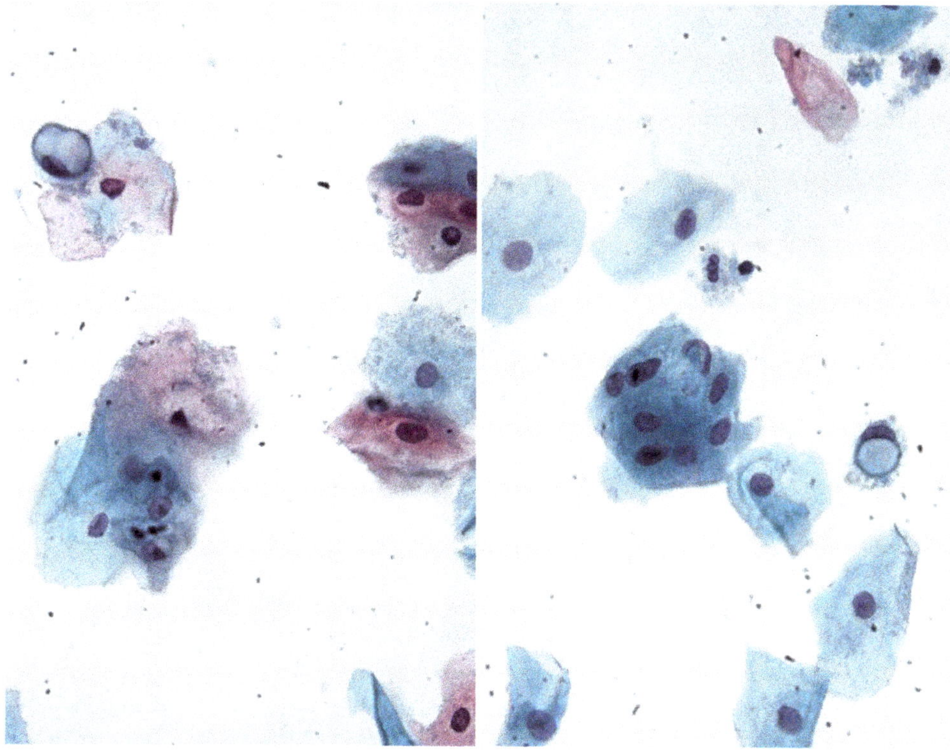

Q-56. The vacuolated cells with signet-ring morphology represent which of the following:

(a) Benign endocervical cells
(b) Adenocarcinoma with signet-ring morphology
(c) Tubal metaplasia
(d) Endometrial cells

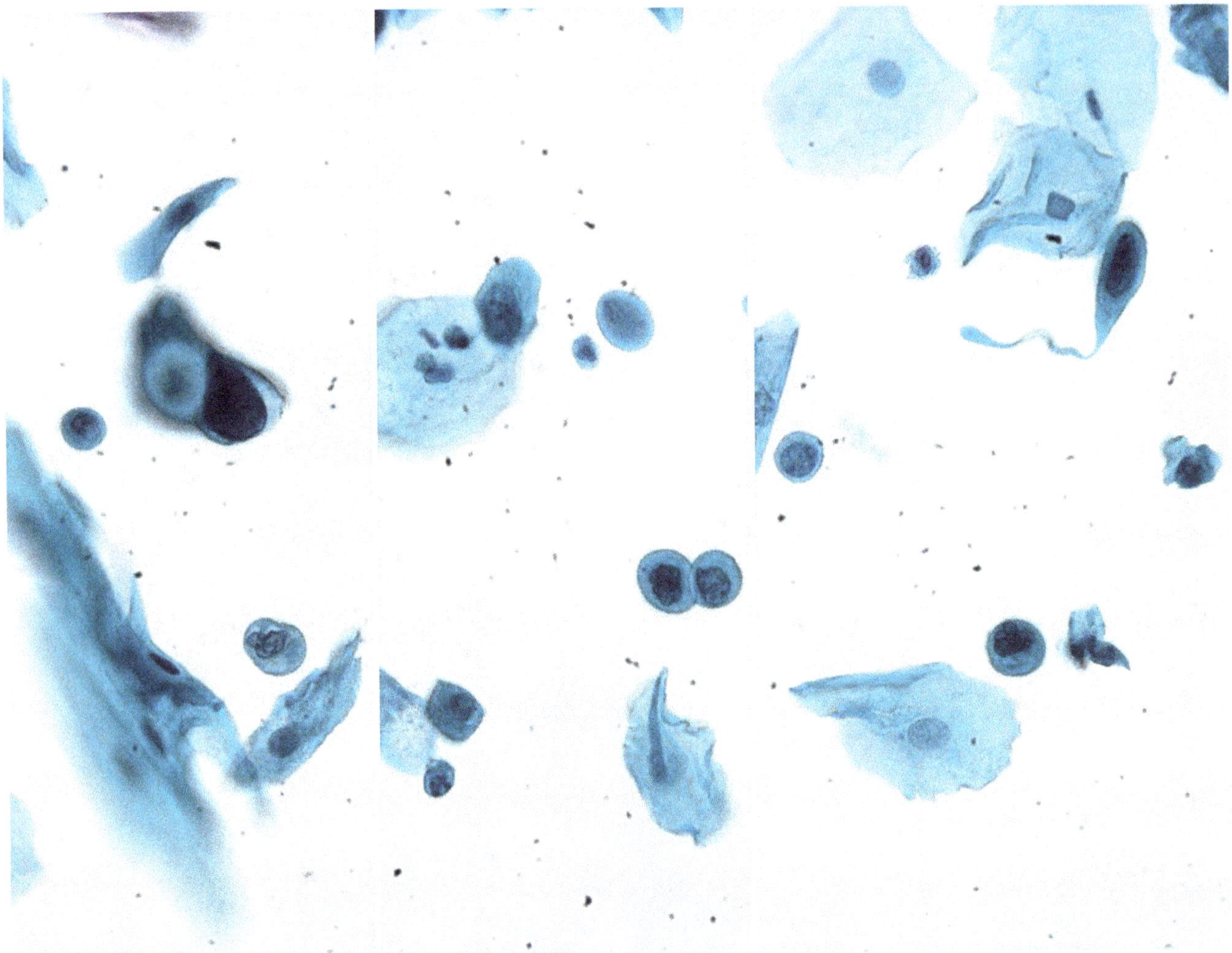

Fig. 5.57

Q-57. This image is of a Pap smear from a 57-year-old woman. What is the most likely diagnosis?
(a) Neoplastic, squamous origin
(b) Neoplastic, glandular
(c) Dysplastic
(d) Benign, reactive, infectious

5.4 Answers and Discussion of Text-Based Questions 1–30

A-1. **(a) The frequency of endocervical adenocarcinoma has been increasing.**
The frequency of endocervical adenocarcinoma has been increasing with doubling of the incidence between early 1970s and mid-1985 in the USA. The differential diagnoses of glandular lesions in liquid-based cytology include reactive conditions, high-grade squamous intraepithelial lesion (HSIL) with glandular involvement, and follicular cervicitis. Low-grade intraepithelial lesions are not in the differential diagnosis of glandular lesions. The majority of adenocarcinoma contains HPV DNA including mucinous adenocarcinoma and adenosquamous carcinomas. Features of AIS include three-dimensional clustering (with continuous depth of focus), variable nuclear size and shape within groups, some alteration in nuclear polarity with feathering, hyperchromatic crowded nuclei, irregular nuclear membranes, uniform stippled chromatin, increased N/C ratio, apoptosis, and presence of few/occasional single atypical cells.

A-2. **(b) The endocervix is a series of deep infoldings of mucosa that tunnel into endocervical stroma forming crypts that secrete mucus.**
The endocervix does not have the classical glandular component of secretory cells that are connected to the surface by a duct lined with ductal cells. Instead, the endocervix consists of a series of deep infoldings of mucosa that tunnel into endocervical stroma forming crypts that secrete mucus. The endocervical mucosa consists of single layer of endocervical columnar cells. Endocervical cells are morphologically different from endometrial cells. The endocervical cells are tall columnar and have basal nuclei and a delicate cytoplasm with an average N/C ratio of 30 %. They are rarely ciliated and can be seen as single or in groups (strips and sheet). They normally do not form acini, papillae, or cell balls. Endometrial cells are smaller than endocervical cells with scant cytoplasm and ill-defined borders. Cytoplasmic vacuoles are infrequent.

A-3. **(b) HPV 16 and 18 have been identified in AIS and adenocarcinomas in similar proportions.**
Endocervical AIS is the known precursor of invasive endocervical adenocarcinoma. Several evidences have been published, such as both are linked to HPV 16 and 18. Furthermore, women with AIS are on average 13 years younger than those with invasive adenocarcinoma (39 vs. 52 years old). Both AIS and adenocarcinoma share several morphological features such as hyperchromatic crowded groups; glandular differentiation; columnar cell morphology, strips, and rosettes; crowding and stratification; apoptosis; and mitosis. However, tumor diathesis and single cells are features of invasive adenocarcinoma. Histological biopsies often AIS coexist with early invasive adenocarcinoma. AIS has been also discovered retrospectively in cervical biopsies that originally called negative in women who later develop invasive adenocarcinoma. The cytologic criteria for AIS were considered reliable to be separated as diagnostic category in the Bethesda System 2001.

A-4. **(c) Invasive adenocarcinoma shows more inflammation, lysed blood, irregular nuclear membranes, nucleoli, and numerous single cells.**
Both AIS and adenocarcinoma share several morphological features such as hyperchromatic crowded groups; glandular differentiation; columnar cell morphology, strips, and rosettes; crowding and stratification; apoptosis; and mitosis. However, tumor diathesis and single cells are features of invasive adenocarcinoma. The average age of AIS is 35–40 years at presentation. It is a precursor to cervical invasive adenocarcinoma. There are acinar three-dimensional groups and feathering of peripheral nuclei. The atypical columnar cells show pseudostratified nuclei and rosette-like arrangement of cells. The cells display enlarged oval nuclei, nuclear hyperchromasia, and granular, evenly distributed chromatin. The oval columnar nuclei in AIS become more round in invasive adenocarcinoma. AIS usually show a clean background with no necrosis. In this case, the background shows some necrosis. Significantly pleomorphic crowded hyperchromatic nuclei with some "drunken honeycomb" morphology are seen. The cells lack the uniformity of nuclear spacing within well-defined, orderly cytoplasmic borders typical of benign groups. AIS usually show small inconspicuous nucleoli, which is prominent, and multiple nucleoli in invasive adenocarcinoma (see right image) are also seen.

A-5. **(b) Diathesis that contains blood with lysed RBCs, inflammation, proteinaceous debris, and degenerated malignant cells**
Tumor diathesis is indicative of invasive cancer. It consists of blood with lysed RBCs, inflammation, proteinaceous debris, and degenerated malignant cells. In conventional Pap test or smears, it shows a dirty background consisting of blood, lysed RBCs, inflammation, nuclear debris, and cellular debris. However, in liquid-based cytology, necrosis is often

patchy displaying discreet aggregates of debris. Clinging necrosis refers to a pattern of necrosis seen in liquid-based cytology where diathesis materials adhere or surround clusters of malignant cells.

A-6. **(c) A group of palisaded strips, complex branched fragments, acinar or rosette architecture, and feathering.**
Tightly crowded hyperchromatic groups can be seen in a wide range of benign, reactive, dysplastic, and neoplastic lesions including AIS. Adenocarcinoma in situ often shows tightly crowded hyperchromatic groups of palisaded strips, complex branched fragments, acinar or rosette architecture, and feathering. These groups are arranged in small sheets, short strips, or large microbiopsy fragments. The three-dimensionality of the groups is often apparent when the field focus is changed.

A-7. **(d) In AGC of endometrial cell origin, nuclear atypia is the most important feature for diagnosis.**
In general, the diagnosis of atypical endometrial cells (AGC of endometrial origin) is based primarily on nuclear atypia, whereas the diagnosis of atypical endocervical glandular cells (AGC of endocervical origin) is based more on architectural atypia and some nuclear atypia. Atypical endometrial cells are usually seen in small groups of cells with enlarged hyperchromatic nuclei and variable prominence of nucleoli. Their distinction from benign endometrial cells is based mainly on the criterion of increased nuclear size. When dealing with LBPs, it is important to know that endometrial cells are often well preserved and may show nuclear size and shape pleomorphism and the presence of nucleoli. The differential diagnosis of atypical endometrial cells is broad and may include endometrial hyperplasia, endometrial polyps, chronic endometritis, IUD-associated changes, and carcinoma. In AGC of endocervical cell origin, the cells are characterized by cellular strips and rosettes demonstrating elongated, overlapping nuclei with moderately coarse chromatin and hyperchromatic nuclei. The peripheral border may show "feathering," with protruding nuclei, in contrast to the smooth communal border typical of benign glandular fragments. In LBPs, cells are more rounded and clustered in three-dimensional configurations. These features may be suspicious for AIS or invasive adenocarcinoma, but they are quantitatively or qualitatively insufficient for such definitive interpretation.

A-8. **(d) The cells have apical "hobnail" nuclei; prominent nucleoli; clear abundant vacuolated cytoplasm; and large, pale, round to irregular nuclei, and naked nuclei are common due the delicate nature of the cytoplasm.**
A, B, and C are characteristics of classical endocervical adenocarcinoma. However, the morphological characteristics of the clear cell carcinoma include cells having apical "hobnail" nuclei, prominent nucleoli, clear abundant vacuolated cytoplasm, and large, pale, and round to irregular nuclei, and naked nuclei are common due the delicate nature of the cytoplasm.

A-9. **(c) Serous adenocarcinoma in Pap test typically shows numerous papillary clusters; coarse to smudgy, dark chromatin; prominent nucleoli; and dense, bulky cytoplasm.**
Serous adenocarcinoma is by definition a high-grade carcinoma with high-grade nuclear features. It is often associated with well-differentiated architectural features such as glands or papillae. This is in contrast to endometrioid carcinoma, which the nuclear and architectural abnormalities are usually concordant. Serous adenocarcinoma shows typically numerous papillary clusters; coarse to smudgy, dark chromatin; prominent nucleoli; and dense, bulky cytoplasm. Bizarre tumor giant cells are characteristic, and psammoma bodies are common.

A-10. **(b) The nuclei are enlarged and irregular, with nucleoli and abnormal chromatin patterns.**
Endometrial adenocarcinoma is typically present in fewer cells and clusters in Pap tests as compared to endocervical carcinoma since it is not directly sampled. The nuclei are enlarged and irregular, with nucleoli and abnormal chromatin patterns. The background is watery or granular/watery diathesis pattern. Foamy histiocytes and epithelial cells with large vacuoles containing neutrophils (so-called oxyphil cells) can be seen and suggest endometrial origin.

A-11. **(c) The cellular abnormalities induced by IUD may mimic glandular or squamous abnormalities.**
The IUD has been noted to cause abnormalities in the glandular or squamous metaplastic cells seen in Pap tests. The origin of the affected glandular cells can be from endometrial origin or from high endocervical canal that exfoliates spontaneously in response to the presence of IUD and the string that extends into the endocervical canal. These changes may mimic either squamous or glandular abnormalities. The abnormal cells may present as single cells of endometrial or squamous metaplastic cells showing high N/C ratio and dark smudged nuclei with smooth nuclear contour that mimics HSIL or in small clusters of rounded cells showing individual cells with large vacuoles that push the uniform nuclei toward the edge of the cluster giving "bubblegum vacuoles" morphology mimicking adenocarcinoma. However, the number of single cells

or small clusters is low with no irregular contour irregularities or significant pleomorphism present. These changes are not specific and can be seen in women without a history of IUD placement.

A-12. **(d) AS-US or LSIL**

Follicular cervicitis is limited to cervical or vaginal submucosa. However, it can be seen in Pap tests when there is erosion or ulceration of overlying cervical or vaginal mucosa. The size of the reactive lymphocytes is similar to intermediate squamous nuclei. The morphology of follicular cervicitis is similar to reactive lymph node. It would show mixture of mature small lymphocytes intermixed with few immature (larger) lymphocytes and histiocytes. The differential diagnosis includes lymphoma which shows predominance of atypical lymphoid cells that are larger than reactive lymphocytes, with more immature chromatin. The differential diagnosis also includes small cell carcinoma which shows highly atypical pleomorphic small cells 2–3 lymphocyte nucleus sizes in background of necrosis. In liquid-based cytology, the lymphocytes particularly from germinal center may clump forming hyperchromatic crowded groups that mimic HSIL, AIS, or adenocarcinoma. AS-US is an atypical intermediate or metaplastic squamous cell that has relatively abundant cytoplasm and low N/C ratio that has some features concerning for LSIL. Therefore, AS-US or LSIL is not in the differential diagnosis of follicular cervicitis. The key features for the diagnosis of follicular cervicitis are in noticing the very small, round lymphocytes within this "pool" of lymphs of a range of maturation. The other helpful features are the presence of occasional tingible body macrophages with lymphocytic nuclear material ingested in the cytoplasm.

A-13. **(a) It is often dense and homogeneous with distinct borders. However, they occasionally become vacuolated and cyanophilic.**

Immature squamous metaplasia shows morphologic spectrum of epithelial changes from a single or multiple layers of reserve cells to an epithelium composed of three or more layers of cells with features of nonkeratinized squamous epithelial cells. Their tendency to occur as single cells is correlated with the degree of maturation to squamous cells. The cytoplasm is dense and homogeneous but can be vacuolated and cyanophilic. Cytoplasmic vacuolation is more observed in the presence of inflammation or as a consequence of degeneration. In Pap test, they often show some degree of atypia (minimal to mild). Cells and nuclei show a slight irregularity in size and shape, which is due to the influence of some irritation. Differential diagnosis with dysplastic changes should be made on the basis of the evenly distributed, finely granular, non-hyperchromatic, or hypochromatic chromatin. Because squamous metaplastic cells are particularly prone to reactive changes, they may show nuclear enlargement and variation in nuclear size (mimicking HSIL) and, occasionally, prominent nucleoli. However, the presence of smooth nuclear membranes and finely textured chromatin is reassuring of the benignity of the cells.

A-14. **(d) The presence of squamous metaplastic cells indicates that the transformation zone (TZ) has been sampled.**

Squamous metaplastic cells have round to oval nuclei that have smooth nuclear contour with fine chromatin and small nucleoli. Cytoplasm is dense and occasionally vacuolated and cyanophilic. They may show cytoplasmic projections with "spider legs" morphology due to sampling. The presence of squamous metaplastic cells indicates that the transformation zone (TZ) has been sampled. In the 2001 Bethesda System, the presence or absence of an endocervical cells or transformation zone component is noted on the report. An endocervical component is considered present if 10 or more endocervical cells or squamous metaplastic cells, either single or in groups, are present.

A-15. **(d) It occurs as single cells of endometrial or high endocervical origin showing dark smudged nuclei with smooth nuclear contour that mimics HSIL.**

The IUD has been noted to cause abnormalities in the glandular or squamous metaplastic cells seen in Pap tests. The origin of the affected glandular cells can be from endometrial origin or from high endocervical canal that exfoliates spontaneously in response to the presence of IUD and its string that extends into endocervical canal. It occurs as single cells of endometrial or endocervical origin showing dark smudged nuclei with smooth (not irregular) nuclear contour that mimics HSIL. It may also show small clusters of rounded cells of glandular or squamous metaplastic cells showing individual cells with large vacuoles that push the uniform nuclei toward the edge of the cluster (bubblegum vacuoles) that mimics adenocarcinoma. However, the number of single cells or small clusters is low with no nuclear contour irregularities or significant pleomorphism present or tumor and diathesis is not present. The presence of actinomyces on the slide is an important clue and seen in 25 % of the cases.

A-16. (**b**) **They are seen more in women who have undergone postoperative radiotherapy**.

Glandular cells in Pap test in women post total hysterectomy are glandular cells resembling normal endocervical cells and are seen in approximately 2 % of vaginal Pap samples. They are more commonly seen in women who have had postoperative radiotherapy and may therefore represent a therapy-induced metaplasia of squamous epithelium. They are entirely benign and should not raise the possibility of an adenocarcinoma, even if the total hysterectomy was carried out for an endocervical adenocarcinoma. A statement in the report such as "benign glandular cells status post-hysterectomy" is appropriate. A careful review of the surgical notes is important since most hysterectomy is supracervical, and therefore, endocervical cells on a vaginal Pap are from the cervical stump.

A-17. (**d**) **Extrauterine carcinoma**

Tumor diathesis in Pap test is seen in invasive malignancies including cervical squamous and adenocarcinoma (>90 % of the cases), endometrial adenocarcinoma (93 % of the cases), and least in extrauterine carcinomas (19.7 % of the cases). Therefore, presence of malignant cells in clean background should raise the possibility of metastasis.

A-18. (**b**) **Feathering refers to cigar-shaped nuclei at the periphery protruding beyond the confines of the cell borders. The nuclei protrude into the free space surrounding the cell group**.

Feathering is a distinctive and nonspecific feature of AIS. It can also be seen in invasive endocervical adenocarcinoma. Feathering refers to cigar-shaped enlarged nuclei at the periphery protruding beyond the confines of the cell due to extreme nuclear crowding and cohesion to the basement membrane. It is produced when the extremely crowded nuclei bounded by basement membrane are released from the confines of cell group upon removal from the glandular crypt attachment point. The nuclei protrude into the free space surrounding the cell group.

A-19. (**d**) **It is a well-differentiated adenocarcinoma, and it has a better prognosis compared to other variants of endocervical adenocarcinoma**.

Adenoma malignum has a worse prognosis than the usual endocervical adenocarcinoma. Furthermore, patients with adenoma malignum tend to present at a more advanced stage than patients with conventional endocervical adenocarcinoma. Analysis of 57 cases of adenoma malignum reported in the literature with follow-up of 2 years revealed an overall survival rate of only 28 % for all stages (see reference below). Furthermore, cases associated with Peutz-Jeghers syndrome (PJS) are also associated with poor prognosis (see reference below).

Adenoma malignum almost exclusively produces neutral mucin and, therefore, shows positivity for PAS-Alcian blue 2.5 stains and NHIK-1083 immunostain. In the majority of reported cases, this rare tumor is negative for high-risk human papillomavirus (HPV) DNA.

A-20. (**a**) **Severe reactive or reparative changes may mimic SIL, AIS, or carcinoma**.

Reactive reparative changes can be caused by several factors such as infection, trauma, polyps, radiation, and IUD. It affects squamous and/or endocervical cells, and in severe changes, they mimic squamous or glandular lesions such as SIL, AIS, or even carcinoma. They can be distinguished from more severe dysplastic or neoplastic lesions by the fact that cells in repair show good cohesion, flat monolayer sheets that maintain polarity and contain pale or hypochromatic nuclei. Furthermore, the nuclei are round, have smooth nuclear membranes, and have evenly distributed pale or hypochromatic chromatin. Prominent or multiple nucleoli and occasional mitoses may also be present.

A-21. (**c**) **Decidual changes are seen in stromal cells, while Arias-Stella changes occur in endocervical or endometrial glandular epithelium**.

Decidual cells are large stromal cells with approximately the size of mature squamous cells that can be seen as isolated or loosely clustered in Pap test due to ulceration or erosion of the overlying mucosa. They can be found in Pap test samples following spontaneous exfoliation or by direct sampling. They are seen in late pregnancy. The cells are large, often degenerated, have abundant granular cytoplasm with distinct cell borders, and contain large bland nuclei with pale chromatin and a prominent nucleolus. Decidual cells can resemble repair, LSIL, HSIL, carcinoma, or sarcoma cells. Arias-Stella changes affect Müllerian epithelium due to pregnancy-related hormone levels (hyperprogestational states). The most common epithelium is endometrial, but it can be seen also in endocervical gland's tubal epithelium. The morphology consists of loosely cohesive cell groups of markedly enlarged glandular cells with abundant clear cytoplasm, eccentric nuclei, nuclear enlargement, prominent nucleoli, prominent nuclear grooves, and inclusions. Binucleation and abundant cytoplasm are also seen. The morphology on both cytological and histological preparations is a known diagnostic pitfall and a source of false-positive diagnoses due to its resemblance to adenocarcinoma especially clear cell adenocarcinoma. Some features such as a relative preservation of nuclear/cytoplasmic ratio, fine chromatin pattern, clean background, cohesiveness of the cells, and the presence of nuclear grooves and inclusions are helpful for accurate diagnosis. There are no single cells and tumor diathesis as it would if it represented cancer.

A-22. (c) **Single and clusters of glandular cells with enlarged nuclei, nuclear membrane irregularity, and prominence of nucleoli**.
Benign endometrial cell balls are often most prominent in days 5–8 of the menstrual cycle. Endometrial epithelial cells are often packed and the nuclear details may be difficult to appreciate. They usually show small glandular cells with round to oval, darkly staining nuclei. Nuclear molding may be seen. Anisocytosis and apoptotic bodies (single cell necrosis) can be present. The cytoplasm is scant and occasionally small vacuoles can be seen. The cytoplasm of the endometrial cells may engulf neutrophils. Other entities that show neutrophils within vacuolated glandular cells are microglandular hyperplasia of the cervix, endocervical polyps, and endometrial adenocarcinoma. In liquid-based preparations, endometrial cell groups appear tighter, isolated cells may be more prominent, the nuclear detail is often better preserved, and the nucleoli may be more prominent. The nuclei may appear as bean shaped with sharper chromatin detail and visible nucleoli. The bloody background of conventional smears is less seen in liquid-based preparations, although stromal cells and histiocytes can still be seen. When endometrial cells show an enlarged nucleus and nuclear atypia such as nuclear membrane irregularity or prominence of nucleoli, they should be categorized as atypical glandular cells (AGC).

A-23. (d) **The TBS 2001 recommended that benign-appearing endometrial cells in postmenopausal women be reported as category "Other," and this was applicable only to exfoliative endometrial cells**.
The Bethesda System for Reporting Cervical Cytology in 1991 (TBS 1991) recommended that benign-appearing endometrial cells in postmenopausal women be reported as an "epithelial cell abnormality" based on the increased risk for endometrial adenocarcinoma (6 %). However, since review of the published literature showed an exceedingly low rate of significant lesions in anyone less than 40 years of age and since cytologists may lack clinical information on menstrual dates/menopausal status, hormone therapy/tamoxifen, abnormal bleeding, and other endometrial carcinoma risk factors, the TBS 2001 created a new category "Other" that was included to report the presence of benign-appearing endometrial cells in women aged 40 years or older. This category should include only exfoliated, intact endometrial cells. These exfoliated groups of endometrial cells may be of epithelial and/or stromal origin, and the morphological distinction of these two cell types is sometimes not possible. Directly sampled lower uterine segment or abraded stromal cells/histiocytes, when present alone, should not be reported under this category.

A-24. (b) **Increased in nuclear size**
Atypical endometrial cells are usually seen in small groups of cells with enlarged nuclei and variable prominence of nucleoli and nuclear hyperchromasia. Their distinction from benign endometrial cells is based mainly on the criterion of increased nuclear size. When dealing with LBPs, it is important to know that endometrial cells are often well preserved and may show nuclear size and shape pleomorphism and the presence of nucleoli. The differential diagnosis of atypical endometrial cells is broad and may include endometrial hyperplasia, endometrial polyps, chronic endometritis, IUD-associated changes, and carcinoma.

A-25. (c) **This category may include cases with AIS**.
The category of atypical glandular cells is new in the Bethesda System (TBS) 2001 for Reporting Cervical Cytology. It includes glandular cells that demonstrate atypical changes beyond those encountered in benign reactive processes yet are insufficient for an interpretation of AIS. In this category, an attempt should be made to further qualify the atypia as endocervical or endometrial origin. This category should also be further subclassified, if possible, to indicate whether a neoplastic process is favored or the changes are nonspecific (NOS). When some features of AIS are present but are inadequate in quantity or quality, AGC may be used.

A-26. (a) **Clear cell carcinoma of the cervix or vagina is a rare malignancy of Müllerian origin**.
It can occur sporadically, but more commonly in daughters of women who took diethylstilbestrol (DES) during pregnancy, before the early 1970s. The age of clear cell carcinoma associated with DES is much younger (14–22 years) than non-DES-associated clear cell carcinoma, which occurs in older age group

(range 13–80 years). It has slightly worse prognosis than classical cervical adenocarcinoma. The majority (>60 %) of clear cell carcinomas are HPV DNA negative; however, HPV DNA has been detected in both DES- and non-DES-associated tumors.

A-27. (**c**) **Pemphigus vulgaris**
Pemphigus vulgaris is an autoimmune disease that can be seen in the Pap test and has cytological features that may mimic adenocarcinoma or squamous cell carcinoma. It is characterized by vesiculobullous lesions of the skin and mucosal membranes with formation of suprabasal acantholytic vesicles and blisters. It has been shown that there is an autoantibody against a cadherin-like cell adhesion molecule on the surface of stratified squamous epithelial cells, resulting in erosions and ulcers. The disease can be seen in the esophagus, oral cavity, conjunctiva, larynx, urethra, vulva, and cervix. The cytomorphological features of pemphigus vulgaris include high cellularity, extremely active nuclear chromatin (mitotic figures and large irregular nucleoli), and marked single cells and clusters mimicking malignancy. The nucleoli may be "bullet-shaped." There is a bloody or inflammatory background (more seen in conventional smears), but there is no true tumor diathesis. The liquid-based preparation will show an inflammatory background only.

A-28. (**d**) **Metastatic serous carcinoma of ovarian origin**
Serous adenocarcinoma is a relatively common malignancy in the ovaries. However, it can be seen also as primary in the cervix, endometrium, or peritoneum. Serous adenocarcinomas are considered high-grade malignant cells and grow in a complex papillary or budding pattern. The nuclei are large, pleomorphic, bizarre, and have macronucleoli. Psammoma bodies, which are concentric ringed calcified material seen within fibrovascular cores of papillae, are characteristic features of serous carcinoma and seen in one third of the cases. However, they are not specific and can be seen in numerous other adenocarcinomas such as thyroid, lung, and others. The tumor cells are cuboidal or hobnail shaped and contain abundant granular eosinophilic or clear cytoplasm. Marked nuclear atypia is always present (required to qualify as serous carcinoma). Lobulated nuclei with smudged chromatin and abnormal mitotic figures are present. Serous adenocarcinomas are aggressive tumors and have a poor prognosis. Necrosis in Pap tests is less likely to be seen if the tumor is metastatic such as in this case.

A-29. (**a**) **ER+, PR+, mammaglobin+, CK7+**
ER+, PR+, mammaglobin+, CK7+ is consistent with breast primary. An ER+, PR+, CEA+, vimentin– would be more consistent with endocervical primary. An ER+, PR+, CK7+, vimentin + would be consistent with endometrial primary. A CK7–, CK20–, CEA+, CDX2+ would be consistent with colorectal primary.

A-30. (**a**) **They may resemble AIS, adenocarcinoma, or HSIL.**
Endometrial cells in Pap test may resemble AIS, adenocarcinoma, or HSIL. They usually demonstrate poorly preserved small, molded, and hyperchromatic nuclei with pyknotic nuclear fragments. The hyperchromasia is degenerative and not neoplastic in nature. Stromal balls or histiocytes are common. Feathering, rosettes, and strips of columnar cells are characteristics of endocervical AIS and not endometrial cells. This case shows an endometrial cell ball or exodus consisting of epithelial and stromal cells. The core of the ball contains condensed stromal cells surrounded by epithelial endometrial cells. Small nucleoli may be present. Endometrial cell balls are often most prominent in days 5–8 of the menstrual cycle. Anisocytosis and apoptotic bodies (single cell necrosis) can be present. The cytoplasm of benign endometrial cells may engulf neutrophils. However, other entities may show neutrophils within vacuolated glandular cells such as microglandular hyperplasia, endocervical polyps, and endometrial adenocarcinoma. The bloody background of conventional smears is less seen in liquid-based preparations, although stromal cells and histiocytes can still be seen.

5.5 Answers and Discussion of Image-Based Questions 31–57

A-31. **(d) Reactive**

This Pap smear is from patient who had squamous cell carcinoma treated with hysterectomy and radiation therapy. The smear shows cytomorphological changes consistent with radiation/treatment changes. One of the most common causes of repair is radiation. The cytomorphology of radiation effects include cellular enlargements (cytomegalic cells) which do not have a significant increase in nuclear/cytoplasmic ratio. The cells, often polychromatic and sometimes having bizarre shapes, may continue for decades after the cessation of radiation therapy. A postradiation dysplasia should be differentiated from repair or radiation effect by the increase in nuclear/cytoplasmic ratio. This finding puts the patient at increased risk for recurrent carcinoma within 3 years of treatment. Recurrent squamous cell carcinoma should have a markedly increased N/C ratio, hyperchromasia, and marked pleomorphic nuclei, and may have nucleoli. A tumor diathesis in the background should be present as well as irregular chromatin patterns. The uniform, streaming cytoplasm; clean background, hypochromatic, finely granular nuclei; numerous PMNs; and absence of single cells can also assist with this differential.

A-32. **(c) Adenocarcinoma in situ (AIS)**

The cells are glandular origin and lack the uniformity of nuclear spacing within well-defined, orderly cytoplasmic borders typical of benign groups. This AIS case shows acinar three-dimensional groups with feathering of peripheral nuclei. The atypical cells show columnar morphology with rosette-like arrangements. The cells have enlarged oval nuclei, nuclear hyperchromasia, and granular, evenly distributed chromatin with a clean background. There is no patchy or clinging necrosis seen. Small inconspicuous nucleoli are also present. Few single atypical cells are also noted in this case. The histological follow-up of this case shows endocervical adenocarcinoma in situ.

A-33. **(d) High-grade squamous intraepithelial lesion (HSIL)**

These cells show rounded, dense, immature cytoplasm with enlarged nuclei. They appear in clusters of cells with syncytial arrangement. These nuclei show a generally finely granular, evenly distributed chromatin pattern and a high N/C ratio. HGSIL would have this scanty amount of cytoplasm and a large, hyperchromatic nuclei which take up over 80–90 % of the cell. Compare the overall cell size and nuclear size with the normal intermediate squamous cells. Especially note the irregular nuclear outlines and signs of clefting and grooving of the nuclei. The background is clean, and the nuclei do not show nucleoli as it would if it represented cancer. These abnormal cells have dense cytoplasm and central nuclei; therefore, they are not glandular origin. Therefore, the best diagnosis for this case would be HGSIL.

A-34. **(d) Negative for intraepithelial lesion or malignancy (NILM)**

This is Arias-Stella reaction (ASR) in Pap Test. The effect was first described in 1954 by Javier Arias Stella. It is a benign cellular proliferative change in Müllerian epithelium due to pregnancy-related hormone levels (hyperprogestational states). The most common epithelium is endometrial, but it can be seen also in endocervical gland's tubal epithelium. The morphology consists of loosely cohesive cell groups of markedly enlarged glandular cells with abundant clear cytoplasm, eccentric nuclei, nuclear enlargement, prominent nucleoli, prominent nuclear grooves, and inclusions. Binucleation and abundant cytoplasm are also seen. The morphology of ASR on both cytological and histological preparations is a known diagnostic pitfall and a source of false-positive diagnoses due to its resemblance to adenocarcinoma. Some features such as a relative preservation of nuclear/cytoplasmic ratio, fine chromatin pattern, clean background, cohesiveness of the cells, and the presence of nuclear grooves and inclusions are helpful for accurate diagnosis. There are no single cells and tumor diathesis as it would if it represented cancer. AIS shows tightly crowded sheets of glandular cells with overlapping stratified, enlarged, coarsely hyperchromatic nuclei, and "ragged-edged" borders.

A-35. **(b) Adenocarcinoma**

This is a case of serous adenocarcinoma of ovarian origin. Cervical serous adenocarcinoma is a rare variant of cervical adenocarcinoma that is similar morphologically to the ovarian or endometrial adenocarcinomas but occurs in bimodal age pattern, with one peak occurring before age 40 and another after age 65. Serous adenocarcinomas are considered high-grade malignant cells and grow in a complex papillary or budding pattern. The nuclei are large, pleomorphic, bizarre, and have macronucleoli. The background is usually bloody and necrotic, and neutrophils may be numerous. Psammoma bodies are uncommon in the cytologic specimens. This tumor is aggressive and has a poor prognosis.

A-36. (**c**) **Adenocarcinoma with clear cell morphology**
This is a case of clear cell carcinoma. The malignant cells are abundant and have apical "hobnail" nuclei, prominent nucleoli, and clear cytoplasm. In Pap test, they are seen singly or in sheets, clusters, or, occasionally, papillae with abundant, delicate, finely granular to vacuolated, glycogen-rich cytoplasm. In occasional cases, the cells may have abundant oxyphilic cytoplasm. Intracytoplasmic mucin can also be present in some cells, resulting in signet-ring morphology. Nuclei are large, pale, round, and irregular, with prominent nucleoli. Naked nuclei are common, owing to the delicate striped cytoplasm, similar to that described in other glycogen-rich tumors such as seminoma and Ewing sarcoma.

A-37. (**d**) **Endocervical cells**
Endocervical cells are simple, columnar, mucus-producing cells that line the endocervical canal. They are epithelial cells that maintain columnar morphology with a frothy mucus cap in Pap test. The nuclei are round to oval, basally located, with smooth contours and evenly distributed finely granular chromatin. The nucleoli are round or may show a characteristic dot-like morphology. When endocervical cells are viewed from the side, they show a picket-fence morphology pattern. However, when viewed on end, they show honeycombing. In honeycombing, the cells are arranged in evenly spaced nuclei with very minimal crowding and overlapping. They show well-defined cytoplasmic borders with mucus cap at different focusing point (3-D-like configuration). Endocervical cells show distinct cytoplasmic borders and may show a honeycomb or picket-fence appearance.

A-38. (**c**) **Recurrent keratinizing squamous cell carcinoma**
Squamous cell carcinoma can be in two morphologic variants, keratinizing and nonkeratinizing. The Bethesda System does not subdivide squamous cell carcinoma into these categories, but the cytologic features are somewhat different. Nonkeratinizing SCC features cells with immature cytoplasm, high N/C ratios, and nuclei with prominent nucleoli, irregular chromatin distribution, and irregular nuclear membranes. These cells may be seen in loose or syncytial groups or as single cells. Associated features may include a tumor diathesis composed of necrotic debris, old blood, and inflammation. Keratinizing SCC (this case) displays all of the cellular characteristics of keratinizing HSIL with the addition of variable numbers of cells demonstrating nucleoli or the addition of a tumor diathesis. Features include marked cellular variation with tadpole, spindle, and caudate shapes; dense eosinophilic cytoplasm; and markedly hyperchromatic, often opaque nuclei with high N/C ratios. Cells may be single or in loose or even thick groups. If an absolute diagnosis of SCC is difficult, then Bethesda System recommends the diagnosis of HSIL with features suggestive of invasive carcinoma. The only difference between keratinizing HSIL and keratinizing SCC is the presence of a tumor diathesis and nucleoli (present in our case, more in left side). A diathesis is often not present, and the dense nuclei make nucleoli difficult to find. A careful search should be made to look for more immature cells with less nuclear opacity to identify the presence of nucleoli.
Radiation-induced epithelial changes include cytomegaly with normal N/C ratios; wispy polychromatic cytoplasm; degenerative cytoplasmic vacuoles; granular, evenly distributed chromatin; and smudged nuclei.

A-39. (**b**) **Carcinoma**
This is a case of small cell squamous carcinoma. The carcinoma has small cell features similar to small neuroendocrine carcinoma (small cells, high N/C ratio, some molding); however, more mature squamous cells with dense cytoplasm, well-defined cell borders, less crush artifact, less nuclear molding, coarse chromatin, and parachromatin clearing nucleoli may be seen. Searching for abnormal keratinized cells or cells with obvious squamous morphology will help in differentiating this neoplasm from small cell neuroendocrine carcinoma. Both small cell neuroendocrine carcinoma and small cell squamous carcinoma are strongly associated with HPV.

A-40. (**b**) **Endometrial**
These are shed endometrial cells (left) and endometrial stromal cells (right). The key features of benign endometrial cells include tight or loose cell clusters, vacuolated cytoplasm, smudged or apoptotic nuclei, and nuclei with size of intermediate squamous cells. However, in LBC, enhanced nuclear detail may confuse benign endometrial cells with a low-grade endometrial adenocarcinoma. If endometrial cells are out of cycle in a woman age 40 years or older, it should be reported, due to presence of very low risk of endometrial adenocarcinoma. However, review of the published literature shows an exceedingly low rate of significant lesions in anyone less than 40 years of age, and since cytologists may lack clinical information on menstrual dates/menopausal status, hormone therapy/tamoxifen, abnormal bleeding, and other endometrial carcinoma risk factors, the TBS 2001 created a new

category "Other" to report the presence of benign-appearing endometrial cells in women aged 40 years or older. This category should include only exfoliated, intact endometrial cells. These exfoliated groups of endometrial cells may be of epithelial and/or stromal origin, and the morphological distinction of these two cell types is sometimes not possible. Directly sampled lower uterine segment or abraded stromal cells/histiocytes, when present alone, should not be reported under this category. Atypical endometrial cells should be reported as an epithelial glandular cell abnormality.

A-41. (**a**) **Adenocarcinoma**

This is a case of endometrial adenocarcinoma in conventional Pap smear. Endometrial cancer cells are typically identified in Pap tests because they spontaneously exfoliate and move through the endocervical mucus to be picked up by the sampling device of Pap test. Because the mucus acts like a liquid suspension, the cells and cell groupings will round up and form three-dimensional clusters. Endometrial cancers in Pap smears will have fewer cells than will endocervical cancers. Endocervical carcinoma is usually highly cellular because it is collected by direct sampling. Nuclei will enlarge, become more irregular, and show nucleoli and abnormal chromatin patterns, often with a background of watery or granular diathesis pattern. This diathesis is distinctive to endometrial tumors because it does not contain the necrotic gritty breakdown material seen in the background of tumors that directly invade the lower genital tract. The cells may be associated with foamy histiocytes and with epithelial cells with large vacuoles containing neutrophils (so-called oxyphil cells).

A-42. (**a**) **Endocervical adenocarcinoma**

The number of malignant cells in endocervical cancer is large as compared to endometrial cancer, due to direct sampling by the sampling devices. These tumor cells often present with mixed "in situ" morphology, as wells as evidence of invasion including tumor diathesis and single cell configurations. The tumor cells are typically in two-dimensional sheets because of their lack of opportunity to "round up" as would be noted in exfoliated samples or in endometrial adenocarcinoma. The nuclei are large (two to three times the size of normal endocervical cells) and have irregular hyperchromatic chromatin, prominent nucleoli, and irregular nuclear contour. The cytoplasm ranges from abundant to scant and may retain a columnar appearance in well-differentiated cases and can show many of the architectural features of in situ adenocarcinoma. This includes honeycombed group configuration, pseudostratified strips of cells, and rosette formation. Invasive endocervical adenocarcinoma always shows a diathesis background pattern which will consist of clumped and clinging granular material in liquid-based specimens and diffuse granular breakdown material in conventional slides.

A-43. (**c**) **Squamous cell carcinoma**

This is a case of invasive squamous cell carcinoma (SCC). Squamous cell carcinoma comes in two morphologic variants, keratinizing and nonkeratinizing. The Bethesda System (TBS) does not subdivide squamous cell carcinoma into these categories, but the cytomorphologic features are somewhat different. Nonkeratinizing variant shows cells with immature cytoplasm, high nuclear/cytoplasmic ratios, and nuclei with prominent nucleoli, irregular chromatin distribution, and irregular nuclear membranes. These cells may be seen in loose or syncytial groups or as single cells. Associated features may include a tumor diathesis composed of necrotic debris, old blood, and inflammation in conventional smear or clinging necrosis in liquid-based preparations. Keratinizing SCC displays all of the cellular characteristics of keratinizing HSIL with the addition of variable numbers of cells demonstrating nucleoli or the addition of a tumor diathesis. Features include marked cellular variation with tadpole, spindle, and caudate shapes (more seen in left image), dense eosinophilic cytoplasm, and markedly hyperchromatic, often opaque nuclei with high N/C ratios. Cells may be single or in loose or even thick groups.

The presence of a tumor diathesis suggests an invasive carcinoma. This finding is still noted on liquid samples but may be somewhat patchy.

A-44. (**c**) **Benign, reactive, infectious**

This is a case showing tubal metaplasia. Tubal metaplasia is a benign, nonneoplastic replacement of the normal endocervical (or endometrial) epithelium with ciliated cells characteristic of the fallopian tube. Tubal metaplasia is common, particularly after age 35, and can be identified histologically in 30–90 % of cervices. Tubal metaplasia usually occurs high in the endocervical canal and can be sampled owing to widespread use of the endocervical brush. It may present challenges in Pap test interpretation because it mimics glandular abnormalities such as adenocarcinoma in situ (AIS). Tubal metaplasia may show crowded sheets or 3-dimensional clusters or may occur as single cells. The cells are columnar with uniform, dense, cyanophilic, or vacuolated cytoplasm. They are usually smaller than normal endocervical cells but can have larger nuclei. The nuclei are round and display finely granular dark chromatin with small or no nucleoli. Mitosis can be seen. The background is usually clean. Tubal metaplasia shares features of glandular neoplasia, presenting as hyperchromatic crowded groups with columnar glandular morphology showing enlarged, pleomorphic nuclei and high N/C ratios. However, the cell groups are more orderly in tubal metaplasia, and the nuclear contour is usually round to oval and more uniform, whereas it is less orderly and with more elongated or irregular nuclei in AIS.

A-45. **(c) Metastatic adenocarcinoma**

This is a case of metastatic breast ductal adenocarcinoma. The diagnosis of metastatic extragenital malignancy to the cervix on a Pap test is rare and challenging often due to the absence of clinical data referring to a previous history of malignancy. In such cases, misinterpretation of these neoplastic elements as primary neoplasms of the cervix can occur. Women with secondary malignancies involving the lower genital tract may present with abnormal vaginal bleeding, ascites, or a rectovaginal fistula. Most patients have a known history of malignancy, the majority of which are poorly differentiated adenocarcinoma or another high-grade malignancy. Approximately 50 % of extrauterine malignancies are from ovarian and fallopian tube malignancies and 50 % from non-gynecological sites.

The most common non-gynecological extrauterine sites are gastrointestinal, breast, pancreas, lung, bladder, and kidney. Extrauterine malignancies in Pap tests are often characterized by a clean background with no diathesis, and the presence of tumor cells that look like them may be "floaters." Therefore, when an obvious malignancy seen in a Pap test is associated with a clean background or when the morphology is unusual, an extrauterine neoplasm should always be suspected. Most metastatic adenocarcinomas, although classifiable as malignant, often cannot be definitively identified by site of origin on cytologic grounds alone. Clinical findings of an extrauterine malignancy, correlation with the histology of the original tumor (if available), and immunostains are usually necessary to confirm the diagnosis.

A-46. **(c) Benign, reactive, infectious**

This is a case of reactive changes due to IUD in Pap test. IUD changes are widely recognized in Pap tests. The cytologic findings include small groups and isolated cells. The cells may display large vacuoles that push the bland uniform nucleus toward the edge of the cluster mimicking adenocarcinoma. A less common finding with IUD-associated change in the Pap test is the presence of small isolated cells with dark, smudged nuclei and smooth nuclear borders that mimic HSIL and/or ASC-H. These cellular changes are thought to represent degenerated high endocervical and/or endometrial cells that exfoliate in response to the IUD and string that extends from the endocervical canal. However, HSIL cells demonstrate variation in nuclear size and shape and show nuclear membrane irregularity and coarse chromatin. Lack of these features and clinical history of an IUD will help in the correct interpretation. The IUD has been noted to cause abnormalities in the glandular or squamous metaplastic cells seen in Pap tests. The origin of the affected glandular cells can be from endometrial origin or from high endocervical canal that exfoliates spontaneously in response to the presence of IUD and its string that extends into endocervical canal. It occurs as single cells of endometrial or endocervical origin showing dark smudged nuclei with smooth (not irregular) nuclear contour that mimics HSIL. It may also show small clusters of rounded cells of glandular or squamous metaplastic cells showing individual cells with large vacuoles that push the uniform nuclei toward the edge of the cluster (bubblegum vacuoles) that mimics adenocarcinoma. However, the number of single cells or small clusters is low with no nuclear contour irregularities or significant pleomorphism present and tumor diathesis is not present. The presence of actinomyces on the slide (right image) is an important clue and seen in 25 % of the cases.

A-47. **(d) Metastatic colonic adenocarcinoma**

This is a case of metastatic colonic adenocarcinoma. The diagnosis of metastatic extragenital malignancy to the cervix on a Pap test is rare and challenging often due to the absence of clinical data referring to a previous history of malignancy. In such cases, misinterpretation of these neoplastic elements as primary neoplasms of the cervix can occur. Women with secondary malignancies involving the lower genital tract may present with abnormal vaginal bleeding, ascites, or a rectovaginal fistula. Most patients have a known history of malignancy, the majority of which are poorly differentiated adenocarcinoma or another high-grade malignancy.

Approximately 50 % of extrauterine malignancies are from ovarian and fallopian tube malignancies and 50 % from non-gynecological sites.

The most common non-gynecological extrauterine sites are gastrointestinal, breast, pancreas, lung, bladder, and kidney. Extrauterine malignancies in Pap tests are often characterized by a clean background with no diathesis, unless the tumor is a direct extension such as this case. The presence of tumor cells with columnar morphology and marked necrosis is characteristic for colonic adenocarcinoma. Immunostains in some cases using CK20 and CDx2 are usually helpful to confirm the diagnosis and can be done on cell block material.

A-48. (c) **High-grade squamous intraepithelial lesion (HSIL)**

This is a case of HSIL with small cell morphology in syncytial-like aggregates.

The category of HSIL encompasses the older categories of moderate and severe dysplasia, CIN II, CIN III, and carcinoma in situ. The cytologic features of HSIL are characterized by cells with immature cytoplasm, abnormal nuclear features, and increased N/C ratios. The two most important differences between LSIL and HSIL are the immaturity of the cytoplasm and the high N/C ratio. The cells are present singly, in sheets, and at the high end of the spectrum may be seen in syncytial-like aggregates. The nuclei of HSIL are most often somewhat smaller than those of LSIL especially in the more severe lesions and may present as small cell morphology mimicking follicular cervicitis. The nuclear size typically ranges from two to five times the size of an intermediate cell nucleus. Of importance, the cytoplasmic area is always decreased yielding a marked increase in the nuclear to cytoplasmic ratio. The nuclei are hyperchromatic with a fine to coarsely granular, evenly distributed chromatin pattern. The nuclear membranes are wrinkled, and there is typically a significant degree of anisonucleosis. Nucleoli are generally absent.

There are variations in the diagnostic criteria for HSIL in liquid-based samples. While the morphologic changes are generally similar for both preparations, HSIL cells from the liquid-based samples may appear to be somewhat smaller than their counterparts in conventional smears. This is especially true in the cells derived from the highest-grade lesions such as carcinoma in situ and is especially marked in ThinPrep™ specimens. The increased nuclear to cytoplasmic ratios seen in moderate and severe dysplasia are evident on LBP. Irregular nuclear contours are clearly seen and may even be accentuated in LBP. Fine to coarse nuclear granularity of the chromatin pattern is preserved. Hyperchromasia may be somewhat decreased in LBP and should be considered to be a minor criterion. Cells from high-grade SIL can be seen singly and in groups. Syncytial aggregates seen in association with carcinoma in situ are clearly identified on LBP. Challenges occur when only a few small high-grade cells are present on the slide. These cells are often small approximating the size of a small histiocyte. In the clean background encountered on LBP, these small cells may be easily missed on routine screening. However, once identified, the abnormal changes such as increased nuclear size, irregular nuclear membranes, and nuclear hyperchromasia should lead the observer to an accurate diagnosis of HSIL.

A-49. (d) **Reactive**

This is a case showing reparative changes in ThinPrep Pap Test. The smear shows clusters of epithelial cells with cytomorphological changes consistent with reparative changes. The cytomorphology includes no significant increase in N/C ratios. The cells are in clusters with no single cells and often polychromatic. The background is clean or inflammatory and no tumor diathesis in the background. The nuclei are relatively uniform, hypochromatic, with finely granular chromatin, and prominent nucleoli. The nuclear contour/envelope is usually smooth. The cytoplasm shows streaming-like morphology. The presence of numerous PMNs and absence of single cells can assist with this differential.

A-50. (d) **Benign/reactive**

These are benign endocervical cells showing cytoplasmic mucus vacuoles. The endocervix does not have the classical glandular component of secretory cells that are connected to the surface by a duct lined with ductal cells. Endocervical cells are morphologically different from endometrial cells. The endocervical cells are tall columnar and have basal nuclei, delicate cytoplasm with an average N/C ratio of 30 %. They are rarely ciliated and can be seen as single or in groups (strips and sheet). They normally do not form acini, papillae, or cell balls. Cytoplasmic vacuoles in endocervical cells can occur. The nuclear size and features should help in avoiding overcalling these cells as dysplastic.

A-51. (a) **Endocervical adenocarcinoma in situ (AIS) vs. invasive endocervical carcinoma**

This case has features of AIS and endocervical adenocarcinoma. The follow-up surgical biopsy confirms presence of both AIS and invasive adenocarcinoma too. The average age of AIS is 35–40 years at presentation. It is a precursor to cervical invasive adenocarcinoma. There are acinar three-dimensional groups and feathering of peripheral nuclei. The atypical columnar cells show pseudostratified nuclei and rosette-like arrangement of cells. The cells display enlarged oval nuclei, nuclear hyperchromasia, and granular, evenly distributed chromatin. The oval columnar nuclei in AIS become more round in invasive adenocarcinoma. AIS usually show a clean background with no necrosis. In this case, the background shows some necrosis. Significantly pleomorphic crowded hyperchromatic nuclei with some "drunken honeycomb" morphology is seen. The cells lack the uniformity of nuclear spacing within well-defined, orderly cytoplasmic borders typical of benign groups. AIS usually shows small inconspicuous nucleoli, which is prominent, and multiple nucleoli in invasive adenocarcinoma (see right image) are also seen.

A-52. (**a**) **Endocervical adenocarcinoma**
Endocervical adenocarcinoma accounts for approximately 25 % of cervical cancers in the USA. However, there is an increasing incidence in both relative and absolute frequency especially in younger women (the patient in this case is young). When endocervical adenocarcinoma is compared to endometrial cancer, endocervical cancer presents with more numerous cells due to direct sampling by the sampling devices. These tumor cells often present with mixed "in situ" morphology, as wells as evidence of invasion including tumor diathesis and single cell configurations. The tumor cells are typically in 2-dimensional sheets because of their lack of opportunity to "round up" as would be noted in exfoliated samples or in endometrial adenocarcinoma. The nuclei are large (two to three times the size of normal endocervical cells or two times the size of neutrophil) and have irregular hyperchromatic chromatin, prominent nucleoli, and irregular nuclear contour. The cytoplasm ranges from abundant to scant and may retain a columnar appearance in well-differentiated cases and can show many of the architectural features of in situ adenocarcinoma. This includes honeycombed group configuration, pseudostratified strips of cells, and rosette formation. Invasive endocervical adenocarcinoma always shows a diathesis background pattern which will consist of clumped and clinging granular material in liquid-based specimens (right side) and diffuse granular breakdown material in conventional slides.

A-53. (**d**) **Benign**
This is an endometrial cell ball/exodus. Cells from the endometrial cavity that can be detected in Pap tests include epithelial, stromal, and histiocytic cells. These cells can be shed or directly sampled from the lower uterine segment using Pap sampling devices. The most typical appearance is that of the endometrial cell ball or exodus or endometrial breakdown that contains a condensed core of stromal cells surrounded by epithelial cells with more abundant paler cytoplasm. Small nucleoli may be present. Endometrial cell balls are often most prominent in days 5–8 of the menstrual cycle. The endometrial cell ball consists of endometrial cells surrounding a stromal cell core. Endometrial epithelial cells are often packed, and the nuclear details may be difficult to appreciate. They have small, round to oval, darkly staining nuclei. Nuclear molding may be seen. Anisocytosis and apoptotic bodies (single cell necrosis) can be present. The cytoplasm is scant, and occasionally small vacuoles can be seen. The cytoplasm of the endometrial cells may engulf neutrophils. Other entities that show neutrophils within vacuolated glandular cells are microglandular hyperplasia of the cervix, endocervical polyps, and endometrial adenocarcinoma. In liquid-based preparations, endometrial cell groups appear tighter, isolated cells may be more prominent, the nuclear detail is often better preserved, and the nucleoli may be more readily visible. The nuclei may appear as bean shaped with sharper chromatin detail and visible nucleoli. The bloody background of conventional smears is less seen in liquid-based preparations, although stromal cells and histiocytes can still be seen.

A-54. (**a**) **Adenocarcinoma**
This case is endometrial adenocarcinoma with clear cell features. The cells have apical "hobnail" nuclei, prominent nucleoli, and clear or granular cytoplasm. The cells are present singly or in sheets or large clusters. They show abundant, delicate, and finely granular to vacuolated, glycogen-rich cytoplasm. Nuclei are large, pale, round to irregular, with prominent nucleoli. Naked nuclei may be present due to the delicate nature of the cytoplasm. The majority (>60 %) of clear cell carcinomas are HPV DNA negative. The round three-dimensional clustering and presence of PMNs within clusters (so-called oxyphil cells) are features that suggest endometrial origin.

A-55. (**c**) **Benign endocervical cells**
Endocervical cells are simple columnar cells that line the endocervical canal. They are epithelial cells that maintain columnar morphology with a frothy mucus cap in the Pap test. The nuclei are round to oval, basally located, with smooth contours and evenly distributed finely granular chromatin. The nucleoli are round or

may show a characteristic dot-like morphology. When endocervical cells are viewed from the side, they show a picket-fence morphology pattern. However, when viewed on end, they show a honeycombing pattern. In the honeycombing pattern, the nuclei of the cells are evenly spaced with very minimal crowding and overlapping. The cells show well-defined cytoplasmic borders with a mucus cap at different focusing points (3-D-like configuration). Endocervical cells show distinct cytoplasmic borders and may show a honeycomb or picket-fence appearance, and they may present as hyperchromatic crowded groups. However, absence of nuclear enlargement, uniform size of the nuclei, and absence of loss of polarity confirm the benign nature of the cells.

A-56. (**a**) **Benign endocervical cells**

These are endocervical cells with degenerative mucinous vacuoles. Endocervical cells are simple, columnar, mucus-producing cells that line the endocervical canal. They may present as single cells, in sheets, or in clusters. They may show mucinous vacuoles or a frothy mucus cap in the Pap test. The nuclei are relatively small, round to oval and basally located, with smooth contours and evenly distributed finely granular chromatin. The nucleoli are round or may show characteristic dot-like morphology. Signet-ring carcinoma shows nuclear enlargement, pleomorphism, and irregular nuclear contour.

A-57. (**d**) **Benign, reactive, infectious**

This is a case of pemphigus vulgaris in a Pap test. Pemphigus vulgaris is an autoimmune disease that can be seen in the Pap test and has cytological features that may mimic adenocarcinoma or squamous cell carcinoma. It is characterized by vesiculobullous lesions of the skin and mucosal membranes with formation of suprabasal acantholytic vesicles and blisters. It has been shown that there is an autoantibody against a cadherin-like cell adhesion molecule on the surface of stratified squamous epithelial cells, resulting in erosions and ulcers. The disease can be seen in the esophagus, oral cavity, conjunctiva, larynx, urethra, vulva, and cervix. The cytological features of pemphigus vulgaris include high cellularity, extremely active nuclear chromatin (mitotic figures and large irregular nucleoli), and marked single cells and clusters mimicking malignancy. The nucleoli may show "bullet-shaped" morphology. There is a bloody or inflammatory background (more seen in conventional smears), but there is no true tumor diathesis. The liquid-based preparation will show inflammatory background only.

Reading List

Clement PB, Young RH. Atlas of gynecologic surgical pathology. Philadelphia: Saunders/Elsevier; 2008.

Covel JL, Wilbur DC, Guidos B, Lee KR, Chhieng DC, Mody DR. Epithelial abnormalities: glandular. In: Solomon D, Nayar R, editors. The Bethesda system for reporting cervical cytology. 2nd ed. New York: Springer; 2004. p. 123–56.

Jiménez-Ayala M, Jiménez-Ayala Portillo B. Cytopathology of the glandular lesions of the female genital tract. Basel: Karger; 2011.

Khalbuss WE, Monaco SE, and Pantanowitz L. Chapter 5, Pap test glandular Abnormalities. In: Khalbuss WE, Monaco SE, Pantanowitz L, editors. In the ASCP quick compendium of cytopathology. Chicago, IL: The ASCP Press; 2013, pp 64–73.

Richard K, Dziura B, Hornish A. Cell block preparation as a diagnostic technique complementary to fluid-based monolayer cervicovaginal specimens. Acta Cytol. 1999;43:69–73.

Solomon D, Nayar R, editors. The Bethesda system for reporting cervical cytology. 2nd ed. New York: Springer; 2004.

Wood MD, Horst JA, Bibbo M. Weeding atypical glandular cell look-alikes from the true atypical lesions in liquid-based Pap tests: a review. Diagn Cytopathol. 2007;35:12–7.

6 Hyperchromatic Crowded Groups (HCGs) in the Pap Test

Marilee Means and Walid E. Khalbuss

Contents

M. Means, PhD, SCT(ASCP) (✉)
School of Health Professions,
University of Kansas Medical Center,
3901 Rainbow Blvd., Mail Stop 4048,
Kansas City, KS 66160, USA
e-mail: mmeans@kumc.edu

W.E. Khalbuss, MD, PhD, FIAC
Director of Cytology and Cytopathology Fellowship Program,
University of Pittsburgh Medical Center Shadyside Hospital,
5150 Centre Avenue, 2, Suite 201,
Pittsburgh, PA 15232, USA
e-mail: khalbussw2@upmc.edu

6.1 Tables and Summary

Table 6.1 Benign or reactive causes of HCGs

Benign or reactive causes of HCGs	Description	Helpful differential features
Endometrial cells vs. CIS or EM neoplasia	3-D clusters, may occur in balls; small, dark degenerated nuclei, scant cytoplasm	Menstrual history; direct sampling (brush) may yield better preserved cells but with very uniform, small nuclei (≤ intermediate nuclei size) too uniform for neoplasia; degeneration in spontaneously shed cells vs. crisp pattern in squamous neoplasia
Atrophy vs. CIS or SCCA	Atrophic syncytial groups of parabasal or basal type cells with dark but smudgy chromatin, may have granular debris-laden background (benign diathesis)	Identifiable parabasal cells at the edges of HCGs in an atrophic background, lack of mitoses, smudgy vs. crisp chromatin pattern, no accompanying dysplasia
Endocervical cells/reactive endocervical cells vs. ECC neoplasia	Orderly architecture, but may become somewhat disordered if reactive due to nuclear enlargement and pleomorphism; upper endocervical canal may be more crowded and enlarged but have bland, round nuclei	Bland vs. irregular nuclear chromatin, lack of true feathering, less elongated nuclei than ECC neoplasia; lacks high N/C ratios, macronucleoli, dirty background of ECC adenocarcinoma
Tubal metaplasia vs. ECC neoplasia	Crowded cuboidal to columnar cells, enlarged nuclei, pleomorphism, high N/C ratios; clear small cytoplasmic vacuoles and terminal bars, cilia, or flat apical cell borders; distorted architecture due to variety of cell types	Cilia and terminal bars are classic differentiating features, but may be degenerated or absent; well-defined apical border; heterogeneity of cell types with intercalated nuclei being smaller, dark, and triangular or elongated with scant cytoplasm

(continued)

W.E. Khalbuss, M. Means (eds.), *Gynecological and Breast Cytopathology Board Review and Self-Assessment*,
DOI 10.1007/978-1-4614-7270-4_6, © Springer Science+Business Media New York 2013

Table 6.1 (continued)

Benign or reactive causes of HCGs	Description	Helpful differential features
Cone biopsy artifact vs. EM neoplasia	Shortens canal so LUS fragments may be sampled; EM cells may show reactive changes but are less crowded than in neoplasia, fine chromatin, rare or absent mitotic figures	Fewer abnormal cells than EM neoplasia, no watery diathesis, no macronucleoli or significant nuclear enlargement

Table 6.2 Neoplastic causes of HCGs

Neoplastic causes of HCGs	Description	Helpful differential features
Carcinoma in situ	Syncytial groups, hyperchromatic nuclei, chromatin may vary from finely granular to coarse and irregular, mitotic figures may occur, scant cytoplasm with increased N/C ratio, may have apparent glandular appearing features (acini or rosettes), large cell type may have more cytoplasm, blander nuclei, and less increase in N/C ratio than usual types; usually occurs with dysplasia, nucleoli rarely occur	Crisp well-preserved chromatin pattern, coexistence of dysplastic cells, high N/C ratio in syncytial groups of cells; note blander chromatin, more cytoplasm, and little or no mitotic activity in large cell type of CIS so as not to misinterpret it; note that some CIS (especially small cell type or in older women) does not have a coexisting dysplasia
Squamous cell carcinoma	May not shed more differentiated cells with identifiable squamous features such as keratinization; mitotic figures; nucleoli; irregular, coarse chromatin patterns; syncytial cell groups; increased N/C ratios; pleomorphism of cells; variations in size and shapes; tumor diathesis	Markedly irregular chromatin patterns which are well preserved, crisp, and hyperchromatic; increase in N/C ratio; nucleoli; mitotic figures; anisonucleosis; raisinoid nuclei with irregular nuclear borders; note that accompanying dysplasia may not be present
ECC adenocarcinoma in situ/ECC adenocarcinoma	Crowded, hyperchromatic groups with feathering, elongated oval nuclei, high N/C ratios, coarse irregular chromatin pattern, pseudopalisading, microacini	Feathering and crowding; coarse, irregular chromatin pattern; invasive adenocarcinoma will have macronucleoli and tumor diathesis
EM adenocarcinoma	Nuclei larger than intermediate cell nuclei, powdery chromatin, nucleoli, 3-D groups, watery tumor diathesis	Variation in nuclear size, nucleoli, enlargement of nuclei over intermediate cell nuclei
Metastatic carcinoma	Appearance depends on type of malignancy; background is usually clean except in case of direct extension of colonic adenocarcinoma	Patient history, clean background, foreign appearing malignant cells

6.2 Text-Based Questions 1–30

Q-1. What approximate percentage of cases with hyperchromatic groups (HCGs) is found to represent benign rather than neoplastic entities?
(a) <10 %
(b) 30 %
(c) 50 %
(d) 75 %
(e) >90 %

Q-2. Which of the following lesions is the LEAST serious neoplastic lesion which is likely to occur as hyperchromatic crowded groups?
(a) ASC-US
(b) LGSIL (slight dysplasia and/or HPV)
(c) HGSIL (moderate to severe dysplasia)
(d) HGSIL (CIS)
(e) Invasive squamous cell carcinoma

Q-3. The neoplastic entity which may occur as hyperchromatic crowded groups includes which of the following?
(a) Atrophy
(b) Tubal metaplasia
(c) Lower uterine segment
(d) Endometrial cells
(e) Adenocarcinoma in situ of the endocervix

Q-4. A feature of neoplastic HCGs which may be more easily identified on low power rather than high power is:
(a) Chaotic architecture
(b) Cytoplasmic vacuolization
(c) Cilia
(d) Fine chromatin
(e) Absence of mitotic figures

Q-5. A feature that is often but not always helpful in distinguishing CIS from benign causes of HCGs is that CIS usually has:
(a) Hypochromasia
(b) Nucleoli
(c) Coexisting dysplasia
(d) Cilia

Q-6. Microacinar-like formations may occur in CIS which is most likely to cause a diagnostic dilemma with which of the following?
(a) Dysplasia
(b) Invasive squamous cell carcinoma
(c) Repair
(d) Endocervical neoplasia

Q-7. A subtype of CIS which is the most likely to have bland chromatin, smooth nuclear membranes, more moderate nuclear/cytoplasmic ratios, and thus be misinterpreted as a benign HCG is:
(a) Small cell CIS
(b) Large cell CIS
(c) Keratinizing CIS
(d) Microinvasive CIS

Q-8. Which of the features of severe atrophy, along with HCGs, is most likely to cause a misinterpretation as invasive carcinoma?
(a) Degenerated cells, fresh or old blood, inflammation, and granular precipitate
(b) Nucleoli
(c) Cytoplasmic streaming
(d) Smudgy chromatin

Q-9. Which group of women is the likeliest to have CIS without evidence of a coexisting dysplasia?
(a) Ages 15–25
(b) Ages 30–45
(c) Postmenopausal women
(d) Pregnant women

Q-10. In the setting of atrophy, the presence of HCGs may interfere with a correct interpretation. Observing the periphery of a group and noting which of the following features would favor the diagnosis of benign atrophy?
(a) Coarse chromatin
(b) Mitotic figures
(c) Crisp distinct chromatin
(d) Chaotic arrangement
(e) Matured parabasal cells

Q-11. Features of endocervical neoplasia which may cause a diagnostic dilemma with benign HCGs include which of the following?
(a) Cilia
(b) Bland, finely granular chromatin
(c) Keratinization
(d) Enlarged elongated nuclei

Q-12. Differentiating benign lower uterine segment (LUS) cells obtained by cytobrush from neoplastic HGCs can best be accomplished by noting which of the following features in LUS?
(a) Coarse chromatin
(b) Uniformity of cell size and shape
(c) Tumor diathesis
(d) Macronucleoli

Q-13. A procedure which may cause the inadvertent sampling of the endometrial cavity and confusion with HCGs is:
(a) Colposcopy
(b) Cervical punch biopsy
(c) Cone biopsy
(d) Acetic acid solution application

Q-14. Important features to note in neoplastic endometrial cell clusters to help differentiate them from benign HCGs include which of the following?
(a) Nuclei larger than intermediate cell nuclei and nucleoli
(b) Bloody, very necrotic diathesis, and uniformity of cell sizes
(c) Picket fence arrangements and nucleoli
(d) 3-D arrangements and nuclei smaller than an intermediate cell nucleus

Q-15. Differentiating tubal metaplasia from neoplastic HCGs may be difficult, but the best feature to confirm tubal metaplasia is the presence of which of the following cellular features?
(a) Enlarged nuclei
(b) Increased N/C ratios
(c) Moderate hyperchromasia
(d) Mitotic figures
(e) Cilia

Q-16. A rare but possible source of neoplastic HCGs in the gynecologic smear is:
(a) Atrophy
(b) Endometrial cells
(c) Endocervical cells
(d) Carcinoma in situ
(e) Metastatic carcinoma

Q-17. Which type of error are HCGs most often responsible for?
(a) Screening error (not seeing the cells)
(b) Interpretive error (incorrectly classifying the cells)
(c) Increase in ASC-US to SIL ratio above suggested levels
(d) Decrease in ASC-US to SIL ratio below suggested levels

Q-18. In the setting of atrophy, the most likely origin of benign hyperchromatic crowded groups is from:
(a) CIS
(b) Parakeratosis
(c) Air-drying artifact
(d) Syncytial groups of parabasal or basal cells

Q-19. A feature of some CIS cases having HCGs which may lead to an incorrect diagnosis of reactive endocervical cells is:
(a) Rosette-like or microacinar structures
(b) Three-dimensional cell balls
(c) Keratinization
(d) Pleomorphic nuclei

Q-20. Although classic CIS is described as having high N/C ratios, scant cytoplasm, and coarse chromatin and occurring in syncytial groups, it should not be misinterpreted as benign HCGs because CIS may also sometimes occur as:
(a) Three-dimensional balls
(b) Cells with rather bland chromatin, smooth nuclear outlines, and more abundant cytoplasm
(c) Sheets of cells with nucleoli and cytoplasmic streaming
(d) Single cells with pleomorphism, keratinization, and nucleoli

Q-21. Atrophic cells may sometimes present as HCGs when they appear as:
(a) Syncytial-like groups of pleomorphic cells with high N/C ratios and hyperchromatic nuclei
(b) Single scattered cells with bland nuclei
(c) Metaplastic cells with sharp cytoplasmic borders
(d) Degenerated cells with bland chromatin

Q-22. A feature which is unlikely to be found in atrophic groups but which should suggest neoplasia is:
(a) Degenerated chromatin
(b) Mitotic figures
(c) Cytoplasmic streaming
(d) Increased nuclear/cytoplasmic ratio

Q-23. For patients with severe atrophy and questionable HCGs, one possible solution to resolving the problem would be to:
(a) Perform an HMB-45 stain on the remaining vial contents
(b) Perform a reticulin stain on the remaining vial contents
(c) Perform a S-100 stain on the remaining vial contents
(d) Request the clinician to perform an estrogen test and repeat the Pap

Q-24. HCGs due to metastatic carcinoma can usually be recognized using both clinical history and:
(a) The presence of many syncytial groups in a dirty background
(b) The absence of mitotic figures

(c) The presence of a clean background and relatively few groups
(d) The presence of orderly architecture

Q-25. Most Pap litigation usually involves interpretation errors concerning which of the following?
(a) Severe atrophy
(b) Tubal metaplasia
(c) LGSIL
(d) CIS
(e) Endometriosis

Q-26. The most reliable manner in which litigation slides can be reviewed and a determination made as to the appropriateness of the original diagnosis is:
(a) Obtain an expert witness, give them the previous slides and reports, and have them render a diagnosis
(b) Have a round table of experts examine the slide and the previous reports and come to a consensus
(c) Have an expert witness review the slide without previous knowledge of the diagnosis and make an interpretation
(d) Have an expert witness review the previous slides and the biopsy and render an opinion as to the diagnosis
(e) Have multiple-slide blinded rescreening in which ten cytotechnologists blindly review the slide within their daily workload of slides. Statistically analyze the results to determine the appropriateness of the original diagnosis.

Q-27. Statistical analysis of the likelihood of a reasonably prudent practitioner calling an "abnormal" slide "normal" uses a value of an "irreducible" false-negative rate of which of the following?
(a) 0.001 %
(b) 0.01 %
(c) 1 %
(d) 5 %
(e) 10 %

Q-28. Retrospective analysis of litigated gynecologic cases shows that the LEAST likely diagnostic category brought to litigation from those listed below is:
(a) LGSIL
(b) HGSIL
(c) Endocervical AIS
(d) Atypical repair vs. carcinoma
(e) Endocervical adenocarcinoma

Q-29. One of the causes for the increase in the litigation of Pap test "errors" is most probably:
(a) The use of multiple experts to review contested slides
(b) The use of the multiple-slide blinded rescreening to review contested slides
(c) The use of the Bethesda System which reduces the traditional number of diagnostic categories
(d) The public's expectation of zero errors in Pap diagnosis

Q-30. One reasonable method to reduce possible risk of litigation of Pap diagnoses is to:
(a) Make follow-up recommendations, especially for glandular lesions
(b) Reduce the use of ASC-H as it is confusing to the clinicians
(c) Have the clinician do colposcopy on all HCGs
(d) Have all cases screened twice using a manual method

6.3 Image-Based Questions 31–60

Fig. 6.31

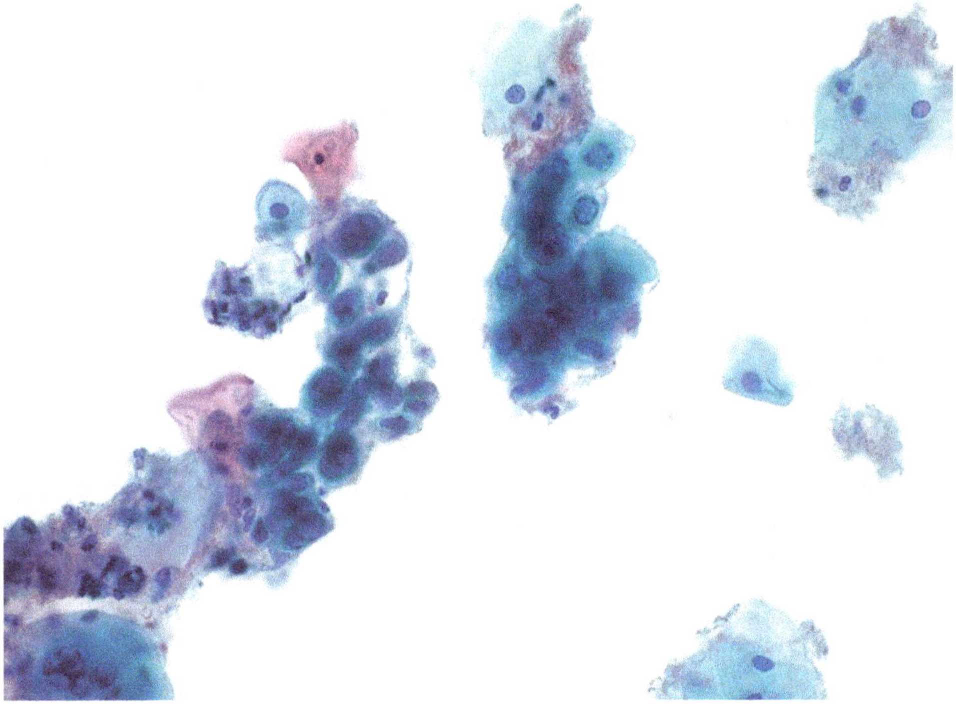

Q-31. These images (right and left, ThinPrep, high power) of hyperchromatic crowded groups (HCGs) are displaying evidence of a benign condition, rather than features of neoplastic HCGs. Of the features listed below, which is evident in these cells and is a general feature of benignity?

(a) Hyperchromasia
(b) Crowding
(c) Multinucleation
(d) Smudgy chromatin

Fig. 6.32

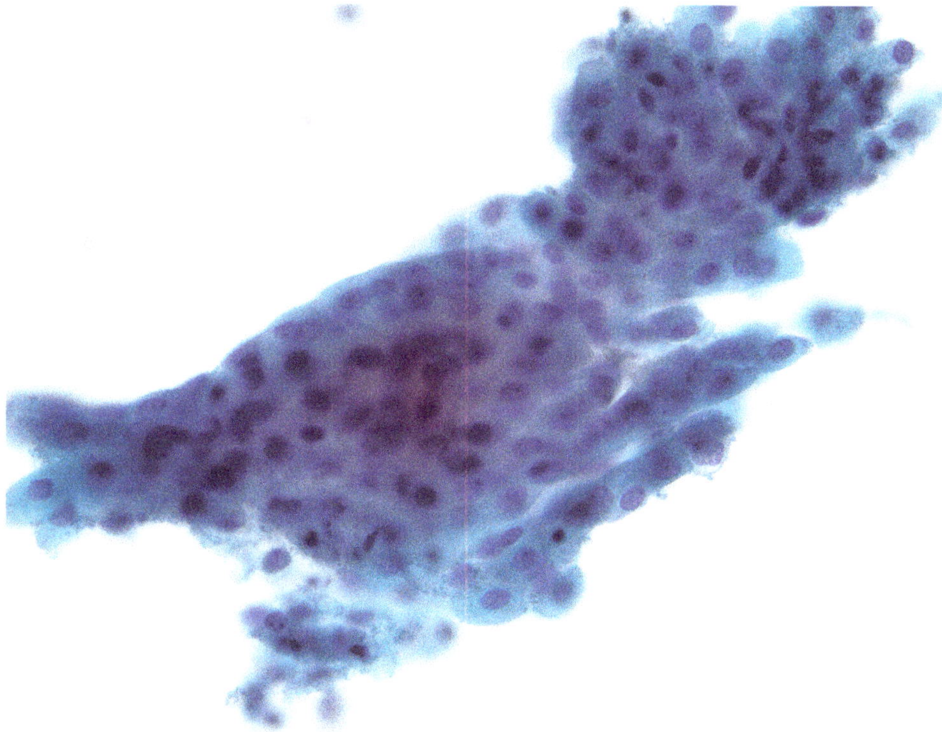

Q-32. This image is from the ThinPrep of a 65-year-old postmenopausal woman (TP, high power). Which type of cells is identified at the edge of the group that provides the greatest assistance in making the correct diagnosis?

(a) Polymorphonuclear leukocytes
(b) Maturing parabasal cells
(c) Syncytia of CIS
(d) Multinucleated histiocyte

Fig. 6.33

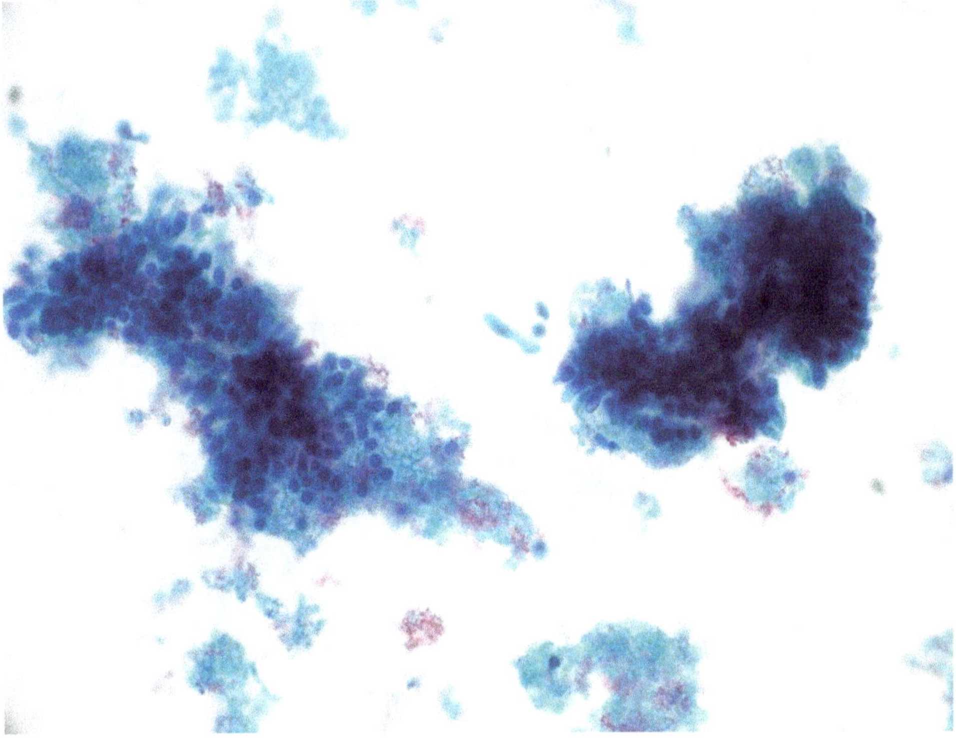

Q-33. These groups of HCGs are most consistent with an interpretation of:
(a) CIS
(b) AGUS, favor endometrial origin
(c) Normal endocervical cells
(d) Endocervical adenocarcinoma

Fig. 6.34

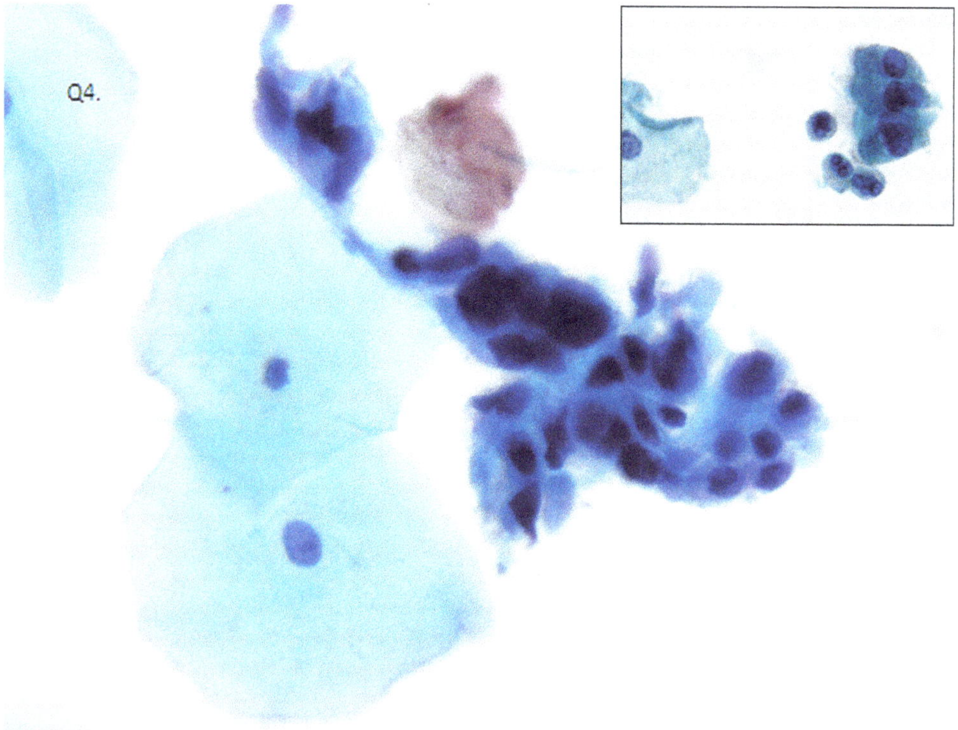

Q-34. These hyperchromatic groups show features of tubal metaplasia, sometimes encountered from specimens from the upper endocervical canal (ThinPrep, high power; inset, ThinPrep, low power). The best feature to assist in calling these cells benign is:

(a) Cilia
(b) Crowding
(c) Feathering of nuclei
(d) Mitotic figures

Fig. 6.35

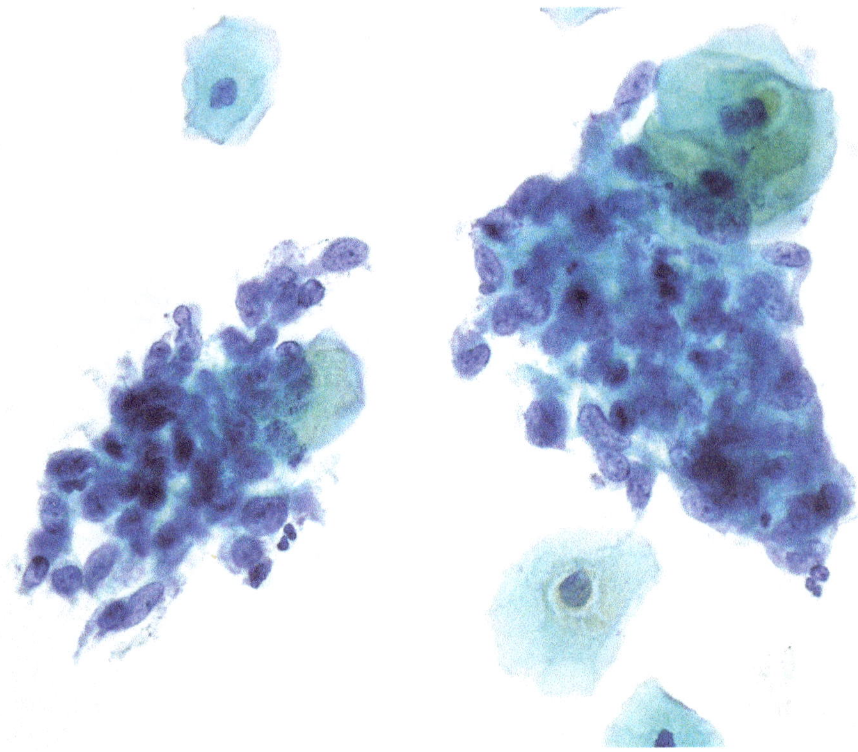

Q-35. These cells were derived from a 29-year-old female, day 10. They are the most consistent with:
(a) CIS
(b) LGSIL
(c) Repair
(d) Endometrial cells

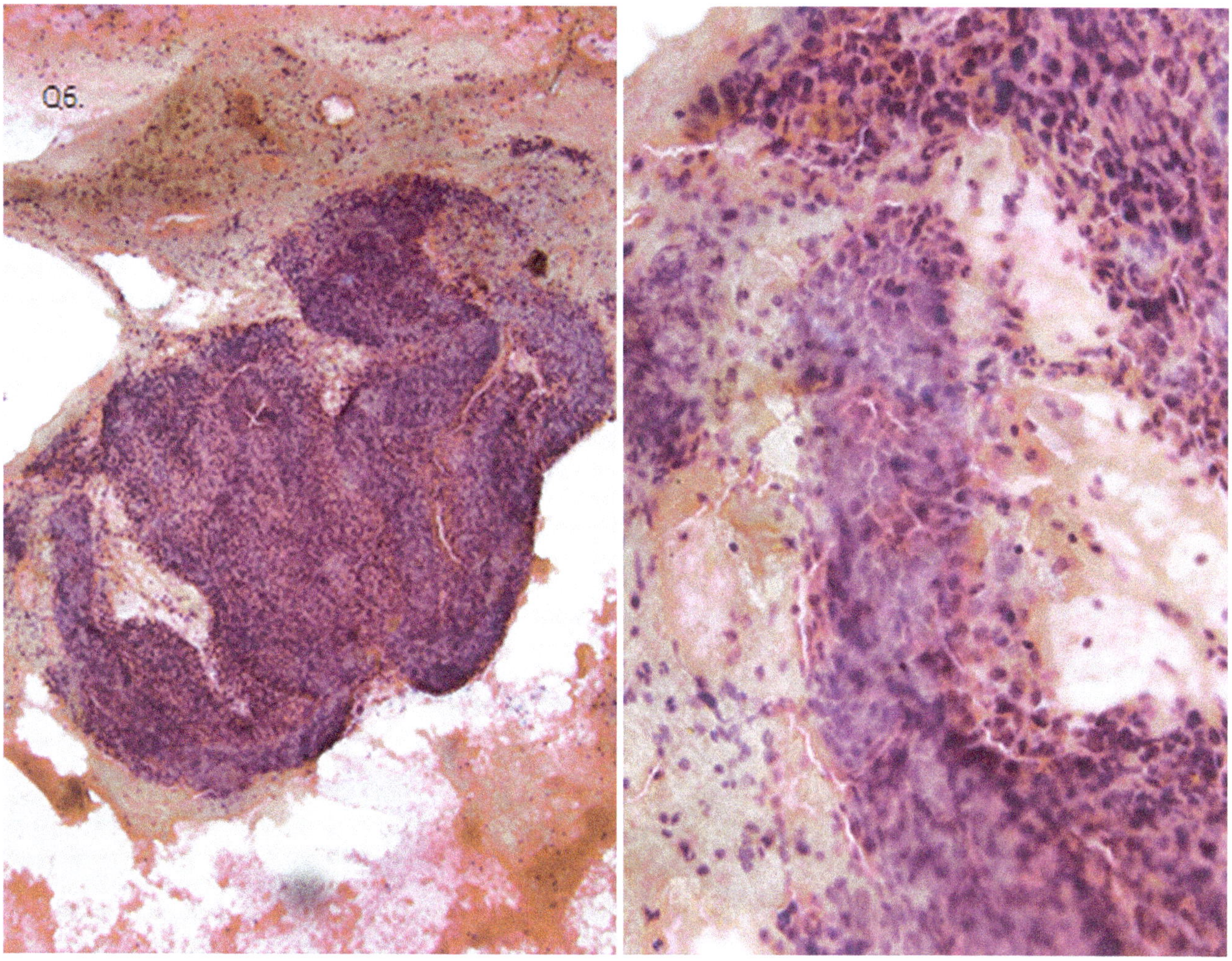

Fig. 6.36

Q-36. In this Pap from a 47-year-old female, hyperchromatic crowded groups (right and left, SurePath, medium and high power) such as these that often occur in small tubular microbiopsies are best interpreted as:

(a) Atrophy
(b) Lower uterine segment
(c) Endocervical adenocarcinoma
(d) Endometrial cells

Fig. 6.37

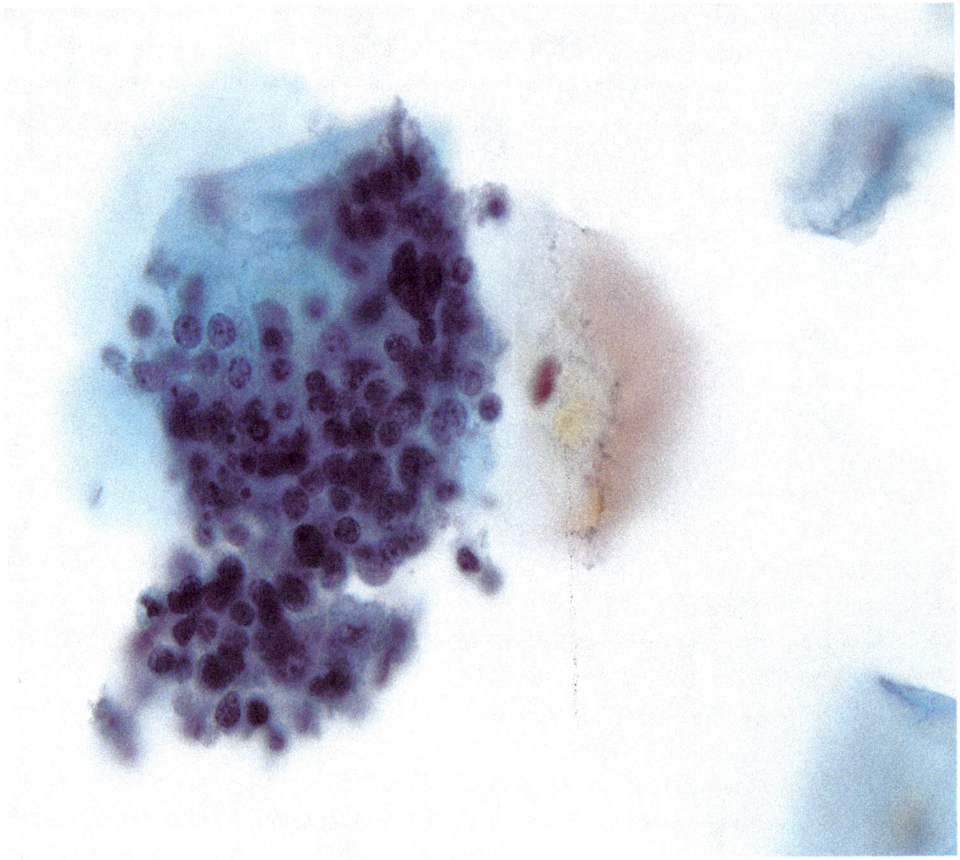

Q-37. This image of a loose cluster of small, round cells is most consistent with an interpretation of:
(a) Small cell CIS
(b) Acute inflammation
(c) LGSIL
(d) Chronic follicular cervicitis

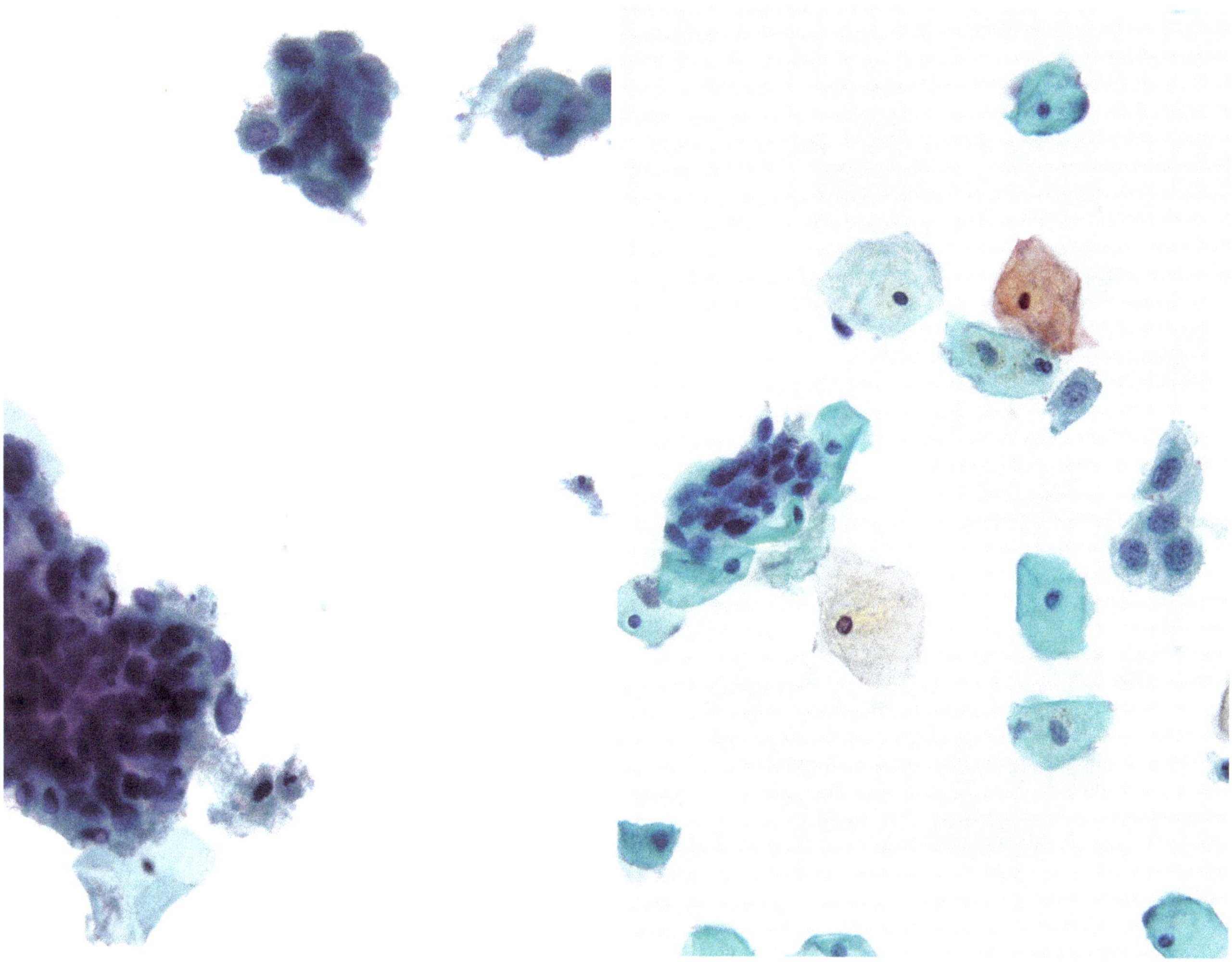

Fig. 6.38

Q-38. (Left and right, low power, ThinPrep) These images of hyperchromatic crowded groups show cells which have coarse chromatin, irregular architecture, and high numbers of abnormal cells. A very useful accompanying feature elsewhere on the slide which may assist in recognizing these cells as neoplastic is:

(a) Regularity of the nuclei
(b) Dysplastic cells
(c) Feathering of the nuclei
(d) Three-dimensional groups

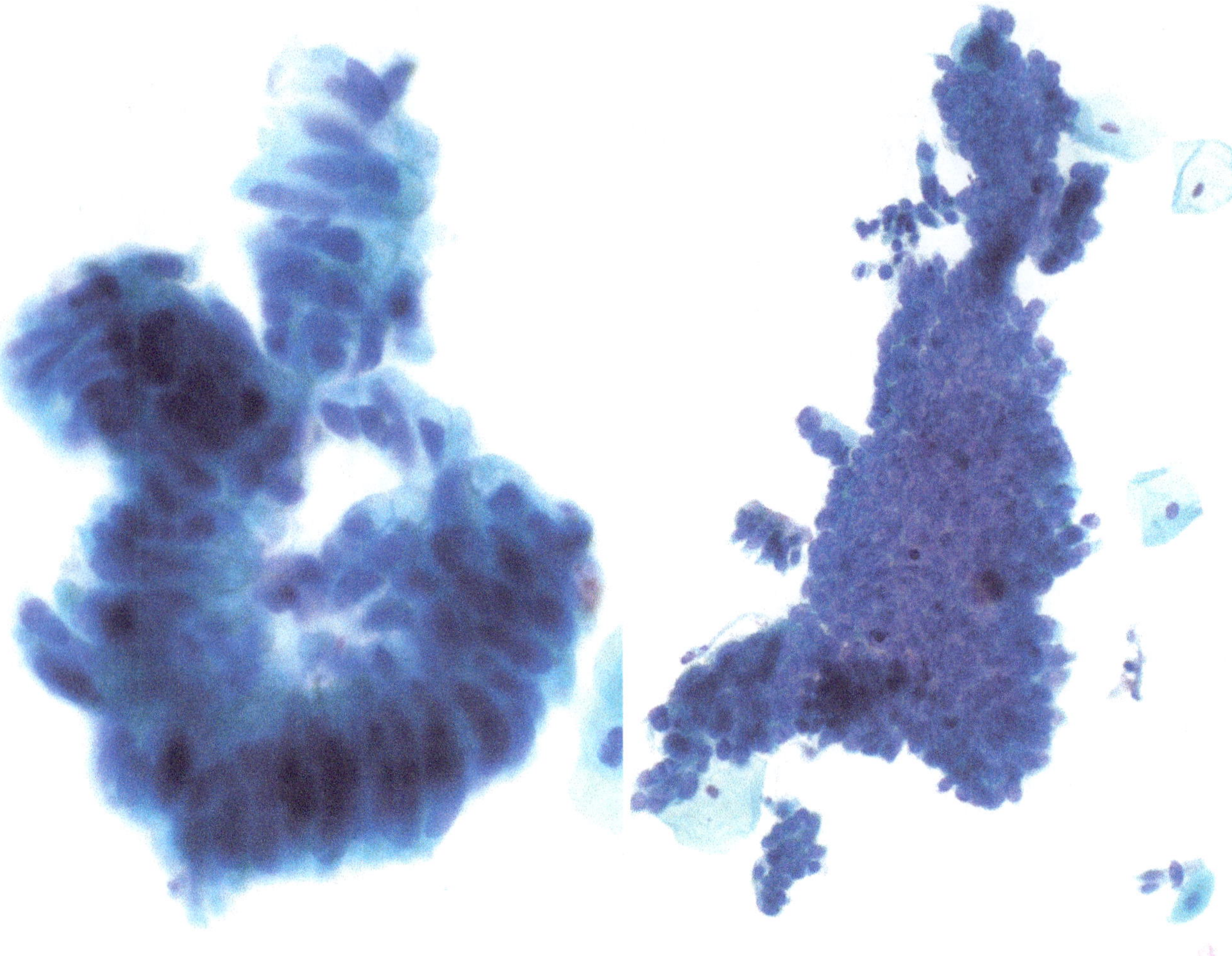

Fig. 6.39

Q-39. Important features useful in classifying this neoplastic HCG lesion (left, SP, high power; right SP, low power) include which of the following?

(a) Coexisting dysplasia
(b) Three-dimensional clusters of cells
(c) Cilia
(d) Hyperchromasia, enlargement, and pseudostratification

Fig. 6.40

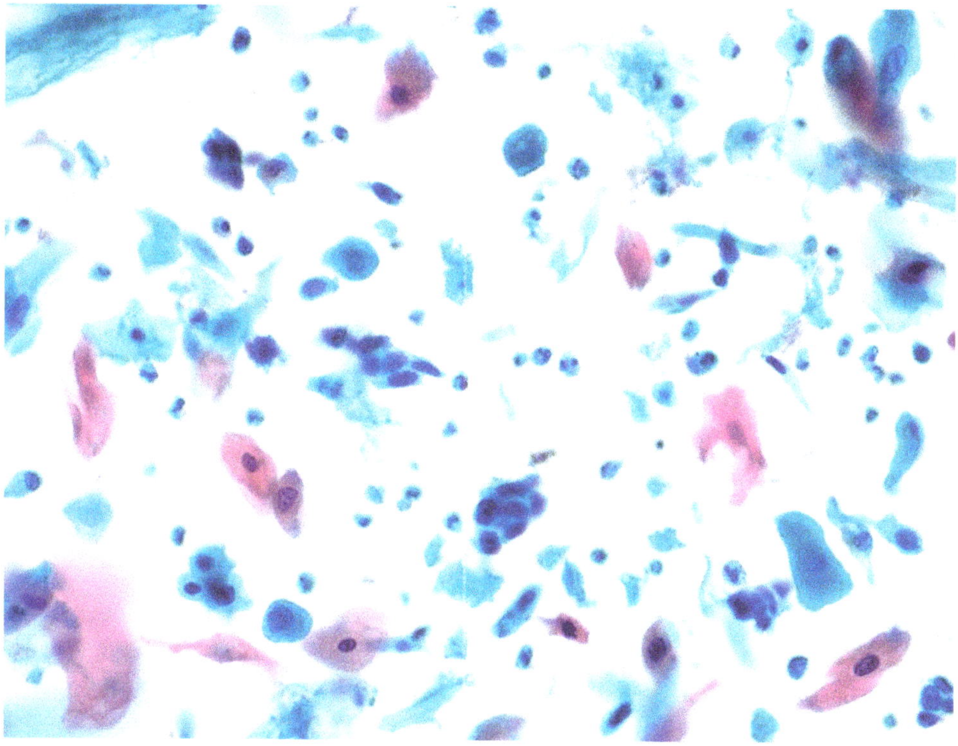

Q-40. Features helpful in correctly interpreting HCGs such as this image include hyperchromasia, irregular and enlarged nuclei, abnormal mitoses, occasional nucleoli, and clinging tumor diathesis (SurePath, low power). The most likely interpretation is which of the following?

(a) Atrophy
(b) Repair
(c) Squamous cell carcinoma
(d) Endometrial adenocarcinoma

Fig. 6.41

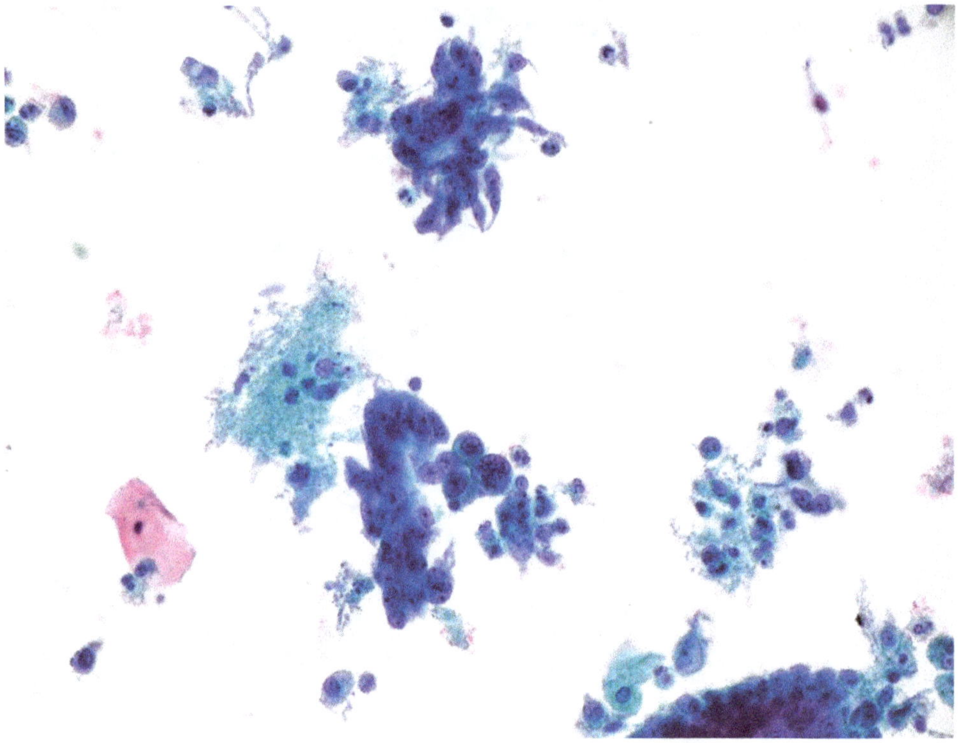

Q-41. Finding high numbers of two-dimensional cell groups with nucleoli, variation in nuclear size, numerous nucleoli, and dark, irregular chromatin patterns such as the cells seen here (ThinPrep, low power) would most likely lead to an interpretation of:

(a) Endometrial adenocarcinoma
(b) Endocervical adenocarcinoma
(c) CIS
(d) Repair

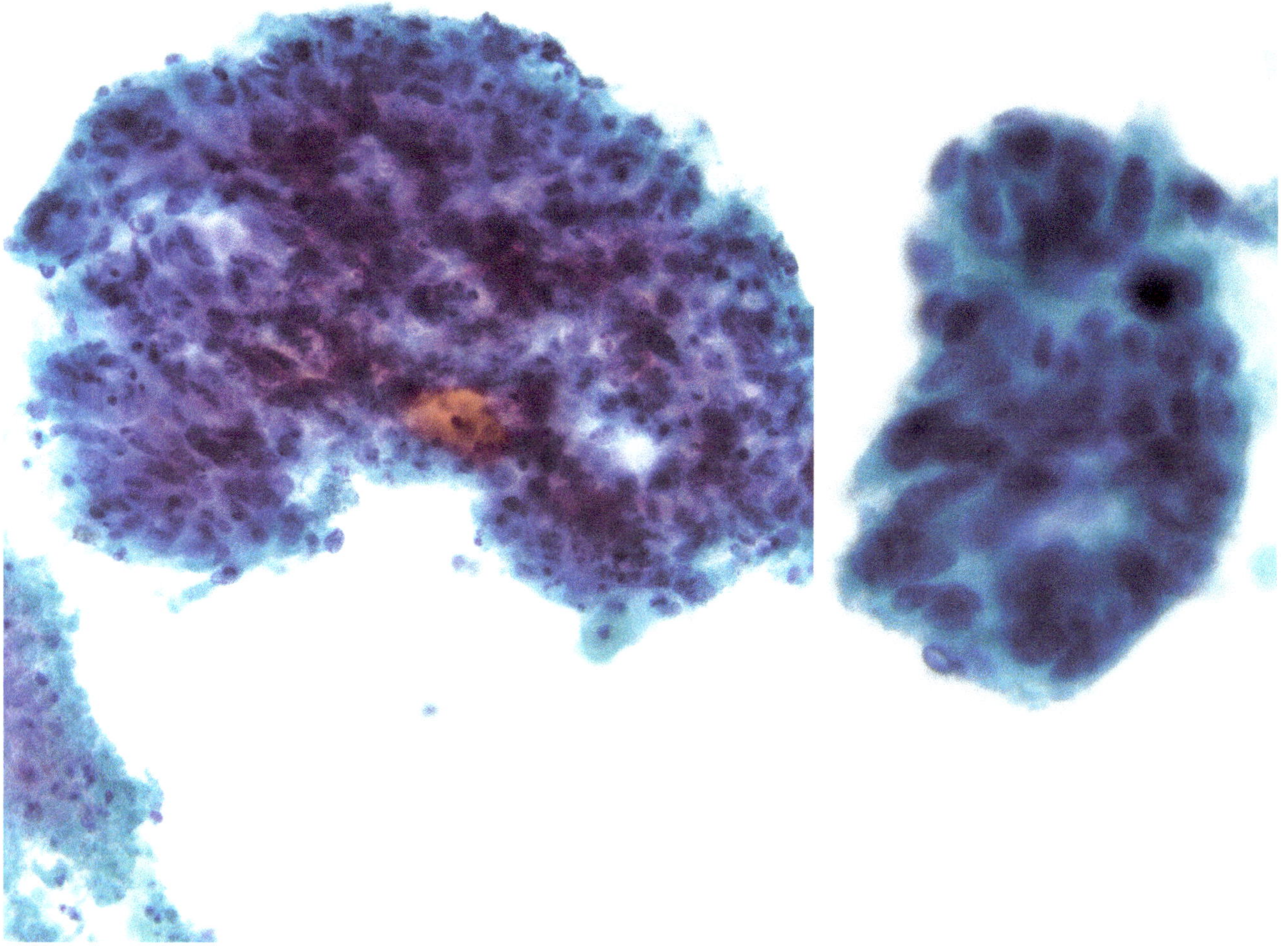

Fig. 6.42

Q-42. The presence of cells such as these (ThinPrep, left, high power; right, low power) in a dirty background might be caused by an adenocarcinoma of the endocervix or less often by which of the following look-alikes?

(a) Ovarian adenocarcinoma
(b) Endometrial adenocarcinoma
(c) Rectal adenocarcinoma
(d) Leukemia

Fig. 6.43

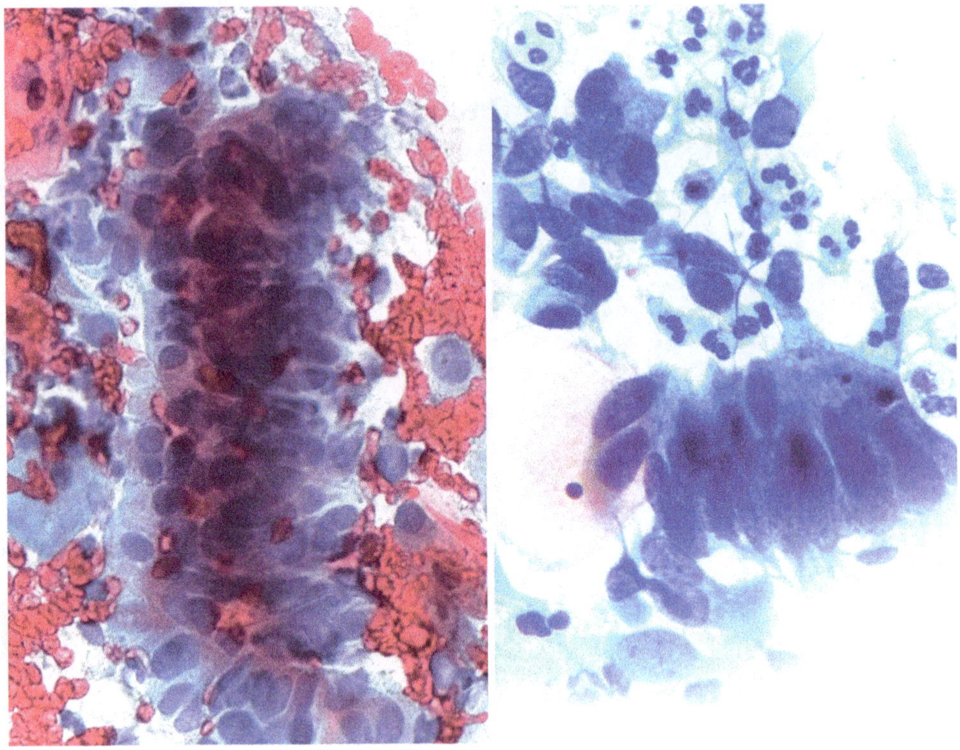

Q-43. A hyperchromatic cell group such as this (ThinPrep, high power) is most likely to correlate with a diagnosis of:

(a) Normal endocervical cells
(b) Endocervical adenocarcinoma in situ
(c) Atrophy
(d) Endometrial adenocarcinoma

Fig. 6.44

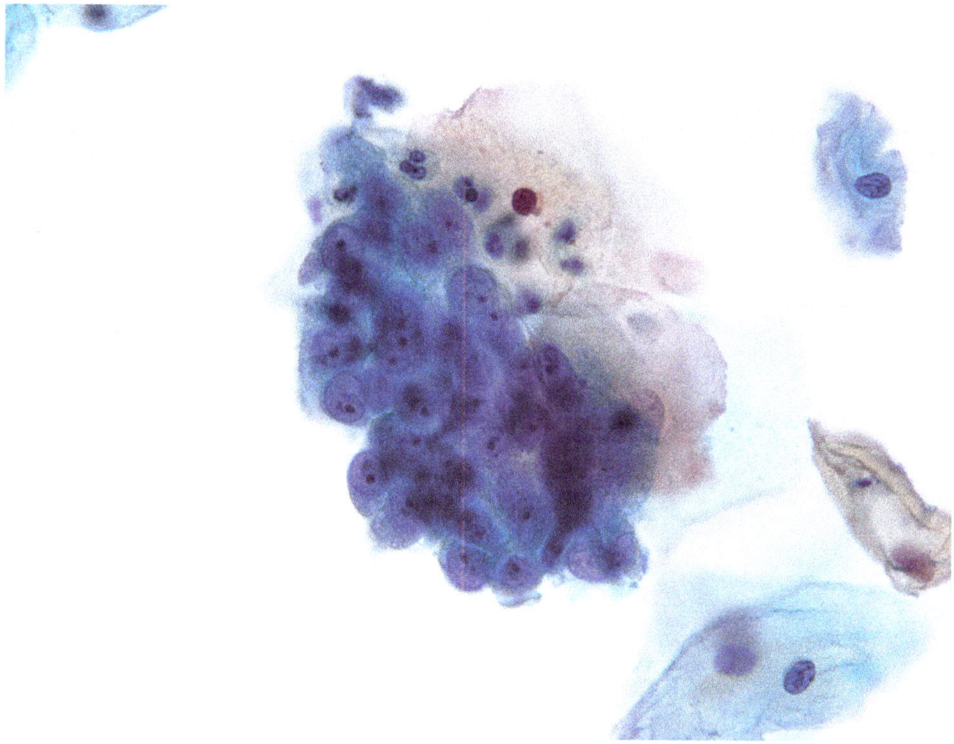

Q-44. (ThinPrep, high power) This HCG can be distinguished from a neoplastic hyperchromatic group of cells by noting the nuclei which appear:

(a) Finely granular with smooth nuclear borders
(b) Coarsely granular with pleomorphism
(c) In a feathering pattern
(d) Loosely cohesive

Fig. 6.45

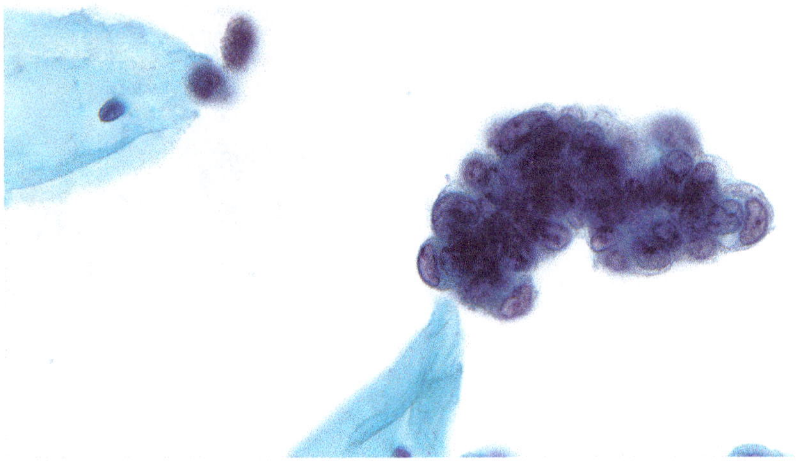

Q-45. The most likely source for these small cells in a HCG (32-year-old female, ThinPrep, high power) is:
(a) Endocervical AIS
(b) Endocervical adenocarcinoma
(c) Endometrial cells
(d) Endometrial adenocarcinoma

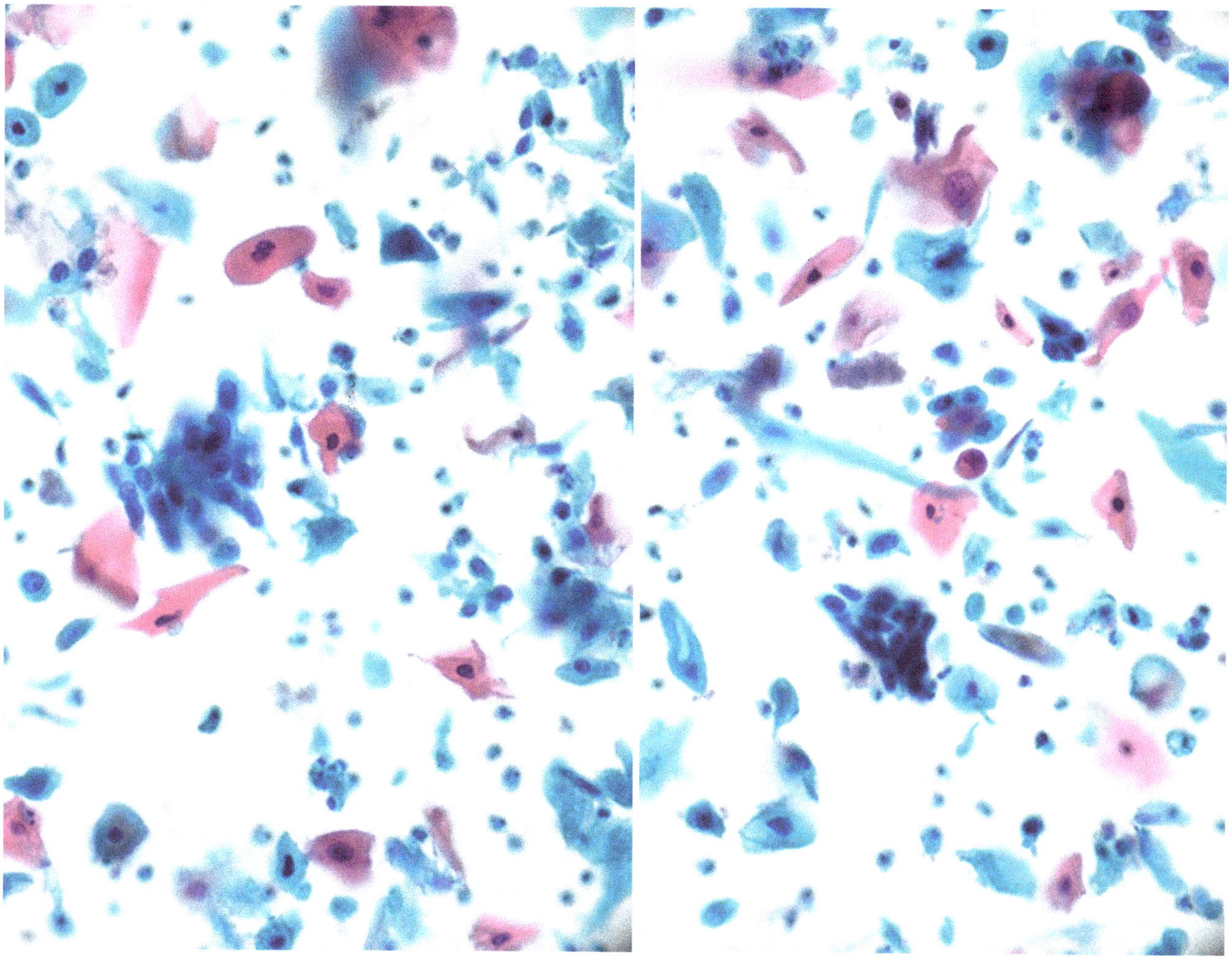

Fig. 6.46

Q-46. (Right and left; SurePath, low power) In this sample from a 59-year-old woman, cells such as these were found in a background of single hyperchromatic small nuclei, cytoplasmic debris, and pleomorphic nuclei. The most likely diagnosis for this case is:

(a) LGSIL
(b) Endometrial adenocarcinoma
(c) Endocervical adenocarcinoma
(d) Squamous cell carcinoma

Fig. 6.47

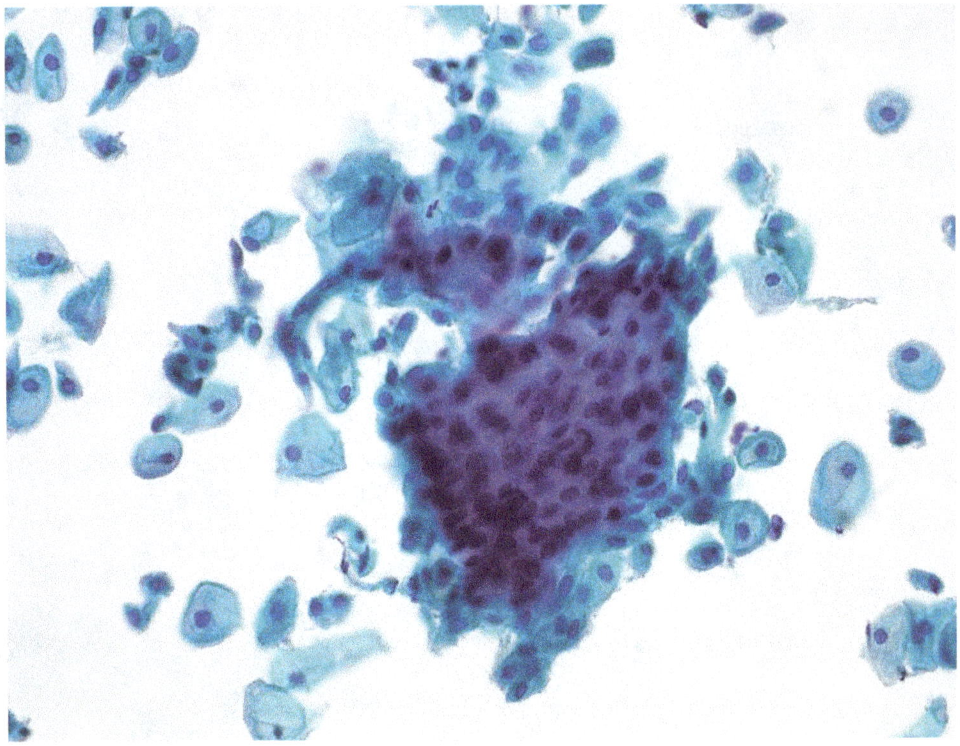

Q-47. Cells such as these were found in the TP sample (low power) from a 61-year-old woman. The most useful clue to their classification as a benign change encountered in atrophy is:
(a) High N/C ratio
(b) Enlarged nuclei
(c) Degenerated chromatin
(d) Mitotic figures

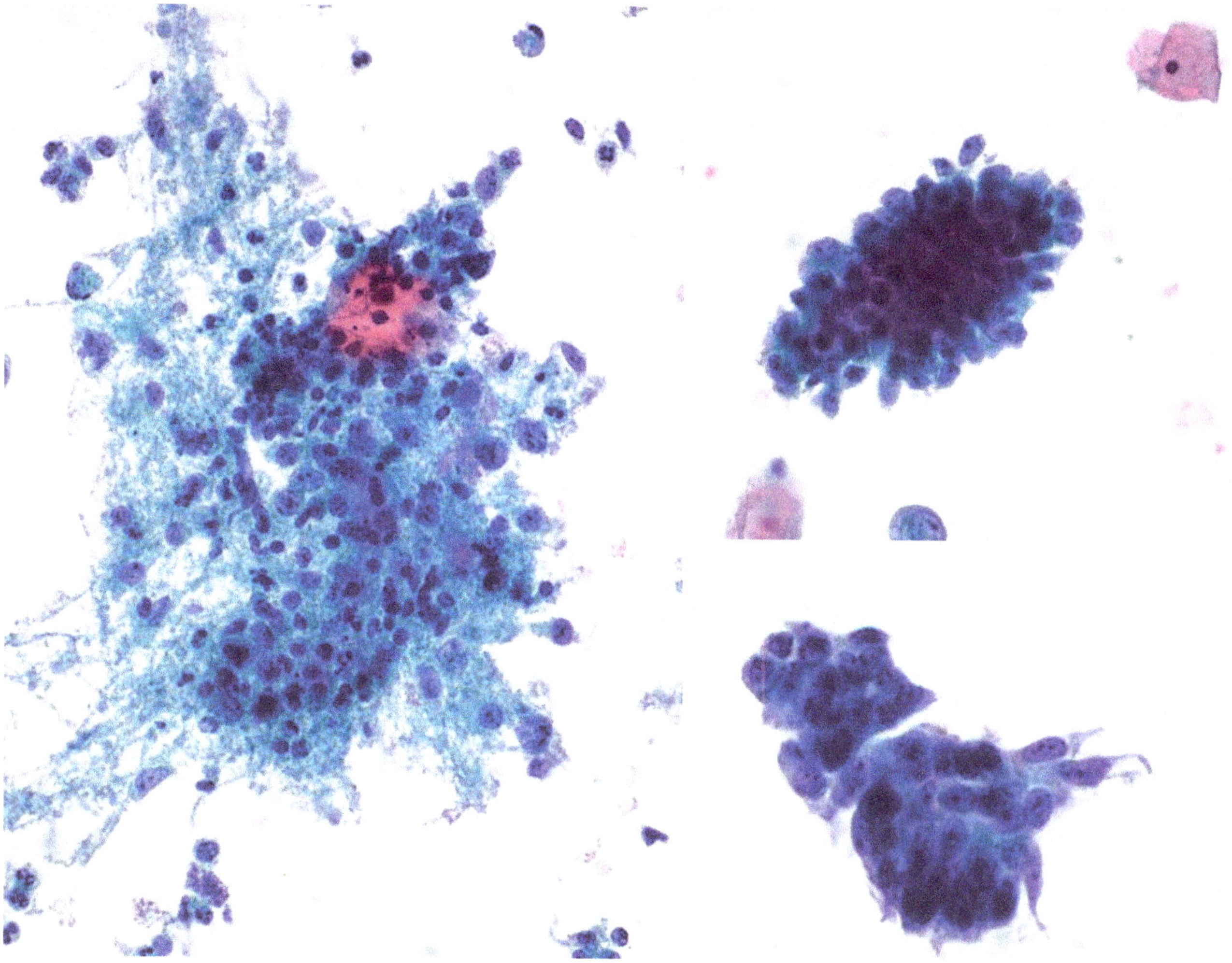

Fig. 6.48

Q-48. These images are from the ThinPrep (right and left, low power) of a 48-year-old woman. Many hyperchromatic crowded groups and a background as noted in these images were found. The most likely interpretation is:

(a) Atrophy
(b) LGSIL
(c) HGSIL
(d) Endocervical adenocarcinoma
(e) Endometrial adenocarcinoma

Fig. 6.49

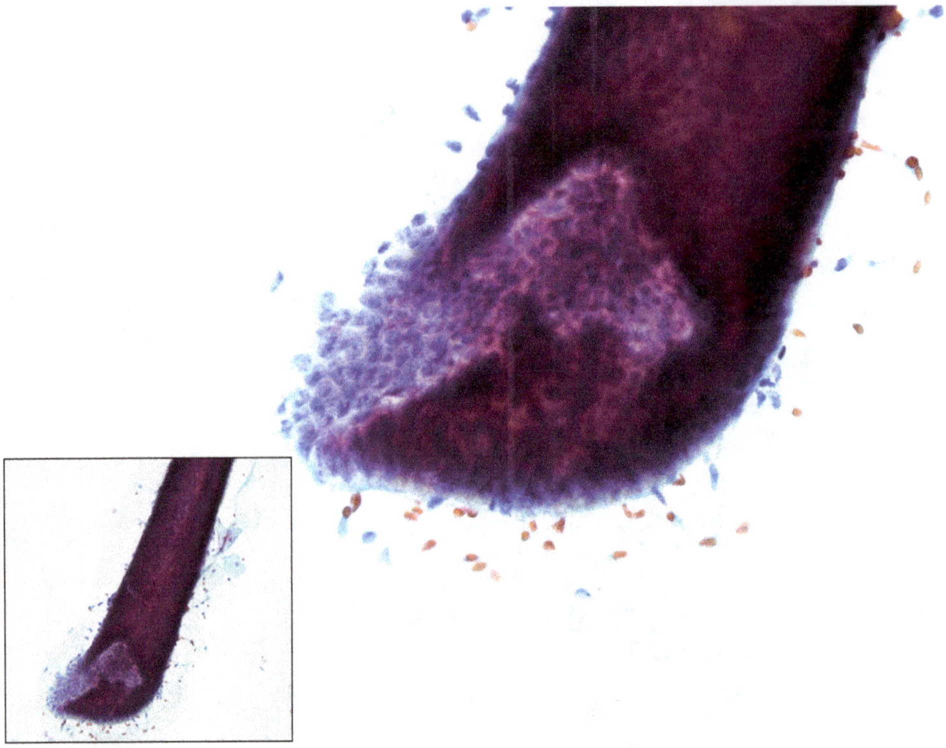

Q-49. Structures such as this (ThinPrep, left inset, low power; right, high power) may display hyperchromasia but can be differentiated from neoplastic HCGs due to their uniformity in cell size, shape, and nuclear outlines, as well as their:

(a) Tubular-shaped architecture
(b) Nucleoli
(c) Irregularity of chromatin
(d) Cohesion

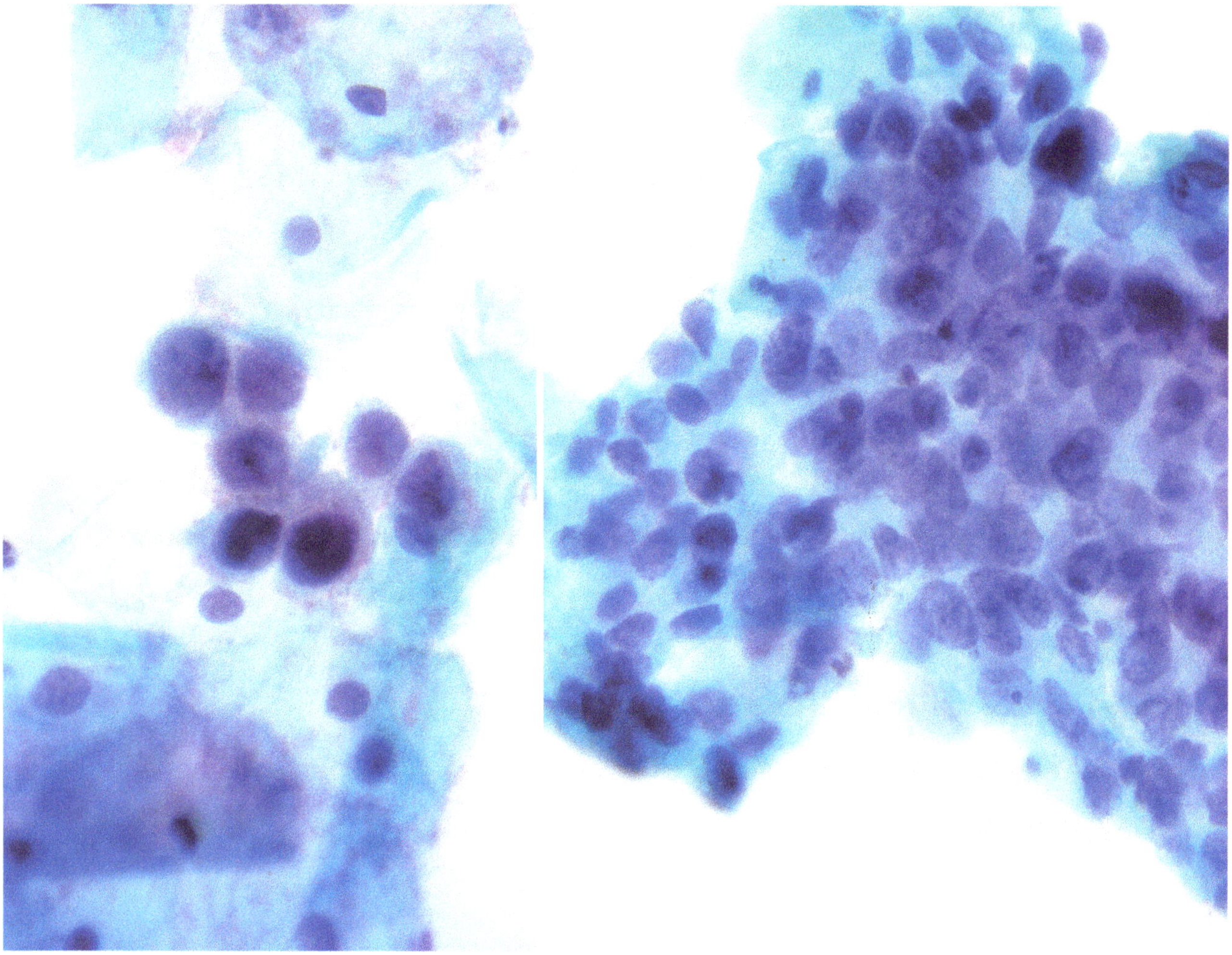

Fig. 6.50

Q-50. This slide illustrates the fact that some HCGs may represent CIS (ThinPrep, left, high power; right, low power), the finding of which of the following may be the most helpful in reaching the correct diagnosis in cases such as these?

(a) Three-dimensional groups
(b) Nucleoli
(c) Variation in nuclear features
(d) Cytoplasmic streaming

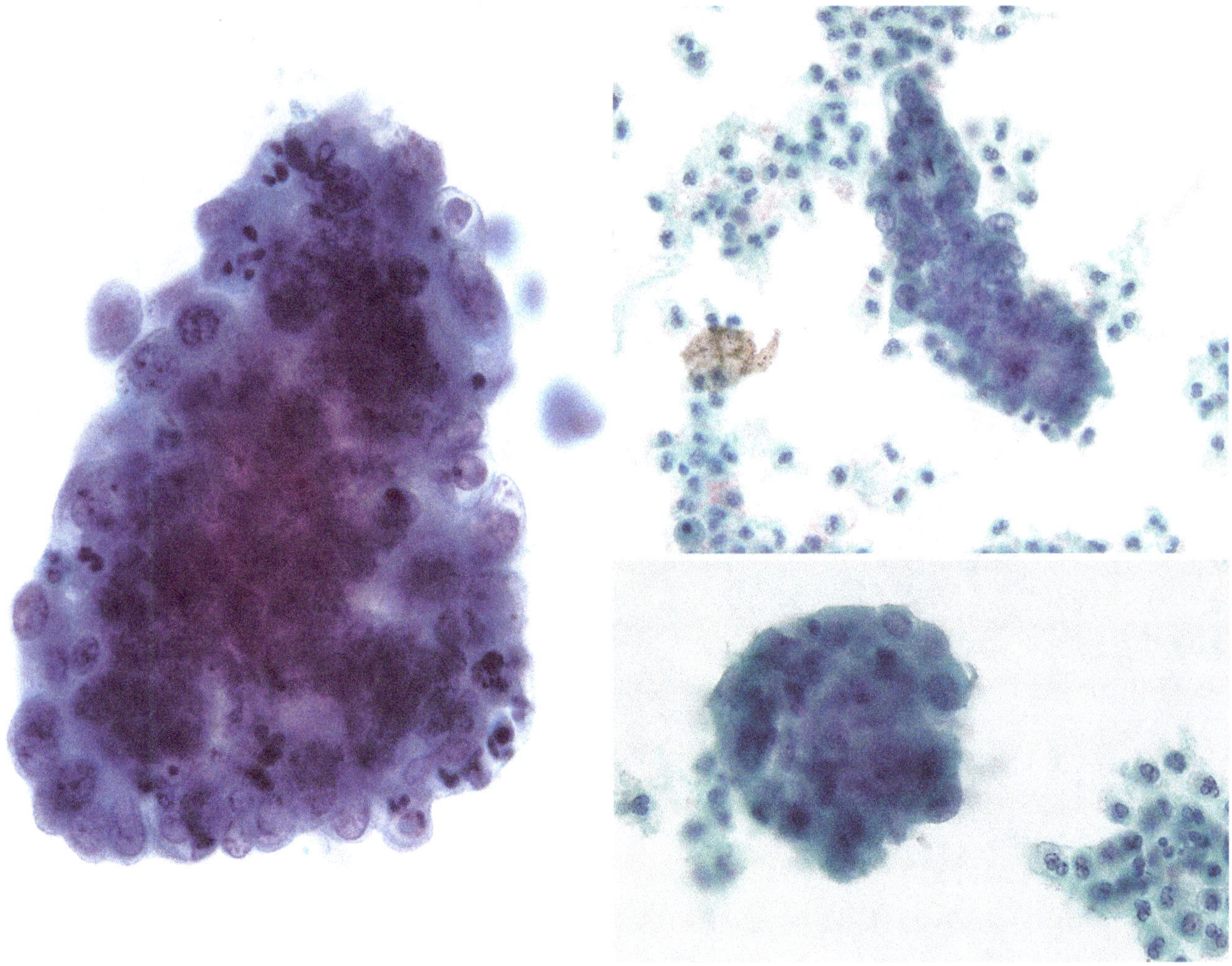

Fig. 6.51

Q-51. Endometrial adenocarcinoma, as seen in this ThinPrep slide (left, high power; right upper and lower, low power) from a 68-year-old woman, is one possible source of neoplastic HCGs. Criteria which may greatly assist in this interpretation include three-dimensional cell groups, nucleoli, and which of the following?

(a) Enlargement of the nuclei beyond the size of an intermediate cell nucleus
(b) Coarse, clumpy chromatin
(c) Abundant, streaming cytoplasm
(d) Evidence of keratinization

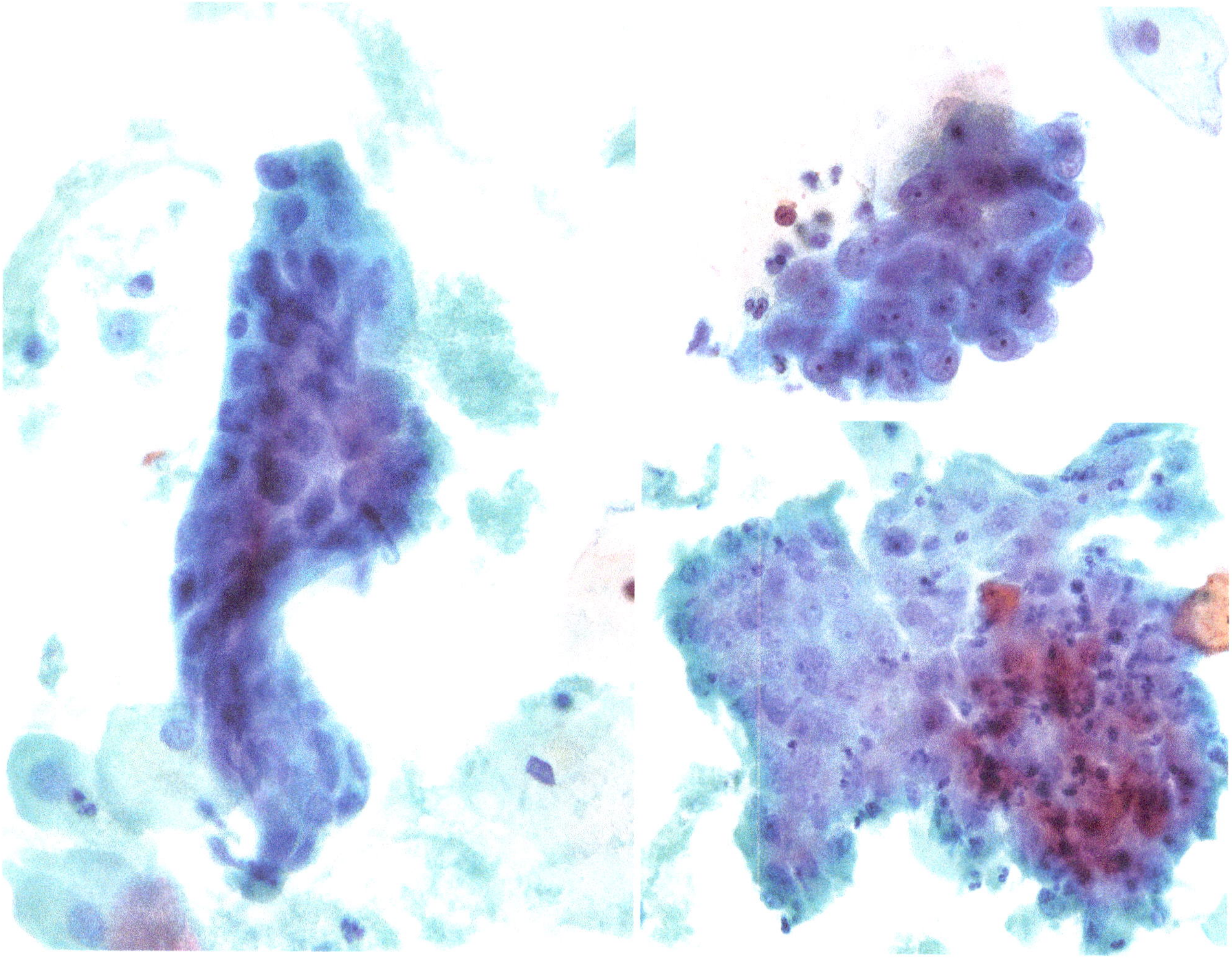

Fig. 6.52

Q-52. (SurePath, left, high power; right, upper and lower, low power) Noting the small nucleoli, the finely granular chromatin, and the "squared off" appearance of many of the ends of the cells in these groups, the best interpretation is that they originate in the _______ and they are _________.

(a) Endometrium; adenocarcinoma
(b) Endocervix; reactive
(c) Ovary; adenocarcinoma
(d) Ectocervix; HGSIL

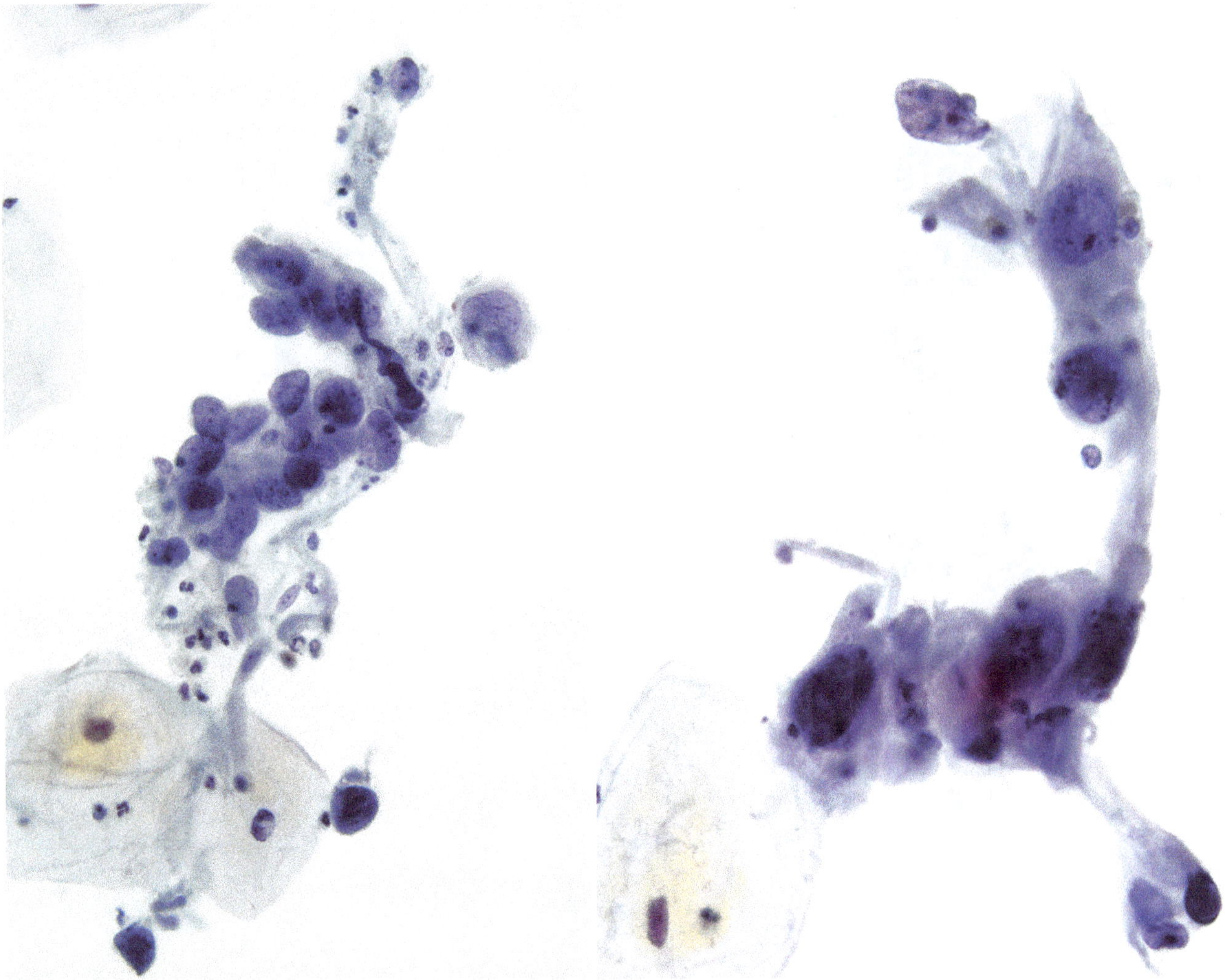

Fig. 6.53

Q-53. This patient's slide revealed several clusters of cells such as these in a clean background. If a previous ECC and endometrial biopsy were negative, what is the most likely source for these cells, given their appearance (right and left, ThinPrep, high power)?

(a) Metastatic small cell carcinoma of the lung
(b) Serous cystadenocarcinoma of the ovary
(c) Metastatic colorectal adenocarcinoma
(d) Carcinoid tumor of the GI system

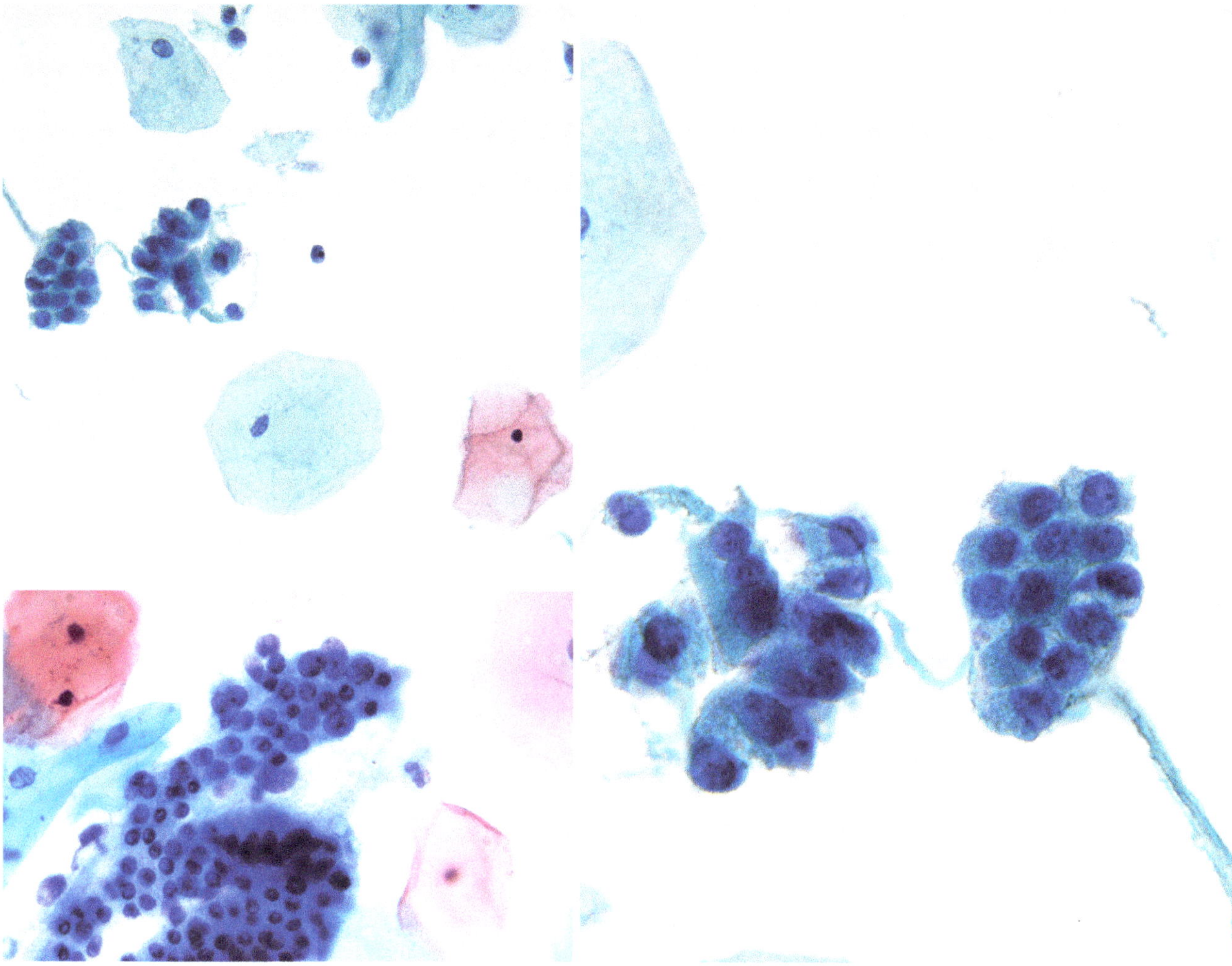

Fig. 6.54

Q-54. Cells such as these may often occur in HCGs (left, upper and lower, ThinPrep, low power; right, ThinPrep, high power). The most likely interpretation of these cells is:

(a) Endocervical adenocarcinoma
(b) Endocervical AIS
(c) Squamous metaplasia in atrophy
(d) Tubal metaplasia

Fig. 6.55

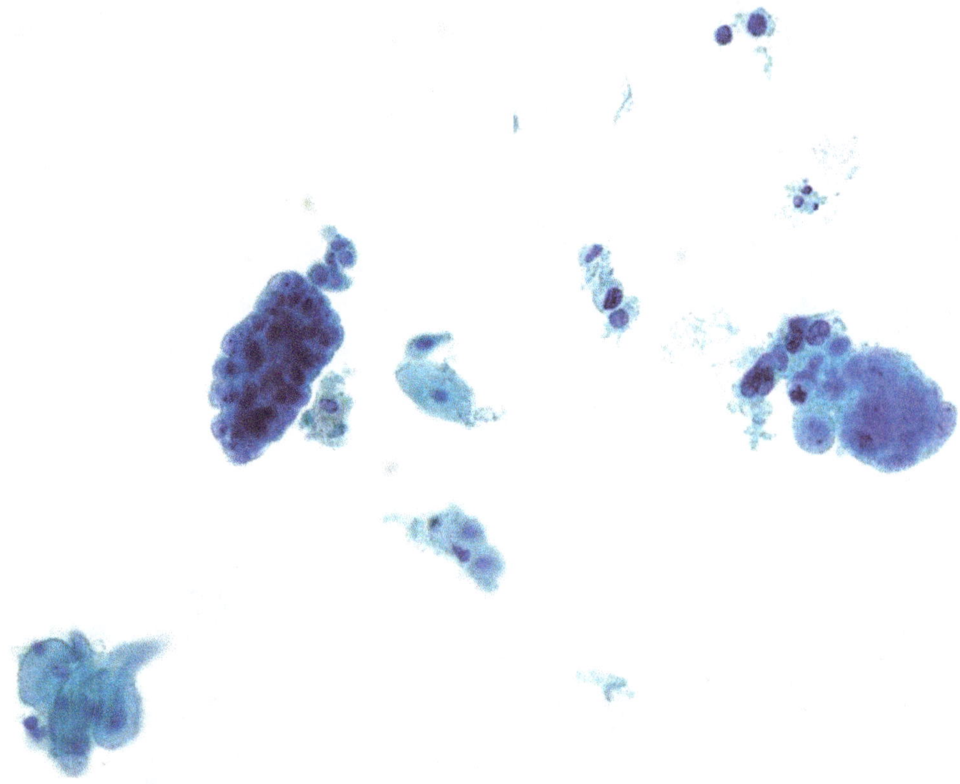

Q-55. These cells were detected in small clusters in the gynecologic sample from a 62-year-old female (ThinPrep, right and left, low power). There was a scant amount of blood and debris in the background. Occasional nucleoli were noted and the chromatin pattern appeared finely granular and powdery. The most likely interpretation of these cells is:

(a) Atrophy
(b) Cytolysis
(c) Squamous cell carcinoma
(d) Endometrial neoplasia

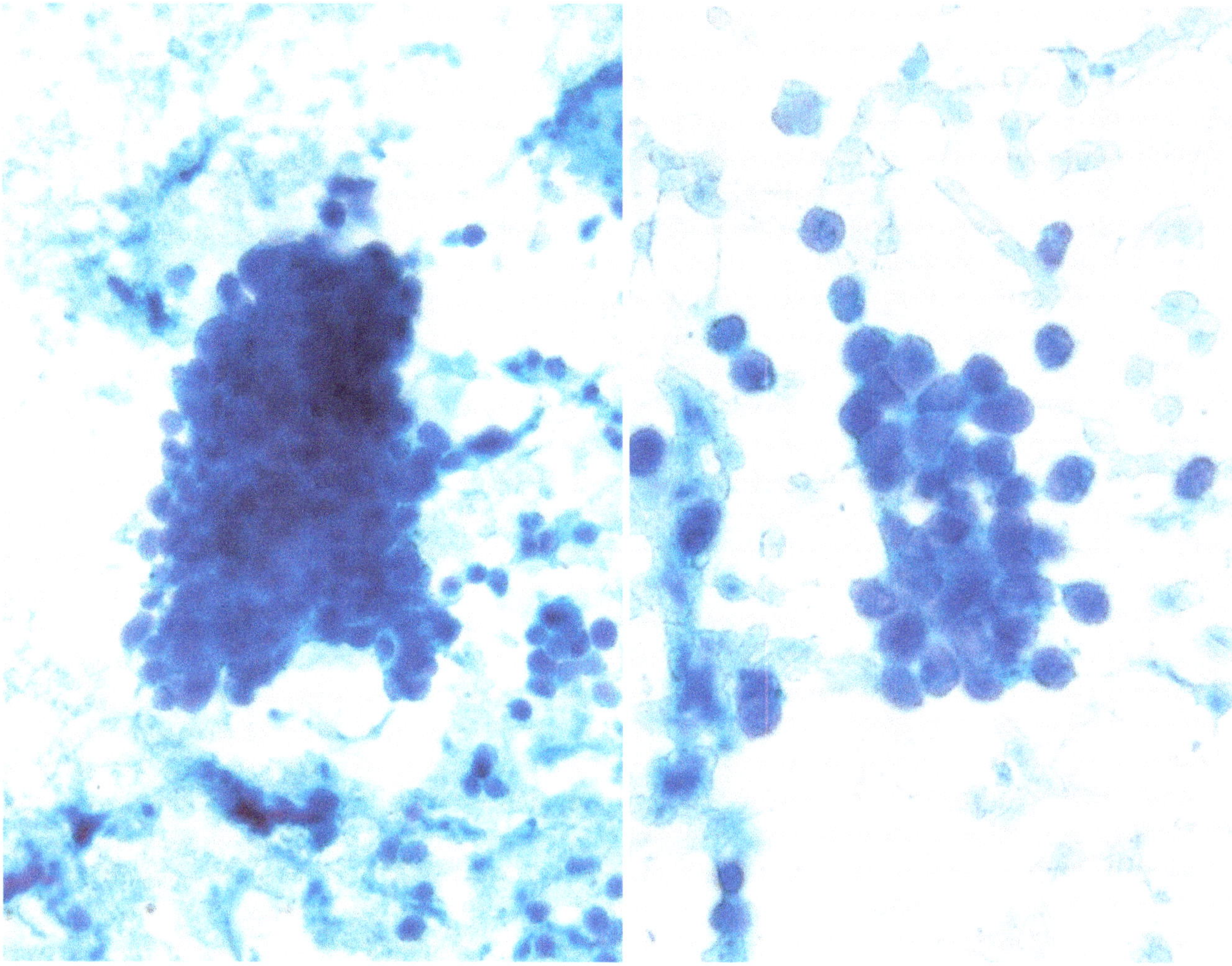

Fig. 6.56

Q-56. Many clusters of cells such as these were detected in the sample from a 36-year-old woman (conventional slide, left, low power; right, high power). There was no coexisting dysplasia. These cells are most consistent with:

(a) Postpartum atrophy
(b) Cytolysis
(c) Endometrial adenocarcinoma
(d) Small cell carcinoma

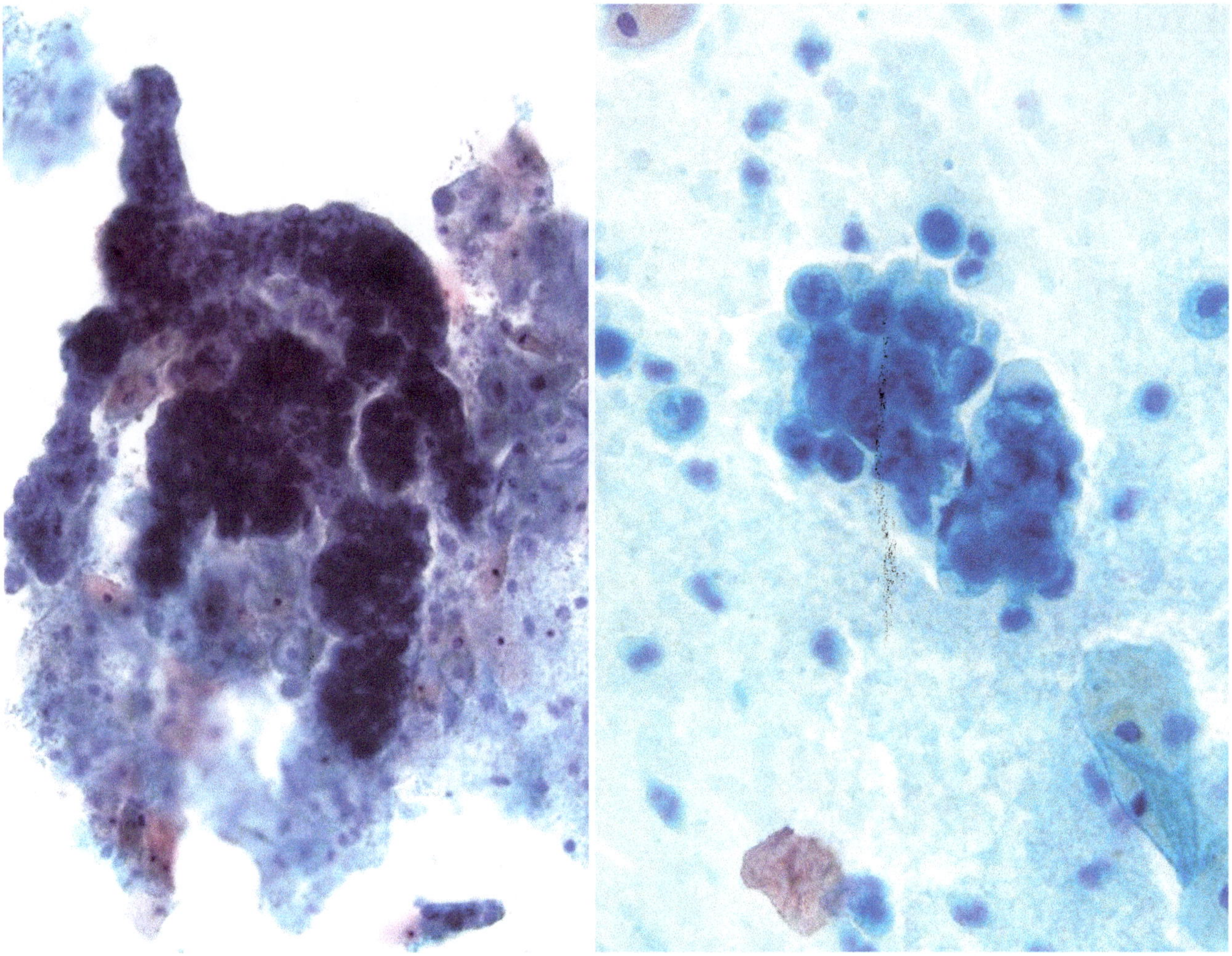

Fig. 6.57

Q-57. These HCGs were found in the conventional slide from a 69-year-old woman (left, low power; right, high power). Features indicative of the correct interpretation include which of the following?

(a) Watery, granular background, three-dimensional groups, and the presence of mature squamous cells
(b) Two-dimensional groups, evidence of keratinization, and macronucleoli
(c) Coarse chromatin, pleomorphic cells, and cytolysis
(d) Salt and pepper chromatin, molding, and lack of nucleoli

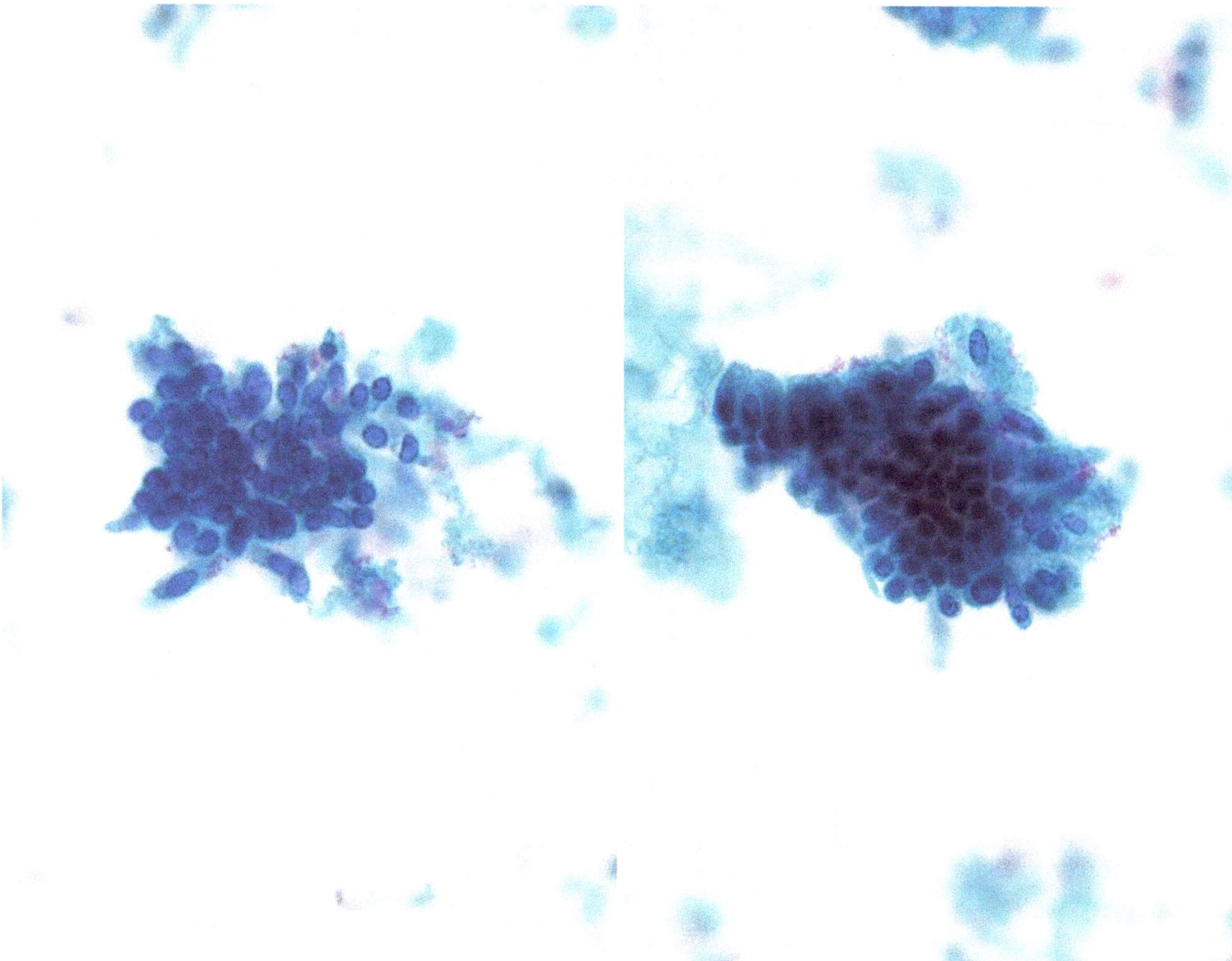

Fig. 6.58

Q-58. These hyperchromatic crowded groups were found in the SurePath sample from a 39-year-old woman (left and right, low power). Careful examination of the cells in these groups reveals that:

(a) There is feathering of the nuclei suggestive of AIS.

(b) There is molding of the nuclei suggestive of small cell carcinoma.

(c) There is uniformity of the cells and nuclei consistent with normal endocervical cells.

(d) There are small nucleoli suggestive of metastatic adenocarcinoma.

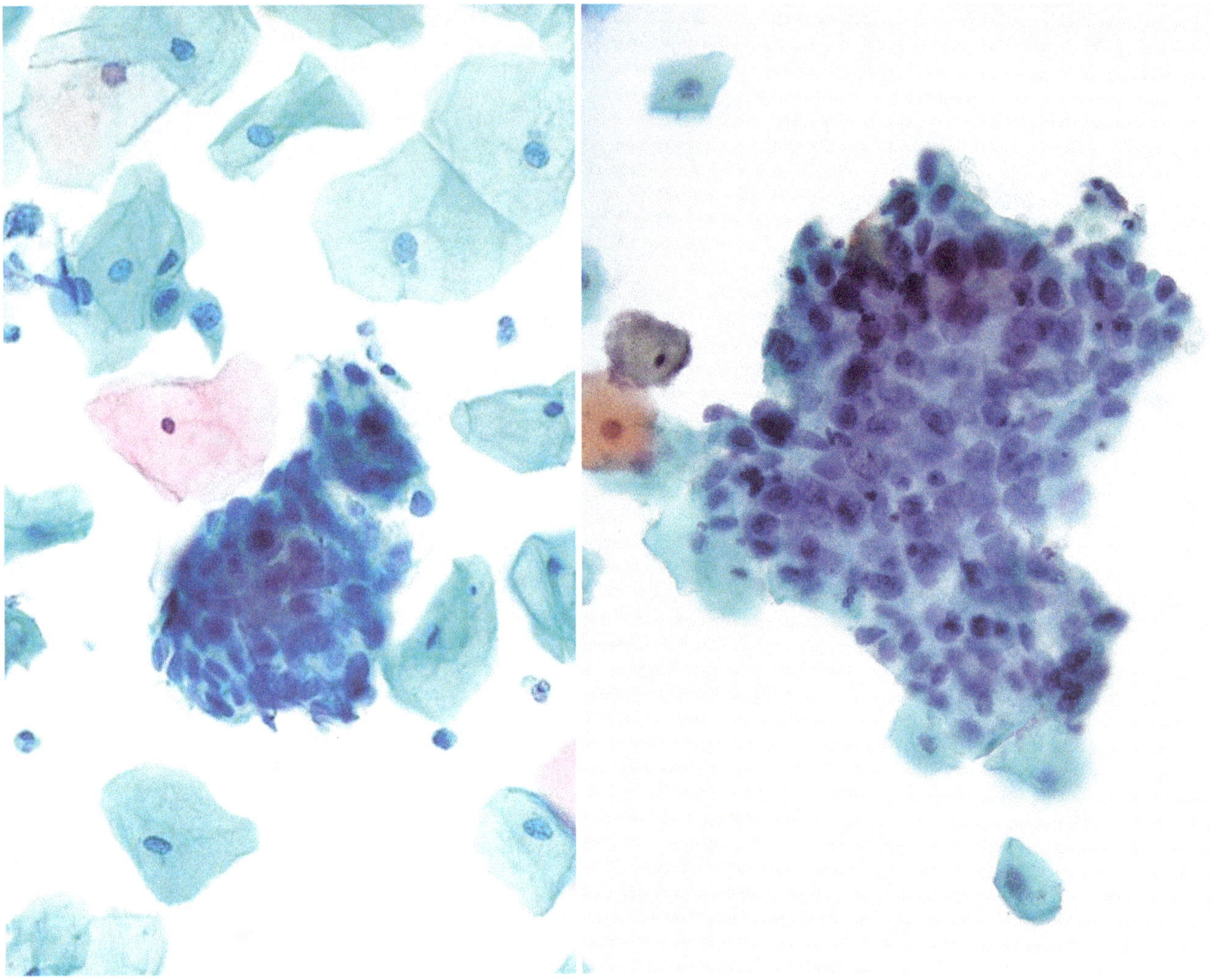

Fig. 6.59

Q-59. Hyperchromatic crowded groups (left, SurePath, high power; right, ThinPrep, medium power) such as these are most consistent with an interpretation of:

(a) CIS
(b) Normal endocervical cells
(c) Tubal metaplasia
(d) Reactive endocervical cells

Fig. 6.60

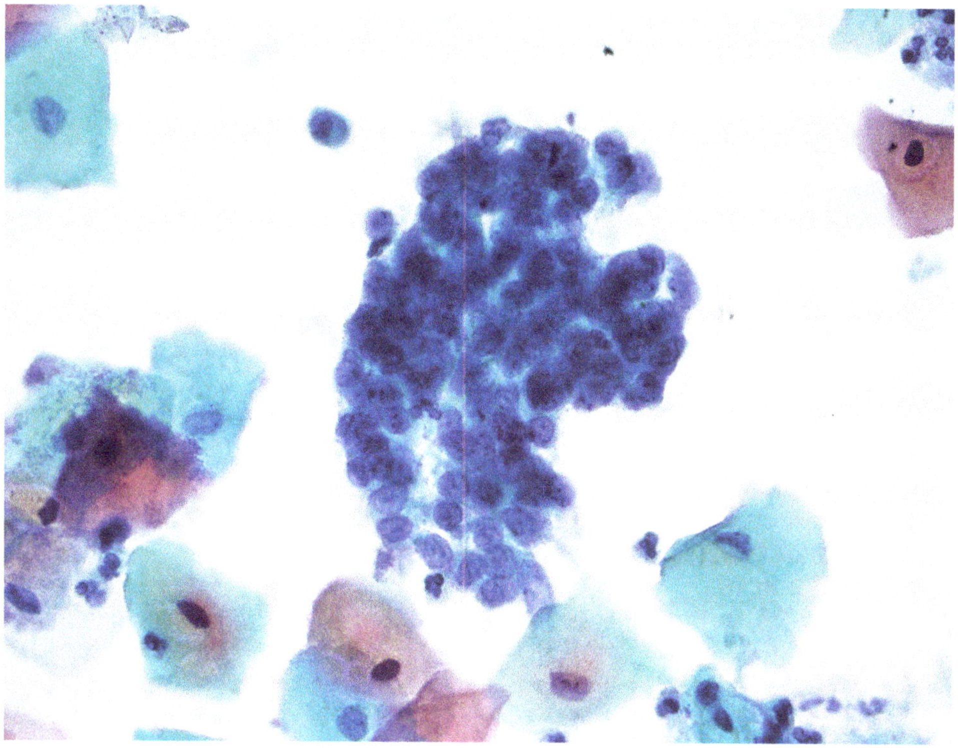

Q-60. This hyperchromatic group was found in the sample from a 33-year-old woman (ThinPrep, high power). Clues to the correct interpretation of these cells may include:

(a) Menstrual history
(b) Macronucleoli
(c) Feathering of the nuclei
(d) Presence of psammoma bodies

6.4 Answers and Discussion of Text-Based Questions 1–30

A-1. **(e) >90 %**
Benign HCGs are quite common, and DeMay estimates that about 99 % of the time, they are benign rather than neoplastic entities.

A-2. **(d) HGSIL (CIS)**
The least serious lesion that HCGs are likely to represent is CIS. Additionally, squamous cell carcinoma, AIS, endocervical or endometrial adenocarcinoma, or metastatic carcinoma may occur as HCGs.

A-3. **(e) Adenocarcinoma in situ of the endocervix**
The only neoplastic entity listed is adenocarcinoma in situ of the endocervix. The other answers are benign causes of HCGs.

A-4. **(a) Chaotic architecture**
Low power may either reveal chaotic architecture (suggestive of neoplasia) or, more orderly, uniform patterns (suggestive of benign causes of HCGs). Cytoplasmic vacuolization is not necessarily a feature of neoplasia and would not be easily identified on low power. Cilia are a feature of benign HCGs, as is fine chromatin and the absence of mitotic figures. Also, these choices would most likely have to be confirmed on high power rather than low power.

A-5. **(c) Coexisting dysplasia**
Most CIS cases usually have a coexisting component of dysplasia which can greatly aid in distinguishing these HCGs as neoplastic. Hypochromasia is not found in hyperchromatic crowded groups. Nucleoli are not a good feature to distinguish CIS from benign HCGs because in the setting of inflammation, either condition may have nucleoli. Cilia are not usually found in CIS and are a sign of benign HCGs.

A-6. **(d) Endocervical neoplasia**
CIS not infrequently may display rosette or microacinar-like formations which may be a result of the primitive reserve cell's capacity to differentiate along either a squamous or glandular pathway. This may be misdiagnosed as endocervical neoplasia, reactive endocervical cells, glandular involvement of the CIS, or even as a mixed squamous and glandular lesion. Microacinar patterns are unlikely to be confused with dysplasia, invasive squamous cell carcinoma, or repair. The most worrisome result is for the cells to be thought of as reactive endocervical cells, in which case they might be signed out as just negative when actually they might represent CIS.

A-7. **(b) Large cell CIS**
The large cell type of CIS is the most likely to have the features described and possibly be misinterpreted as a benign HCG. In these cells the chromatin may be bland, the N/C ratio only moderately increased, the membranes smooth and regular, and the cytoplasm may be unexpectedly more abundant than the classical patterns described in texts. It is important to recognize these more unusual patterns of CIS so that they are not dismissed as only benign HCGs. Small cell CIS does not have the described pattern, and keratinizing CIS and microinvasive CIS are not terms which are recognized and are therefore incorrect.

A-8. **(a) Degenerated cells, fresh or old blood, inflammation, and granular precipitate**
The only choice which is present in atrophy as well as one which might mislead the observer into a diagnosis of invasive carcinoma is "a." This "dirty" appearing background is sometimes termed "benign diathesis." Nucleoli are not typically present in atrophy, nor is cytoplasmic streaming which is more often found in repair. Smudgy chromatin is an indication of degeneration seen in atrophy but invasive carcinoma should have crisp, sharply defined chromatin.

A-9. **(c) Postmenopausal women**
Although most CIS cases have a coexisting dysplasia, an important feature in helping to correctly recognize neoplastic HCGs, it is important to note that the most common population to have CIS cells without a coexisting dysplasia are postmenopausal women. The other three groups are more likely to have the usual pattern of CIS mixed with dysplastic cells.

A-10. **(e) Matured parabasal cells**
Carefully observing the edge of a group of hyperchromatic, crowded cells in an atrophic smear, one may note cells which appear to have undergone some maturation to parabasal-type cells, and this can help to correctly identify the group as benign atrophy. The other choices are all features of neoplastic HCGs.

A-11. **(d) Enlarged elongated nuclei**
Enlarged, oval nuclei are the only feature listed which overlaps in appearance with endocervical neoplasia and benign, reactive endocervical cells. Cilia are a not a feature of neoplasia and would actually rule out its

presence. Bland, fine chromatin is not consistent with the usual endocervical AIS or adenocarcinoma chromatin pattern. Keratinization is a feature seen in well-differentiated keratinizing dysplasias or carcinomas. Thus, the best answer is "d."

A-12. (b) **Uniformity of cell size and shape**
The nuclei from the cells of lower uterine segment are bland, more uniform, and have a more regular shape than the cells of endocervical neoplasia. Although they may appear somewhat more crowded with a higher N/C ratio than usual, their lack of feathering, marked hyperchromasia, and coarse chromatin rules out consideration of endocervical neoplasia. Tumor diathesis and macronucleoli are more often found in invasive endocervical lesions.

A-13. (c) **Cone biopsy**
Samples taken post cone biopsy may inadvertently sample the lower uterine segment due to shortening of the endocervical canal. The other procedures would not have this effect.

A-14. (a) **Nuclei larger than intermediate cell nuclei and nucleoli**
The standard nuclear size with which to compare endometrial cells is the size of an intermediate cell nucleus. Endometrial cells larger than this, especially if they contain nucleoli, should be strongly considered as neoplastic. Endometrial lesions usually do not have a bloody necrotic background; the diathesis is more usually watery. Picket fence arrangements are more often found in endocervical adenocarcinomas or AIS cases. While 3-D arrangements are more common in endometrial clusters, whether benign or malignant, the nuclear size should be larger than an intermediate cell nucleus, not smaller.

A-15. (e) **Cilia**
Cilia are a practical indicator to distinguish a benign HCG such as tubal metaplasia from glandular neoplasia. Although the cilia may be degenerated or somewhat difficult to recognize, they are more reliable than enlarged nuclei, which may occur in both benign and neoplastic HCGs. Also, increased N/C ratios or moderate hyperchromasia may also occur in both conditions. Mitotic figures may also be found in either tubal metaplasia or in glandular neoplasia.

A-16. (e) **Metastatic carcinoma**
The only two neoplastic conditions listed are CIS and metastatic carcinoma. CIS is a rather common source of neoplastic HCGs, but metastatic carcinoma is rarely found in the gynecologic sample.

A-17. (b) **Interpretive error (incorrectly classifying the cells)**
Since the cells of HCGs are both hyperchromatic and crowded, they are usually fairly easily seen. The difficulty is in correctly interpreting them, since they occur very frequently but most often are benign. Thus, the correct answer is "b," interpretive error. Neither an increase nor a decrease in ASC-US to SIL ratios would usually be caused by HCGs.

A-18. (d) **Syncytial groups of parabasal or basal cells**
The most common cause of benign hyperchromatic crowded groups in atrophic smears is syncytial groups of parabasal or basal cells. CIS is not a benign cause of HCGs; parakeratosis is unlikely to cause HCGs as the cells are small and orangeophilic and have polygonal cytoplasm. Air-drying artifact may occur in atrophic smears (although much less often since the advent of liquid-based preparation methods); however, the cells are usually pale, uniform, and have more abundant cytoplasm than is seen in HCGs.

A-19. (a) **Rosette-like or microacinar structures**
Reactive endocervical cells would be most likely to be confused with the occasional occurrence of rosette-like HCGs in CIS. This is an important differential since confusing reactive endocervical cells with CIS might lead to a failure to appropriately follow-up the patient. These glandular appearing cells may derive from the potential of the reserve cells to differentiate along either glandular or squamous lines. Three-dimensional cell balls are more commonly associated with endometrial cells, while keratinization and pleomorphic nuclei are associated with well-differentiated squamous dysplasias. Thus, the best answer is "a."

A-20. (b) **Cells with rather bland chromatin, smooth nuclear outlines, and more abundant cytoplasm**
The correct answer is "b." Large cell CIS is the most likely subtype to occur as described, and the bland chromatin and more abundant cytoplasm should also be recognized as consistent with CIS and not misinterpreted as benign HCGs. Finding coexisting dysplasia may assist in the correct interpretation. Three-dimensional balls of cells are likely to derive from an endometrial origin. Sheets of cells with nucleoli and cytoplasmic streaming are associated with repair. Single cells with pleomorphism, keratinization, and nucleoli are associated with invasive squamous cell carcinoma.

A-21. **(a) Syncytial-like groups of pleomorphic cells with high N/C ratios and hyperchromatic nuclei**
HCGs found in atrophy are most likely to appear as syncytial-like groups of cells with hyperchromasia and high N/C ratios. Single scattered cells with bland nuclei are unlikely to be considered as HCGs since they are not in groups. Metaplastic cells with sharp borders are likely to be correctly interpreted as consistent with atrophy, and degenerated cells with bland chromatin are not likely to be considered in the differential with hyperchromatic groups since their chromatin is so bland it is not worrisome.

A-22. **(b) Mitotic figures**
Mitotic figures are not expected in atrophic groups and should therefore be a feature concerning for neoplasia. Degenerated chromatin is more often found in atrophic cells than in neoplastic cells which should display crisp, well-preserved chromatin. Cytoplasmic streaming is usually associated with repair, not neoplasia. Increased N/C ratio can be found in atrophy due to the absence of estrogen causing immaturity of the squamous cells.

A-23. **(d) Request the clinician to perform an estrogen test and repeat the Pap**
The best answer is to have the clinician administer a short-term course of estrogen to the patient and then to repeat the Pap smear. If there were HCGs which were merely caused by atrophy, the administration of estrogen would cause the cells to mature and the diagnostic dilemma would be resolved. If, however, the HCGs were actually neoplastic cells, the surrounding background of immature cells would mature but the groups would remain unchanged, eliminating the diagnostic difficulty. None of the special stains listed are useful in detecting likely gynecologic neoplasia.

A-24. **(c) The presence of a clean background and relatively few groups**
Metastatic carcinomas in the gynecologic tract are unlikely to occur without previous sites of metastatic disease and a well-known clinical history. Typically metastatic carcinoma will occur with a clean background and have relatively rare tumor cells which seem unrelated to the surrounding normal cells. The finding of a dirty background with abundant cells is not typical for metastatic carcinoma. The absence of mitotic figures is more of a benign sign but may also be seen in neoplasia. It would not be a good indicator either way for the presence or absence of metastatic carcinoma. Orderly architecture is a feature of benignity. The best answer is "c."

A-25. **(d) CIS**
Benign conditions such as severe atrophy, tubal metaplasia, and endometriosis are seldom involved in litigation involving interpretation errors of Pap samples. LGSIL, although important to diagnose, usually has little to no severe long-term consequences if left undiagnosed since many patients clear the disease even without treatment and because there is usually a rather longtime period prior to the development of invasive carcinoma often allowing detection of the lesion on the next examination. CIS, on the other hand, may go undetected, especially if its presentation is unusual or if its hyperchromatic crowded groups are misinterpreted as benign in origin. This lesion may have a relatively more rapid development into invasive carcinoma and thus is involved in litigation more frequently than the other entities.

A-26. **(e) Have multiple-slide blinded rescreening in which ten cytotechnologists blindly review the slide within their daily workload of slides. Statistically analyze the results to determine the appropriateness of the original diagnosis.**
Multiple-slide blinded rescreening (MSBR) is the preferred method to resolve possible cases of misdiagnosis and/or misinterpretation of litigated cases. It has the advantage of having multiple cytotechnologists review the case in a blinded fashion, without knowing previous reports or subsequent events, and so helps to eliminate "witch hunts" for the occasional questionable cell. It places the supposedly "abnormal" slide in question among a set of other, similar review slides and is done within a normal workday, in a fashion similar to the original laboratory. The results of at least ten cytotechnologists are then compared to the original diagnosis. If at least two of the ten report the slide as negative, then it can be statistically proven to be within the "irreducible" false-negative rate of 5 %. In other words, that finding would not support the idea that any reasonably prudent practitioner would have found the slide abnormal. All of the other scenarios, although perhaps more expedient, will unduly bias the cytologist, will give special importance to the slide prior to examination, and will not take into account the usual number of slides screened and the amount of time spent with a routine slide in the laboratory. Prior knowledge of subsequent history cannot help but bias the observer so the elimination of that factor helps to create a more reliable, reproducible, and accurate method of fairly adjudicating a questionable result.

A-27. **(d) 5 %**
5 % is the figure used in the statistical analysis of multiple-slide blinded rescreening as the figure representing

an "irreducible" false-negative rate. Smaller figures than this are unreasonable and would require thousands of cytotechnologists to achieve (0.01 % would require 369,000 cytotechnologists to review the slide to achieve a p value of <0.05). 10 % is a much higher value than that which is used.

A-28. **(a) LGSIL**
LGSIL is not often brought to litigation for a variety of reasons. One reason is that the plaintiff must show significant harm caused by a failure to accurately diagnose the lesion correctly on the slide. LGSIL often resolves by itself, even without treatment, and so significant harm is not caused. Additionally, it often requires several years for a LGSIL to evolve into a more serious lesion, during which time there are more opportunities for the abnormality to be detected. Finally, LGSIL lesions have been found to represent the most reproducible and reliable of all common cytologic diagnoses. This may be because these are common lesions, with large, usually dark nuclei which are fairly easily seen and recognized, and so these cases are not often represented in the litigated pool of cases. HGSIL is a commonly litigated diagnostic category, as well as endocervical AIS and adenocarcinoma. Finally, a carcinoma may simulate atypical repair so that the case is misdiagnosed. All of these possibilities are more common than LGSIL.

A-29. **(d) The public's expectation of zero errors in Pap diagnosis**
It is the public's expectation that a diagnostic "test" will never have errors that has been a significant factor in the increase in litigation of gynecologic results. Only increased communication with clinicians and the public will help clients to realize that the Pap is a screening test and cannot be equated with a 100 % accuracy rate. None of the other choices would lead to an increase in litigation.

A-30. **(a) Make follow-up recommendations, especially for glandular lesions**
Adding follow-up recommendations for the clinicians is the most reasonable method to try to avoid errors and reduce possible litigation risk. Especially for those diagnoses which may be less familiar to clinicians (e.g., AGUS vs. ASC-US), recommendations for follow-up included within the report may serve to provide guidance to clinicians and reduce false-negatives and, therefore, litigation. Reducing the use of ASC-H is not a reasonable option, as it is specified in The Bethesda System classification. Colposcopy on all cases displaying HCGs might reduce false-negative cases but would be an expensive and unwieldy option since these occur so often but are so often benign. Double screening using usual methods also would be an overly time-consuming and expensive alternative to reduce risk of litigation.

6.5 Answers and Discussion of Image-Based Questions 31–60

A-31. (**d**) **Smudgy chromatin**

These cells are showing evidence of infection by herpes virus. In the lower left corner, there is a multinucleated cell showing the typical molding, ground glass chromatin, and thickened nuclear membranes of nuclei infected with herpes. The remaining cells are somewhat more difficult to see; however, the absence of crisp chromatin indicates a benign rather than neoplastic origin for hyperchromatic crowded groups (HCGs). This lack of crisp chromatin, despite the hyperchromasia seen, helps in the evaluation of many types of benign HCGs such as in cases of atrophy, crowded but benign reactive endocervical cells, tubal metaplasia, and lower uterine segment. Degeneration as seen in atrophy, for example, may display dark nuclei, but the cells will lack the crisp chromatin of true neoplasia, such as seen in CIS. Thus, hyperchromasia, by itself, may be seen in either benign or neoplastic cells. Crowding may also be seen in both types of HGCs. Multinucleation is a feature of some benign HCGs, but is not a general feature of benignity.

A-32. (**b**) **Maturing parabasal cells**

This cell group is made up of parabasal cells from an atrophic woman. The finding of more mature appearing parabasal cells at the edge of a group such as this helps to indicate the benign nature of the entire group. Again, note the smooth-bordered, finely granular nuclei which help to exclude a neoplastic origin of these cells. Polymorphonuclear leukocytes are not useful in this case. The cells are not in a syncytial arrangement, as would be expected in CIS. Multinucleated histiocytes are also not useful in the case. The best answer is therefore “b.”

A-33. (**c**) **Normal endocervical cells**

Groups of normal endocervical cells often occur in HCGs, and they can be troublesome. The best evaluation should include a close examination of at least some of these groups in order to rule out a neoplastic origin. Examination of the edges of these groups reveals their columnar orientation, honeycomb architecture, and uniformity of nuclear size. Also, in the visible areas, there is a lack of feathering of the nuclei, an absence of nucleoli, and morphologic uniformity from cell to cell that helps to exclude an endocervical neoplasia. CIS is ruled out by the endocervical appearance of the cells and by their lack of pleomorphism. The cells are not in a three-dimensional arrangement which excludes an endometrial origin for the cells.

A-34. (**a**) **Cilia**

Tubal metaplasia can be difficult as it may occur in hyperchromatic crowded groups and can be confused with endocervical neoplasia or other significant squamous lesions. It occurs as a combination of ciliated, secretory, or intercalated cells with round to slightly oval nuclei which are usually less coarsely granular than endocervical neoplasia and less elongated. The groups may appear architecturally “clumsy” due to a variation in the size of the nuclei and due to the variety of the types of cells which disrupts the orderly honeycomb pattern. Sharp apical borders are another clue to the correct interpretation of the cells as well as the presence of very small, clear cytoplasmic vacuoles. In the large group, note the smaller, dark, triangular nuclei which may correspond to the intercalated cells. Also, note the distinct cilia in both groups of cells. This is a very useful finding but unfortunately may be degenerated and less distinct than seen here. This finding virtually excludes a neoplastic source for these cells. Crowding is not a useful distinguishing feature as it may be present in both neoplastic and benign HCGs. Feathering can occasionally be present in tubal metaplasia and is a significant source of difficulty with endocervical neoplasia. Mitotic figures would not normally be found in tubal metaplasia.

A-35. (**d**) **Endometrial cells**

These clusters of cells are consistent with normal shedding endometrial cells. Note the loose three-dimensional cluster; the irregular, raisinoid shapes of the nuclei; the scant cytoplasm; and the relatively uniform size of the cells. These nuclei should not exceed the size of intermediate cell nuclei. CIS would be more hyperchromatic; would have coarse, irregular chromatin patterns; and would usually be larger in nuclear size than these endometrial cells. LGSIL would have much more cytoplasm and much larger nuclei and would not occur in the three-dimensional group seen here. Finally, repair would have much more abundant, streaming cytoplasm, pale nuclei with nucleoli in almost every cell, and retained polarity.

A-36. (**b**) **Lower uterine segment**

The advent of the cervical brush collection device has resulted in an increase in the number of specimens obtained from the lower uterine segment. On conventional slides, these groups usually are larger with a complex-branched appearance. Liquid-based preparations usually have smaller groups with frayed edges. The combinations of the tubular glandular components and the stromal elements are both seen in this image. Liquid-based preparations show both components less frequently. The stromal components are made up of elongated and bland oval nuclei which may appear disordered. The presence of both components helps to confirm the benign nature of these cells. Atrophy would not display this branched and biphasic appearance. Differentiation from endocervical neoplasia can sometimes be difficult in cases in which the stromal component is scant or missing. The regularity of the size of the cells and the bland chromatin help to rule out neoplasia. Normal shedding of endometrial cells would not occur in such a well-formed branching group and would not be accompanied by the epithelial glandular cells seen here.

A-37. (**d**) **Chronic follicular cervicitis**
Chronic follicular cervicitis will present as a loose cluster of lymphocytes of varying degrees of maturity. Therefore, there will be some variation in the size of the nuclei which ranges from very small and round to somewhat larger, more immature appearing lymphs. The clusters of these cells usually appear in smaller groupings on liquid-based preparations but occur in pools on conventional slides. Tingible body macrophages may or may not be present. Since the cells are so hyperchromatic, they might be confused with small cell CIS. But the cells of small cell CIS show more variation; have coarser, more irregular chromatin; and show more variation in size and shape than chronic follicular cervicitis. Acute inflammation would have polymorphonuclear leukocytes, not lymphocytes. The cells have too little cytoplasm, and the nuclei are too small to be considered LGSIL.

A-38. (**b**) **Dysplastic cells**
CIS can occur in hyperchromatic crowded groups which may cause a diagnostic problem with the many benign causes of HCGs. One helpful feature which is usually present, and is seen in this image, is the presence of clearly dysplastic cells accompanying the HCGs of CIS. These cells are by definition larger, have larger dark nuclei, and have clearly squamous-type cytoplasm with an increase in N/C ratio. If dysplastic cells are found, the HCGs present on the slide should be carefully examined for the presence of cells which would meet the criteria for CIS. The nuclei of CIS will usually vary in uniformity of size, shape, and chromatin pattern, so regularity of nuclei is not a useful feature. Feathering of nuclei is a diagnostic feature of AIS of the endocervix and would not be useful in this case. Three-dimensional cell groups are found in shedding endometrial cells and would not be useful in correctly interpreting the CIS seen here.

A-39. (**d**) **Hyperchromasia, enlargement, and pseudostratification**
These cells seem to be clearly derived from the endocervix and the important features seen here include nuclear crowding, elongation and enlargement of the nuclei, hyperchromasia, and pseudostratification. Thus, these groups are indicative of endocervical neoplasia, most likely AIS. A coexisting dysplasia would more likely be seen in a case of squamous CIS. Three-dimensional clusters of cells are associated with endometrial cells. Cilia, when present, are a clear indication of a benign source of the hyperchromatic crowded group, such as tubal metaplasia. AIS would also usually show more variation in the size of the nuclei and the nuclear chromatin pattern than tubal metaplasia.

A-40. (**c**) **Squamous cell carcinoma**
Hyperchromatic crowded groups can occur in squamous cell carcinoma alongside other features of invasive squamous cell carcinoma, such as single, pleomorphic cells with evidence of keratinization, dirty background, and very dark, irregular chromatin. These other features are very useful in assisting with the correct interpretation. Atrophy may show dark, smudgy, degenerated nuclei, but will lack the keratinization, pleomorphism, and dirty background seen here. Repair would show enlarged cytoplasm and hypochromatic nuclei with nucleoli. Endometrial adenocarcinoma would not show the dark, keratinized, pleomorphic cells seen here. Usually endometrial adenocarcinoma will show three-dimensional loose groups with powdery, enlarged nuclei, and nucleoli in a watery tumor diathesis.

A-41. (**b**) **Endocervical adenocarcinoma**
The presence of two-dimensional groups, abnormal cells, and the elongated, columnar cell shapes helps to lead one to a diagnosis of neoplasia of endocervical origin. The hyperchromasia, nucleoli, and dirty background also assist in this interpretation. Endometrial adenocarcinoma would have more three-dimensional groups, powdery chromatin, and a watery tumor diathesis. CIS should have a clean background and only rare or absent nucleoli and would not have cells of a columnar configuration. These cells are too dark are irregular and show too much loss of polarity to be considered for repair.

A-42. (**c**) **Rectal adenocarcinoma**
The typical, tall columnar look of these cells brings to mind an endocervical adenocarcinoma. When cells such as these are accompanied by a dirty background, this interpretation is further strengthened. However,

one exception to the general rule of metastatic carcinomas occurring in a clean background may occur with metastatic colonic or rectal adenocarcinomas which invade by direct extension from the colorectal area. This causes a very dirty background and may be a potential source of error. However, note the gland-like spaces reminiscent of colonic histologic patterns. These lesions may also demonstrate vegetable material from rectovaginal fistulas which may occur. Obtaining a complete clinical history is always a valuable adjunct to microscopic examination. Ovarian adenocarcinoma would likely have more abundant cytoplasm, macronucleoli, and vacuolization which are not evident in these images. Endometrial adenocarcinoma would not likely be confused with an endocervical adenocarcinoma since endometrial adenocarcinoma cells usually occur in three-dimensional groups, are not so hyperchromatic, and are not tall columnar shapes. Leukemia would have discohesive, smaller cells with scant cytoplasm and would not form the cohesive group seen here.

A-43. (**b**) **Endocervical adenocarcinoma in situ**

These nuclei are exhibiting pseudostratification, enlargement, abnormal elongation of the nuclei, and crowding. The size of these nuclei can be compared to the normal squamous cells in the image. The irregularities in the nuclei and the abnormal architectural pattern exclude normal endocervical cells from consideration. Atrophy is not a consideration as mature squamous cells are seen in the background and these cells are clearly from the endocervix. Endometrial adenocarcinoma is also not the best interpretation since the cells are in a two-dimensional configuration rather than a three-dimensional group. Two-dimensional groups are the most common in cells of endocervical origin.

A-44. (**a**) **Finely granular with smooth nuclear borders**

These cells were interpreted as reactive endocervical cells. Note on the left edge of the group as well as at the bottom of the group are distinct terminal bars, indicating the endocervical origin of these cells. Small nucleoli might be worrisome unless one notes the very smooth nuclear borders and finely granular chromatin of the cells. This helps to establish the benign nature of these cells, especially when noting the uniformity of the cells and nuclei. The cells are not coarsely granular, in a feathering pattern, nor are they loosely cohesive. Coarsely granular chromatin would imply a neoplastic HCG. A feathering pattern would suggest AIS of the endocervix and discohesion might also lead one away from a benign interpretation.

A-45. (**c**) **Endometrial cells**

Endometrial cells are often found in three-dimensional groups with scant cytoplasm. Note the quite uniform size range of these cells which are oval or may have slightly pointed ends. Normal endometrial cells may appear somewhat hyperchromatic, especially if they have not degenerated. However, the regularity of the nuclear size, which should not exceed the size of an intermediate cell nucleus, helps to confirm their benign nature. These cells are not displaying the tall, columnar look of endocervical cells, so choices "a" and "b" must be excluded. Endometrial adenocarcinoma would display cells with more variation in size and nucleoli and would occur with a watery tumor diathesis.

A-46. (**d**) **Squamous cell carcinoma**

The correct interpretation of these HCGs is made easier by the background of abnormal keratinized cells, debris, and pleomorphic cell shapes. Any dark groups such as these found in this type of background should be carefully examined for the possibility of malignancy. The cells are not large enough for a diagnosis of LGSIL. Endometrial adenocarcinoma would be less hyperchromatic, usually occurring as pale, powdery nuclei within enlarged cells of endometrial origin. Endocervical adenocarcinoma is not a likely diagnosis due to the lack of two-dimensional cell groups and the coexisting pleomorphism and keratinization.

A-47. (**c**) **Degenerated chromatin**

Atrophy can sometimes contain HCGs which may be a source of concern. However, the nuclear features of these cells, although dark, are also smudgy and degenerated. Actual neoplastic HCGs will usually have crisp, well-defined chromatin which is also hyperchromatic. Basing a diagnosis on nuclei in which the particles of chromatin seem fused together, or washed out, or degenerated is unwise. Note also the parabasal cells surrounding the group in question. They help to suggest the true nature of the dark group. Also note the uniformity of the nuclei which argues against a neoplastic origin for these cells. The N/C ratio is not really enlarged given their parabasal origin. Mitotic figures are a worrisome feature when discovered but they are not noted in this image.

A-48. (**d**) **Endocervical adenocarcinoma**

These images are most consistent with an interpretation of endocervical adenocarcinoma. Careful examination of the cells at the edges of the groups will reveal eccentric nuclei which seem to be so crowded that the cells lose their normal architecture. A bloody tumor diathesis is often found with endocervical adenocarcinoma and high numbers of abnormal cells are often found, due to the proximity to the area of direct sampling. Atrophy, LGSIL, and HGSIL would not have a dirty background nor the nucleoli seen here. Endometrial adenocarcinoma is not a consideration due to the columnar morphology and the eccentric nuclei seen in the lower right image.

A-49. (a) **Tubular-shaped architecture**
Tubular-shaped structures of glandular cells such as these are found in liquid-based preparations from lower uterine segment. The HCGs in LUS on liquid-based preparations are usually smaller and less complex than on conventional slides, in which the microbiopsies are large and often show complex branching. Note also the uniformity of the glandular cells which helps to differentiate them from neoplastic HCGs. Nucleoli and irregular chromatin are features of neoplasia. Cohesion may be present in both neoplastic and benign HCGs, so it is not a useful discriminating feature.

A-50. (c) **Variation in nuclear features**
HCGs may occur in CIS and variation in the size and shape of the nuclei, as well as an extremely high N/C ratio of the cells assists in the correct interpretation. CIS also often has syncytial groups with hyperchromasia and irregular chromatin patterns. Benign HCGs usually have uniformity of the cells with little variation, although there are some exceptions such as tubal metaplasia. Three-dimensional groups are usually associated with cells of endometrial origin, and these cells are much too large and hyperchromatic for such an interpretation. Nucleoli are not seen in these images. Although CIS may rarely have nucleoli, it is an uncommon finding. Cytoplasmic streaming usually occurs in repair with abundant cytoplasm, nucleoli, and maintained polarity.

A-51. (a) **Enlargement of the nuclei beyond the size of an intermediate cell nucleus**
The finding of three-dimensional groups with nuclei enlarged beyond the size of intermediate cell nuclei is indicative of an endometrial adenocarcinoma. Note the finely vacuolated cytoplasm with ingested polymorphonuclear leukocytes and small nucleoli. The chromatin pattern is usually finely granular and powdery, rather than coarsely granular and hyperchromatic as in HGSIL lesions. Abundant streaming cytoplasm is common in repair. Evidence of keratinization would be more likely to be found in dysplastic or invasive keratinizing squamous cell lesions.

A-52. (b) **Endocervix; reactive**
The "squared off" appearance of the columnar cells corresponds with the apical portion of the endocervical cells. Often terminal bars and/or cilia may also be observed on these cells at the apical portion of the cell. Note also the nucleoli, the orderly architecture of the cells, and the hypochromasia of the nuclei. In some areas one can also notice PMNs within the reactive groups of endocervical cells. The streaming cytoplasm, finely granular nuclei, and orderly architecture rule out endometrial adenocarcinoma. Ovarian adenocarcinoma would have abundant cytoplasm and macronucleoli and may have psammoma bodies as well. HGSIL should have hyperchromatic nuclei with high N/C ratios and sharp-edged, squamous appearing cytoplasm.

A-53. (c) **Metastatic colorectal adenocarcinoma**
Of the choices given and in light of the negative results from investigation of the endometrium and endocervix, the most likely source is metastatic colorectal adenocarcinoma. These cells have a columnar appearance, and the left image shows a gland-like space that would be consistent with colonic origin. The cells are tall columnar but are quite variable in appearance. Metastatic small cell carcinoma of the lung would have molding, small cells, and little cytoplasm. Serous cystadenocarcinoma of the ovary would have abundant cytoplasm, macronucleoli, and enlarged nuclei. Carcinoid tumor of the GI tract would have the classic "salt and pepper" look to the nuclei, with very small amounts of cytoplasm, and no nucleoli.

A-54. (d) **Tubal metaplasia**
These groups are showing variation in nuclear size, as well as cilia, indicating a benign cause for this HCG. Tubal metaplasia is made up of several types of cells, including ciliated, nonciliated, and intercalated cells. The latter have smaller, darker, more triangular nuclei than the others, and this variation in nuclear size may help to correctly classify the cells. Note also some pseudostratification which also suggests this diagnosis. The chromatin pattern is however rather bland, and the sharp apical cell borders also lead to this interpretation. Endocervical AIS or adenocarcinoma might be a consideration, but the cilia argue against a neoplasia. The background cells are mature, and the groups of cells seen here are not parabasal cells but are glandular in origin. Thus, atrophy is not a consideration.

A-55. (**d**) **Endometrial neoplasia**
The clusters of cells in the image, as well as the description of finely granular, powdery chromatin, should lead one to an interpretation of endometrial neoplasia in this patient. The cells are too small and too clustered in a three-dimensional group to be considered as atrophy. Cytolysis is also not an attractive interpretation as it does not account for these clusters of cells of endometrial origin. Squamous cell carcinoma is not consistent with these glandular appearing cells. Additionally, the chromatin pattern in this image is not consistent with the hyperchromatic, irregular chromatin pattern and pleomorphism usually seen in squamous cell carcinoma. Careful evaluation of crowded groups of cells, especially noting those cells at the edges, is important so that abnormalities are not missed.

A-56. (**d**) **Small cell carcinoma**
These cells are quite small and have scant cytoplasm, slight variation in nuclear size, and subtle molding of the nuclei. Additionally, they are hyperchromatic and found in a very dirty background. Irregularities in the nuclear shape may also be noted. These features are consistent with small cell carcinoma, a rare type of carcinoma of the cervix which may not be accompanied by a coexisting dysplasia. Additionally, these carcinomas can occur in women who are relatively younger than cervical cancer patients in general. Atrophy such as would occur in a postpartum patient is not consistent with the images seen here, as these cells have too little cytoplasm even for very immature parabasal-type cells. Cytolysis is also inconsistent with this image as these cells are not lysed, but still have identifiable intact cytoplasm with abnormal nuclei. The groups are not consistent with an endometrial adenocarcinoma, being too hyperchromatic, more in a syncytial group than a three-dimensional cluster, and lack nucleoli.

A-57. (**a**) **Watery, granular background, three-dimensional groups, and the presence of mature squamous cells**
The high- and low-power images of these cells are consistent with an endometrial adenocarcinoma. The low-power image shows a branching papillary architecture which is most consistent with a glandular lesion. The high-power image shows cells with finely vacuolated cytoplasm and a nuclear size which is enlarged beyond the size of intermediate cell nuclei. Nucleoli are also present. Therefore, the cytologic features described in choice "a" best fit an interpretation of endometrial adenocarcinoma. Two-dimensional groups would more likely be associated with endocervical adenocarcinoma, as would macronucleoli. But keratinization is not a feature of endocervical adenocarcinoma; choice "b" does not fit with the image of more cuboidal glandular cells in a three-dimensional group. Coarse chromatin and pleomorphic cells would fit with a diagnosis of squamous cell carcinoma, but that is not a good fit with the images. Salt and pepper chromatin, molding, and lack of nucleoli would be more likely found in a neuroendocrine small cell carcinoma but that does not match the image seen here.

A-58. (**c**) **There is uniformity of the cells and nuclei consistent with normal endocervical cells.**
One of the most common causes of hyperchromatic crowded groups is normal endocervical cells. The danger lies in merely accepting these groups as the norm and not evaluating them carefully for neoplasia. However, close examination of these images shows the normal architectural pattern of honeycomb and picket fence that is characteristic of normal endocervical cells. Also, there is no variation or enlargement of the nuclei, nor is there feathering or coarse chromatin. Therefore, AIS is not a correct interpretation. The cells are small but clearly can be seen to have eccentric nuclei, consistent with an endocervical cell origin. Small cell carcinoma is therefore not a consideration. Nucleoli are not seen in these images, and the cells are very regular both in their architecture and their morphology, so a metastatic adenocarcinoma is not a correct interpretation.

A-59. (**a**) **CIS**
These groups show dark, coarse nuclei which appear to be in syncytial arrangements. Particularly in the right image, significant variation in the nuclear size and morphology can be seen. The background appears clean and no nucleoli are visible. These features are most consistent with CIS. The architecture of normal endocervical cells is not seen in these groups. Tubal metaplasia should show the sharp apical edges of the cells, cilia, or terminal plates and should be composed of several cell types giving a "clumsy" appearance to the architecture due to nuclear variation. Finally, reactive endocervical cells should retain their normal endocervical architecture and usually have prominent nucleoli. Neither of these features is seen in these images.

A-60. (**a**) **Menstrual history**
These cells, although somewhat hyperchromatic, are normally shed endometrial cells which can often have well-preserved, crisp, somewhat dark chromatin as seen here. This is especially true early in the menstrual

cycle in which the cells are not degenerated. Therefore, the patient's menstrual history can be a useful clue in the interpretation of these hyperchromatic groups.

Note that the nuclei of the cells are the same size as the normal intermediate cell nuclei in the image. They show very little variation and have a somewhat "raisinoid" appearance. They should always be carefully examined to differentiate them from the rare small cell CIS or carcinoma which will have more variation in nuclear size and more coarse, hyperchromatic chromatin and will occur in syncytial arrangements. Macronucleoli are not present in this image. The nuclei are not feathering so that AIS is not a consideration. Psammoma bodies are also not seen; ovarian adenocarcinoma is the most likely to have them and would have abundant cytoplasm, much larger, more variable nuclei, and macronucleoli.

Reading List

Cibas ES. Cervical and vaginal cytology. In: Cibas ES, Ducatman BS, editors. Cytology diagnostic principles and clinical correlates. Philadelphia: Saunders Elsevier; 2009.

DeMay RM. The Pap test. In: DeMay RM, editor. The art and science of cytopathology. 2nd ed. Chicago: ASCP Press; 2012.

Wilbur DC, Henry MR. College of American pathologists. College of American pathologists practical guide to gynecologic cytopathology: morphology, management, and molecular methods. Northfield: CAP Press; 2008.

Challenging and Uncommon Lesions in the Pap Test

7

Jing Yu, Pamela Michelow, and Walid E. Khalbuss

Contents

J. Yu, MD, PhD (✉)
Department of Pathology, University of Pittsburgh Medical Center,
300 Halket Street, Pittsburgh, PA 15213, USA
e-mail: yuj@upmc.edu

P. Michelow, MBBCh, MSc
Cytology Unit, Department of Anatomical Pathology,
National Health Laboratory Service, University of the Witwatersrand,
Corner Hospital Hill, Dekone St.,
Johannesburg, Gauteng 2000, South Africa
e-mail: pamela.michelow@nhls.ac.za

W.E. Khalbuss, MD, PhD, FIAC
Director of Cytology and Cytopathology Fellowship Program,
University of Pittsburgh Medical Center Shadyside Hospital,
5150 Centre Avenue, 2, Suite 201,
Pittsburgh, PA 15232, USA
e-mail: khalbussw2@upmc.edu

7.1 Tables and Summary

Table 7.1 Cytomorphology of pemphigus versus malignancies in Pap test

	Pemphigus	Squamous cell carcinoma	Adenocarcinoma
Cellular arrangement	Loose flat sheet or single cells	Syncytial flat sheet	2D crowded groups, rosettes
Cell shape	Uniform, round	Pleomorphic	Variable pleomorphism
Nuclear contour	Smooth	Irregular	Variably irregular
Chromatin	Fine, pale	Coarse, dark	Coarse, dark
Nucleoli	Multiple, irregular (bullet shaped)	Sometimes, single	Usually single, prominent
Cytoplasm	Dense	Dense	Vesicular

Table 7.2 Common culprits of uncommon female neoplasms in Pap test

Small cell neuroendocrine carcinoma
Malignant lymphoma and leukemia
Malignant melanoma
Uterine sarcoma (leiomyosarcoma, endometrial stromal sarcoma, carcinosarcoma)
Gestational trophoblastic diseases

Table 7.3 Cytomorphology of small cell carcinoma in liquid-based cytology (LBC)

Singly or in small clusters
Hyperchromatic nucleus with fine dark chromatin
Scant cytoplasm
Inconspicuous nucleoli
Mitoses
Nuclear molding is less prominent in LBC
Crush artifact (nuclear smearing) is absent in LBC

W.E. Khalbuss, M. Means (eds.), *Gynecological and Breast Cytopathology Board Review and Self-Assessment*, DOI 10.1007/978-1-4614-7270-4_7, © Springer Science+Business Media New York 2013

Table 7.4 Differential diagnosis of small cell carcinoma

Poorly differentiated squamous cell carcinoma
Poorly differentiated adenocarcinoma
Lymphoma
Sarcoma
Melanoma

Table 7.5 Differential diagnosis of lymphoma and leukemia

Follicular cervicitis
Poorly differentiated carcinoma
Small cell carcinoma
High-grade squamous dysplasia (CIN 3)
Endometrial stromal sarcoma

Table 7.6 Cytomorphology of melanoma

Dissociated single cells
Round to oval or spindle nuclei with prominent nucleoli
Intracellular melanin in some cases
S-100, HMB-45, and other melanoma markers positive

Table 7.7 Metastatic malignancies in Pap test

Most have known primary
Common sites: ovary, breast, GI, lung, etc.
Most common type: adenocarcinoma
Clean background (no diathesis except for direct invasion by colorectal carcinoma)

Table 7.8 Pearls of wisdom for the selected uncommon tumors in Pap test

Small cell carcinoma	Lymphoma	Sarcoma	Metastasis
• Most common neuroendocrine carcinoma of cervix	• Produces a detectable tumor mass at cervix	• Usually easy to recognize as malignant but hard to classify	• Typically malignant-appearing tumor cells in a clean background (no tumor diathesis)
• Strong association with HPV 18 • Associated with squamous or glandular neoplasias in half of the cases	• Most cases have a well-documented history of lymphoma	• Tumor diathesis is common because the surface must be ulcerated to exfoliate the stromal tumor cells	• Ovary followed by breast and GI tract are the most common sources • Tumors that invade directly, e.g., colorectal carcinomas, often have marked tumor diathesis

7.2 Text-Based Questions 1–37

Q-1. Small cell carcinoma of the cervix is associated with:
(a) HPV 16
(b) HPV 16 and 18
(c) Negative HPV
(d) HPV 18
(e) HPV 6 and 11

Q-2. Which of the following statements is true?
(a) Metastatic breast carcinoma in a Pap test demonstrates a marked tumor diathesis.
(b) A Pap test containing metastatic tumor cells of ovarian serous carcinoma shows a clean background.
(c) Colorectal carcinoma directly invading the cervix is ironically associated with a clean background.
(d) A Pap test with evidence of malignant lymphoma lacks a tumor diathesis.
(e) The clue to metastatic adenocarcinoma of stomach in a Pap test is signet ring cells in a dirty necrotic background.

Q-3. The following statements are true about pemphigus vulgaris in Pap test EXCEPT:
(a) Tzanck cells are large pleomorphic cells characteristic in the Pap test of a patient with pemphigus vulgaris.
(b) Tzanck cells may mimic repair except for the predominance of single cells.
(c) Clinical history is the most important clue in the diagnosis of pemphigus vulgaris.
(d) Coarse dark chromatin and a necrotic background are not features of pemphigus cytology.
(e) Follow-up biopsy and high-risk HPV DNA test are advisable management.

Q-4. The presence of psammoma bodies on Pap test is:
(a) A common benign finding
(b) Irrelevant to tumors
(c) Diagnostic for neoplasm
(d) Worrisome and should prompt a search for neoplasm
(e) Contaminant

Q-5. Tumors involving cervix or vagina by direct extension can be distinguished from those metastasizing from distant sites by:
(a) Mucinous background in tumors involving cervix via direct extension
(b) Clusters of cells through direct extension versus single cells from distant metastasis
(c) Abundant tumor diathesis in tumors from direct extension
(d) The presence of psammoma bodies in tumors from distant metastasis
(e) Distinct “floater” morphology in distant metastases

Q-6. The following statements are true regarding lymphoma of the cervix on Pap test *except*:
(a) As part of a disseminated disease, lymphoma of the cervix may not have any clinically detectable local signs.
(b) Most patients with evidence of lymphoma on their Pap tests have a well-documented history of the disease.
(c) Dirty inflammatory/hemorrhagic background is characteristic in Pap tests with evidence of lymphoma.
(d) The major differential diagnosis of lymphoma on Pap test is follicular cervicitis.
(e) Nuclear “nipples” may occur in lymphoma cells.

Q-7. Psammoma bodies may be seen in all the situations EXCEPT:
(a) Endosalpingiosis
(b) Granulosa cell tumor of ovary
(c) Use of intrauterine device
(d) Borderline tumor of ovary
(e) Serous carcinoma of fallopian tube

Q-8. The following cervical tumors are associated with high-risk HPV infection EXCEPT:
(a) Adenocarcinoma
(b) Small cell carcinoma
(c) Squamous cell carcinoma
(d) Large cell neuroendocrine carcinoma
(e) Lymphoma

Q-9. The following statements are true about sarcomas in Pap test *except*:
(a) The tumor cells are often easy to recognize as malignant.
(b) Carcinosarcoma (MMMT) is often diagnosed as adenocarcinoma on Pap tests.
(c) Routine Pap test rarely attributes to the primary diagnosis of these tumors.
(d) They occur in postmenopausal women, presenting as abnormal vaginal bleeding.
(e) A tumor diathesis is not common in Pap tests of sarcomas.

Q-10. The most common extrauterine malignancy that appears in the Pap test is from:
(a) Breast
(b) Colon and rectum
(c) Ovary and fallopian tube
(d) Lung
(e) Kidney

Q-11. Choose the correct statement regarding *Molluscum contagiosum*:
(a) It is caused by a herpes virus.
(b) In immunocompromised patients, the infection can become widely disseminated.
(c) A prominent intranuclear inclusion is seen on cytologic evaluation.
(d) Marked inflammation is usually seen in the background of a smear with *Molluscum contagiosum*.
(e) This virus is not a sexually transmitted disease.

Q-12. All of the following statements regarding mycobacterial infection of the cervix are correct *except*:
(a) Tuberculosis of the female genital tract usually involves the fallopian tubes and endometrium rather than the cervix.
(b) Mycobacterial cervicitis is often clinically misdiagnosed as carcinoma of the cervix due to the clinical presentation and presence of necrosis.
(c) Most mycobacterial infections of the cervix are due to *M. tuberculosis* rather than atypical mycobacteria.
(d) Mycobacterial infections of the cervix usually indicate primary infection.
(e) As there are several causes of granulomas in the cervix, ancillary investigations are required for definitive diagnosis.

Q-13. Choose the correct statement regarding schistosomiasis:
(a) *S. haematobium* usually infects the bowel and is best diagnosed on specimens from the colon and rectum.
(b) Schistosomiasis of the female genital tract is most likely due to *S. mansoni*.
(c) Schistosomiasis of the cervix may be associated with an increased risk of cervical squamous carcinoma.
(d) A cervix infected with schistosomiasis bleeds on contact but does not become ulcerated, friable, and/or mimic malignancy.
(e) Schistosomiasis of the female genital tract is not associated with an increased risk for spread of sexually transmitted infection.

Q-14. All of the following statements regarding parasitic infection of the cervix are correct *except*:
(a) Microfilariae are thin worms, 1–4 cm in length, and can provoke a severe cervicitis.
(b) Both *Entamoeba histolytica* and *Entamoeba gingivalis* can be found on cervical smear.
(c) In infection with *Trypanosoma cruzi*, giant cells with amastigotes are noted.
(d) In Taeniasis, the female worm can travel up the vaginal canal, causing infection of the vagina and cervix, and can even enter the uterus, resulting in endometritis and endosalpingitis.
(e) Detection of *Taenia* ova on cervical smear indicates true infection of the cervix.

Q-15. The following statements regarding high-grade squamous intraepithelial lesion of small cell type are correct *except*:
(a) These cells are derived from reserve or basal cells of the endocervical epithelium.
(b) This lesion may be the precursor of small cell carcinoma of the cervix.
(c) Pap tests show single cells and clusters of small dysplastic cells with scant, often barely visible basophilic, or rarely eosinophilic, cytoplasm.
(d) Necrosis and apoptosis are prominent features.
(e) The cells have hyperchromatic, coarsely granular nuclei with irregularity of the nucleus contour and may show prominent nucleoli.

Q-16. The differential diagnosis of high-grade squamous intraepithelial lesion of small cell type includes:
(a) Atypical squamous cells of undetermined significance
(b) Low-grade squamous intraepithelial lesion
(c) Reparative changes
(d) Inflammatory changes
(e) Follicular cervicitis

Q-17. Choose the correct statement regarding neuroendocrine tumors of the cervix:
(a) These are seen most frequently in women under the age of 40 years.
(b) They are not associated with human papillomavirus (HPV) infection.
(c) Paraneoplastic syndromes such as Cushing's syndrome, SIADH, hypercalcemia, or hypoglycemia may be seen.
(d) The prognosis is generally good.
(e) TTF1 positivity on immunostaining suggests metastases from the lung rather than a primary cervical tumor.

Q-18. Choose the correct statement regarding adenoma malignum of the cervix:
(a) The cervix, in adenoma malignum, is grossly indurated and barrel shaped.
(b) They are associated with human papillomavirus (HPV) infection.
(c) They are seen most frequently in postmenopausal women.

(d) Positive immunostaining for estrogen (ER) and progesterone receptors (PR) is usually seen.
(e) These tumors produce an equal amount of neutral and acidic mucin.

Q-19. The following statement regarding the cytomorphology of adenoma malignum is correct:
(a) Polygonal-shaped cells
(b) Fine brownish cytoplasmic pigment
(c) Pleomorphic cells arranged in 3D clusters and papillary fragments
(d) Syncytial arrangements
(e) Closely resembles benign endocervical cells

Q-20. The following cytomorphologic feature favors a diagnosis of adenoma malignum over endocervical adenocarcinoma in situ:
(a) Lack of single-lying cells
(b) Feathering at the edges of cell groups
(c) Loss of polarity within cell groups
(d) Tightly crowded sheets of glandular cells with overlapping nuclei
(e) Loss of cytoplasmic mucin

Q-21. Choose the correct statement regarding extramammary Paget's disease:
(a) Extramammary Paget's disease is confined to the vulva.
(b) Extramammary Paget's disease manifests as burning or itchy pink-to-red vulvar lesions.
(c) Extramammary Paget's disease describes an invasive malignancy.
(d) Extramammary Paget's disease usually affects women in their third and fourth decade.
(e) Extramammary Paget's disease does not metastasize.

Q-22. Choose the correct statement regarding the cytomorphology of extramammary Paget's disease:
(a) Extramammary Paget's disease is usually associated with a background tumor diathesis.
(b) The cells are large with hyperchromatic nuclei and macronucleoli.
(c) The cytoplasm often contains ingested neutrophils.
(d) Single-file formations, seen in lobular carcinoma of the breast, may also be noted.
(e) If a cell-in-cell arrangement is seen, a diagnosis of squamous carcinoma should rather be made.

Q-23. On immunostaining, the cells in extramammary Paget's disease stain positively for the following stain:
(a) CK20
(b) GCDP-15
(c) HMB45
(d) Leu M1
(e) Melan A

Q-24. Choose the correct statement regarding metastatic malignancies to the cervix:
(a) Approximately 80 % of extrauterine malignancies are from ovary and fallopian tube.
(b) Extrauterine malignancies in Pap tests, occasionally have an associated tumor diathesis.
(c) The most common nongynecological extrauterine sites are breast, lung, and bladder.
(d) Tumors metastatic to the cervix usually appear morphologically different to primary cervical carcinoma.
(e) Metastatic tumors to the cervix occur more frequently than primary carcinoma in countries with well-organized cervical screening programs.

Q-25. Psammoma bodies may mimic the following structures *except*:
(a) Blue blobs of atrophy
(b) Inspissated mucus
(c) Calcified fragments of intrauterine contraceptive devices
(d) Taenia ovum
(e) Lubricant

Q-26. Choose the correct statement regarding metastatic breast carcinoma to the cervix:
(a) The most likely type of breast cancer to metastasize to the cervix is duct carcinoma.
(b) The frequency of cervical metastasis of breast cancer is estimated to be <1 %.
(c) Potential routes of dissemination include transcoelomic, lymphatic, and vascular spread.
(d) Cervical metastases of breast carcinoma are amenable to treatment with a good prognosis.
(e) Metastatic breast cancer is easily distinguishable from primary cervical adenocarcinoma.

Q-27. Choose the correct statement regarding hematolymphoid malignancies of the cervix:
(a) The cervix may be involved by primary or secondary lymphoma or leukemia.
(b) The exfoliation of malignant cells, in patients with cervical involvement by lymphoma/leukemia, is extensive in most patients.
(c) The age range of women with cervical involvement by lymphoma/leukemia is usually 50–70 years.
(d) Most lymphoma involving the cervix is of T-cell type.
(e) The 5-year survival is less than 10 %.

Q-28. The differential diagnosis of non-Hodgkin lymphoma on cervical smear includes all of the following *except*:
(a) Follicular cervicitis
(b) Endometrial stromal sarcoma
(c) Granulocytic sarcoma
(d) Small cell carcinoma
(e) Hodgkin lymphoma

Q-29. Choose the correct statement regarding primary urothelial carcinoma of the cervix:
(a) This tumor has a good prognosis.
(b) They are unrelated to HPV infection.
(c) They are associated with JC virus infection.
(d) They usually have an exophytic-papillary growth pattern.
(e) On immunostaining, they are CK7 positive and CK20 positive.

Q-30. Choose the correct statement regarding malignant mixed Mullerian tumor (MMMT) of the endometrium:
(a) This is an indolent tumor with a good prognosis.
(b) It is associated with HPV infection.
(c) They are seen, most often, in younger, premenopausal women.
(d) Predisposing factors include multiparity and malnutrition.
(e) The most common presenting symptom is vaginal bleeding.

Q-31. The epithelial component of a malignant mixed Mullerian tumor (MMMT) is usually:
(a) Endometrioid carcinoma
(b) Squamous carcinoma
(c) Papillary carcinoma
(d) Clear cell carcinoma
(e) Undifferentiated carcinoma

Q-32. Choose the correct statement regarding MMMT:
(a) If the malignant stromal component consists of smooth muscle, it is called "homologous."
(b) If the malignant stromal component consists of fat, it is called "homologous."
(c) If the malignant stromal component consists of endometrial stroma, it is called "heterologous."
(d) The differential diagnosis includes IUCD changes.
(e) Most Pap tests with MMMT comprise very few cells.

Q-33. Choose the correct statement regarding cervicovaginal malignant melanoma:
(a) They arise more frequently in the cervix than the vagina.
(b) They are seen most often in younger, premenopausal women.
(c) The cell of origin of malignant melanoma, in the cervicovaginal region, is the basal cell.
(d) The cytomorphologic findings may comprise either epithelioid or spindled features.
(e) The prognosis is generally good.

Q-34. Choose the correct statement regarding uterine sarcoma:
(a) Uterine sarcomas make up 20–25 % of all uterine malignancies.
(b) Signs and symptoms resemble uterine leiomyoma, but leiomyosarcoma occur more frequently.
(c) Some endometrial stromal sarcomas carry the t(7;17) translocation with involvement of JAZF1 and JJAZ1.
(d) Uterine leiomyosarcomas express estrogen, progesterone, and androgen receptors in 0–10 % of cases.
(e) Most endometrial stromal tumors show negative immunostaining for CD10.

Q-35. The following benign lesion of the cervix is associated with psammoma bodies:
(a) Follicular cervicitis
(b) Reparative change
(c) *Trichomonas* infection
(d) Lower urinary tract infection
(e) Ovarian inclusion cyst

Q-36. Choose the correct statement regarding metastatic ovarian carcinoma to the cervix:
(a) Spread from the ovary to the cervix occurs primarily via lymphatic spread.
(b) Metastatic ovarian carcinoma, on a Pap test, has neoplastic cells, ± clean background, and ± psammoma bodies.
(c) The most common ovarian tumor, metastatic to the cervix, is mucinous carcinoma.
(d) If cytoplasmic vacuoles are seen, the diagnosis is likely to be endometrial rather than metastatic ovarian, carcinoma.
(e) In most instances of ovarian carcinoma metastatic to the cervix, an extensive exfoliation of malignant cells is seen.

Q-37. Choose the correct statement regarding metastatic colorectal carcinoma to the cervix:
(a) The background often shows a tumor diathesis
(b) Tumor spread is through either lymphatics or hematogenous
(c) The cells have a polygonal shape with a large, hyperchromatic nucleus
(d) Extracellular collagen globules are noted
(e) Syncytial arrangements are seen

7.3 Image-Based Questions 38–63

Fig. 7.38

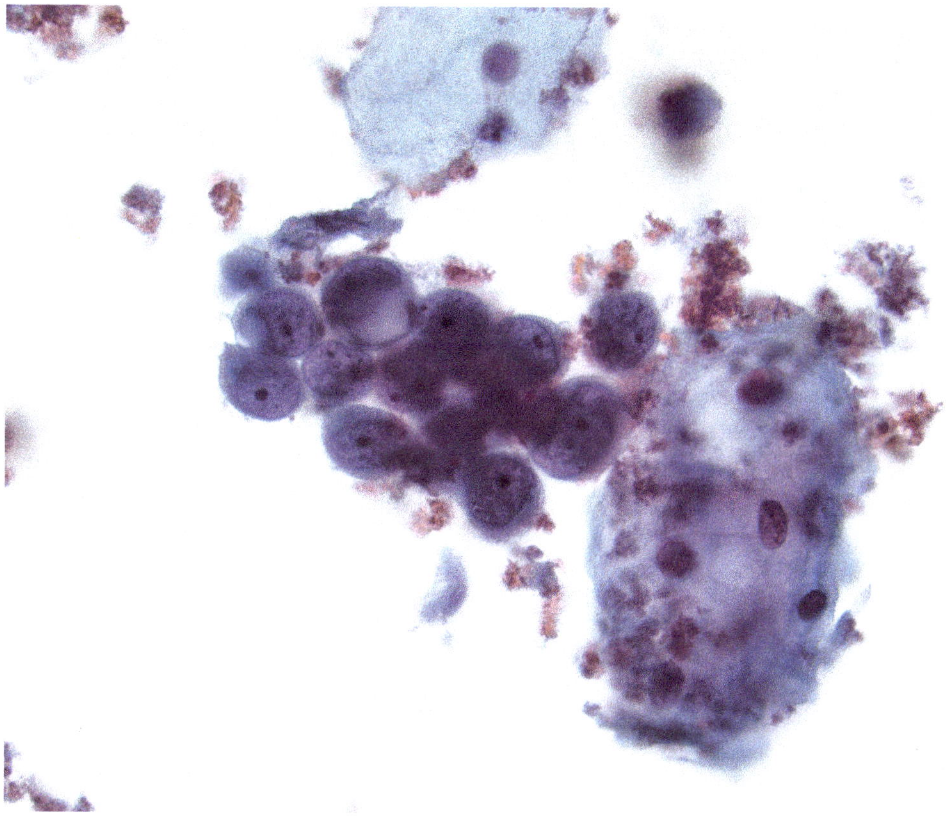

Q-38. This Pap test of a 70-year-old woman with a remote history of cancer who presents with abnormal bleeding most likely represents a diagnosis of:
(a) Poorly differentiated squamous cell carcinoma
(b) Metastatic adenocarcinoma of colon
(c) Metastatic carcinoma of breast
(d) Atypical endometrial cells
(e) Adenocarcinoma of endocervix

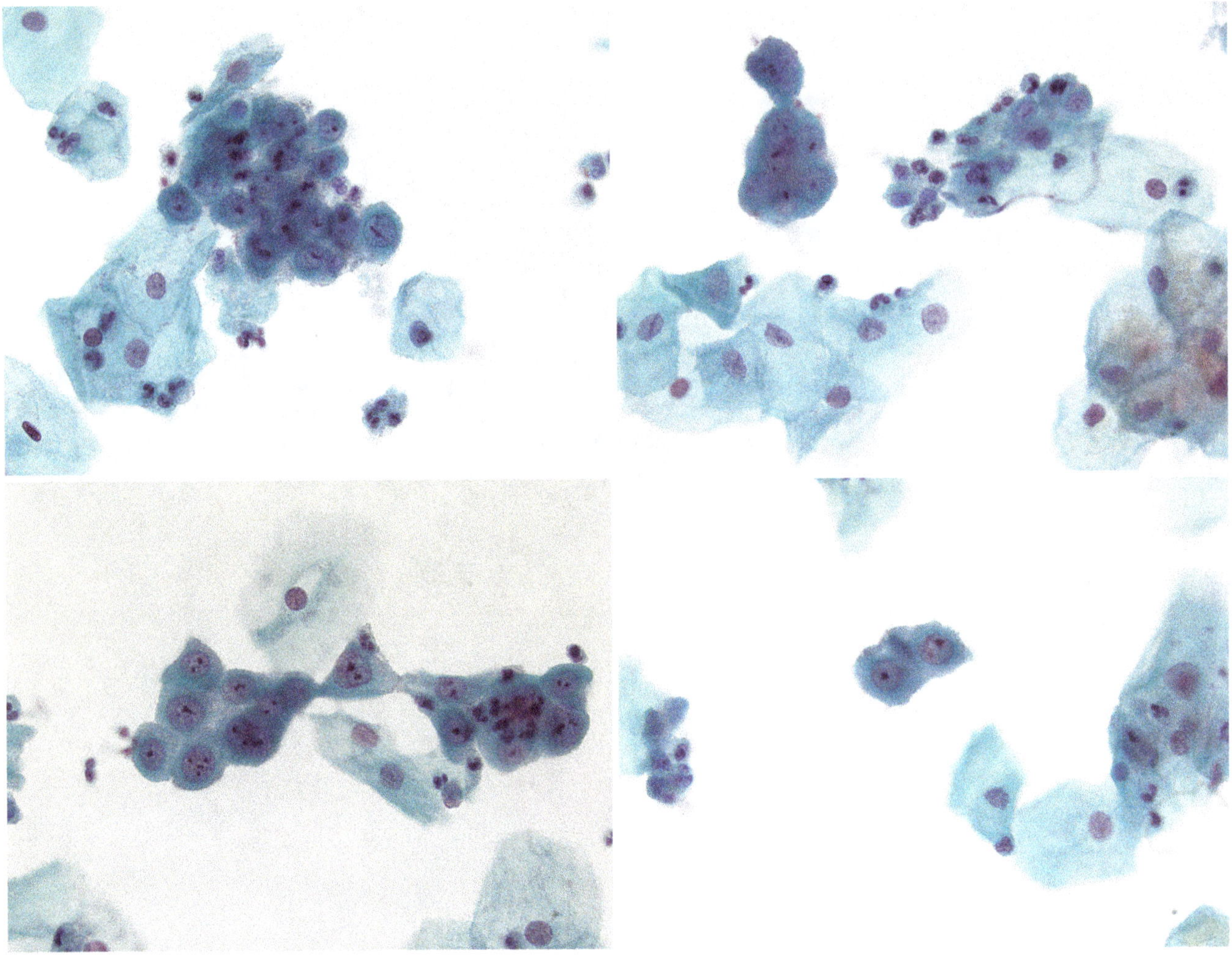

Fig. 7.39

Q-39. These images of a Pap test from a 58-year-old woman with a history of an autoimmune disease *most likely* represent:

(a) Squamous cell carcinoma
(b) Adenocarcinoma
(c) Repair/reactive change
(d) Pemphigus vulgaris
(e) Malignant melanoma

Fig. 7.40

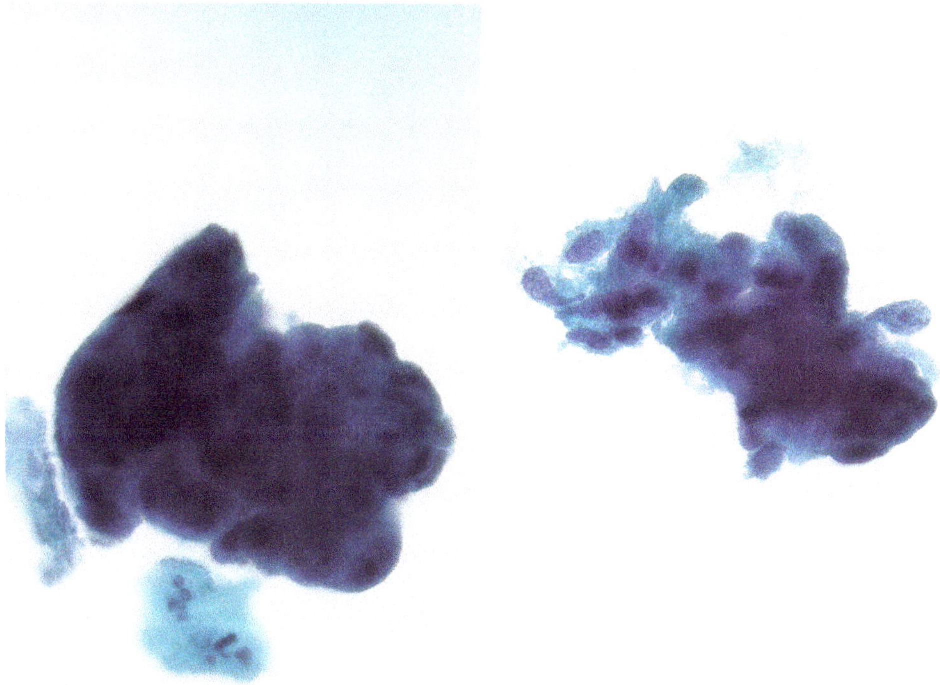

Q-40. These images of a Pap test from a 73-year-old woman presenting with postmenopausal bleeding most likely represent a diagnosis of:
(a) HSIL
(b) Malignant mixed Mullerian tumor/carcinosarcoma
(c) Squamous cell carcinoma
(d) Atypical glandular cells
(e) Adenocarcinoma of endocervix

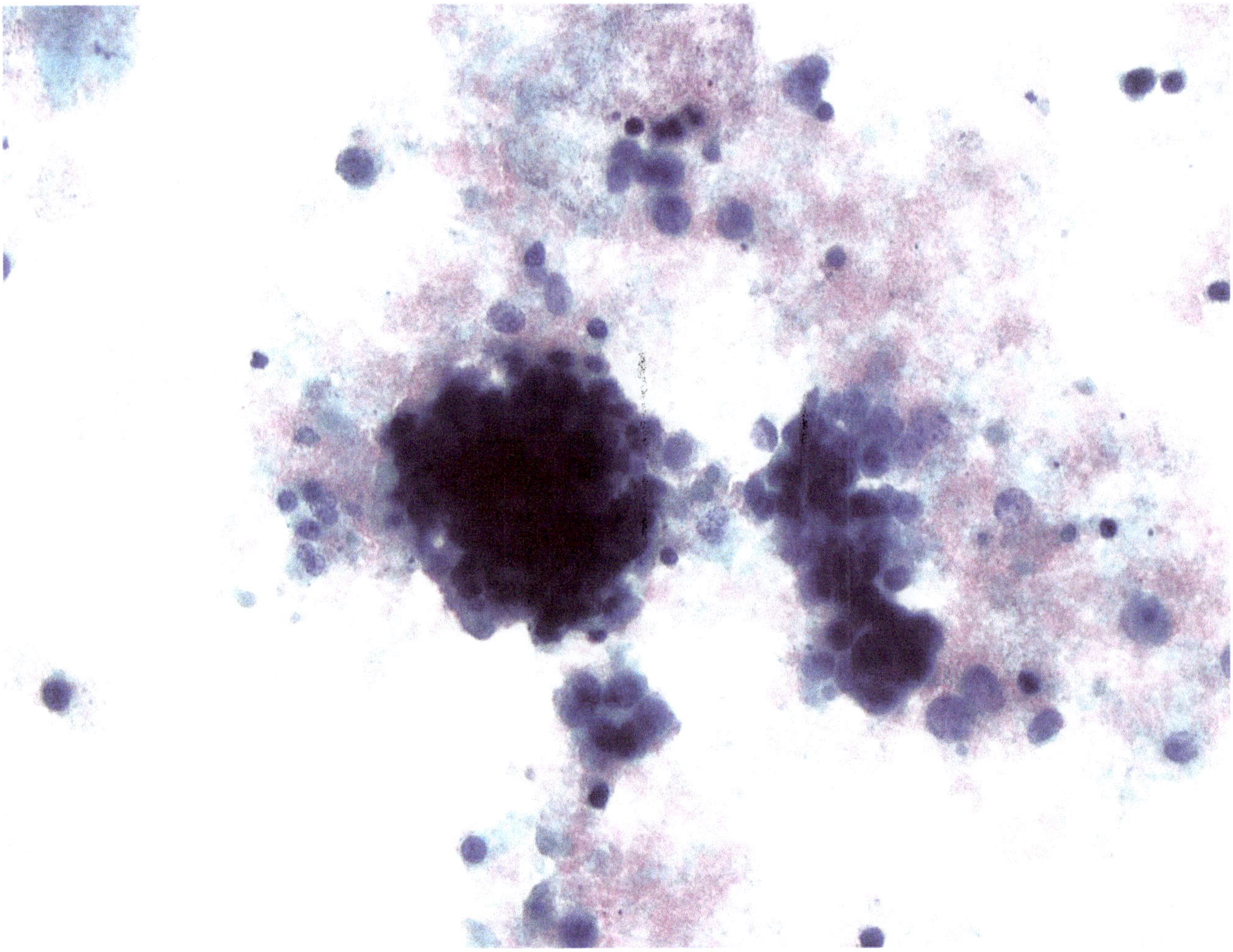

Fig. 7.41

Q-41. This 40-year-old woman had a history of atypical Pap tests. The current liquid-based annual Pap test revealed:
(a) Follicular cervicitis
(b) Benign endometrial cells
(c) Squamous cell carcinoma
(d) Small cell carcinoma
(e) HSIL

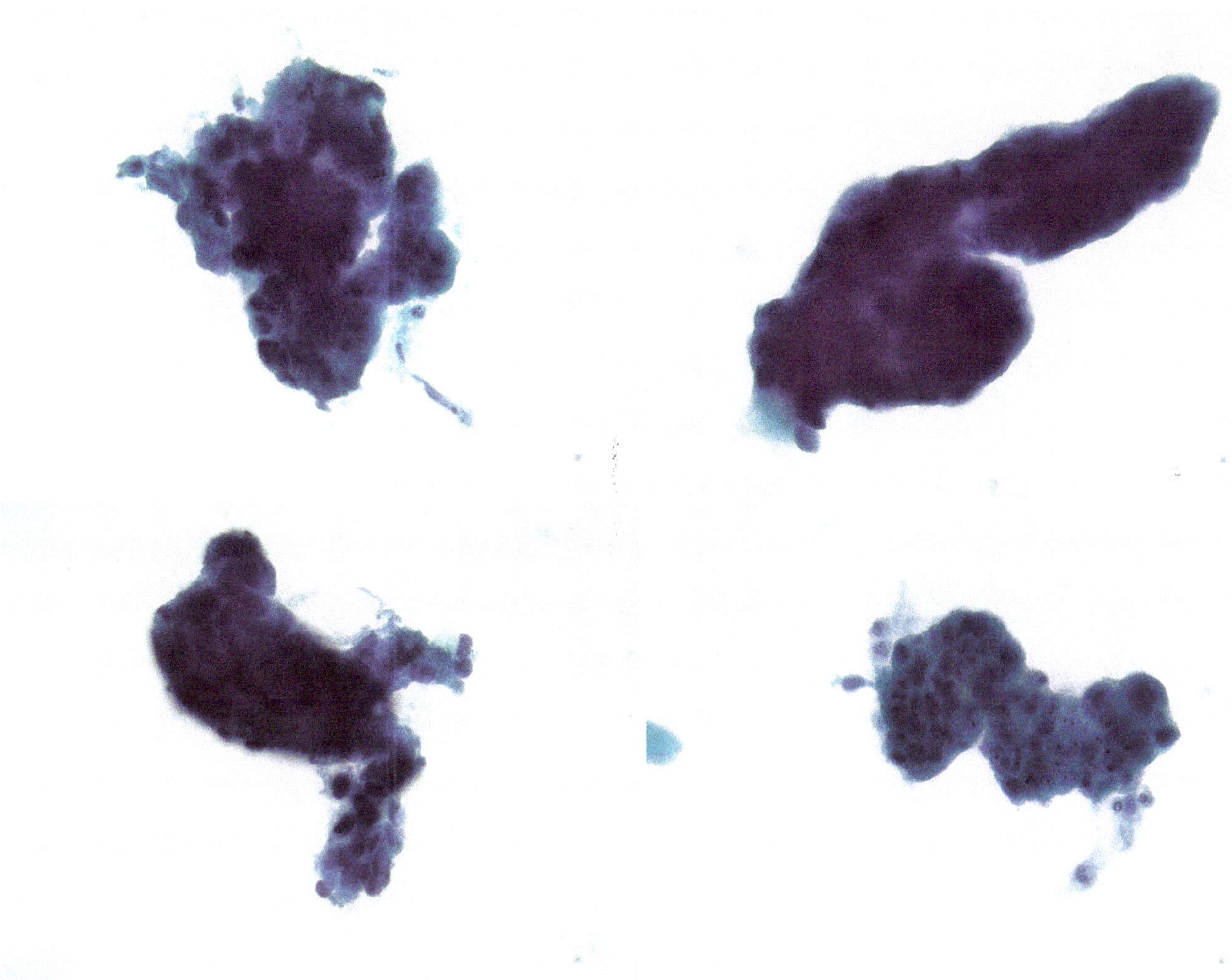

Fig. 7.42

Q-42. The Pap test from a 54-year-old woman showed the cells seen in this image. Her follow-up endocervical and endometrial biopsies were both negative for malignancy. The most likely source of the cells is:

(a) Endometrium
(b) Breast
(c) Colon
(d) Ovary
(e) Endocervix

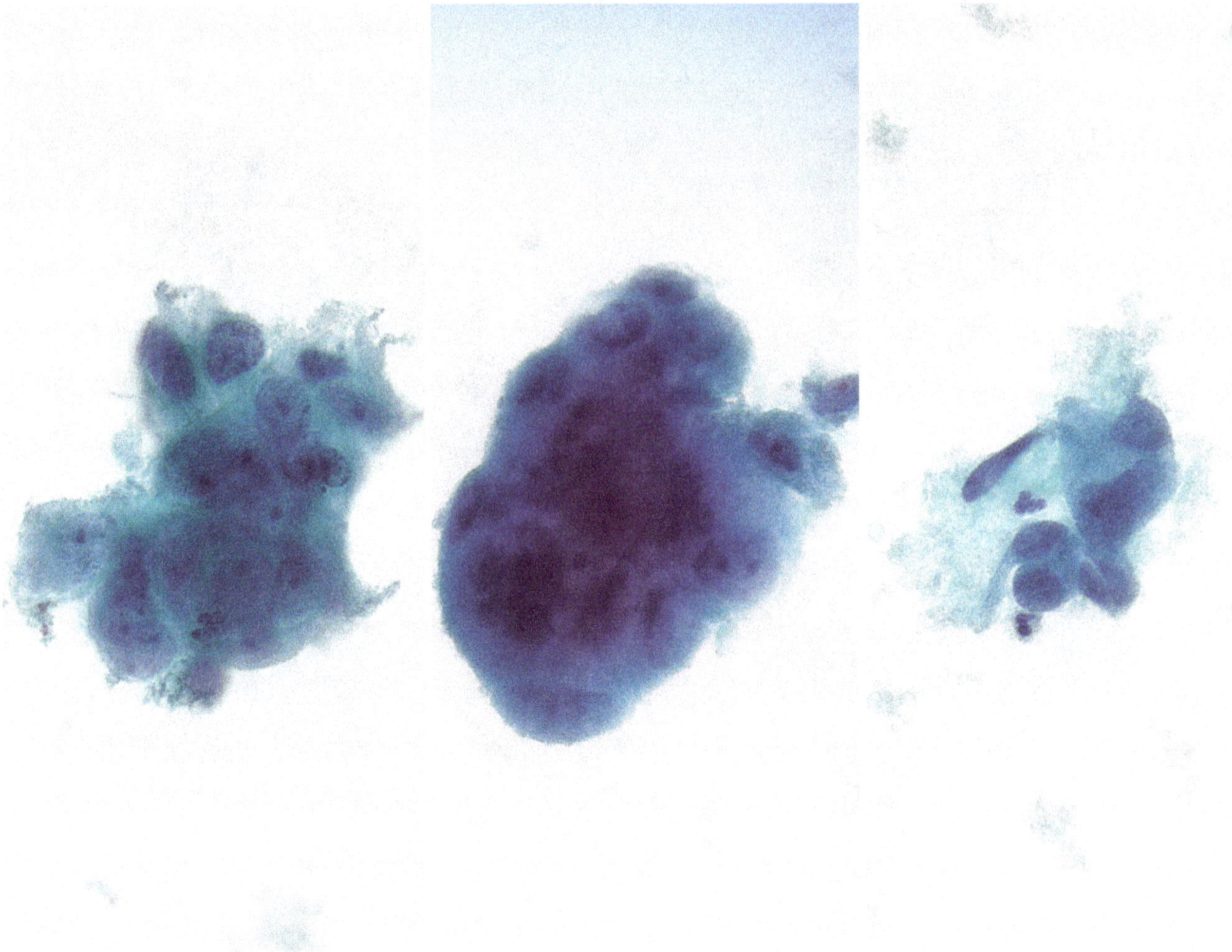

Fig. 7.43

Q-43. These are the images of a Pap test from an 80-year-old woman who developed postmenopausal bleeding. The most appropriate next step in management is:

(a) HPV DNA test
(b) Colposcopy
(c) LEEP cone biopsy
(d) Endocervical curettage
(e) Endometrial curettage

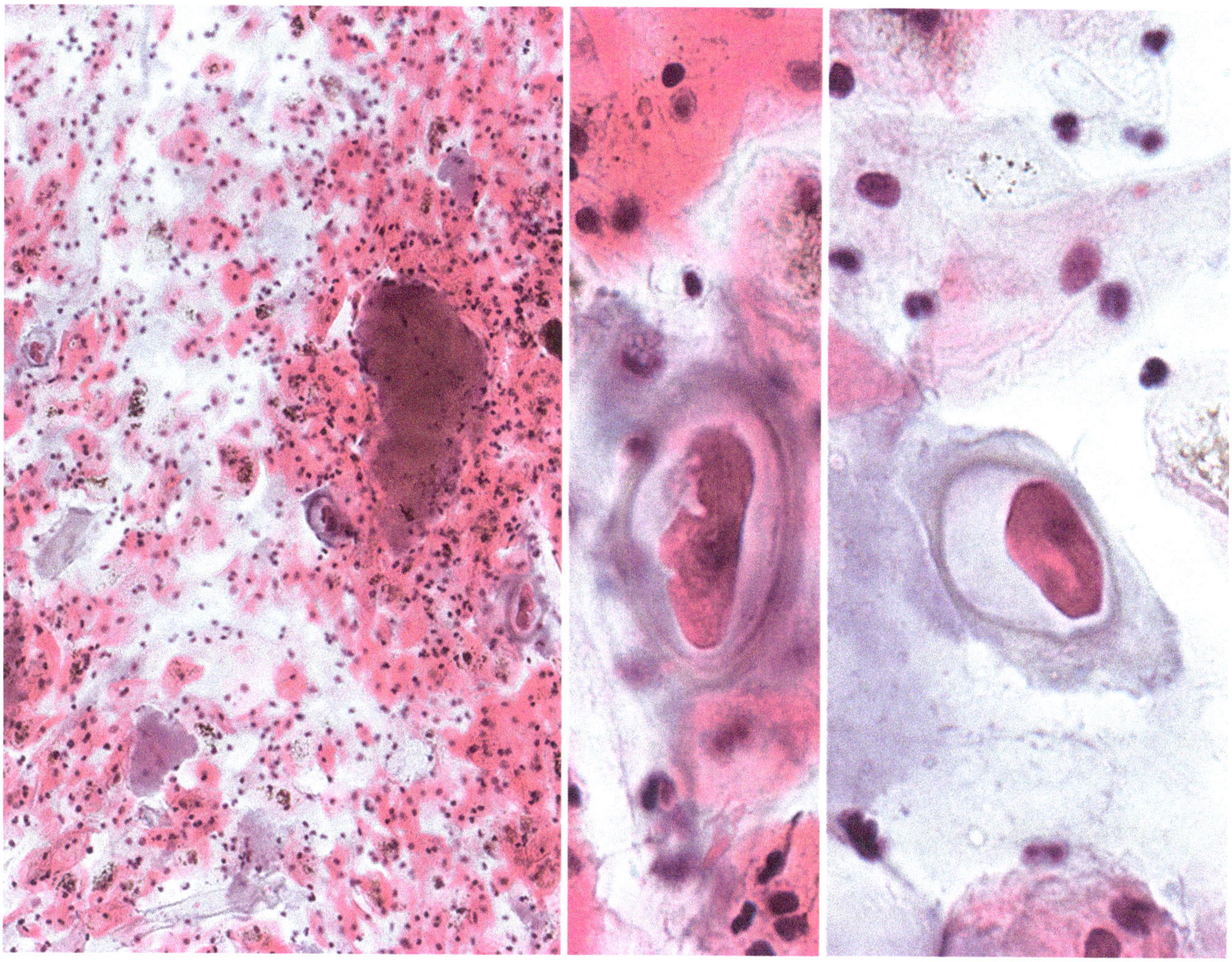

Fig. 7.44

Q-44. These images of a Pap test from a 21-year-old woman *most likely* represent:

(a) *Molluscum contagiosum* body like
(b) Squamous cell carcinoma
(c) LSIL
(d) CMV
(e) HSV

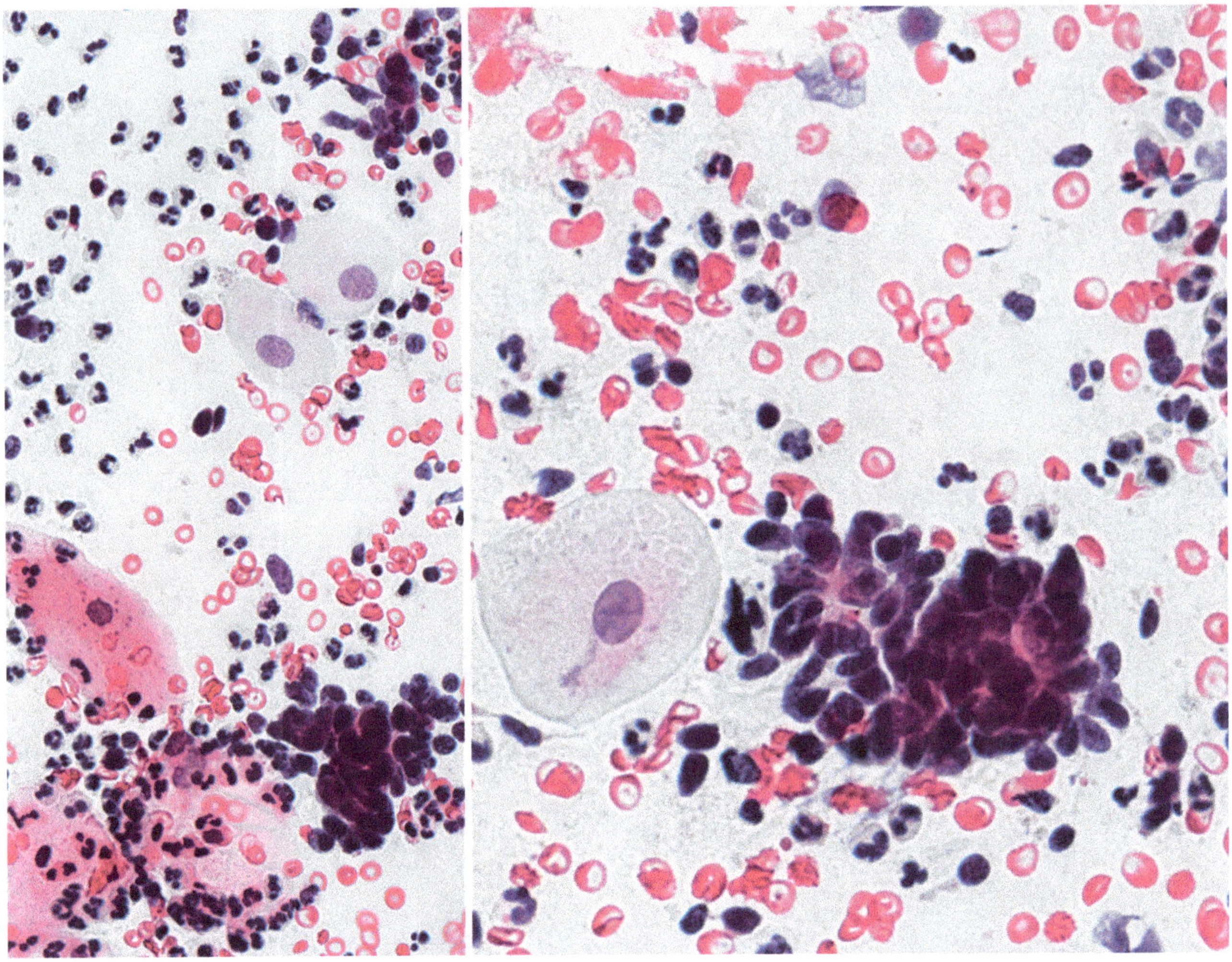

Fig. 7.45

Q-45. These images of a routine conventional Pap test of 35-year-old woman revealed:

(a) Adenocarcinoma in situ (AIS) of endocervix
(b) Small cell carcinoma
(c) HSIL
(d) Benign endometrial cells
(e) Atypical endometrial cells

Fig. 7.46

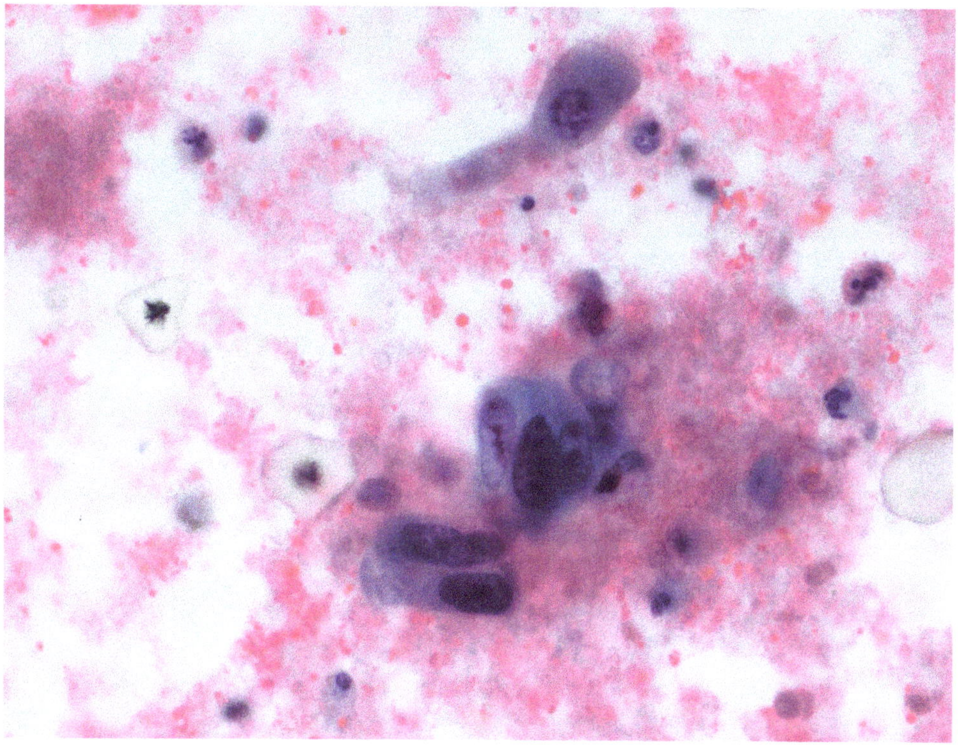

Q-46. This image of a Pap test from a 70-year-old woman presenting with postmenopausal bleeding most likely represents a diagnosis of:

(a) Adenocarcinoma of endocervix
(b) Metastatic adenocarcinoma of colon
(c) Squamous cell carcinoma
(d) Atypical glandular cells
(e) Adenocarcinoma of endometrium

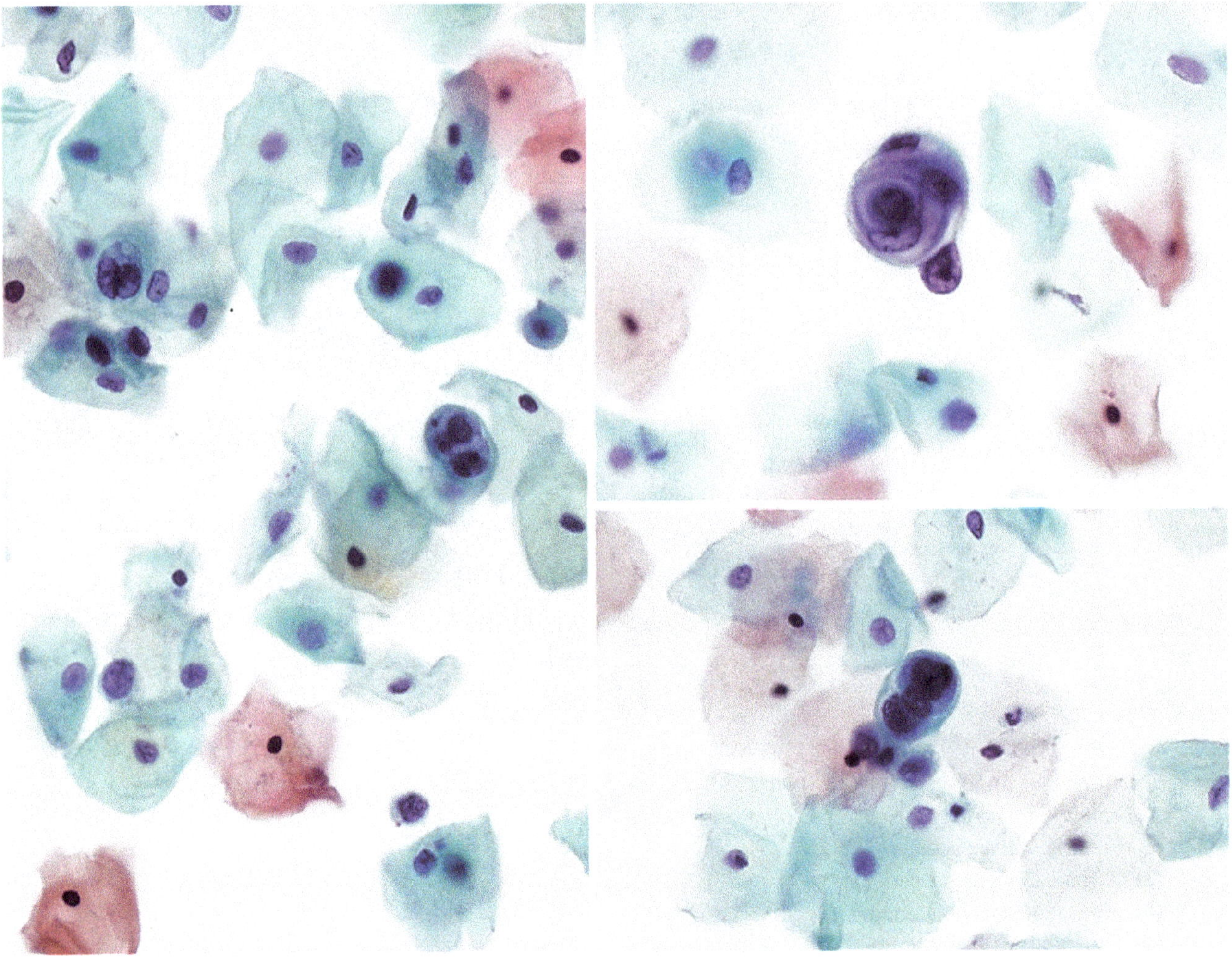

Fig. 7.47

Q-47. These images of a Pap test from a 68-year-old woman with prior negative Pap tests *most likely* represent:
(a) Squamous cell carcinoma
(b) Adenocarcinoma
(c) Metastatic carcinoma
(d) Reactive cellular change
(e) Paget's disease

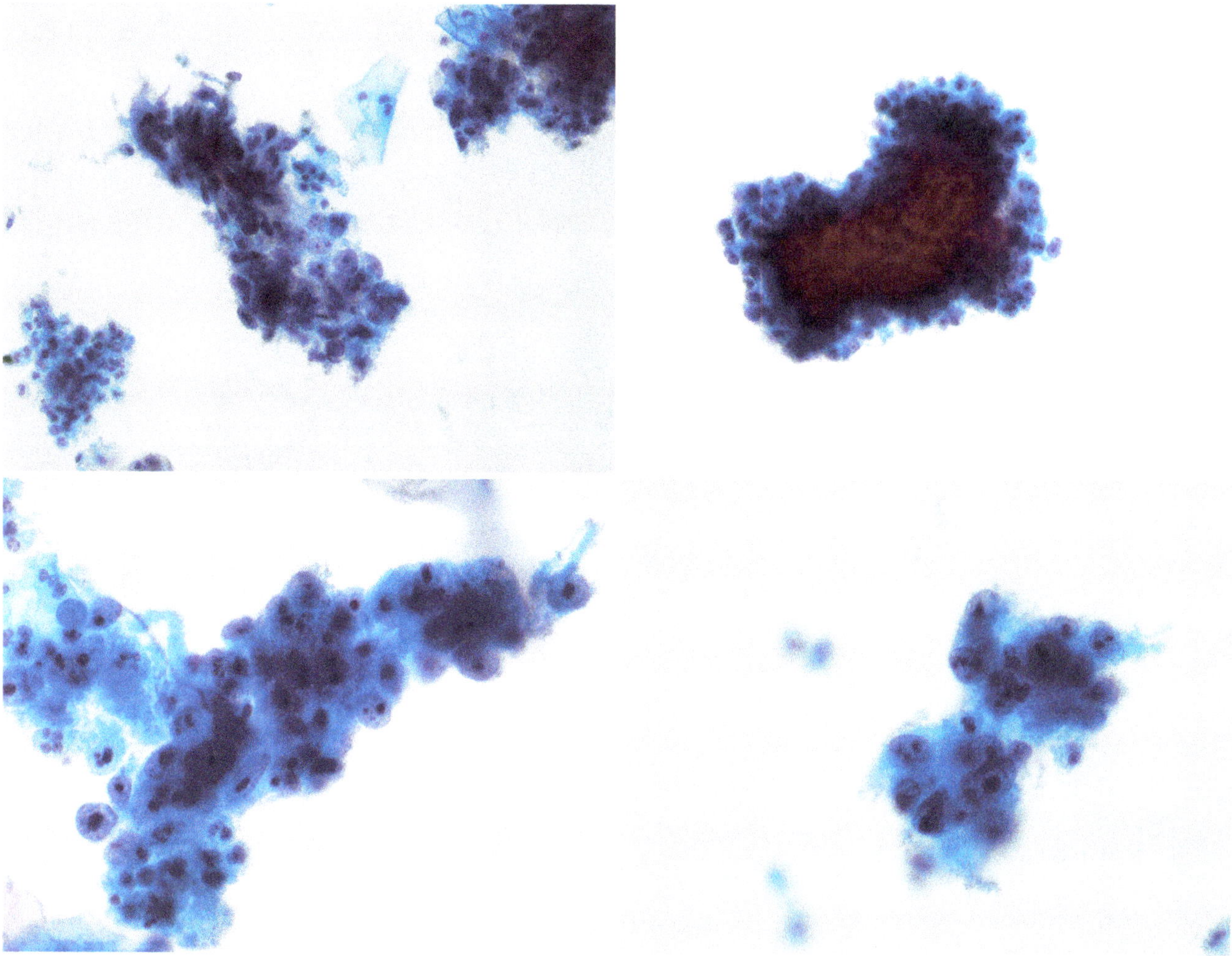

Fig. 7.48 Include credit (*Image courtesy*: *Dr. R. Marshall Austin*)

Q-48. This is a routine Pap test of a 36-year-old woman 1 year after the birth of her child. The current liquid-based annual Pap test revealed:

(a) Adenocarcinoma of cervix
(b) Benign endometrial cells
(c) Squamous cell carcinoma
(d) Placental site trophoblastic tumor
(e) HSIL

Fig. 7.49

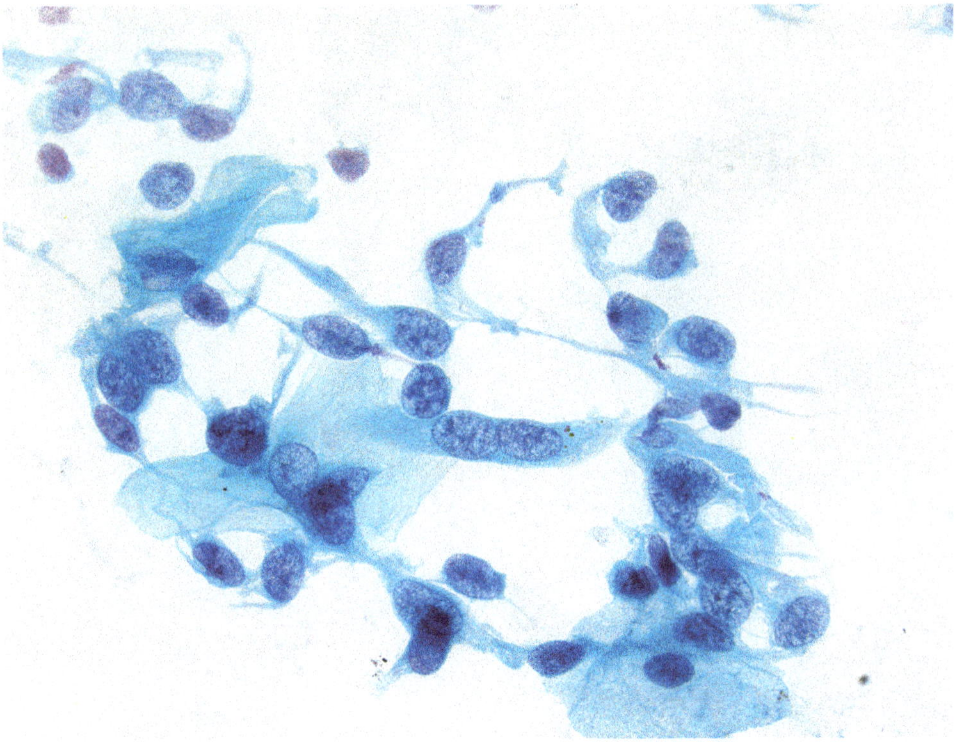

Q-49. The ThinPrep image from a 66-year-old woman most likely represents a diagnosis of:
(a) Atypical repair
(b) HSIL
(c) Squamous cell carcinoma
(d) Leiomyosarcoma
(e) Melanoma

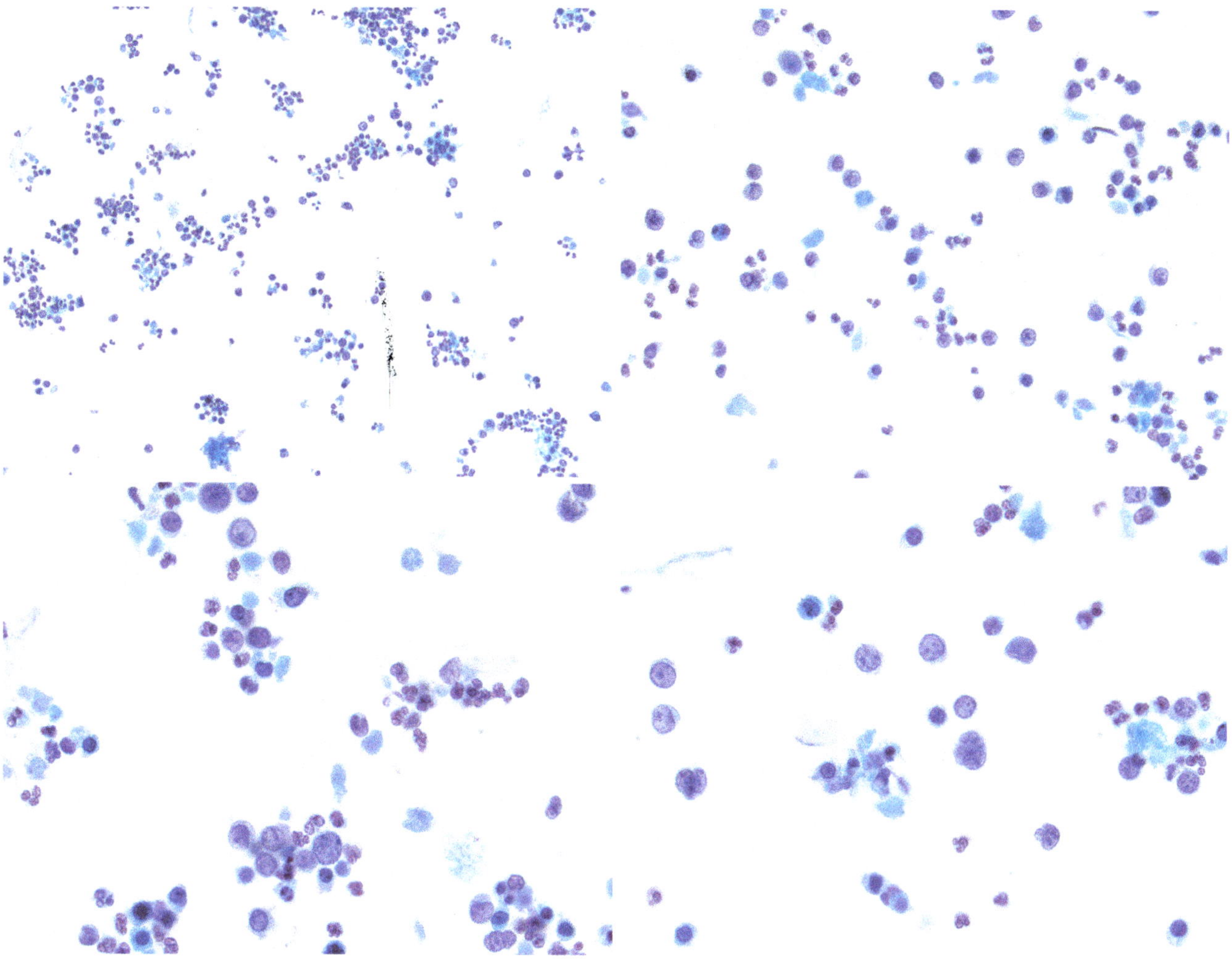

Fig. 7.50

Q-50. This image of a Pap test from a 65-year-old woman presenting with a cervical mass *most likely* represents a diagnosis of:
(a) Follicular cervicitis
(b) Small cell carcinoma
(c) Squamous cell carcinoma
(d) Atypical endometrial cells
(e) Lymphoma

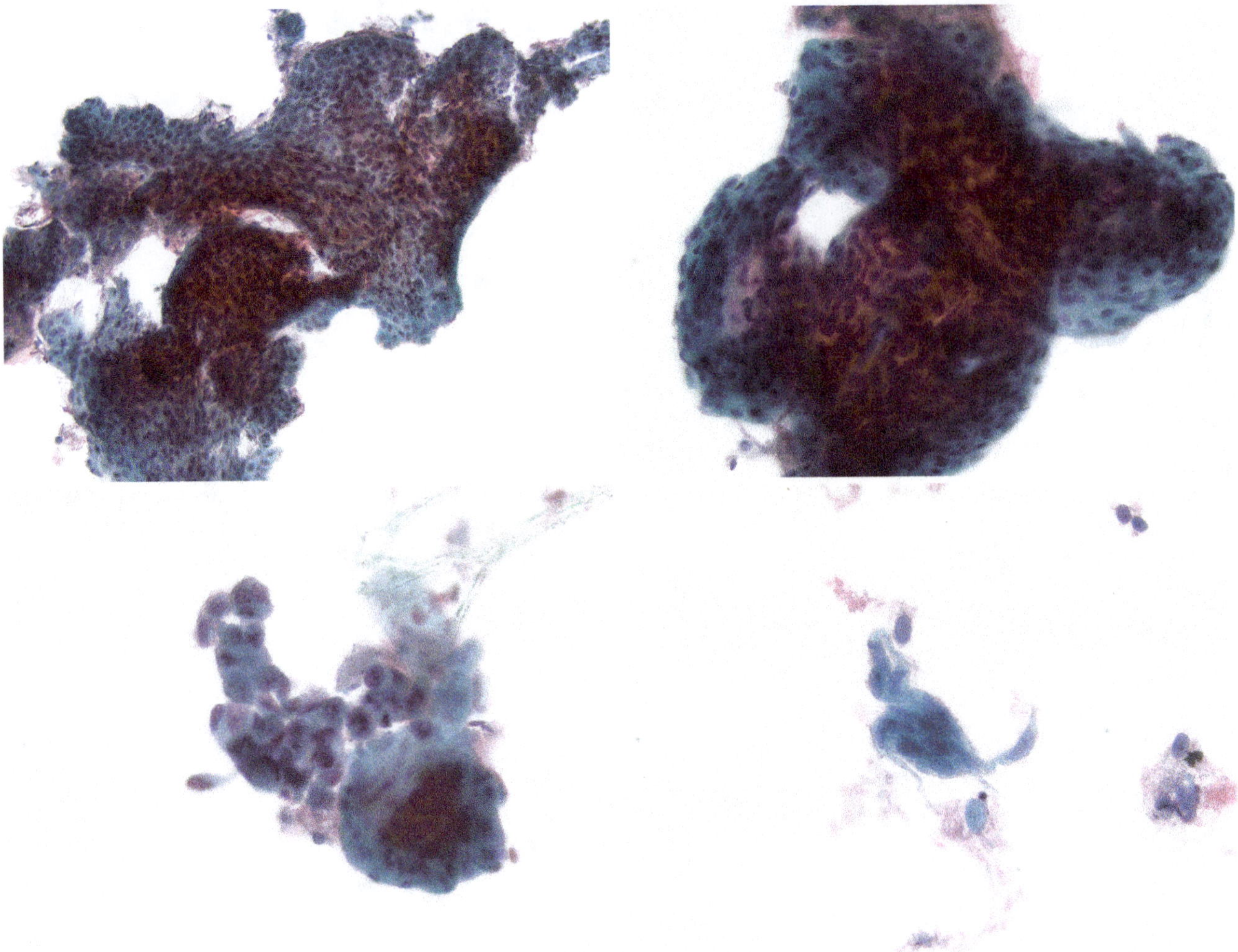

Fig. 7.51

Q-51. These images of a Pap test from a 58-year-old woman with vaginal bleeding and hematuria *most likely* represent:

(a) Squamous cell carcinoma
(b) HSIL
(c) Metastatic urothelial carcinoma
(d) Atrophy
(e) Reactive cellular changes

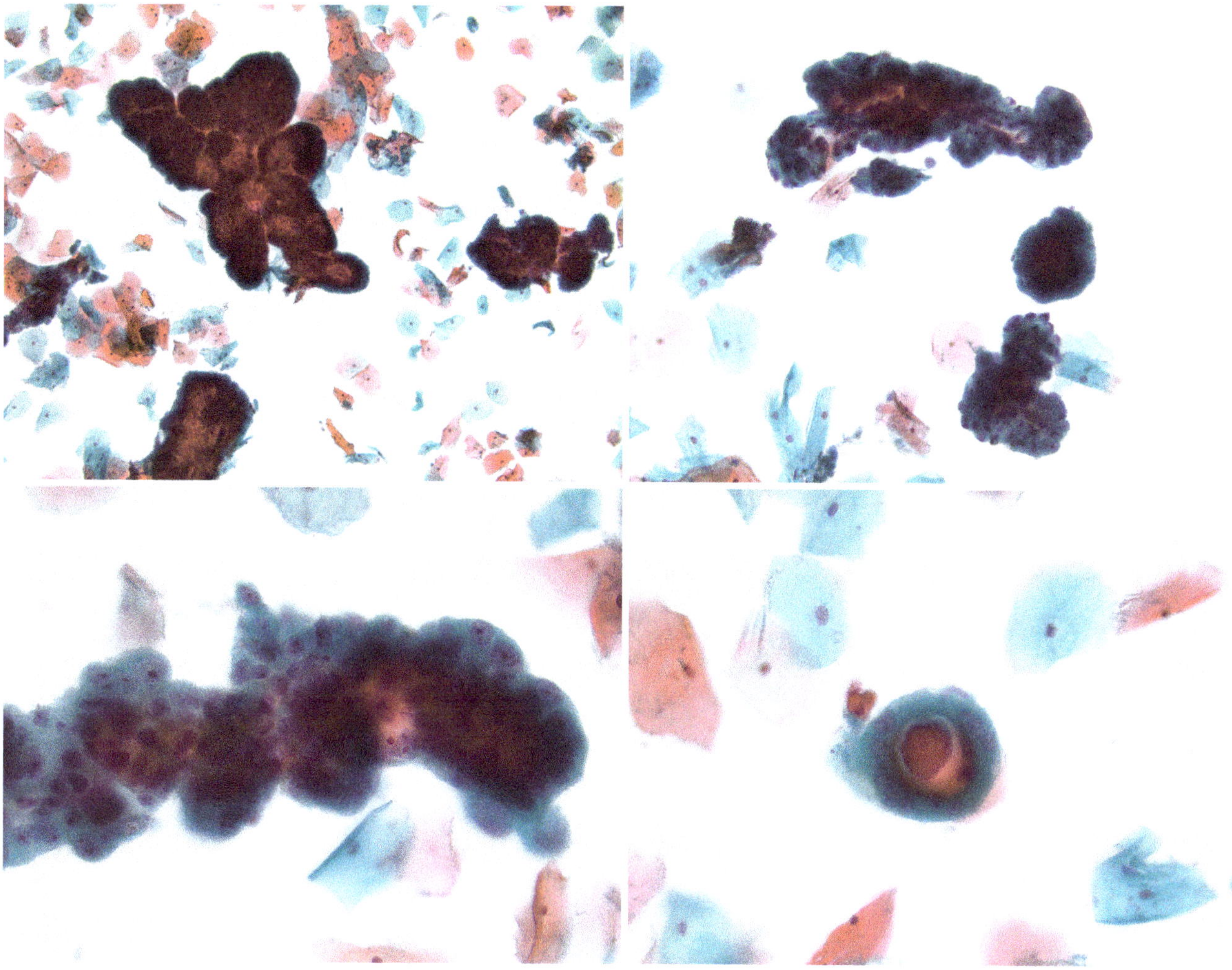

Fig. 7.52

Q-52. These images of Pap test from a 51-year-old woman MOST LIKELY represent:

(a) Endometrioid adenocarcinoma
(b) Endocervical adenocarcinoma
(c) Metastatic ovarian papillary serous carcinoma
(d) Metastatic urothelial carcinoma
(e) Endometrial polyp

Fig. 7.53

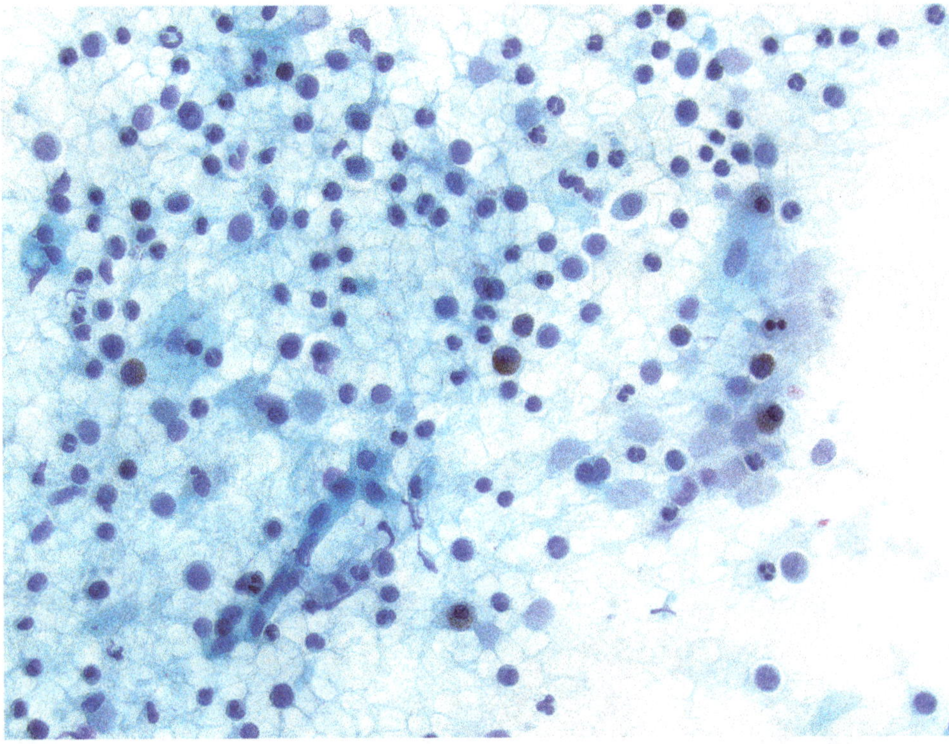

Q-53. This 46-year-old woman most likely has:

(a) Follicular cervicitis
(b) Endometrial cells in woman >40 years old
(c) HSIL
(d) Metastatic carcinoma
(e) Leukemia

Fig. 7.54

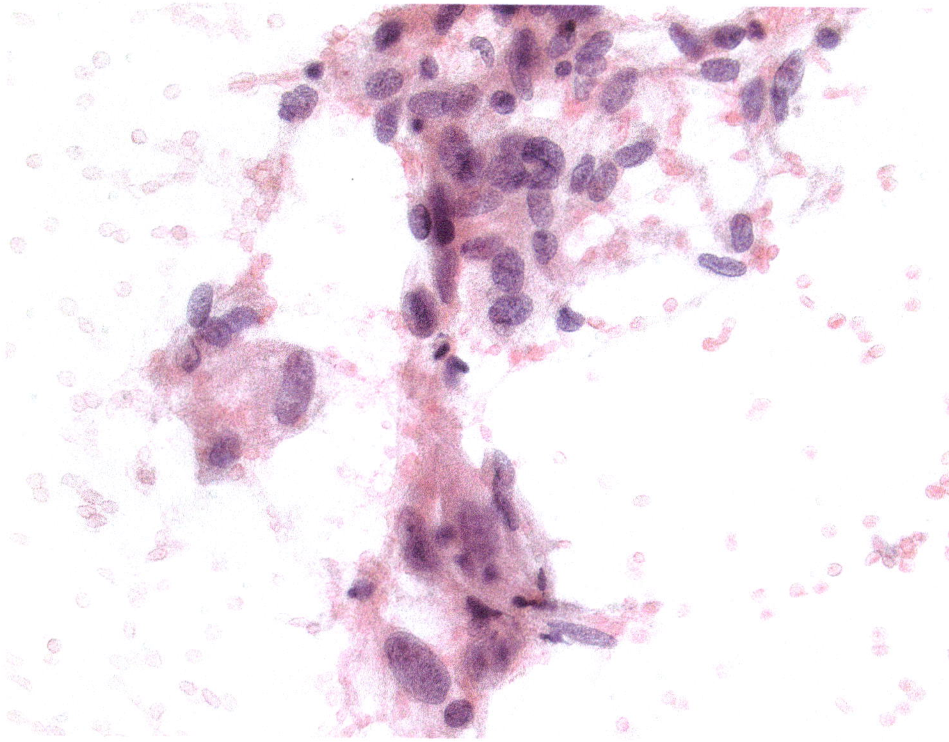

Q-54. This conventional Pap smear from a 56-year-old woman with a large pelvic mass MOST LIKELY represents:
(a) Reactive cellular change
(b) LSIL
(c) Leiomyosarcoma
(d) Atypical repair
(e) Melanoma

Fig. 7.55

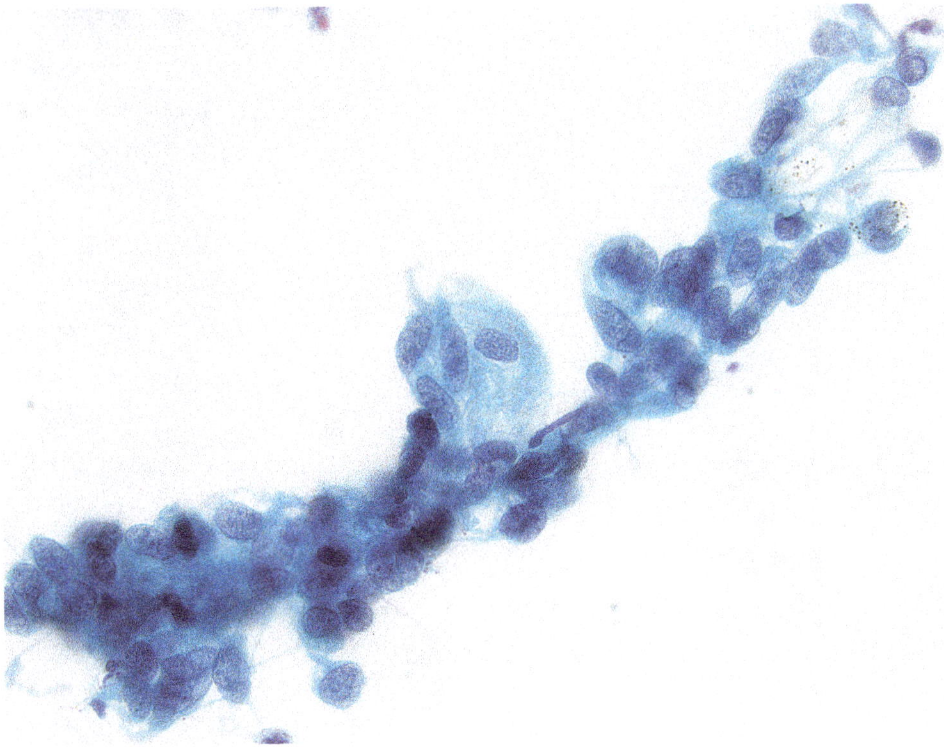

Q-55. The Pap test image from a 45-year-old woman most likely represents a diagnosis of:
- (a) Leiomyosarcoma
- (b) Melanoma
- (c) Squamous cell carcinoma
- (d) Atypical repair
- (e) HSIL

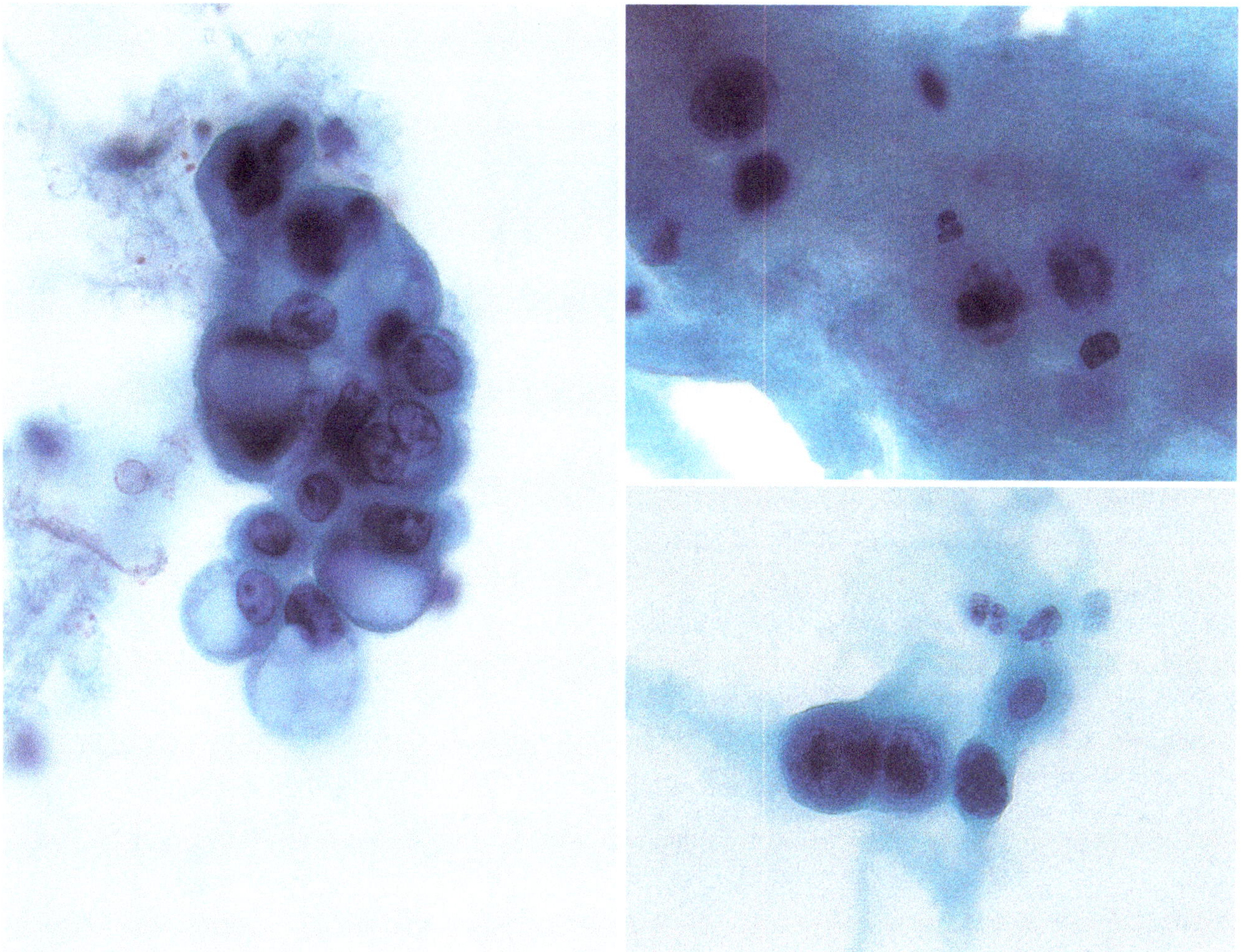

Fig. 7.56

Q-56. These ThinPrep images from an 82-year-old woman with postmenopausal bleeding *most likely* represent:

(a) Squamous cell carcinoma
(b) HSIL
(c) Endometrial adenocarcinoma
(d) MMMT of endometrium
(e) Adenosquamous carcinoma of endocervix

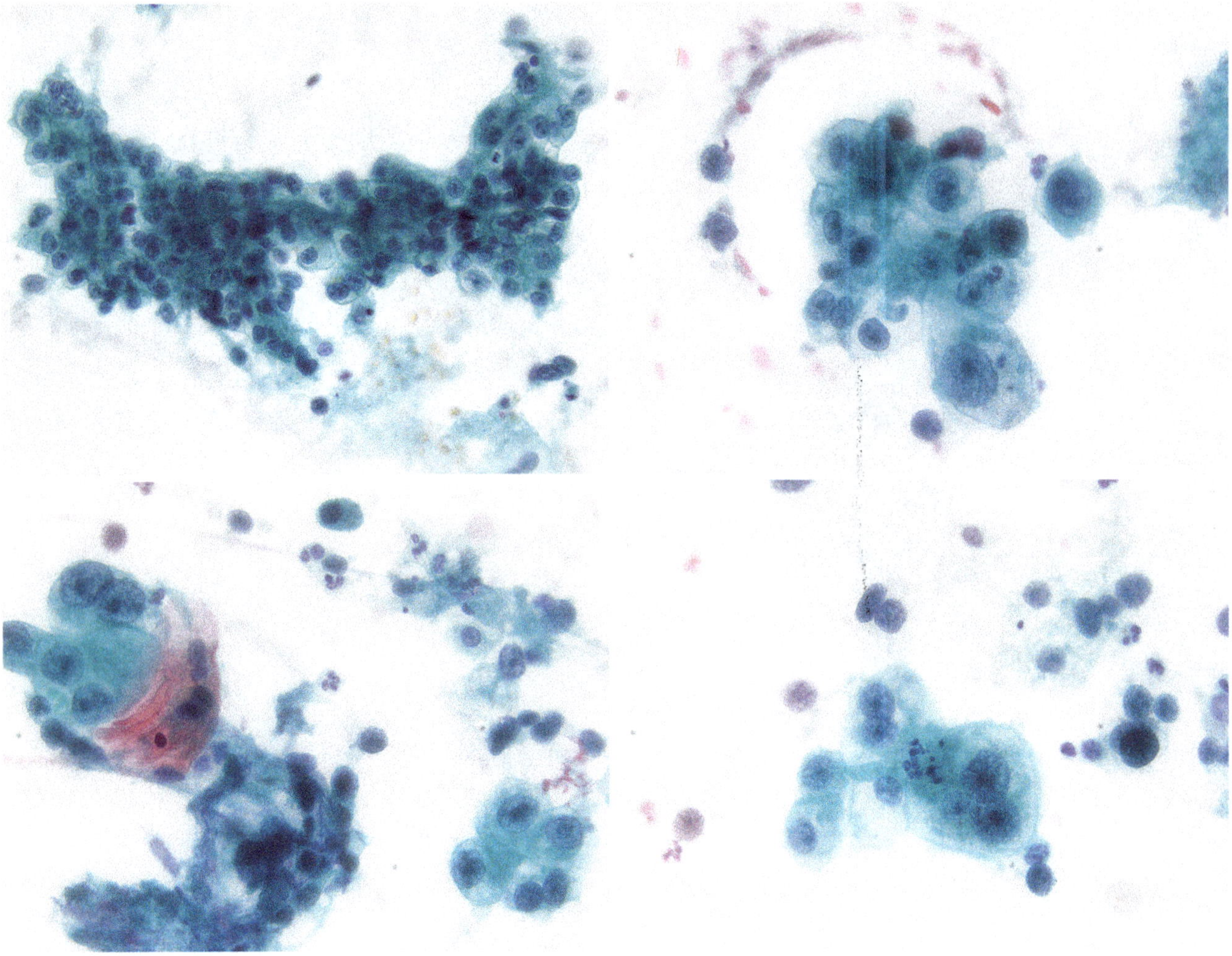

Fig. 7.57

Q-57. The images of this conventional Pap smear from a 76-year-old woman *most likely* represent:
(a) Reactive endocervical cells
(b) Atypical repair
(c) Endocervical adenocarcinoma
(d) Endometrial adenocarcinoma
(e) Metastatic clear cell carcinoma

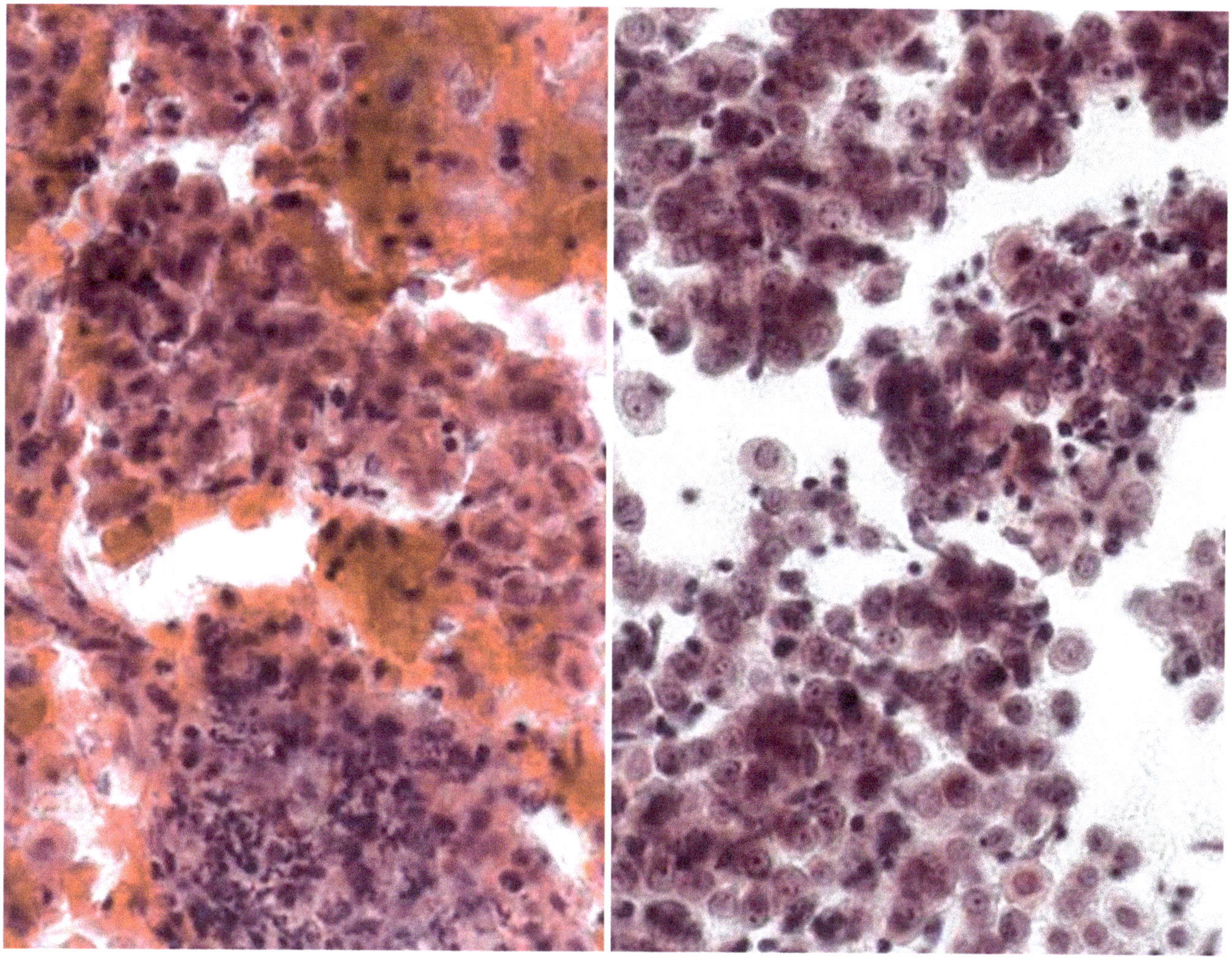

Fig. 7.58

Q-58. The following image is from a conventional Pap smear. What is the most likely diagnosis?
(a) Endocervical adenocarcinoma
(b) Endocervical adenocarcinoma in situ
(c) Squamous carcinoma
(d) Pemphigus vulgaris
(e) Cytomegalovirus

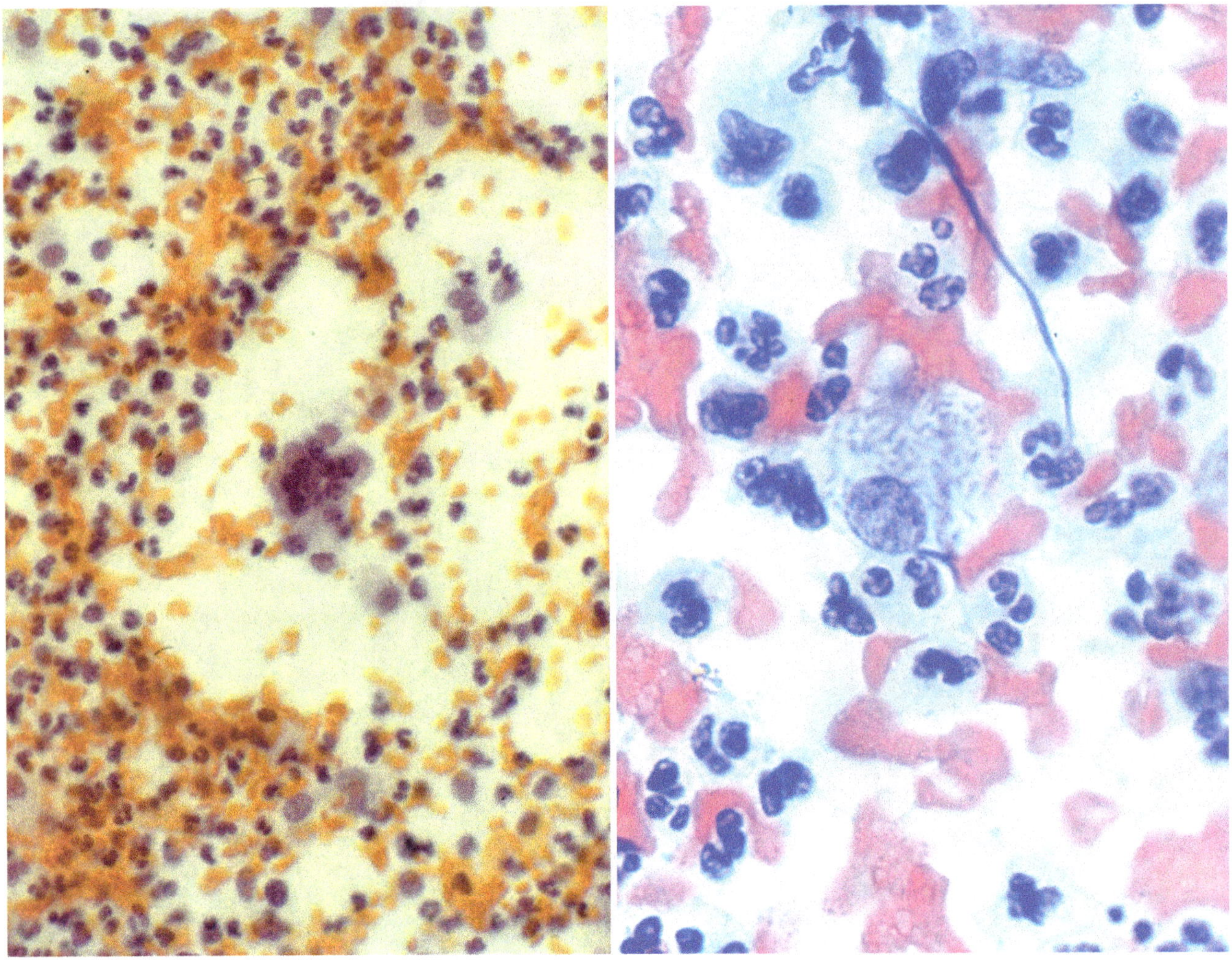

Fig. 7.59

Q-59. This image is from a 38-year-old female with a vaginal discharge. The most likely causative organism is:

(a) Herpes simplex virus
(b) Cytomegalovirus
(c) *Treponema pallidum*
(d) *Mycobacterium tuberculosis*
(e) *Klebsiella granulomatis*

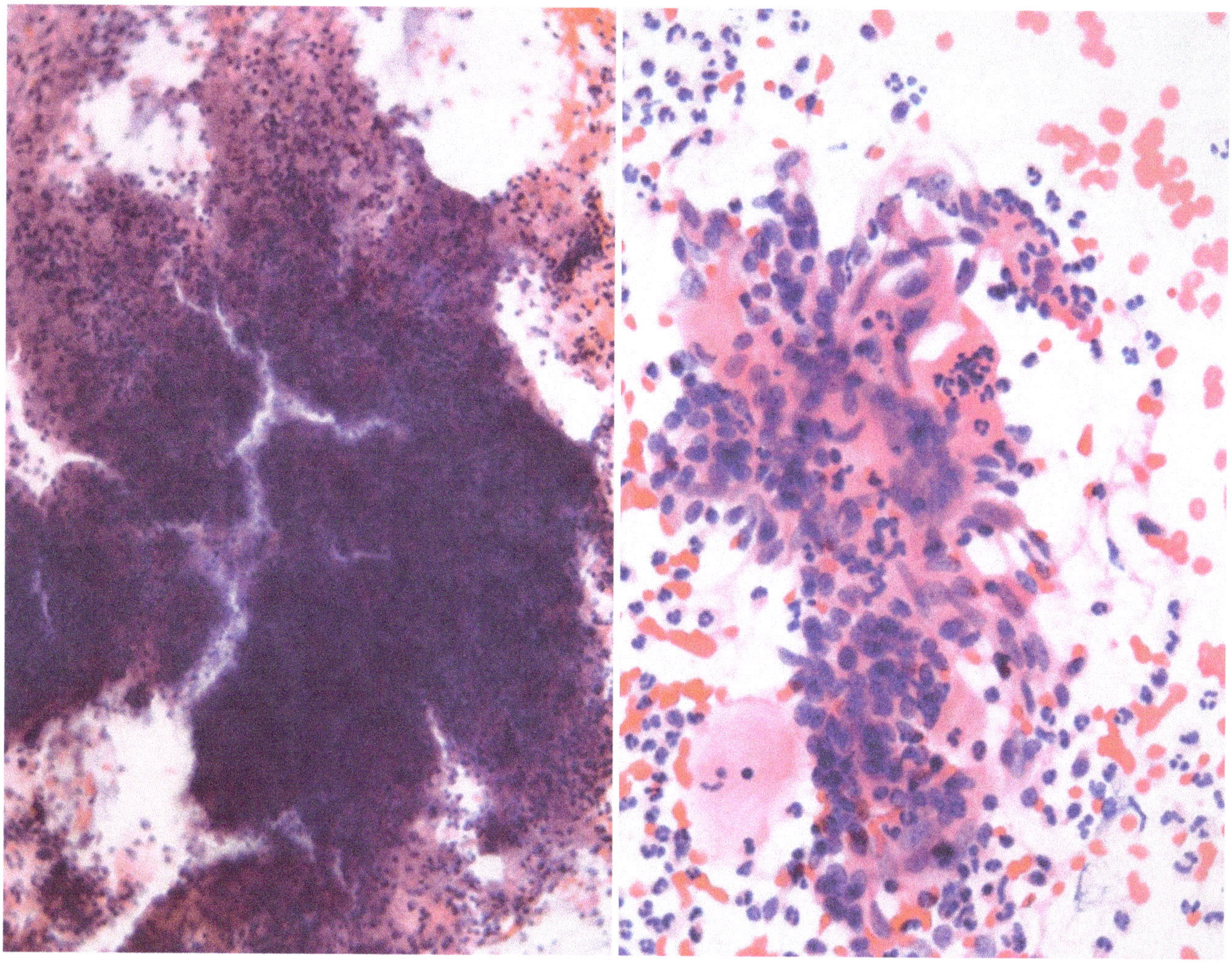

Fig. 7.60

Q-60. This Pap smear is from a 35-year-old asymptomatic woman who underwent a routine conventional Pap smear. On examination, the cervix appeared suspicious. The most likely diagnosis is:

(a) Tuberculosis
(b) Squamous carcinoma
(c) Granuloma inguinale
(d) High-grade squamous intraepithelial lesion
(e) Leiomyosarcoma

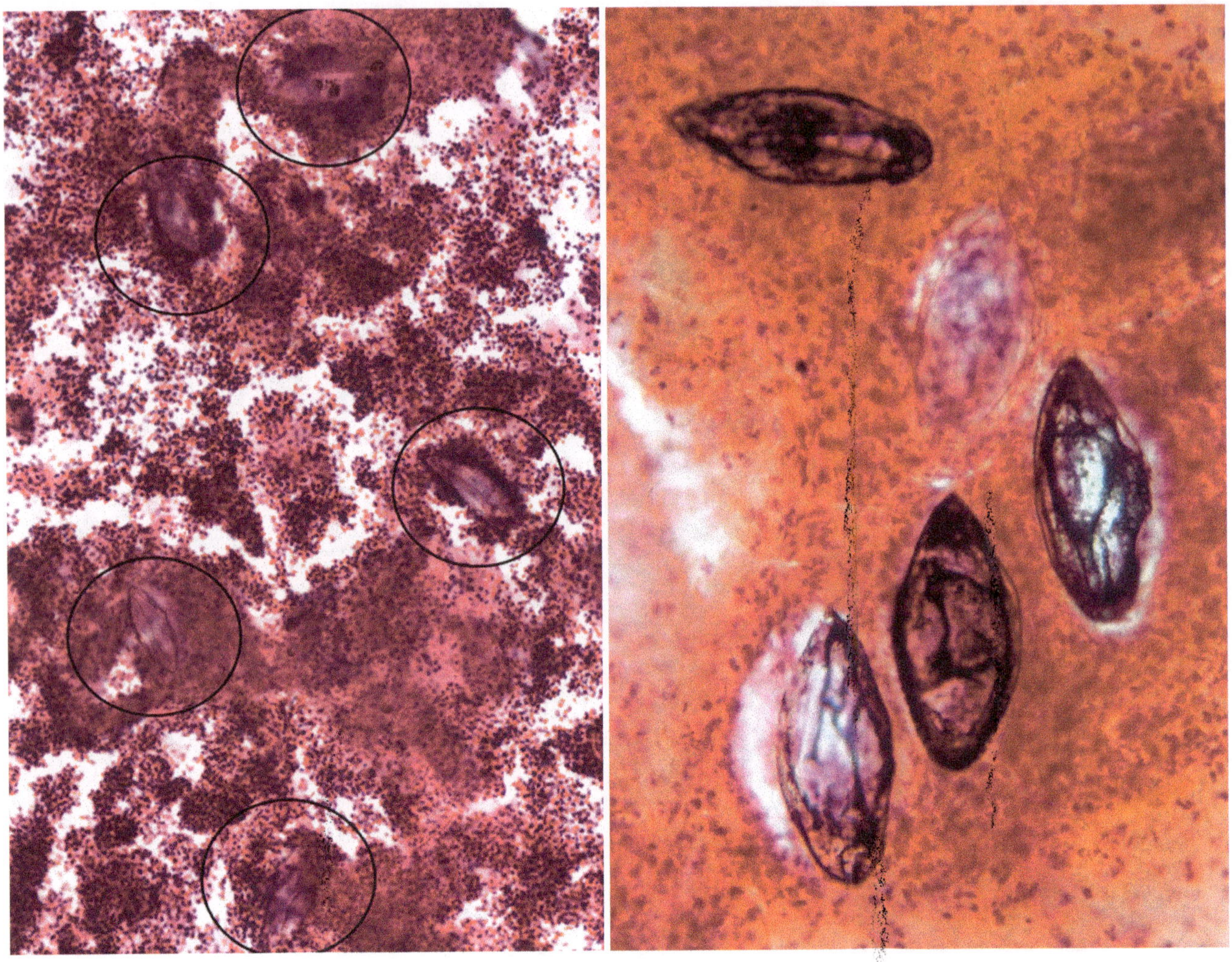

Fig. 7.61

Q-61. The following image is from a 40-year-old female who underwent routine cervical smear. On examination the cervix looked suspicious. A Pap test was performed. What is the most likely diagnosis?

(a) *Schistosomiasis haematobium*
(b) *Ascaris lumbricoides*
(c) *Trichuris trichiura*
(d) *Taenia solium*
(e) Enterobius vermicularis

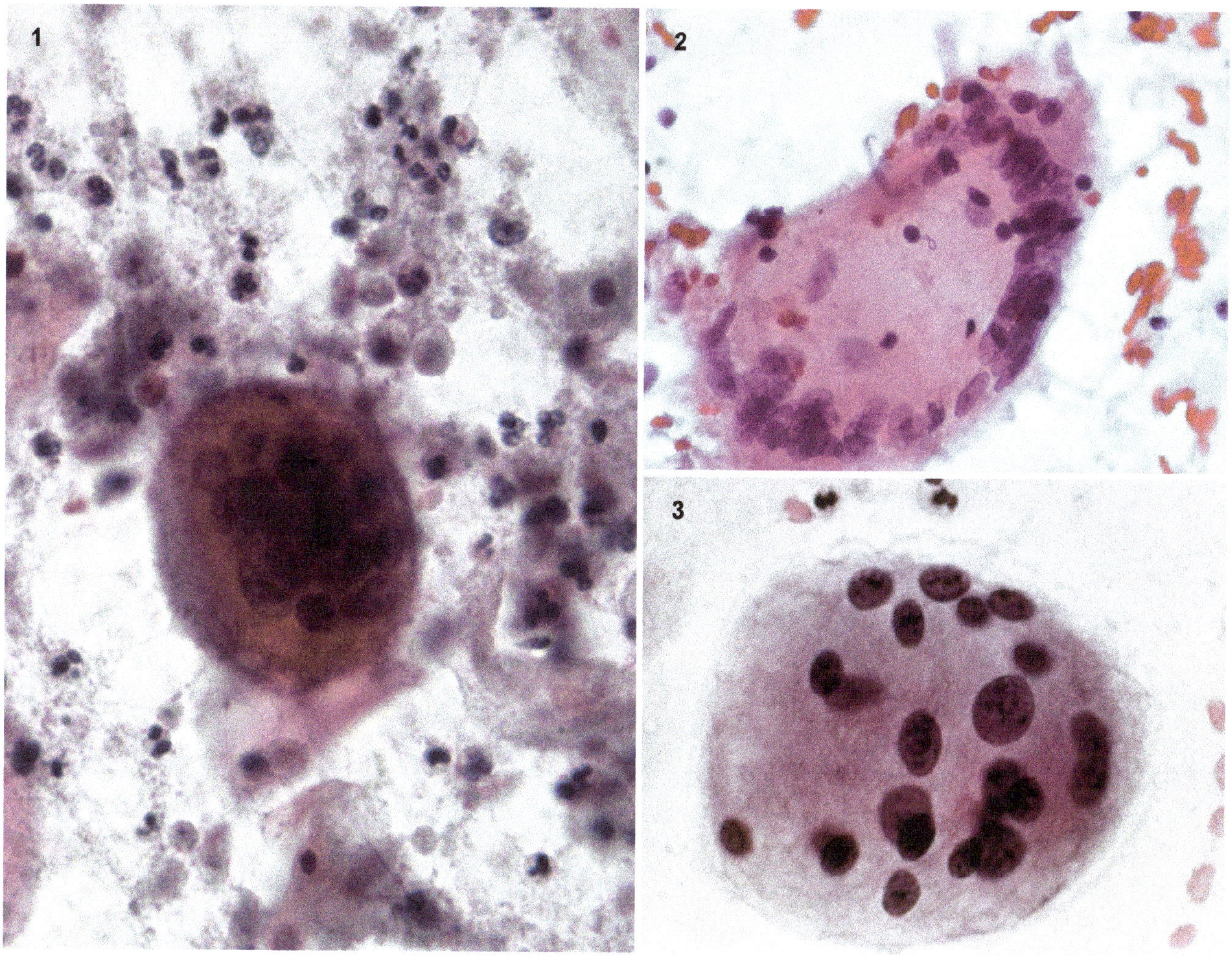

Fig. 7.62

Q-62. Choose which answer best corresponds to the order of the images:

(a) 1. Reactive multinucleated endocervical cell; 2. Langerhans-type giant cell; 3. multinucleated histiocyte
(b) 1. Syncytiotrophoblast; 2. Langerhans-type giant cell; 3. multinucleated histiocyte
(c) 1. Syncytiotrophoblast; 2. foreign body-type giant cell; 3. tumor giant cell
(d) 1. Schistosoma ova; 2. foreign body-type giant cell; 3. emperipolesis
(e) 1. Herpes simplex multinucleated cell; 2. Langerhans-type giant cell; 3. tumor giant cell

Fig. 7.63

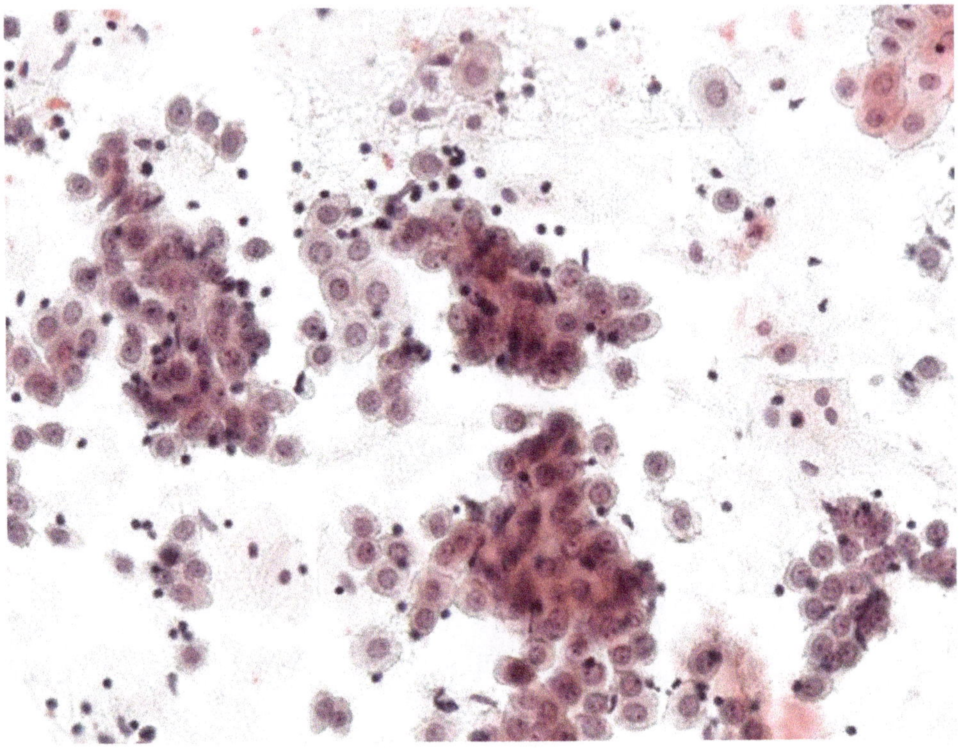

Q-63. What is the cause of the lesion in question 1?
(a) Human papillomavirus (HPV)
(b) Herpes simplex virus (HSV)
(c) Autoimmune
(d) Radiation therapy
(e) Folate deficiency

7.4 Answers and Discussion of Text-Based Questions 1–37

A-1. **(d) HPV 18**

Small cell neuroendocrine carcinoma of the cervix is strongly associated with HPV 18, while the pulmonary counterpart is only rarely HPV positive. Small cell carcinoma of the cervix is associated with squamous or glandular neoplasia in about half of the cases, possibly due to shared viral etiology. Therefore, even though there is no known precursor lesion for small cell carcinoma and the Pap test cannot prevent the occurrence of this tumor, the common association with SIL may lead to early detection in some cases.

A-2. **(b) A Pap test containing metastatic tumor cells of ovarian serous carcinoma shows a clean background.**

Metastatic tumors generally shed fewer tumor cells than primary tumors and lack a tumor diathesis. The typical finding on Pap test is a "second population" or "floater" occurring in a clean background. Tumors that directly invade cervix or vagina, such as colorectal carcinomas, often show marked tumor diathesis. The most common sources of extrauterine malignancies are ovarian carcinomas, followed by breast (more often lobular), and gastrointestinal tract (colon, rectum, stomach). The lymphoma cells will not be sampled in Pap test unless the surface is ulcerated. A dirty inflammatory or hemorrhagic background is typical in Pap tests with evidence of lymphoma.

A-3. **(a) Tzanck cells are large pleomorphic cells characteristic in the Pap test of a patient with pemphigus vulgaris.**

Pemphigus vulgaris is a rare autoimmune disease manifested by Tzanck cells in cytology specimens. Tzanck cells are parabasal-sized cells, often present singly or in loose clusters, characterized by uniform round nuclei with a smooth nuclear membrane, pale and fine chromatin, and prominent nucleoli (often multiple and classically bullet shaped). The characteristic perinuclear acidophilia (red-staining cytoplasm around the nucleus) described on conventional smears is not apparent on liquid-based ThinPrep. The background is normally clean with inflammatory cells admixed with atypical Tzanck cells, mimicking repair in Pap test. Nevertheless, high N/C ratio and prominent nucleoli often lead to misdiagnosis of malignancy. Clinical history is critical in reaching the correct diagnosis. Irregular, hyperchromatic nuclei, coarse chromatin, and necrotic background are indicative of malignancy. However, malignant neoplasm and pemphigus may occur in the same patient. Follow-up biopsy and high-risk HPV DNA test are advisable management options.

A-4. **(d) Worrisome and should prompt a search for neoplasm**

Psammoma bodies are concentrically laminated calcifications. They rarely occur in Pap tests, roughly 1 in every 100,000 cases. They can be found in association with both benign and malignant conditions. When they are associated with atypical epithelial cells, it should prompt a search for neoplasm. Benign conditions associated with psammoma bodies include pregnancy, IUD use, oral contraceptives, endometriosis, and endosalpingiosis. Malignant conditions associated with psammoma bodies include ovarian or fallopian tube serous carcinoma, ovarian borderline tumor, and endometrial malignancy. Keep in mind while evaluating psammoma bodies in Pap tests: malignant cells are not always present in the Pap tests of patients who are found to have tumors; atypical epithelial cells are commonly present in the Pap tests of women who do not have cancers; in many women no cause is ever identified.

A-5. **(c) Abundant tumor diathesis in tumors from direct extension**

The typical finding of metastatic tumor on Pap test, regardless of the route of involvement, is a "second population" or "floater," either singly or in clusters. Metastatic tumors from distant sites often lack a tumor diathesis and show a clean background. Tumors that directly invade cervix or vagina, such as colorectal carcinomas, often show marked tumor diathesis. The presence of psammoma bodies in Pap test is a nonspecific finding that may occur in both benign and malignant conditions, even though their presence, especially in association with atypical epithelial cells, should prompt a search for neoplasm.

A-6. **(a) As part of a disseminated disease, lymphoma of the cervix may not have any clinically detectable local signs.**

In contrast to follicular cervicitis, lymphoma of the cervix produces a clinically detectable tumor mass in most cases. One should be extremely cautious of making a diagnosis of lymphoma in the absence of a mass lesion. The neoplastic cells will not be sampled in Pap test unless the surface is ulcerated. A dirty inflammatory or hemorrhagic background is typical. The lymphoma cells are small and dispersed. Occasionally, the nuclei may form small "nipple"-like protrusions. The major differential diagnosis of lymphoma on Pap test is follicular cervicitis, a common inflammatory condition characterized by polymorphous lymphocytes in various stages of maturation, tingible body macrophages, and plasma cells. Other differential diagnoses include poorly differentiated squamous cell carcinoma, small cell carcinoma, and HSIL (CIN 3). In most cases, immunohistochemical stains or biopsy confirmation is needed.

A-7. **(b) Granulosa cell tumor of ovary**
Psammoma bodies are concentrically laminated calcifications. In rare cases, they may be found in the Pap test. The presence of psammoma bodies is nonspecific in diagnosis. They can be associated with both benign and malignant conditions, including pregnancy, IUD use, oral contraceptives, endometriosis, endosalpingiosis, ovarian or fallopian tube serous carcinoma, ovarian borderline tumor, endometrial malignancy, and other nongynecologic metastases.

A-8. **(e) Lymphoma**
The majority of squamous cell carcinoma and adenocarcinoma of cervix are associated with high-risk HPV infection, especially HPV 16 and 18. Small cell as well as large cell neuroendocrine carcinomas of the cervix can be associated with squamous or glandular dysplasia, and high-risk HPV has been reported in neuroendocrine tumors, suggesting a common etiology.

A-9. **(e) A tumor diathesis is not common in Pap tests of sarcomas.**
The malignant mesenchymal tumors arise in the stroma. They do not usually exfoliate until the overlying surface is ulcerated. Therefore, routine Pap test cannot detect sarcomas until they produce a surface ulceration, and a tumor diathesis is common in Pap tests of sarcomas when they are identifiable. MMMT is an uncommon but highly aggressive malignancy occurring in postmenopausal women who present as abnormal vaginal bleeding. When tumor cells of MMMT exfoliate, the adenocarcinomatous component is more likely than the sarcomatous component to shed characteristic cells, so the primary diagnosis on Pap test is frequently adenocarcinoma only. When the malignant spindle cells are present in Pap test, as a minor component, they often look ugly and are easy to recognize as malignant.

A-10. **(c) Ovary and fallopian tube**
The most common sources of extrauterine malignancies in Pap tests are stage III or IV ovarian and fallopian tube carcinomas, followed by breast (more often lobular) and gastrointestinal tract (colon, rectum, stomach). The metastatic ovarian carcinomas are typically serous type, resembling the serous carcinoma of endometrium. Metastatic malignancies generally shed fewer tumor cells than primary tumors and lack a tumor diathesis. Adenocarcinoma is by far the most common type of metastatic malignancy detected in the Pap test. Cases of metastatic tumor cells may often be interpreted as atypical glandular cells in the Pap test. In general, specific characterization of the primary site is not possible without the clinical history and previous biopsy specimen for comparison. Immunocytochemistry can sometimes be helpful in differential diagnosis by highlighting the tumor markers.

A-11. **(b) In immunocompromised patients, the infection can become widely disseminated.**
Molluscum contagiosum infection is caused by a double-stranded DNA virus of the poxvirus family. In immunocompromised patients such as those with AIDS, the infection can become widely disseminated. Cytology specimens show single and multiple clusters of squamous cells with waxy-appearing eosinophilic intracytoplasmic inclusion bodies (molluscum bodies). Large inclusions tend to push the nucleus toward the periphery. Inclusions may be eosinophilic or basophilic in appearance. The background rarely shows inflammation. This virus is identified as a sexually transmitted disease, and the smear should be thoroughly screened to determine if other sexually transmitted diseases are present.

A-12. **(d) Mycobacterial infections of the cervix usually indicate primary infection.**
Tuberculosis of the female genital tract usually involves the fallopian tubes and endometrium. Infection of the cervix is rare even where mycobacterial infection is prevalent. Mycobacterial infection of the cervix is usually secondary from pulmonary infection or direct spread from higher up in the genital tract. It has been suggested that occasionally cervical TB may even be sexually transmitted from a partner with tuberculous epididymitis. The vast majority are due to *M. tuberculosis*. Mycobacterial cervicitis is often clinically misdiagnosed as carcinoma of the cervix due to the clinical presentation and presence of necrosis. As granulomas of the cervix are seen in other conditions, ancillary tests, e.g., acid-fast stains, autofluorescence, culture, and PCR, are required to confirm the diagnosis.

A-13. **(c) Schistosomiasis of the cervix may be associated with an increased risk of cervical squamous carcinoma.**
S. haematobium causes bladder disease and can be isolated from the bladder by cytology or biopsy. *S. mansoni* and *S. japonicum* are more commonly seen in the bowel and are therefore diagnosed by intestinal/rectal biopsy or stool samples. Involvement of the female genital tract, most commonly by *S. haematobium*, is seen mainly in the vagina and cervix. However, parasite eggs can also be found in the uterus, ovary, and fallopian tubes. Schistosomiasis of the cervix may be associated with an increased risk of cervical squamous carcinoma, increased risk for spread of sexually transmitted infection, and infertility. A cervix infected with schistosomiasis can be vascular and demonstrates significant contact bleeding. The cervix can also be ulcerated and friable, mimicking carcinoma.

A-14. **(e) Detection of *Taenia* ova on cervical smear indicates true infection of the cervix.**
Microfilariae are thin worms, 1–4 cm in length, include several nuclei along their length, and can provoke a severe cervicitis. Both *Entamoeba histolytica* and Entamoeba gingivalis can be found on cervical smear, although *Entamoeba histolytica* is seen more frequently. *Entamoeba* may colonize tumors such as squamous cell carcinoma of the cervix. In infection with *Trypanosoma cruzi* (Chagas disease), giant cells with typical amastigotes are noted. Taeniasis is a parasitic infection caused by the tapeworm species. Eggs of these various tapeworms can be distinguished by detailed morphologic examination. In female patients, the female worms can travel up the vaginal canal causing infection of the vagina and cervix and can enter the uterus causing endometritis and endosalpingitis. The presence of *Taenia* ova on Pap smear usually indicates contamination from the perianal region or feces and not true infection of the cervix.

A-15. **(d) Necrosis and apoptosis are prominent features.**
These cells are derived from reserve or basal cells of the endocervical epithelium and may be the precursor of small cell carcinoma of the cervix. On a Pap test, single cells and clusters of small dysplastic cells with scant, often barely visible basophilic, or rarely eosinophilic, cytoplasm is seen. The cells have hyperchromatic, coarsely granular nuclei with irregularity of the nucleus contour. Some cases may show prominent nucleoli, and rarely even cytoplasmic vacuoles may be seen. HSIL of small cell type is a frequent cause of false-negative diagnoses.

A-16. **(e) Follicular cervicitis**
Pap tests of small cell HSIL show single cells and clusters of small dysplastic cells with scant, often barely visible basophilic, or rarely eosinophilic, cytoplasm. Follicular cervicitis exfoliates as a range of small and large lymphoid cells admixed with tingible body macrophages. High-grade squamous intraepithelial lesion (HSIL) of small cell type does not show the range of cell size seen in follicular cervicitis, nor associated tingible body macrophages. Cells showing ASCUS, LSIL, and reparative and inflammatory changes are not small and have much more abundant cytoplasm than HSIL. The differential diagnosis of HSIL includes microglandular hyperplasia, transitional cell metaplasia, endometrial cells (benign and malignant), small cell neuroendocrine carcinoma, non-Hodgkin lymphoma, and small clusters of benign metaplastic cells.

A-17. **(c) Paraneoplastic syndromes such as Cushing's syndrome, SIADH, hypercalcemia, or hypoglycemia may be seen.**
Small cell or neuroendocrine tumors of the uterine cervix have been described over a wide age range (21–94). They are associated with HPV type 16 or 18. Most patients present with vaginal bleeding, discharge, or postcoital spotting. However, paraneoplastic syndromes such as Cushing's syndrome, SIADH, hypercalcemia, or hypoglycemia may be seen. The prognosis is generally poor and is related to the degree of differentiation. TTF-l immunopositivity has been reported in rare small- and large-cell neuroendocrine carcinomas of the cervix. Other positive immunostaining includes neuron-specific enolase (NSE), chromogranin, synaptophysin, cytokeratin, and CEA. Immunoreactivity for serotonin, intestinal polypeptide, and somatostatin is variable.

A-18. **(a) The cervix, in adenoma malignum, is grossly indurated and barrel shaped.**
Adenoma malignum is a rare variant of endocervical adenocarcinoma. It occurs in women of reproductive age (ranges from 34 to 42 years). The cervix in adenoma malignum is grossly indurated and barrel shaped (diffusely enlarged). They are not associated with human papillomavirus (HPV) infection. Ancillary studies can be performed on cell block material or on biopsy. Adenoma malignum exclusively produces neutral mucin. This differs from normal endocervical glands or the other endocervical adenocarcinomas that usually produce an equal amount of neutral and acidic mucin. Neutral mucin can be seen as red-stained material on PAS–Alcian blue pH2.5 stains. On

immunostaining, adenoma malignum is positive for CEA, Ki67 (>50 % of tumor nuclei), and p53, while it is negative for ER and PR.

A-19. **(e) Closely resembles benign endocervical cells**
Cytomorphology of adenoma malignum comprises a large number of abnormal glandular cells that closely resemble benign endocervical cells. They are arranged in clusters, strips, and isolated cuboidal to columnar cells. The abnormal clusters exhibit loss of polarity with a disorganized "drunken" honeycomb sheet arrangement, and the glandular strips have pseudostratification, not syncytia. The presence of "golden yellow" intracytoplasmic mucin reflects the production of neutral, gastric/pyloric-type phenotypic mucin. Although the number of abnormal glandular clusters is large, frankly malignant cells are only seen in a minority of these cell groups. Their nuclei are enlarged (two to three times the size of intermediate squamous nuclei) and pleomorphic with visible nucleoli. If pleomorphic cells arranged in 3D clusters and papillary fragments are noted, endometrial adenocarcinoma should be considered.

A-20. **(c) Loss of polarity within cell groups**
Endocervical adenocarcinoma in situ (AIS) shows loss of mucin and lacks abnormal single cells, which are both present in adenoma malignum. The main architectural features that are helpful in recognizing AIS are tightly crowded sheets of glandular cells with overlapping nuclei and "ragged-edged" borders. The honeycomb pattern and palisaded edge seen in clusters of normal endocervical cells are absent in AIS. In AIS, the clusters of endocervical cells may also show pseudostratification with nuclei seen at different levels within the groups. However, polarity of cells in AIS is maintained. Cells in AIS clusters may arrange in a circular pattern with peripheral location of nuclei. Feathering is another distinctive feature of AIS. Also, there is no "golden yellow" mucin and no tumor diathesis in AIS.

A-21. **(b) Extramammary Paget's disease manifests as burning or itchy, pink-to-red vulvar lesions.**
Extramammary Paget's disease of the vulva may extend into the vagina and present as an adenocarcinoma on Pap smear. This disease usually occurs in Caucasian women in their fifth to sixth decade. Clinical symptoms and signs include a burning or itchy, pink-to-red vulvar lesions which may have white hyperkeratotic patches that can be confused with eczema, especially if it extends into the groin area. Extramammary Paget's disease is an intraepithelial adenocarcinoma derived from the apocrine or sebaceous glands around the anogenital area. This lesion is usually a noninvasive adenocarcinoma of the epidermis and skin appendages; however, in 10–20 % of cases, an underlying invasive adenocarcinoma is present. Extramammary Paget's disease can metastasize.

A-22. **(b) The cells are large with hyperchromatic nuclei and macronucleoli.**
Ancillary investigations are useful in extramammary Paget's disease (EMPD) to exclude other primary and metastatic adenocarcinoma and malignant melanoma. The cytoplasm of tumor cells contains mucopolysaccharide that stains positively with PAS digest, Alcian blue, and mucicarmine. IHC stains are frequently used in the histologic evaluation of EMPD. Most Paget's cells stain positively for CEA and cytokeratin (CK) 7, and 60 % are positive for gross cystic disease fluid protein (GCDFP). They also stain positively for CAM5.2, B72.3, MUC1, and MUC5AC and 30 % are positive for S-100. They usually stain negatively for HMB45, Melan A, and Leu M1. The cells are usually negative for CK20 but can be positive if the extramammary Paget's disease is secondary to urothelial carcinoma.

A-23. **(c) HMB45**
Approximately 50 % of extrauterine malignancies are of upper gynecological origin (ovary and fallopian tubes) and 50 % from nongynecological sites. The most common nongynecological extrauterine sites are gastrointestinal, breast, pancreas, lung, bladder, and kidney. Malignancies metastatic to the cervix are often characterized by a clean background with no tumor diathesis. Most metastatic adenocarcinomas, although classifiable as malignant, often cannot be definitively identified by site of origin on cytologic grounds alone. On the Pap test, they often appear morphologically similar to endometrial or endocervical adenocarcinoma. The diagnosis of metastatic extragenital malignancy to the cervix on a Pap test is extremely rare, even in countries with well-organized cervical screening programs.

A-24. **(b) Extrauterine malignancies in Pap tests, occasionally have an associated tumor diathesis.**
Ovarian carcinoma mainly involves the cervix and vagina by spreading down the endometrial cavity. Metastatic ovarian carcinoma, on a Pap test, has neoplastic cells associated with possible psammoma bodies and a clean background. A tumor diathesis may occasionally be seen in metastatic disease if the cervix contains substantial necrotic tumor implants. The

most common metastatic ovarian tumor seen is serous carcinoma. Cytoplasmic vacuoles may be seen in both endometrial carcinoma and metastatic ovarian carcinoma, and this feature cannot be used to make this distinction. The quantity of abnormal cells is usually less than that seen with endometrial or endocervical adenocarcinomas.

A-25. (**d**) ***Taenia* ovum**
Psammoma bodies are round, calcific collections with concentric laminations. If psammoma bodies are seen in a Pap test, the possibility of endometrial or metastatic carcinoma should be considered. However, there are mimics of psammoma bodies. Round, basophilic formations called "blue blobs" are sometimes seen in atrophic smears and are thought to be degenerated cells. They are amorphous and lack the concentric laminations of psammoma bodies. Inspissated mucus and lubricant can form dense, round structures but lack the form of psammoma bodies. Calcified fragments of intrauterine contraceptive devices are unstructured, and concentric laminations are not obtained. Ova from *Taenia* species have a thick wall with radial, not concentric, striations.

A-26. (**b**) **The frequency of cervical metastasis of breast cancer is estimated to be <1 %.**
Metastatic extragenital malignancy to the cervix on Pap test is extremely rare (<1 %). Most patients have known history of malignancy. The most common non gynecological extrauterine sites are gastrointestinal, breast, and pancreas. Breast lobular carcinoma is more common than ductal carcinoma. They often shows a clean background (no diathesis), and looks like "floater". Most metastatic adenocarcinomas, although classifiable as malignant, cannot be definitively identified by site of origin on cytologic grounds alone. Metastatic lobular adenocarcinomas, the cells may be small and bland, rather than poorly differentiated. Metastatic breast cancer cells may resemble histiocytes.

A-27. (**a**) **The cervix may be involved by primary or secondary lymphoma or leukemia**.
The female genital tract may be involved by primary or secondary lymphoma or leukemia. The age range of afflicted patients with cervical lymphoma is 20–80 years, and the majority is premenopausal. The utility of cytology in this clinical setting is limited as most lesions are submucosal. Malignant cells will be seen if ulceration of the mucosa occurs with subsequent extension of malignant cells into the mucosa. B-cell non-Hodgkin lymphoma of the cervix is much more common than T-cell lymphoma with diffuse large B-cell lymphoma and follicular lymphoma the most common types. The prognosis depends if the non-Hodgkin lymphoma is low or high grade.

A-28. (**e**) **Hodgkin lymphoma**
Follicular cervicitis may show mixed inflammatory cells with tingible body macrophages and neutrophils. Poorly differentiated and small cell carcinomas that present with dispersed highly atypical cells should be carefully examined for some degree of cohesion and nuclear molding as evidence of their epithelial nature. Endometrial stromal sarcoma presents as small malignant cells that may on occasion be highly pleomorphic with visible nucleoli lying in a tumor diathesis. Granulocytic sarcoma comprises immature myeloid cells that are medium to large. The presence of eosinophilic myelocytes and staff/band cells should alert one to the diagnosis. In Hodgkin lymphoma, Reed–Sternberg cells, with a distinctive binucleated appearance and giant nucleoli, present in a background of mixed inflammatory cells including eosinophils. In many of these conditions, the cellular monotony associated with B-cell non-Hodgkin lymphoma is lacking.

A-29. (**d**) **They usually have an exophytic-papillary growth pattern**.
Primary urothelial carcinoma of the cervix is a rare tumor. It has been described in other areas of the female genital tract including ovary, fallopian tube, broad ligament, and endometrium. It usually has an exophytic papillary growth pattern. Morphologically, these tumors resemble urothelial carcinoma of the urinary tract. These tumors are often HPV 16 positive. They do not appear to be related to infection with the JC virus. They are aggressive tumors and show metastases and recurrences. Unlike urothelial carcinoma of the urinary tract, urothelial carcinoma of the female genital tract is CK7 positive and CK20 negative.

A-30. (**e**) **The most common presenting symptom is vaginal bleeding**.
Malignant mixed Mullerian tumor (MMMT) is also called carcinosarcoma, sarcomatoid carcinoma, malignant mesodermal mixed tumor, and metaplastic carcinoma. MMMT is an aggressive tumor with a poor prognosis. These tumors are usually seen in postmenopausal women with a history of bleeding. Examination reveals uterine enlargement. A soft mass protruding through the cervical os is seen in many women with an MMMT. They originate mainly from the endometrium but can, on occasion, arise from the cervix, vagina, peritoneum, or extragenital sites.

Predisposing factors include a history of radiation therapy and chronic estrogen stimulation. Other predisposing factors include nulliparity, diabetes, and obesity. They do not appear to be associated with HPV infection.

A-31. (**a**) **Endometrioid carcinoma**
Malignant mixed Mullerian tumor (MMMT) is a biphasic, high-grade tumor with malignant epithelial and stromal components. The epithelial component is most often an endometrioid carcinoma, but squamous carcinoma, papillary carcinoma, clear cell carcinoma, and undifferentiated carcinoma may be seen. About 50 % of uterine MMMT cases may exhibit malignant or abnormal findings on Pap test, and an accurate diagnosis is based on identification of the two malignant components, i.e., carcinoma and sarcoma. However, most cases usually lack the sarcoma component on Pap tests. Therefore, a poorly differentiated carcinoma or malignant neoplasm is the most rendered diagnosis for these cases.

A-32. (**a**) **If the malignant stromal component consists of smooth muscle, it is called "homologous**."
If the malignant stromal component of a malignant mixed Mullerian tumor MMMT is composed of cells native to the uterine corpus such as endometrial stroma or smooth muscle, then the stroma is said to be "homologous." If the malignant stromal component comprises fat, cartilage, skeletal muscle, it is referred to as "heterologous." The Pap test in MMMT is usually hypercellular and shows high-grade malignant tumor cells composed of malignant epithelial or glandular cells admixed with malignant spindle cells. The differential diagnosis includes stromal repair, botryoid rhabdomyosarcoma (seen in children/adolescents), teratoma, and metastatic ovarian serous cystadenocarcinoma.

A-33. (**d**) **The cytomorphologic findings may comprise either epithelioid or spindled features**.
Malignant melanoma of the lower female genital tract is most common in the vulva, then the vagina, and least common in the cervix. Primary melanoma of the cervix or vagina occurs predominantly in postmenopausal women and likely originates from melanocytes in this region. The cytomorphological findings of melanoma in a Pap test are similar to those seen in other sites in the body. The cytology includes discohesive large malignant cells with abundant dusty cytoplasm and a round to ovoid nucleus with a prominent nucleolus. Since melanoma may present with either epithelioid or spindled features, the differential diagnosis, on Pap test, usually includes poorly differentiated carcinoma and sarcoma. These are aggressive tumors with a poor prognosis.

A-34. (**c**) **Some endometrial stromal sarcomas carry the t(7;17) translocation with involvement of JAZF1 and JJAZ1**.
Uterine sarcoma is very uncommon and comprises 3–7 % of uterine malignancies. The signs and symptoms of uterine leiomyoma and uterine leiomyosarcoma are similar, viz., vaginal bleeding, pelvic pain, and pelvic mass; however, leiomyoma occurs more frequently than leiomyosarcoma. Uterine leiomyosarcomas express smooth muscle markers such as desmin, h-caldesmon, and smooth muscle actin. They sometimes express CD10, keratin, and EMA on immunostaining. In addition, uterine leiomyosarcomas are estrogen, progesterone, and androgen receptor positive in 30–40 % of cases. On immunostaining, most endometrial stromal tumors are positive for CD10. However, leiomyosarcomas and MMMT may express CD10 as well. Some endometrial stromal sarcomas carry the t(7;17) translocation with involvement of JAZF1 and JJAZ1.

A-35. (**e**) **Ovarian inclusion cyst**
Although the presence of psammoma bodies may indicate a malignant process within the cervix, they are seen, on a Pap test, in several benign lesions. These include endosalpingiosis, endometrial tuberculosis, ovarian cystadenoma, ovarian inclusion cyst, and intrauterine contraceptive device. Psammoma bodies have not been described in follicular cervicitis, reparative change, *Trichomonas* infection, and lower urinary tract infection. In benign lesions with psammoma bodies, a tumor diathesis is lacking and many of the psammoma bodies are lying stripped of cells compared to malignancy where psammoma bodies are usually incorporated in malignant cell groups, although stripped psammoma bodies may occasionally be seen.

A-36. (**b**) **Metastatic ovarian carcinoma, on a Pap test, has neoplastic cells, ± clean background, and ± psammoma bodies**.
Ovarian carcinoma mainly involves the cervix and vagina by spreading down the endometrial cavity. Metastatic ovarian carcinoma, on a Pap test, has neoplastic cells associated with possible psammoma bodies and a clean background. A tumor diathesis may occasionally be seen in metastatic disease if the cervix contains substantial necrotic tumor implants. The most common metastatic ovarian tumor seen is serous

carcinoma. Cytoplasmic vacuoles may be seen in both endometrial carcinoma and metastatic ovarian carcinoma, and this feature cannot be used to make this distinction. The quantity of abnormal cells is usually less than that seen with endometrial or endocervical adenocarcinomas.

A-37. (**a**) **The background often shows a tumor diathesis**.

Although the majority of metastatic adenocarcinoma to the cervix is associated with a clean background, an exception is metastatic rectal or colonic adenocarcinoma that is often associated with a necrotic background. Adenocarcinomas of the colon and rectum can spread directly to the cervix. The cells have a columnar shape with a large, hyperchromatic nucleus. Strips of cells with a luminal border may be obtained, in addition to cellular arrangements comprising papillary or acinar architecture. Colonic tumors may also show cells with more mucinous differentiation including cells with a signet ring appearance. Ancillary investigations including immunocytochemistry may be required to make the distinction between a primary adenocarcinoma of the cervix and metastatic colorectal adenocarcinoma. Extracellular collagen globules are noted in gastrointestinal stromal tumors.

7.5 Answers and Discussion of Image-Based Questions 38–63

A-38. **(c) Metastatic carcinoma of breast**

The image shows a small, loose cluster of large, round nuclei that have irregular nuclear contours, prominent nucleoli, very scant foamy cytoplasm, and intracytoplasmic vacuoles without associated neutrophils. The background reveals fresh blood; however, no apparent tumor diathesis is present. The morphologic features combined with patient's known history of cancer are consistent with metastatic carcinoma of breast. Metastatic carcinomas usually shed fewer tumor cells than primary tumors of female genital tracts. They typically lack tumor diathesis, unless the metastasis is locally invasive or involves the cervix by direct extension. Metastatic breast carcinoma, even though not pathognomonic, characteristically shows intracytoplasmic lumens (targetoid mucin vacuoles) or single files arrangement. Metastatic colorectal carcinoma often shows tall columnar cells with terminal bars, goblet cells, and dirty necrosis in the background. A known history of cancer is the key to diagnosis and is present in most patients. Squamous cell carcinoma usually demonstrates dense cytoplasm, variation in nuclear size and shape, hyperchromasia, coarse chromatin or parachromatin clearing, and tumor diathesis. Adenocarcinoma of cervix generally shows marked cellular crowding with microacini, rosettes, and feathery edges. High-risk HPV DNA testing is useful in assessing the likelihood of cervical carcinomas.

A-39. **(d) Pemphigus vulgaris**

This case stresses the importance of differentiating benign mimics of malignancy in Pap tests. The images showed Tzanck (acantholytic) cells of Pemphigus vulgaris, a rare autoimmune blistering disease. Tzanck cells are parabasal-sized cells which have atypical features that could be misinterpreted as malignant, including high nuclear to cytoplasmic ratio and prominent irregular nucleoli, as well as occasional single cells on liquid-based cytology. The dense cytoplasm and accompanying dyskaryotic cells may result in a misdiagnosis of squamous cell carcinoma. The prominent nucleoli, vesicular chromatin, and round nuclear shape may erroneously suggest an atypical glandular lesion or adenocarcinoma. The features favoring a benign process include clean background, admixed inflammatory cells, generally loose and flat cellular arrangement without nuclear overlapping, uniform round cells with smooth nuclear contour, fine and pale chromatin, and characteristic multiple "bullet-shaped" nucleoli. Tzanck cells may also mimic repair in the Pap test, except that the abundance of single cells or small clusters is not a feature of repair and the "streaming" pattern seen in repair is not present in pemphigus. Nevertheless, clinical history is critical in reaching the correct diagnosis. High-risk HPV DNA test could also help assess the risk of significant squamous or glandular lesions.

A-40. **(b) Malignant mixed Mullerian tumor/carcinosarcoma**

Malignant mixed Mullerian tumor (MMMT), also called carcinosarcoma, is an uncommon metaplastic epithelial malignancy that is composed of both malignant epithelial and stromal elements. It usually occurs in postmenopausal women. A precise diagnosis of carcinosarcoma on cytology specimen is rarely made, because a dual malignant cell population is usually not present or appreciated. Most commonly, the cytologic diagnosis rendered is adenocarcinoma or carcinoma owing to the fact that, when tumor cells are exfoliated, the adenocarcinomatous component is more likely than the sarcomatous component to shed representative cells. The carcinomatous tumor cells have the usual malignant features, including pleomorphism, coarse chromatin, and prominent nucleoli. Looking for the sarcomatous component, such as atypical spindle cells, bizarre tumor cells, smooth or striated muscle cells, cartilage, or osteoid, may assist in a more specific interpretation.

A-41. **(d) Small cell carcinoma**

The small, dark, round tumor cells form crowded groups or scattered single cells, in a background of necrosis and blood. The tumor cells have a very high N/C ratio with scant cytoplasm, hyperchromatic nuclei, and indistinct nucleoli. An atypical mitosis is present in between the two big tumor clusters. In liquid-based cytology, molding is usually not a prominent feature of small cell carcinoma, and crush artifact is absent. The hyperchromatic crowded groups may mimic various other malignancies, such as poorly differentiated squamous cell carcinoma, endometrial carcinoma, and lymphoma, or some benign conditions like follicular cervicitis and menstrual phase endometrial shedding. Squamous cell carcinoma often has more and denser cytoplasm. Atypical mitosis is uncommon in benign endometrial cells. Small cell carcinoma of the cervix has a strong association with HPV 18 and is frequently present along with squamous or glandular neoplasia.

A-42. **(d) Ovary**
Even though not specific, the finding of papillary groups of tumor cells on Pap test of a woman with negative endometrial and endocervical biopsies suggests an ovarian origin. Metastatic carcinoma often lacks tumor diathesis on Pap test, unless it becomes locally invasive. Papillary groups may also be present in renal cell carcinoma, urothelial carcinoma, fallopian tube carcinoma, mesothelioma, pancreatic carcinoma, etc. Immunocytochemical stains could be of value in characterizing the origin of tumor.

A-43. **(e) Endometrial curettage**
The images show 2D and 3D crowded groups of large nuclei with irregular contours, coarse chromatin and prominent nucleoli, in a background of tumor diathesis. A rare atypical spindle cell is also present (right panel). In an elderly woman with postmenopausal bleeding, the top line differential diagnosis for malignant cells with glandular configuration would be endometrial malignancy. The diagnosis in this case was malignant mixed Mullerian tumor (MMMT). The most commonly exfoliated malignant cells of MMMT on Pap test are the carcinoma cells, usually adenocarcinomas, and occasionally serous carcinomas or other high-grade carcinomas. Finding the sarcomatous component, such as atypical spindle cells or bizarre mesenchymal cells, is helpful to reach a more specific diagnosis.

A-44. **(a) *Molluscum contagiosum* body like**
Molluscum contagiosum (MC) is a poxvirus that may infect the vulva and vagina via sexual transmission. It is characterized by large intracytoplasmic inclusions that are homogenous, dense, and deeply pink (molluscum bodies). The differential diagnosis may include koilocytes in low-grade squamous intraepithelial lesion (LSIL). However, koilocytes characteristically demonstrate a wrinkled nuclear membrane, dark and granular or smudged chromatin. In contrast, MC cells have degenerated nuclei that are pushed to the periphery of the cells by the large homogenous intracytoplasmic inclusions (*Image courtesy*: *Dr. Walid Khalbuss*).

A-45. **(b) Small cell carcinoma**
The images of the conventional Pap smear showed crowded groups of small, dark cells (compared to adjacent squamous intermediate cell nucleus and background red blood cells). The lesional cells have very high N/C ratio, remarkably hyperchromatic nuclei, inconspicuous nucleoli, and apparent nuclear molding. AIS of the endocervix typically shows enlarged nuclei with characteristic feathering on conventional smears. HSIL cells present with prominent irregularity of nuclear membrane, coarse chromatin, and less nuclear molding. The disorganized arrangement, irregular nuclear contour, and nuclear molding are unlikely features of endometrial cells (*Image courtesy*: *Dr. Walid Khalbuss*).

A-46. **(b) Metastatic adenocarcinoma of colon**
Unlike the clean background on Pap tests of most metastatic carcinomas, carcinomas of colon and rectum often spread to the vagina via direct extension and show dirty tumor necrosis. The tumor cells have a characteristic columnar shape with large, hyperchromatic, cigar-shaped nuclei, and sometimes discernable terminal bars. In contrast, adenocarcinomas of endocervix or endometrium typically form 2D or 3D clusters with round or pleomorphic nuclei and occasional intracytoplasmic vacuoles.

A-47. **(e) Paget's Disease**
Extramammary Paget's disease of the vulva is an uncommon entity that usually occurs in postmenopausal women. The diagnosis is almost always made through biopsy specimen. The tumor cells are rarely seen in Pap smears, often with disease involving the vagina or cervix. The most consistent cytomorphologic features include cells-within-cells arrangement (pseudocannibalism), intracytoplasmic vacuoles and signet ring cells to indicate the glandular nature of the tumor cells, and basophilic cytoplasm resembling squamous metaplasia. Definitive diagnosis is based on histologic examination and sometimes also immunohistochemical studies. Clinical history is also important in helping make an accurate cytologic diagnosis (*Image courtesy*: *Dr. Walid Khalbuss*).

A-48. **(d) Placental site trophoblastic tumor**
Placental site trophoblastic tumor (PSTT) is a rare form of trophoblastic tumor, composed of intermediate trophoblasts, without cytotrophoblasts. Intermediate trophoblasts are large, mononucleated, round or polygonal cells and have abundant cytoplasm, irregular and dark nuclei, but scant mitoses. The tumor cells are often positive for human placental lactogen (hPL), but serum β-HCG is usually low.

A-49. **(e) Melanoma**
The cytomorphology of melanoma varies from case to case and misinterpretation is common. They often present as discohesive groups or isolated cells, which is a helpful pattern to differentiate from carcinomas. The tumor cells are frequently epithelioid or spindled,

with varying size from small to large. The nuclei are round to oval, pale or dark, and may have occasional intranuclear cytoplasmic invaginations (pseudoinclusions). Melanin pigment is the most characteristic feature. However, it is not always present and may sometimes be mistaken for hemosiderin.

A-50. (e) **Lymphoma**
The dominant population in this Pap test is monomorphic small round blue cells, predominantly in single cell pattern. The lesional cells are round with occasional nuclear contour irregularity and have fine chromatin. The differential diagnoses include follicular cervicitis, small cell carcinoma, poorly differentiated squamous carcinoma, or adenocarcinoma, including endometrial carcinoma. In contrast to lymphoma, follicular cervicitis does not produce a cervical mass lesion and is usually characterized by polymorphous lymphocytes mixed with tingible body macrophages. Poorly differentiated carcinomas often form aggregates, and the tumor cells show coarse chromatin, hyperchromasia, or nuclear molding. Biopsy and immunophenotyping are almost always necessary in rendering a definitive diagnosis for lymphoma.

A-51. (c) **Metastatic urothelial carcinoma**
The specimen contains large papillary fragments of crowded oval cells. The nuclear pleomorphism and irregularity are more prominent in the small clusters of cells, which also occasionally reveal tadpole cells. Metastatic urothelial carcinoma presenting in Pap tests is rare, often via direct extension (notice the tumor diathesis). The differential diagnosis includes high-grade dysplasia of cervical squamous cells, squamous cell carcinoma, and atrophy. Clinical presentation of hematuria or history of urothelial carcinoma is helpful in directing the diagnosis. Clues to the diagnosis are a hypercellular specimen consisting of large papillary fragments of crowded oval cells and characteristic so-called cercariform cells (tadpole or pollywog forms).

A-52. (c) **Metastatic ovarian papillary serous carcinoma**
Large and small 3D papillary groups along with psammoma bodies in a clean background highly suggest metastatic papillary serous carcinoma of ovarian origin, even though neither is specific. The tumor cells are large and round, with prominent nucleoli and cytoplasmic vacuoles. In contrast to endometrial and endocervical adenocarcinomas, which normally show tumor diathesis on Pap test, metastatic tumors often occur in a clean background. Ovary is the most common source of metastatic tumor in the Pap test.

A-53. (e) **Leukemia**
This conventional Pap test contains dissociated atypical hematopoietic cells, morphologically compatible with myeloblasts, eosinophilic myelocytes, and nucleated red cells. Extramedullary immature myeloid tumor, also known as granulocytic sarcoma or chloroma, can develop in about 3–5 % of patients with acute or chronic myeloid leukemia. The diagnosis of this rare entity poses even more of a challenge on liquid-based Pap tests (ThinPrep and SurePath) as the background inflammatory cells, tumor necrosis, and apoptotic debris are reduced by the preparation. Relatively well-differentiated tumors may show eosinophilic myelocytes that contain distinct cytoplasmic eosinophilic granules. Poorly differentiated tumors can be easily misinterpreted as inflammatory cells, lymphoma, and poorly differentiated carcinoma.

A-54. (c) **Leiomyosarcoma**
Even though leiomyosarcoma accounts for half of uterine sarcomas, it is not easily detected on Pap tests, mainly because it arises in the stroma and will only exfoliate when the surface epithelium is ulcerated. When the tumor cells are present on Pap test, they usually form small loosely cohesive groups or a single-cell pattern. The tumor cells are spindle or epithelioid with cigar-shaped nuclei as well as variable pleomorphism and mitotic activities. The differential diagnosis may include atypical repair, low-grade squamous intraepithelial lesion, and metastatic tumors, such as melanoma. The final diagnosis depends on histologic evaluation of cellularity, nuclear atypia, mitosis, and tumor necrosis.

A-55. (b) **Melanoma**
The cytomorphology of melanoma varies from case to case. They often present as discohesive groups or isolated cells, which is a helpful pattern to differentiate from carcinomas. However, they do occasionally form cohesive clusters. The tumor cells are frequently epithelioid or spindled, with varying size from small to large. The nuclei are round to oval, pale or dark, and may have occasional intranuclear cytoplasmic invaginations (pseudoinclusions). The differential diagnosis covers a wide range of lesions and tumors, including nonkeratinizing squamous cell carcinoma, leiomyosarcoma, atypical repair, and squamous intraepithelial lesions. Melanin pigment is the most characteristic feature (right upper corner in the above image).

A-56. (d) **MMMT of endometrium**
In addition to the tight clusters of apparent adenocarcinoma component (left panel), malignant

chondrocytes are present singly and in small loose clusters embedded in chondromyxoid matrix (right panel). The malignant chondrocytes are round, with dense and well-defined cytoplasm. Binucleation is readily seen. The differential diagnosis includes other tumors with biphasic pattern, such as adenosquamous carcinoma.

A-57. (**e**) **Metastatic clear cell carcinoma**
The apparently malignant tumor cells have large nuclei and prominent nucleoli. In contrast to the cytoplasmic vacuoles seen in adenocarcinoma, the most distinctive feature of clear cell carcinoma is the overall clear cytoplasm with sharply defined border. Clear cell carcinoma can be renal in origin; however, a primary tumor of Mullerian origin (ovarian or endometrial) must be excluded.

A-58. (**d**) **Pemphigus vulgaris**
Pemphigus vulgaris is a bullous skin condition that may also involve mucus membranes. In this smear that is very cellular, the cells lie in loosely cohesive clusters and have a high nuclear: cytoplasmic (N/C) ratio. The nuclei show extremely active nuclear chromatin with large irregular nucleoli that can be "bullet-shaped." There are several single cells and clusters mimicking malignancy. There is no background tumor diathesis. The cells are uniform. The presence of uniform cells, characteristic nucleoli, and lack of tumor diathesis makes the diagnosis of malignancy unlikely. The cytopathic effect of cytomegalovirus (CMV) is a large intranuclear inclusion surrounded by a clear zone of chromatin.

A-59. (**e**) ***Klebsiella granulomatis***
The smear is markedly inflamed with a dearth of epithelial cells. Histiocytes with thin-walled intracytoplasmic vacuoles are seen. Within the vacuoles, small organisms are noted. The cytomorphology is that of granuloma inguinale. Please note that in a smear containing granuloma inguinale, acute inflammation tends to mask the lymphocytes and plasma cells seen on cervical biopsy. Granuloma inguinale is caused by *Klebsiella granulomatis*, intracellular Gram-negative bacteria, sometimes referred to as a Donovan body. This organism is sexually transmitted. Herpes simplex virus and cytomegalovirus cause a characteristic cytopathic effect. Syphilis (caused by *Treponema pallidum*) leads to nonspecific inflammatory changes including granulomas, lymphocytes, and plasma cells. Epithelioid histiocytes, caseous necrosis, and inflammatory cells are found in tuberculosis of the cervix.

A-60. (**a**) **Tuberculosis**
Present on this smear is a group of caseous necrosis (left image) and epithelioid histiocytes (right image). The most likely diagnosis is mycobacterial infection. The diagnosis of *Mycobacterium tuberculosis* was confirmed on cervical biopsy with the use of acid–fast stains and polymerase chain reaction (PCR). Patients with cervical mycobacterial infection may be asymptomatic or complain of amenorrhea, menstrual irregularities, infertility, vaginal discharge, and postmenopausal bleeding. On examination, an ulcer, polyp, or lesion suspicious for cervical cancer may be seen. Epithelioid granulomas are seen in other conditions such as syphilis, granuloma inguinale, amebiasis, schistosomiasis, foreign body granulomas, radiation reaction, invasive squamous carcinoma, and malakoplakia.

A-61. (**a**) ***Schistosomiasis haematobium***
These are ova from *Schistosoma haematobium* lying in a hemorrhagic background. The ova are large measuring 112×170 μm by 40×70 μm and nonoperculate and have a transparent shell with a characteristic prominent terminal spine. Ova from *Trichuris trichiura* are 25 μm×50 μm, barrel shaped with protuberances on either end called "polar plugs." Ova from *Enterobius vermicularis* are ovoid, measure 20 μm × 60 μm with a double-walled shell that is flattened on one side. The ova of *Taenia solium* have a round shape with a radially striated shell and a diameter of 35 μm. Ova from *Ascaris lumbricoides* are oval, 30–40 μm×75–90 μm in size with a thick external layer that may contain large protuberances or none at all. Aside from schistosomiasis, these other parasites are contaminants when seen on Pap smear.

A-62. (**b**) **1. Syncytiotrophoblast**; **2. Langerhans-type giant cell**; **3. multinucleated histiocyte**
Various lesions of the cervix are associated with multinucleated giant cells. Syncytiotrophoblasts have numerous nuclei with dense cytoplasm and a cytoplasmic tail (arrow). Langerhans-type giant cells usually have a peripheral rim of nuclei. Multinucleated histiocytes are of variable size and have nuclei with fine, pale chromatin and delicate cytoplasm that may be vacuolated or contain phagocytosed debris. Reactive multinucleated endocervical cells maintain their columnar shape. Foreign body-type giant cells vary in size but can be very large with many nuclei and dense cytoplasm in which ingested material may be noted. Viable *Schistosoma* ova contain miracidia with multiple nuclei and a chitinous shell. In emperipolesis, the histiocytes are large with abundant

vacuolated cytoplasm in which lymphocytes are engulfed. Multinucleated herpes simplex-infected cell have nuclei that are molded rather than overlapped, pale nuclei, and a large intranuclear inclusion.

A-63. (c) **Autoimmune**

Pemphigus vulgaris is an autoimmune condition. There is an autoantibody against a cadherin-like cell adhesion molecule on the surface of stratified squamous epithelial cells causing the cells to separate from one another. The etiology is unknown in the majority of patients, but it can be caused by certain medication (e.g., penicillamine, ACE inhibitors). Human papillomavirus is associated with epithelial lesions, e.g., squamous and glandular lesions of the cervix. Herpes simplex virus is not oncogenic but produces a typical cytopathic effect. Radiation therapy to the cervix and folate deficiency cause enlarged squamous cells, cytoplasmic vacuoles, multinucleation, and enlarged nucleus and cytoplasm, so although the nucleus is enlarged, the N/C ratio is maintained. Hypersegmented neutrophils (5–6 lobes) are seen in folate deficiency.

Reading List

Akhyani M, Chams-Davatchi C, Naraghi Z, Daneshpazhooh M, Toosi S, Asgari M, et al. Cervicovaginal involvement in pemphigus vulgaris: a clinical study of 77 cases. Br J Dermatol. 2008;158:478–82.

Bibbo M, Wilbur D. Chapter 8: Benign proliferative reactions, intraepithelial neoplasia, and invasive cancer of the uterine cervix. In: Comprehensive cytopathology. 3rd ed. Philadelphia: Saunders/Elsevier; 2008.

Cibas ES. Chapter 1: Cervical and vaginal cytology. In: Cibas ES, Ducatman BS, editors. Cytology: diagnostic principles and clinical correlates. Philadelphia: Saunders/Elsevier; 2009. p. 1–66.

Cox JT, Solomon D, Schiffman M. Prospective follow-up suggests similar risk of subsequent CIN 2 or 3 among women with CIN 1 or negative colposcopy and directed biopsy. Am J Obstet Gynecol. 2003;188:1406–12.

DeMay RM. Chapter 1: The Pap test. In: DeMay RM, editor. The art and science of cytopathology. 2nd ed. Chicago: ASCP Press; 2012. p. 2–199.

Grayson W, Rhemtula HA, Taylor LF, Allard U, Tiltman AJ. Detection of human papillomavirus in large cell neuroendocrine carcinoma of the uterine cervix: a study of 12 cases. J Clin Pathol. 2002;55:108–14.

Gu M, Ghafari S, Lin F. Pap smears of patients with extramammary Paget's disease of the vulva. Diagn Cytopathol. 2005;32(6): 353–7.

Hanley KZ, Tadros TS, Briones AJ, Birdsong GG, Mosunjac MB. Hematologic malignancies of the female genital tract diagnosed on liquid-based Pap test: cytomorphologic features and review of differential diagnoses. Diagn Cytopathol. 2009;37(1):61–7.

Ishi K, Suzuki F, Saito A, Koyatsu J, Akutsu S, Kubota T. Cytodiagnosis of placental site trophoblastic tumor. A report of two cases. Acta Cytol. 1998;42(3):745–50.

Klapsinou E, Terzakis E, Arnogiannaki N, Daskalopoulou D. Paget's disease of the vulva detected in vulvar and vaginal brushing smears: a case report. Acta Cytol. 2010;54((5 Suppl)):898–902.

Khalbuss WE, Michelow P, Benedict C, Monaco SE, and Pantanowitz L. A Cytomorphology of Unusual Infectious Entities in the Pap Test. CytoJournal, 2012;9(15):1–8.

Onuma K, Kanbour-Shakir A, Modery J, Kanbour A. Pemphigus vulgaris of the vagina–its cytomorphologic features on liquid-based cytology and pitfalls: case report and cytological differential diagnosis. Diagn Cytopathol. 2009;37:832–5.

Wang KL, Yang YC, Wang TY, Chen JR, Chen TC, Chen HS, et al. Neuroendocrine carcinoma of the uterine cervix: a clinicopathologic retrospective study of 31 cases with prognostic implications. J Chemother. 2006;18:209–16.

Management Issues and Quality Assurance (QA) in the Pap Test

8

Asif Loya, Noreen Akhtar, Marilee Means, and Walid E. Khalbuss

Contents

A. Loya, MD, MBBS (✉) • N. Akhtar, FCPS, MBBS
Department of Pathology, Shaukat Khanum Memorial Cancer Hospital and Research Centre,
7-A/R-3, M.A Johar town, Lahore, Punjab 13041, Pakistan
e-mail: asifloya@skm.org.pk; noriaakhter@yahoo.com

M. Means, PhD, SCT(ASCP)
School of Health Professions, University of Kansas Medical Center,
3901 Rainbow Blvd., Mail Stop 4048, Kansas City, KS 66160, USA
e-mail: mmeans@kumc.edu

W.E. Khalbuss, MD, PhD, FIAC
Director of Cytology and Cytopathology Fellowship Program,
University of Pittsburgh Medical Center Shadyside Hospital,
5150 Centre Avenue, 2, Suite 201,
Pittsburgh, PA 15232, USA
e-mail: khalbussw2@upmc.edu

8.1 Tables and Summary

Table 8.1 Quality control (QC) vs. quality assurance (QA)

Quality control (QC) procedures help ensure that the preparation, interpretation, and reporting of cytology specimens meets specified quality criteria
Quality assurance (QA) is a retrospective tool that measures the success of specific processes

Table 8.2 The Clinical Laboratory Improvement Amendments (CLIA) of 1988

In the United States, the Clinical Laboratory Improvement Amendments (CLIA) of 1988 standards serve as the foundation of cytology QC/QA
A CLIA certificate is required in order for a laboratory to receive Medicare or Medicaid payments
To obtain a CLIA certificate, a laboratory must be accredited (and inspected) by the Joint Commission or College of American Pathologists (CAP)
CLIA 1988 deals with workload limits for cytotechnologists, addresses certain quality indicators (5-year retrospective rescreening, cytologic-histologic correlation) and states that a pathologist must review all abnormal Pap tests and stress proficiency testing
CLIA 1988 requires the cytology laboratory to provide and document whether alert information (e.g., medical director letter) was sent to providers, with regard to all patients with a Pap test diagnosis of HSIL (or carcinoma) in which there is no record of further patient follow-up in the pathology or hospital information system. This ensures that those patients at high risk for cervical cancer get appropriate and timely intervention and treatment

W.E. Khalbuss, M. Means (eds.), *Gynecological and Breast Cytopathology Board Review and Self-Assessment*, DOI 10.1007/978-1-4614-7270-4_8, © Springer Science+Business Media New York 2013

Table 8.3 Coding and billing

There are two billing coding components: Part A: technical component billing for procedures performed by lab personnel (e.g., making slides, performing stains) which is largely automated Part B: a professional component that is typically and manually coded according to the interpretation/diagnosis given by pathologists
A physician interpretation charge can only be billed if a pathologist personally reviews a slide and provides an interpretation (i.e., signs the case out). This does not include slide review for QA purposes
In order to bill for a test, the following codes are required: Procedure code according to Current Procedural Terminology (CPT) or, for Medicare purposes, the Healthcare Common Procedure Coding System (HCPCS) International Classification of Diseases (ICD)-9 or ICD-10 code supplied by the referring physician to justify the medical necessity of the diagnostic test (e.g., ICD-9 code V15.89 is used for a screening Pap in a woman at high risk for developing cervical or vaginal cancer)

Table 8.4 The most common CPT codes for Pap tests

CPT code	Component	Description (assigned service/task)
88164	Technical	Conventional Pap smear
88142	Technical	Non-imaged liquid-based Pap (manual screening)
88175	Technical	Imaged liquid-based Pap (automated screening)
87621	Technical	HPV testing
88141	Professional	Pathologist-interpreted Pap

Table 8.5 Pap test categories according to medical indication

Category	Medicare definition	Beneficiary coverage
Screening (routine) Pap test	No current complaint/symptom or sign related to the cervix No prior abnormal Pap No high-risk factors for cervical cancer	Only one test every 2 years is covered
Screening (high-risk) Pap test	Early onset of sexual activity (<16 years) Multiple sexual partners (≥5 in a lifetime) STD history (which includes HIV) Less than three negative Paps in the past 7 years Abnormal Pap in the last 3 years in women of childbearing age DES exposure	Only one test every 11 months is covered
Diagnostic Pap test	Cancer diagnosis of cervix, vagina, or uterus Prior abnormal Pap test Current abnormal female genital tract findings or complaint Any gynecologic symptom or sign	Unlimited coverage

Table 8.6 Pap proficiency testing (PT)

Per CLIA 1988, the cytology lab must participate in a Pap proficiency testing (PT) program approved by the Centers for Medicare & Medicaid Services (CMS)
Proficiency testing should be performed annually, proctored on-site, during which participants are allowed 2 h to evaluate ten gynecologic slides prepared in a similar manner (smear versus liquid-based) to that which the lab customarily uses. Pathologists are permitted to examine slides prescreened by a cytotechnologist.
There are only four possible answers in a Pap PT: unsatisfactory, negative (including non-HPV infections), LSIL and HSIL, or cancer. The scoring system is different for cytotechnologists and cytopathologists
If a passing score of ≥90 % is not achieved, participants are asked to retake another 10-slide test. If they also fail this retest, they will need to undergo documented remedial training, now have all of their screened Pap slides reevaluated and take another 4-h 20-slide test. If they fail this third test, the individual will have to stop examining Pap slides until they participate in ≥35 h of continuing education and successfully pass another 20-slide proficiency test

Table 8.7 Workload limits for different Pap tests

Pap test type	Workload limit (slides/day)
Conventional Pap smear	100
LBC Pap smear	100
ThinPrep Imaging System™	170
BD FocalPoint™ GS Imaging System	200

Table 8.8 The ASC guidelines for review of Pap tests for litigation purposes

The finding of a false-negative sample is not necessarily an evidence of practice below the standard of care
Atypical cells of undetermined significance represent an equivocal interpretive category with poor inter/intra-observer reproducibility. Therefore, disputed cases of ASC or AGC are not likely to represent reasonable grounds for allegations of practice below the standard of care
Pap test slides being assessed for possible litigation should be reviewed without knowledge of clinical outcome and in an environment that stimulates the normal screening practice as closely as possible
The standard of care should be that of the reasonable and prudent practitioner
Professional expert witnesses who do not have significant experience in cytopathology are not qualified to express an expert opinion on the standard of care
Compensation of the physician-witness should reasonably reflect the time and effort expended by the witness in preparation, depositions, and trial
The state should adopt a mechanism by which nonbinding arbitration would be required before the filing of any civil action alleging negligence in the taking, examining, or reviewing of a Pap test or the reporting of its results

Table 8.9 Commonly used ICD-9 codes for Pap tests

Code	Definition
V76.2	Screening Pap of cervix in the absence of signs, symptoms, or history
V72.31	Screening Pap of cervix in the absence of signs, symptoms, or history, collected as part of gynecologic examination
V76.47	Screening Pap of vagina in the absence of signs, symptoms, or history
V76.49	Screening Pap in the absence of signs, symptoms, or history in woman without a cervix
V15.89	Screening Pap in woman at high risk for developing cervical or vaginal cancer
616.0	Cervicitis
616.10	Vaginitis
622.10	Histologic CIN, unspecified
622.11	Histologic CIN I (mild dysplasia)
622.12	Histologic CIN II (moderate dysplasia)
233.1	Histologic CIN III (severe dysplasia)
795.00	Abnormal glandular Pap (cervix)
795.01	Abnormal cervical Pap—ASCUS
795.02	Abnormal cervical Pap—ASC-H
795.03	Abnormal cervical Pap—LSIL
795.04	Abnormal cervical Pap—HSIL
795.05	High-risk HPV DNA positive (cervix)
795.06	Malignant cells (cervical Pap) without histologic confirmation
795.08	Unsatisfactory cervical Pap
795.09	Other abnormal cervical Pap (includes reactive or reparative changes)
112.1	Candidiasis
623.5	Vaginal discharge
626.2	Menometrorrhagia
626.4	Irregular menstrual cycle
626.6	Metrorrhagia
626.8	Dysfunctional uterine bleeding
627.1	Postmenopausal bleeding

Abbreviation: *ASC-H* atypical squamous cells, cannot exclude HSIL, *ASCUS* atypical squamous cells of undetermined significance, *CIN* cervical intraepithelial neoplasia, *HPV* human papillomavirus, *HSIL* high-grade squamous intraepithelial lesion, *LSIL* low-grade squamous intraepithelial lesion

Table 8.10 Maslow's law of hierarchy (pyramid)

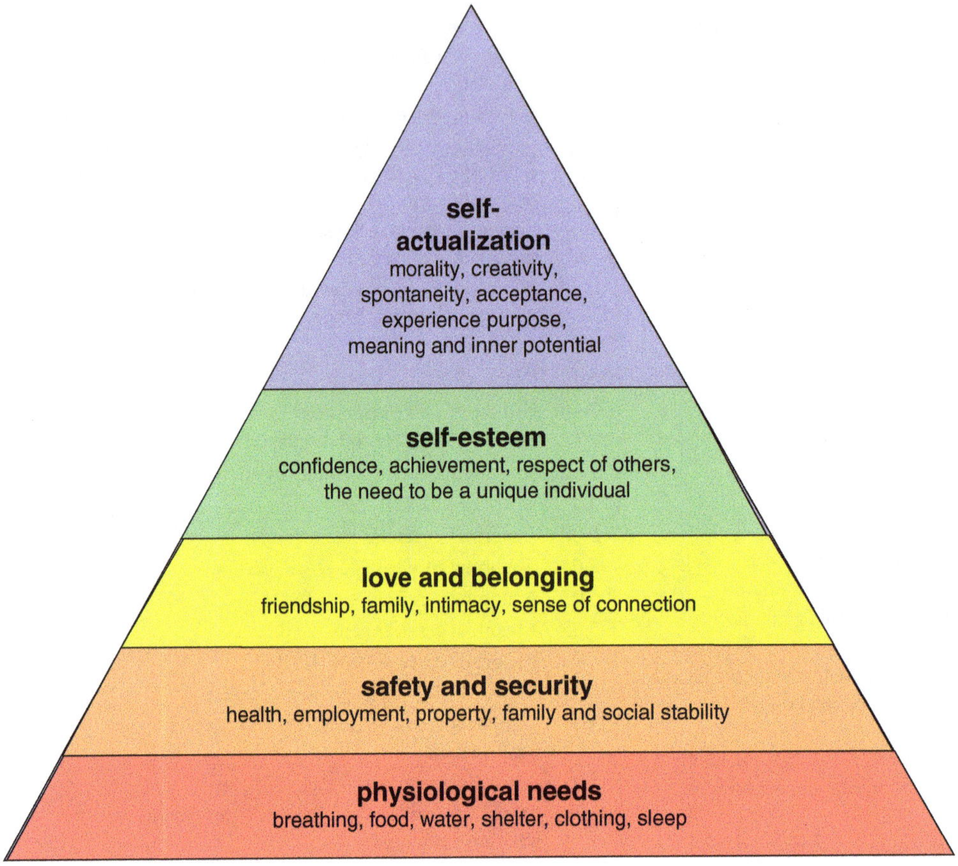

Table 8.11 CPT code, tech code, and billing fee code description

CPT	Tech code	Billing fee code description
88108	22800146	Concentration tech., smears, and interp. (cyto)
88112	22800147	Selective cellular enhancement tech. (cyto)
88172	22800505	FNA evaluation on-site (cyto)
88173	22800506	FNA interp and report (cyto)
88104	22803000	Fluid urine (cyto)
88104	22803010	Fluid gastric (cyto)
88104	22803035	Fluid other (cyto)
88104	22804000	Smear breast (cyto)
88104	22804005	Smear upper resp (cyto)
88104	22804015	Smear other (cyto)
88305	22805000	Cell block (cyto)
10021	22805015	FNA collect by path (cyto)

Table 8.12 Rating system for cytotechnologist system false-negative fraction

FNF (%)	Evaluation	Action
<5	Superior	Commendation
5–10	Excellent	Commendation
10–15	Good	Review w/supv.
15–20	Fair	Review w/supv. Vol. restriction
20–25	Marginal	Quality alert/100 % resc.
>25	Unsatisfactory	Probation

8.2 Text-Based Questions 1–100

Q-1. The maximum # of slides allowed per 24-h period (primary and rescreen) for a pathologist under CLIA 1988 is:
(a) 80
(b) 100
(c) 120
(d) 140
(e) 200

Q-2. The CLIA regulations stipulate that negative gynecologic glass slides must be kept for a minimum of:
(a) 2 years
(b) 5 years
(c) 10 years
(d) 15 years
(e) 20 years

Q-3. CLIA 1988 requires which of the following:
(a) 10 % review of focused or high-risk cases as well as random review
(b) 10 % random review only
(c) 10 % focused or high risk only
(d) 10 % review of abnormal diagnoses
(e) 20 % focused or high risk only

Q-4. Quality assurance is defined as:
(a) Use of collected data to determine trends in test accuracy
(b) Reexamination of abnormal material
(c) Reexamination of negative material
(d) Performing a 10 % review on all gynecologic cases
(e) Cytology/histology correlation

Q-5. The 100-slide primary workload manual screening limit equates to a maximum screening rate of how many slides per hour?
(a) 10.5
(b) 11.0
(c) 11.5
(d) 12.0
(e) 12.5

Q-6. Manually screened gynecologic slides count as:
(a) ½ slide
(b) 1 slide
(c) 1.5 slides
(d) 2 slides
(e) 2.5 slides

Q-7. What common term is defined as the official acknowledgment of professional competence?
(a) Guideline
(b) Credentialing
(c) Registration
(d) Regulation
(e) Bylaw

Q-8. Which federal agency regulates market entry of medical devices, laboratory instruments, reagents, and systems?
(a) National Cancer Institute
(b) Environmental Protection Agency
(c) Food and Drug Administration
(d) Occupational Safety and Health Administration
(e) Risk Management Agency

Q-9. This international nonprofit organization was founded in 1896 and represents approximately 100 nations. It is:
(a) College of American Pathologists
(b) American Cancer Society
(c) Clinical Laboratory Improvement Advisory Committee
(d) Occupational Safety and Health Administration
(e) National Fire Protection Association

Q-10. What year was the cytology proficiency testing (PT) program approved?
(a) 2002
(b) 2003
(c) 2004
(d) 2005
(e) 2006

Q-11. The cytotechnologist is able to screen this many slides under CLIA 1988:
(a) 80
(b) 90
(c) 100
(d) 110
(e) 120

Q-12. The Current Procedural Terminology (CPT) code for the professional component (pathologist-interpreted Pap test) is:
(a) 88140
(b) 88141
(c) 88142
(d) 88144
(e) 88175

Q-13. A physician interpretation charge can be billed:
(a) When quality control is performed
(b) On all negative gynecologic cases
(c) On LSIL and ASCUS cases
(d) On ASCUS and AGUS cases
(e) On all cases reviewed and interpreted by the pathologist

Q-14. An Advanced Beneficiary Notice (ABN) allows:
(a) The lab to bill the submitting physician
(b) The lab to bill Medicare
(c) The lab to bill the patient's insurance
(d) The lab to bill the patient directly if Medicare does not cover a service
(e) The lab to bill the patient directly if the test is abnormal

Q-15. How many categories of Pap tests are available that impact coding and Medicare payment?
(a) Two
(b) Three
(c) Four
(d) Five
(e) Six

Q-16. Who is qualified to classify Pap tests for medical indication?
(a) Patient
(b) Nurse practitioner
(c) Physician's assistant
(d) Receptionist
(e) Physician

Q-17. Regardless of the result of the Pap test, which of the following will pay the lab directly for a diagnostic Pap test?
(a) Primary insurance
(b) Secondary insurance
(c) Medicaid
(d) Medicare
(e) Tricare

Q-18. The current CLIA maximum workload for computer-assisted slides reviewed on the ThinPrep Imaging System allows for how many slides screened by the 22 fields of view review process?
(a) 80 slides
(b) 100 slides
(c) 150 slides
(d) 200 slides
(e) 250 slides

Q-19. The technical supervisor of the cytopathology laboratory must set individual workload limits based on the ability of each individual technologist. The workload limit for each screener must be reassessed every:
(a) 3 months
(b) 6 months
(c) 9 months
(d) 12 months
(e) 18 months

Q-20. The laboratory cannot bill for a Pap test slide in which of the following situations?
(a) If the slide was prepared, reviewed, and unsatisfactory
(b) If the slide was prepared, reviewed, and negative
(c) If the slide was prepared, reviewed, and abnormal
(d) If the slide was submitted and broken beyond repair
(e) If the slide was prepared, review, and less than satisfactory

Q-21. Medicare beneficiary coverage provides testing for routine screening Pap test every:
(a) 2 years
(b) 3 years
(c) 4 years
(d) 5 years
(e) 6 years

Q-22. A high-risk screening Pap test involves which of the following conditions?
(a) DES exposure
(b) No symptoms related to the cervix
(c) Late onset of sexual activity
(d) One sex partner
(e) Three negative Pap tests within 5 years

Q-23. Beneficiary coverage for a diagnostic Pap test is:
(a) Every year
(b) Every 2 years
(c) Every 3 years
(d) Every 5 years
(e) Unlimited

Q-24. This not-for-profit organization evaluated and has accredited hospitals for more than 50 years and has accredited hospital laboratories since 1979. It is:
(a) Health Insurance Portability and Accountability Act (HIPPA)
(b) The Joint Commission
(c) The Centers for Medicare & Medicaid Services (CMS)

(d) Clinical Laboratory Improvement Amendments (CLIA)
(e) American Medical Association (AMA)

Q-25. Which of the following represents the professional society that offers a laboratory accreditation program and inspects over 6,000 cytopathology laboratories in the United States?
(a) Centers for Medicare & Medicaid Services (CMS)
(b) US Department of Health and Human Services
(c) Food and Drug Administration
(d) Council for Accreditation of Allied Health Education Programs
(e) College of American Pathologists

Q-26. Glass slide material needs to be kept for a minimum number of years according to federal regulations. Both gynecologic and non-gynecologic slides must be kept for:
(a) 2 years
(b) 3 years
(c) 5 years
(d) 7 years
(e) 10 years

Q-27. Cytopathology reports interpreted in the cytopathology laboratory need to be retained for:
(a) 2 years
(b) 3 years
(c) 5 years
(d) 7 years
(e) 10 years

Q-28. This division of the Department of Labor was established by Congress in 1971 to a response to public outcry in the 1960s against rising injuries and deaths in the workplace:
(a) Health Insurance Portability and Accountability Act of 1996 (HIPAA)
(b) Clinical Laboratory Improvement Amendments of 1988 (CLIA 1988)
(c) Occupational Safety and Health Administration (OSHA)
(d) National Fire Protection Association
(e) DHHS Office of Civil Rights

Q-29. Which of the following is the US government's principal agency for protecting essential human services?
(a) DHHS Office of Civil Rights
(b) Occupational Safety and Health Administration
(c) Central Intelligence Agency
(d) Department of Health and Human Services
(e) National Institute of Health

Q-30. The federal regulation requirement for cytology laboratory test requisitions retention is:
(a) 2 years
(b) 3 years
(c) 5 years
(d) 7 years
(e) 10 years

Q-31. Worksheets required by federal regulations such as quality control, quality assurance, and proficiency testing results need to be retained in the cytopathology laboratory for:
(a) 2 years
(b) 3 years
(c) 5 years
(d) 7 years
(e) 10 years

Q-32. When a cytopathology final report is amended, which of the following needs to be stated on the report?
(a) The original date
(b) The reason for the correction
(c) The issued date
(d) The clinical history
(e) The specimen source

Q-33. The CPT code for HPV testing is a technical component. Which of the following represents the correct CPT code?
(a) 88164
(b) 88142
(c) 88175
(d) 87621
(e) 88141

Q-34. The CPT code for image-guided liquid-based Pap test (automated screening) is:
(a) 88164
(b) 88142
(c) 88175
(d) 87621
(e) 88141

Q-35. Which CPT modifier denotes that only the physician professional component of the service is being billed?
(a) Modifier 26
(b) Modifier 52
(c) Modifier 59
(d) Modifier GY
(e) Modifier GA

Q-36. Proficiency testing must be performed every:
(a) Year
(b) 2 years
(c) 3 years
(d) 5 years
(e) 10 years

Q-37. Proficiency testing (PT) is performed annually, proctored on-site. How many hours are cytotechnologists and cytopathologists given to perform the exam?
(a) ½h
(b) 1 h
(c) 1½h
(d) 2 h
(e) 2½h

Q-38. If a cytotechnologist fails an initial 10-slide PT exam, then fails the subsequent 10-slide PT exam, what is the next exam they have to take after documented remedial training is complete?
(a) 10-slide gynecologic examination
(b) 15-slide gynecologic examination
(c) 20-slide gynecologic examination
(d) 25-slide gynecologic examination
(e) 30-slide gynecologic examination

Q-39. For quality control purposes, which type of specimen is often regarded as the gold standard?
(a) Pap test specimen
(b) HPV test specimen
(c) Fine-needle aspiration specimen
(d) Microbiology specimen
(e) Histopathology specimen

Q-40. Laboratories surveyed under the Joint Commission or the College of American Pathologists (CAP) have been deemed certifiable under:
(a) American Medical Association
(b) Health Insurance Portability and Accountability Act
(c) National Institute of Health
(d) Clinical Laboratory Improvement Amendments
(e) Centers for Disease Control and Prevention

Q-41. To maintain accreditation from the Joint Commission, hospitals are surveyed every:
(a) Year
(b) 2 years
(c) 3 years
(d) 4 years
(e) 5 years

Q-42. Surveys by both the Joint Commission and the College of American Pathologists have been unannounced since this year:
(a) 2004
(b) 2005
(c) 2006
(d) 2007
(e) 2008

Q-43. Which of the following conducts inspections in response to reports of employee complaints or serious accidents?
(a) The Joint Commission
(b) Occupational Safety and Health Administration
(c) College of American Pathologists
(d) American Society for Clinical Pathology
(e) Clinical Laboratory Improvement Amendments

Q-44. Specialized surveys are required by CLIA 1988 on a small proportion of cytology laboratories with CLIA certificates. These surveys are conducted by:
(a) The Joint Commission
(b) College of American Pathologists
(c) American Society for Clinical Pathology
(d) American Medical Association
(e) American Society for Cytotechnology

Q-45. This committee was appointed to advise CMS and other government agencies on the need for revisions in laboratory testing. It is:
(a) The National Safety Committee
(b) The Laboratory Ethics Committee
(c) The Clinical Laboratory Oversight Committee
(d) The Clinical Laboratory Improvement Advisory Committee
(e) The National Cancer Registry Committee

Q-46. Who is responsible for implementing the new ruling on comprehensive privacy legislation that took effect in April 2001 and required compliance by healthcare providers by April of 2003?
(a) DHHS Office of Civil Rights
(b) Clinical Laboratory Improvement Amendments
(c) Environmental Protection Agency
(d) Risk Management Agency
(e) National Safety Institute

Q-47. The International Classification of Disease, Clinical Modification is based on the official version of:
(a) International Disease Registry
(b) Healthcare Common Procedural Coding System

(c) National Cancer Institute Disease Registry
(d) American Medical Association Disease Classification
(e) World Health Organization International Classification of Diseases

Q-48. If a Pap test is submitted for follow-up of a prior Pap test with ASCUS and the current finding is LSIL, what ICD-9 code should be used?
(a) ICD-9 code 795.02 (ASC-H)
(b) ICD-9 code 795.05 (cervical high-risk HPV test positive)
(c) ICD-9 code 795.00 (atypical glandular cells)
(d) ICD-9 code 795.01 (ASCUS)
(e) ICD-9 code 795.03 (LSIL)

Q-49. Which of the following represents the code that is considered acceptable for documentation of payment to laboratories for a routine cervical Pap smear, intact cervix?
(a) V76.49
(b) V76.47
(c) V76.2
(d) V15.89
(e) V76.1

Q-50. Which of the following generations represent the group of employees that were born between 1965 and 1980?
(a) Veterans
(b) Baby boomers
(c) Generation X
(d) Generation Y
(e) Nexters

Q-51. This is the process where all individuals are treated equally in the hiring process, training, and promotion:
(a) Needs assessment
(b) Family Leave Act
(c) Equal employment opportunity
(d) Workman's compensation
(e) Affirmative action

Q-52. This is the process of gathering information to assist in making data-driven decisions and recommendations about staffing levels and skills:
(a) Needs assessment
(b) Equal employment opportunity
(c) Affirmative action
(d) Job description
(e) Staff competency assessment

Q-53. What is the current OSHA PEL for xylene for an 8-h time-weighted average?
(a) 10 ppm
(b) 25 ppm
(c) 50 ppm
(d) 75 ppm
(e) 100 ppm

Q-54. False-negative Pap tests are largely due to which of the following?
(a) Staining errors
(b) Preparation errors
(c) Sampling errors
(d) Interpretation errors
(e) Screening errors

Q-55. The false-negative rate (FNR) is defined as the proportion of abnormal Pap tests that are falsely negative. FNR equals:
(a) False positives ÷ true positives + false negatives
(b) False positives ÷ true negatives + false positives
(c) False positives ÷ true positives + false positives
(d) False negatives ÷ true positives + false negatives
(e) False negatives ÷ true positives = false positives

Q-56. Pap tests for possible litigation are recommended to be reviewed:
(a) In the lawyer's office
(b) In a laboratory setting
(c) In the courtroom
(d) In a home office
(e) Through a legal app on the iPad

Q-57. Retrospective rescreening is performed on Pap tests which are interpreted as:
(a) NILM
(b) ASCUS
(c) ASC-H
(d) LSIL
(e) Cancer

Q-58. Who must be notified when a significant discrepancy is found on a Pap test retrospective review which will affect patient care?
(a) Patient
(b) Medicare
(c) Medicaid
(d) Referring physician
(e) CMS

Q-59. CLIA 1988 requires the cytology laboratory to compile statistics for review. Which of the following are required?
(a) Number of Pap tests that are reclassified as normal
(b) Number of HPV tests ordered
(c) Number of Pap tests that are reclassified as abnormal
(d) Number of Pap tests with Candida spp.
(e) Number of Pap tests with herpes simplex virus

Q-60. Which of the following ICD-9 CM codes represent a cervical high-risk human papillomavirus (HPV) test positive?
(a) 795.02
(b) 795.03
(c) 795.04
(d) 795.05
(e) 795.06

Q-61. For Advance Beneficiary Notice (ABN) signatures, the laboratory generally relies on:
(a) Patient
(b) Relatives of the patient
(c) Referring physician
(d) Medical director
(e) Cytotechnician

Q-62. The screening (high-risk) Pap test is defined by Medicare as follows:
(a) Previous Pap smear was abnormal.
(b) Any sign or symptom that might be related to a gynecological disorder.
(c) No current sign and symptoms.
(d) Multiple sexual partners (five in lifetime).
(e) Normal Pap smear.

Q-63. One can bill for an unsatisfactory Pap smear under the following circumstance:
(a) Broken beyond repair
(b) Insufficient identifying information
(c) Obscuring blood
(d) Obscuring inflammation
(e) Both c and d

Q-64. Separate professional fee is billable by the pathologist:
(a) If pathologist interpretation is precipitated by finding of abnormal, atypical, or reactive cells by the cytotechnician
(b) Normal Pap smear reported by the cytotechnician
(c) Pathologist review of high-risk patient smear judged to be normal by the cytotechnician
(d) Pathologist's review of laboratory quality assurance and quality control program
(e) Abnormal Pap smear reported by cytotechnician

Q-65. The ICD-9 codebook includes series of "health status" codes called "V" codes which are used when:
(a) If a cytology specimen is interpreted as positive for malignancy
(b) If patients have only clinical symptoms
(c) If cytology specimen is reported as "suspicious for malignancy"
(d) When patient has no current sign or symptom of disease or injury
(e) When the cytology specimen is reported negative

Q-66. Potential sampling error in false-negative Pap interpretations includes:
(a) Screening
(b) Interpretation (misinterpreted)
(c) Inefficient transfer of lesional cell from collection device to glass slide
(d) CT screening the slide
(e) TS screening the side

Q-67. The prospective rescreening of 10 % of negative Pap has been a QC requirement of all laboratories in the United States. The only exception being:
(a) Government sector laboratories with pathologists and CT
(b) Laboratories with pathologist and CT
(c) Laboratories with pathologist, fellow, and CT
(d) Laboratories with a solo pathologists and no CT
(e) Laboratories with pathologists, residents, fellow, and CT

Q-68. The 10 % rescreening of negative Paps must be done by a Technical Supervisor (TS), General Supervisor (GS), or Cytotechnologist (CT) with:
(a) 3 years full-time experience in past 10 years
(b) 3 years full-time experience in past 20 years
(c) 2 years full-time experience in past 20 years
(d) 2 years full-time experience in past 10 years
(e) 2 years full-time experience in past 30 years

Q-69. The positive predictive value (PPV) of the Pap test of which reported abnormality is highest?
(a) ASCUS
(b) ASC-H
(c) LSIL
(d) SIL
(e) Squamous cell carcinoma

Q-70. The most common cause of discrepancies in cytologic-histologic correlation in QC of cytology is:
(a) Error in cytologic interpretation
(b) Screening error
(c) Sampling error
(d) Error in histologic interpretation
(e) CT screening the sample

Q-71. Slides that typically count as half slides:
(a) Direct smear
(b) ThinPrep slides (gynecologic cases)
(c) Cytocentrifuge preparation
(d) SurePath slides (gynecologic case)
(e) FNA slides

Q-72. The CLIA 1988 regulations allow how many number of slides of CT to examine in 24 h?
(a) 100
(b) 50
(c) 150
(d) 125
(e) 200

Q-73. According to CLIA 1988 for cytology proficiency testing, each participant must evaluate how many gynecologic slides?
(a) 25
(b) 20
(c) 10
(d) 15
(e) 30

Q-74. How many slide-testing events does an individual get when taking the proficiency test before ceasing to examining Pap slides?
(a) 2
(b) 1
(c) 3
(d) 4
(e) 6

Q-75. A CT's screening skills can be assessed from:
(a) False-negative detected during rescreening of 10 % of negative PAPs
(b) False-negative retrospective rescreen
(c) Number of screening hours
(d) Number of screening slides in 24 h
(e) Smear preparation by CT

Q-76. The percentage of abnormal cases (ASC, AGS, SIL, and carcinoma) diagnosed by a CT divided by the total number of cases examined is:
(a) False-negative rate
(b) Abnormal rate
(c) True-positive rate
(d) Unsatisfactory rate
(e) Normal rate

Q-77. A proposed upper limit ratio of atypical squamous cell to squamous intraepithelial lesion to measures of cytopathologist's performance should not exceed:
(a) 1:1
(b) 3:1
(c) 2:1
(d) 2:2
(e) 3:2

Q-78. The probability of given test result if disease is present divided by the probability of the same result if disease is absent is known as:
(a) Likelihood ratio (LR)
(b) Unlikelihood ratio (ULR)
(c) FNR
(d) Positive predictive value
(e) Negative predictive value

Q-79. The performance evaluation of cytopathologist is required by:
(a) AMA
(b) CLIA 1988
(c) CAD
(d) HIPPA
(e) TJC

Q-80. A document containing list of all job classifications in which all employees have occupational exposure and a list of all job classifications in which *some* employees have exposure is known as:
(a) Exposure control
(b) Exposure determination
(c) Post exposure disease
(d) Exposure assessment
(e) Occupational exposure list

Q-81. To maintain accreditation, unannounced survey by CAP is performed after how many years?
(a) 3 years
(b) 2 years
(c) 4 years
(d) 1 year
(e) 6 years

Q-82. In order to obtain CLIA 1988 certificate, a laboratory must be accredited by which approved accrediting organization:
(a) American Society for Cytotechnologists
(b) American Society of Cytopathology
(c) Council for Accreditation of Allied Health Education
(d) Joint Commission
(e) Centers for Medicare & Medicated Services (CMS)

Q-83. According to federal retention requirement for cytology laboratories, reports must be retained for how many years?
(a) 5 years
(b) 2.5 years
(c) 10 years
(d) 15 years
(e) 7 years

Q-84. According to CLIA 1988, the reporting system used in a cytology report must use:
(a) Numerical reporting system (e.g., class IV)
(b) Photographic format
(c) May be in electronic format
(d) Hard copy format
(e) Narrative, descriptive terminology

Q-85. A uniform language which describes all medical, surgical, and diagnostic services and provides effective communication between physicians, patients, and third parties is:
(a) ICD-9 coding system
(b) CPT codes
(c) HCPC codes
(d) Bar codes
(e) ICD8 codes

Q-86. The HCPCS (Healthcare Common Procedure Coding System) is administered by:
(a) AMA
(b) CLIA 1988
(c) CAP
(d) TJC
(e) CMS

Q-87. Which CPT modifier is used when only the physician professional component of the service is being billed?
(a) CPT modifier 52
(b) CPT modifier 59
(c) CPT modifier 26
(d) CPT modifier GC
(e) CPT modifier 62

Q-88. The steps in the flow of work of cytology laboratory are in the following order:
(a) Accessioning specimen collection and transportation, slide preparation, slide examination, report results, and retention
(b) Specimen collection and transportation, accessioning, slide preparation, slide examination, report results, and retention
(c) Specimen collection and transportation, accessioning, slide preparation, slide examination, report retention, and report result
(d) Specimen collection and transportation, accessioning, slide examination, slide preparation, report retention, and result
(e) Specimen collection and transportation, slide preparation, slide examination, report result, and retention

Q-89. The laboratory procedure manual must include:
(a) The name and address of the laboratory
(b) Specimen labelling policies
(c) Criteria for specimen rejection
(d) Specimen preservation policies
(e) Conditions for transportation

Q-90. Records of discontinued procedures must be kept for:
(a) 3 years
(b) 5 years
(c) 6 months
(d) 2 years
(e) 1 month

Q-91. Publications like Standard for Health Care Facilities for cytology laboratories are published by:
(a) CLIA 1988
(b) Health Insurance Portability and Accountability Act
(c) OSHA laboratory standard
(d) CAP
(e) National Fire Protection Association

Q-92. A specialized survey conducted by American Society of Cytotechnologist randomly at laboratories reviews at least:
(a) 100 body fluids
(b) 50 body fluids
(c) 100 FNAC
(d) 100 Pap tests
(e) 50 FNAC

Q-93. Clinical Laboratory Improvement Advisory Committee (CLIAC) consists of:
(a) 15 members
(b) 20 members
(c) 5 members
(d) 30 members
(e) 26 members

Q-94. A cytotechnologists must have graduated from a school of cytotechnology accredited by:
(a) CLIA 1988
(b) CAP
(c) IJC
(d) CMS
(e) CAAH EP

Q-95. Which type of service is not included in Part A of Medicare plans:
(a) Inpatient services
(b) Home health services
(c) Skilled nursing facility
(d) Outpatient laboratory
(e) Physician administrative activities

Q-96. Physician professional fees are calculated using a formula based on standard expense variables and local expense factors known as:
(a) Expense-based value scale
(b) Resource-based value scale
(c) Net present value
(d) Gross present value
(e) Account factor

Q-97. In which of the following scenarios must the patient be notified in advance that the test will likely to be denied payment:
(a) Medicare is primary payer.
(b) Medicare is secondary payer.
(c) Lab is a Medicare beneficiary.
(d) Test is covered by Medicare.
(e) Test ordered is experimental.

Q-98. According to the elements of CLIA 1988 regulations, labelling of reagents, controls, and calibration must not be outside expiration date comes under:
(a) Quality program
(b) Quality assurance
(c) Quality control
(d) Quality systems
(e) Laboratory protocols

Q-99. Health Insurance Portability and Accountability Act determines:
(a) Workload limits for cytotechnologists
(b) QC procedures
(c) Privacy of medical information
(d) Statistical records
(e) Proficiency testing

Q-100. According to national patient safety goals to improve the accuracy of patient identification, JCAHO requires the use of:
(a) One identifier
(b) Three identifiers
(c) Two identifiers
(d) Four identifies
(e) Five identifies

8.3 Answers and Discussion 1–100

A-1. **(b) 100**

CLIA 1988 requires that all gynecologic slides should be thoroughly screened by a cytotechnologist/pathologist in a CLIA-certified laboratory. CLIA 1988 allows a maximum primary manual screening workload of 100 slides per day, over no less than 8 h. Some states have lower workload limits, and laboratories must adhere to the most restrictive limit in effect. Pathologists who function as primary screeners are subject to the workload limit, and compliance must be documented. Cases prescreened by a cytotechnologist are not counted as part of the pathologist's workload.

A-2. **(b) 5 years**

Previously negative cytologic and relevant histologist material should be reviewed to correlate results whenever current samples show a significant abnormality that could have been overlooked in the prior specimen. The degree of abnormality that causes a review is determined by the laboratory; however, CLIA 1988 stipulates that negative or normal cytologic specimens obtained within the previous 5 years, either on-site or in storage, should be reviewed whenever a high-grade squamous intraepithelial lesion or malignant process is detected on the subsequent cytology specimen.

A-3. **(a) 10 % review of focused or high-risk cases as well as random review**

CLIA1988 regulations specify that at least 10 % of negative gynecologic specimens in cytology from the primary screener should be rescreened. Both randomly selected cases and those from focused or high-risk individuals based on available patient information are included in the rescreened cytologic specimens. The review must be performed by a supervisor-qualified cytotechnologist or pathologist and needs to be completed prior to final reporting. Written documentation of all rescreening should be maintained.

A-4. **(a) Use of collected data to determine trends in test accuracy**

Quality assurance (QA) refers to the planned and systemic activities implemented in a quality system so that quality requirements for a product or service are fulfilled. Collected data is used to determine trends in test accuracy. This contrasted with quality control (QC) which focuses primarily on process outputs. Two principles included in QA are that the product should be suitable for the intended purpose and mistakes should be eliminated. QA includes management of the quality of materials, products, services related to production, management, and inspection processes.

A-5. **(e) 12.5**

The CLIA 1988 100 glass slide workload limit applies to both previously unscreened gynecologic and non-gynecologic glass slides. The limit equates to a maximum screening rate of 12.5 glass slides per hour. Slides manually rescreened for quality control are also included in this workload limit of 100 glass slides.

A-6. **(b) 1 slide**

Manually screened slides count as one slide. The workload limit set by CLIA 1988 allows a maximum primary manual screening of 100 slides per day, over no less than 8 h. The workload limit applies to both previously unscreened gynecologic and non-gynecologic slides. Slides manually rescreened for quality control are also included in this workload limit. Pathologists who function as primary screeners are subject to the same workload limitations. All gynecological slides (manual screened) count as 1 slide. However, non-gynecologic slides of 1/2 of a slide or less (ThinPrep, SurePath, or cytospin preparations) may be counted as 1/2 slide.

A-7. **(b) Credentialing**

Credentialing is the process of establishing qualifications of licensed professionals, organizational members, or organizations and assessing their background and competence. Many healthcare institutions and provider networks conduct their own credentialing with review by medical staff or a credentialing committee. The process is usually an objective evaluation of a subject's current licensure, training experience, competence, and ability to provide a particular service or perform particular procedures.

A-8. **(c) Food and Drug Administration**

The Food and Drug Administration (FDA) is the federal agency that regulated market entry of medical devices, laboratory instruments, reagents, and systems. If an instrument has been cleared or approved by the FDA, the laboratory must document and report any adverse event or failure. Specifically, the FDA states, "user facilities must establish and maintain MDR (medical device report) event files." MDR event files are written or electronic files maintained by the user facility.

A-9. (**e**) **National Fire Protection Association**
The National Fire Protection Association (NFPA) is an international nonprofit organization which was founded in 1896. It represents close to 100 nations and serves as the premier advocate of fire safety and prevention. Its safety codes influence the design and construction of all building in the United States. The cytopathology professional must be familiar with all applicable safety codes to be sure they are observed, especially when renovations occur within the laboratory.

A-10. (**c**) **2004**
Despite provisions of CLIA 1988 for cytology proficiency testing (PT), a national cytology PT program was not approved until the year 2004. CMS approved an examination offered by the state of Maryland, but this test was only offered to those who practiced in the state. The first version of a national PT program was the Midwest Institute for Medical Education (MIME). Approval of the MIME program was granted in the year 2004, and testing began in 2005.

A-11. (**c**) **100**
Cytotechnologists are allowed to manually screen 100 slides under CLIA 1988. The cytotechnologist needs to document slide interpretation results and record the number screened per day. The maximum of 100 slides per 24 h is not intended as a performance target but as an absolute maximum number allowed by law. If the cytotechnologist works at another lab that day, the hours spent working at the other lab and the number of slides screened at that laboratory must also be recorded and taken into account by the technical supervisor of the primary laboratory of employment to ensure the total number of slides at all laboratories does not exceed the maximum allowed.

A-12. (**b**) **88141**
A medical bill submitted to an insurer for payment needs to describe the procedure of service that is being billed. The Current Procedural Terminology (CPT) code for the pathologist-interpreted Pap test is 88141. CPT codes are the foundation for determining facility (technical) and physician (professional) payments in conjunction with Medicare's resource-based relative value system (RBRVS). CPT codes are a registered trademark of the American Medical Association (AMA).

A-13. (**e**) **On all cases reviewed and interpreted by the pathologist**
A physician-interpreted Pap test (CPT code 88141) can be billed on all cases reviewed and interpreted by the pathologist. When a pathologist interprets or reviews a Pap, their signature must appear on the report (handwritten or electronic). There is a separate professional billable fee submitted by the pathologist if his or her interpretation is due to a finding of abnormal, atypical, or reactive cells by the cytotechnologist. A pathologist's professional fee is legitimate in this case even if the Pap test is determined to be normal.

A-14. (**d**) **The lab to bill the patient directly if Medicare does not cover a service**
By signing an Advanced Beneficiary Notice (ABN), usually on the requisition form, a patient can authorize a lab to directly bill her if Medicare does not cover a service. The laboratory generally relies on the referring physician to obtain the ABN signatures it needs because it almost never has direct contact with the patient in advance of a Pap test. Medicare states that an ABN is valid, and the patient is financially liable for the service only if the ABN is signed in advance for the test. Posttest ABN signatures are not valid or binding on the beneficiary.

A-15. (**b**) **Three**
There are three categories of Pap tests based on their medical indication that impact coding and Medicare payment. Only the referring physician can classify Pap tests. The three categories include a screening (routine) Pap test, a screening (high-risk) Pap test, and a diagnostic Pap test. All three categories have different beneficiary coverage.

A-16. (**e**) **physician**
Only the referring physician can classify Pap tests. Unlike a screening Pap test, Medicare will always cover (direct Pap test in the laboratory) for a diagnostic Pap test regardless of the interpreted results. It is important to recognize the distinction between screening and diagnostic Pap tests, as this will determine CPT or HCPCS codes for Medicare. For diagnostic (medical) Medicare Pap and for most third-party payer Pap tests, CPT codes are used exclusively. The designation of a Pap test as diagnostic is based on information provided by the referring physician. This may be in the ICD-9 codes, signs or symptoms data, or a written narrative.

A-17. (**c**) **Medicaid**
Regardless of the result of the Pap test, Medicaid will pay the lab directly for a diagnostic Pap test. The designation of a Pap test as diagnostic is based on information provided by the referring physician. Diagnostic

Paps are not limited by frequency and are payable as submitted as long as information that documents medical necessity is included (proper ICD-9 code). CMS has designated ICD-9 as the coding system physicians must use. It is important to assign the correct and most specific ICD-9 code, as this documents medical necessity for the procedure. In the absence of such information, it may be necessary to access the patient's medical record and or contact the physician's office.

A-18. **(d) 200 slides**
The workload limit for the ThinPrep Imaging System has been established at 200 slides in no less than an 8-h workday for review of the 22 fields of view review process. For slides that are triaged to full manual review, the workload cannot exceed 100 slides in an 8-h workday. Some state may have more stringent regulations, and the technologist will need to follow those. Any combination of field of view only and full manual reviews must be combined with the total number of slides not to exceed the limits. These values can be used to count workload, not exceeding the CLIA maximum limit of 100 slides, in no less than an 8-h day. Full manual review (FMR) = 1 slide, field of view (FOV) review = 0.5 slide, and FMR + FOV = 1.5 slides. Upper limit = 100 slides.

A-19. **(b) 6 months**
The laboratory director must ensure that competent personnel are employed to perform and report tests. The technical supervisor is responsible for evaluating competency and conducting performance evaluations for new employees and annually thereafter. The technical supervisor has responsibility for evaluating the performance of all cytotechnologists every 6 months and determining the actual workload limit of each cytotechnologist for the next 6-month period. These assessments must be based on the results from the 10 % rescreen of negative Paps and level of pathologist concordance with the cytotechnologist's interpretation on the cases referred to the cytopathologist for review.

A-20. **(d) If the slide was submitted and broken**
The laboratory cannot bill for a Pap test if a glass slide was submitted broken beyond repair or if insufficient identifying information was available. The slide would be unsatisfactory before review, and a charge should not be submitted on that case. If, however, the slide was reviewed and deemed unsatisfactory because of obscuring blood, insufficient squamous cells, or inflammation, then a charge should be reported accompanied by the appropriate ICD-9 code.

A-21. **(a) 2 years**
Routine screening Pap tests are covered every 2 years. The Pap test is considered a screening routine Pap test is ordered solely as part of a preventative healthcare visit annual or periodic checkup. If the woman has not had a Pap paid for by Medicare within the last 2 years, then the laboratory can expect a payment by Medicare and can post one of the four accepted ICD-9 codes, V72.31, V76.2, V76.47, or V76.49, as it has been supplied by the ordering physician.

A-22. **(a) DES exposure**
The screening of a high-risk Pap test is defined by Medicare as follows: early onset of sexual activity (under 16 years of age), multiple sex partners (≥5 in a lifetime), history of sexually transmitted disease (including HIV), fewer than three negative Pap tests in the previous 7 years, daughter of a woman who was given diethylstilbestrol (DES) during pregnancy, or a woman of childbearing age who has had an abnormal Pap test in the past 3 years.

A-23. **(e) Unlimited**
As defined, a diagnostic Pap test is always covered by Medicare, whether or not it is abnormal, if the clinical ICD-9 code provided by the referring physician is on the local Medicare Part B carrier's limited coverage list. A diagnostic Pap test has unlimited beneficiary coverage.

A-24. **(b) The Joint Commission**
The Joint Commission is an independent, not-for-profit organization that evaluates and accredits more than 15,000 healthcare organizations in the United States. It is governed by a Board of Commissioners that include physicians, consumers, and administrators. It was founded in 1959 and has developed standards for evaluating hospitals, assisted living facilities, outpatient services, and clinical laboratories. It has been accrediting hospitals for more than 50 years and laboratories since 1979.

Laboratories surveyed by the Joint Commission have been deemed certifiable under Clinical Laboratory Improvement Amendments of 1988 (CLIA 1988) requirements. To earn accreditation, a hospital or laboratory undergoes an on-site survey.

A-25. **(e) College of American Pathologists**
The College of American Pathologists (CAP) is a professional society of pathologists that offers a laboratory accreditation program that inspects more than 6,000 laboratories in the United States. Surveys are performed every 2 years and have been unannounced

since 2006. Volunteer surveyors use inspection checklists that undergo regular revision to reflect the federal regulations and professional standards. Like the laboratories inspected by the Joint Commission, CAP-inspected laboratories are also eligible for CLIA certificates.

A-26. **(c) 5 years**
Glass slide material needs to be kept for a minimum of 5 years. This includes both gynecologic and non-gynecologic samples. Both negative and abnormal glass slides must be kept for 5 years. FNA slides should be kept for minimum of 10 years. Certain states may have more stringent regulations for cytology records and slides.

A-27. **(e) 10 years**
Reports interpreted in the cytopathology laboratory need to be kept for further review for a minimum of 10 years. This may be in an electronic or hard copy format. This is a federal regulation; some states may require more stringent regulations.

A-28. **(c) Occupational Safety and Health Administration (OSHA)**
The Occupational Safety and Health Administration (OSHA) established guidelines and monitors compliances with chemical and biohazardous regulations. OSHA recognizes hazards in the laboratory, often referred to as the "laboratory standard," for occupational exposure to hazardous chemicals. All labs are required to produce a chemical hygiene plan that addresses the hazards in the cytopathology laboratory. Violations of standards can result in stiff monetary penalties.

A-29. **(d) Department of Health and Human Services**
The Department of Health and Human Services is the United States government's principal agency for protecting the health of all Americans and providing essential human services, especially for those who are at least able to help themselves. It comprises the Office of the Secretary and 11 operating divisions. The agencies perform a wide variety of tasks and services, including research, public health, food and drug safety, grants and other funding, and health insurance.

A-30. **(a) 2 years**
To ensure proper handling of specimens and documentation, CLIA 1988 regulation specifies certain mandatory procedures. Original test requisitions must be kept on hand for a minimum of 2 years. These test requisitions can be electronic, scanned into a system for retrieval, microfilmed, or hard copy. The requisition form must be completed by a physician or authorized individual.

A-31. **(a) 2 years**
Quality control worksheets including retrospective review and discrepancies between Pap and biopsy results need to be kept in the cytopathology laboratory for a minimum of 2 years similar to test requisitions. They can be kept as a hard copy, in electronic format, or scanned into a system for easy retrieval.

A-32. **(b) The reason for the correction**
If a corrected or amended report needs to be issued in the cytology laboratory, the corrected report must state the reason for the correction. For example, a pleural fluid cytology sample was interpreted as malignant for adenocarcinoma, and the report was issued. The referring physician asked for additional immunohistochemical stains to be performed on the case. An amended report needs to be issued stating the reason for the correction (i.e., immunohistochemical stains were requested by the referring physician. TTF-1 and napsin A immunostains were positive, and p63 immunostain was negative with adequate controls. The immunostains support an adenocarcinoma consistent with lung primary).

A-33. **(d) 87621**
The Current Procedural Terminology or CPT is a registered trademark of the American Medical Association (AMA). CMS which administers Medicare program for DHHS uses CPT codes as the main source of codes and descriptors for processing medical claims. These codes help determine technical (facility) and professional (physician) payments. HPV testing is technical, and the CPT code for billing is 87621.

A-34. **(c) 88175**
The CPT code for image-guided liquid-based Pap test (automated screening) is 88175. It is a technical component billing for procedures performed by laboratory personnel which is largely automated (i.e., making slides performing stains). A CPT code has been assigned to virtually every type of physician and laboratory service, including cytologic slide preparation and interpretation. CPT codes describe even the most complex medical procedures in the form of a five-digit code.

A-35. **(a) Modifier 26**
In some circumstances, CPT and HCPCS codes require the use of modifiers to avoid filing a false claim and to assure prompt payment by payers. Some

commonly used modifiers include CPT code modifier 26, 52, and 59. CPT modifier 26 is the most widely used in pathology. It denotes that only the physician professional component of the service is being billed.

A-36. (**a**) **year**
Per CLIA 1988, the cytology laboratory must participate in the Pap proficiency testing (PT) program approved by the Centers for Medicare & Medicaid Services (CMS).

PT should be performed annually. It is administered on-site and is an announced test. Each participant evaluates ten gynecologic slides, and a score of 90 % is needed to pass.

A-37. (**d**) **2 h**
PT should be performed annually, proctored on-site, during which participants are allowed 2 h to evaluate ten gynecologic slides prepared in a similar manner to what the laboratory is used to reviewing (smear versus liquid based). Pathologists are permitted to examine slides prescreened by a cytotechnologist.

A-38. (**c**) **20-slide gynecologic examination**
There are four possible answers in the PT examination: unsatisfactory, negative, LSIL and HSIL, or cancer. If a passing score of ≥90 % is not achieved, participants are asked to retake another 10 slide exam. If they fail this test, they need to undergo documented remedial training, have all Pap test slides they examined reevaluated, and take a 4-h 20-slide examination.

A-39. (**e**) **Histopathology specimen**
Cytologic-histologic correlation is the mainstay of QC in the cytology laboratory and is the foundation for developing and refining diagnostic criteria. Histologic outcome is a common gold standard against which cytologic gynecologic and non-gynecologic interpretations are measured. Discrepancies between Pap tests and biopsies are not uncommon. The majority of discrepancies are from sampling errors.

A-40. (**d**) **Clinical Laboratory Improvement Amendments**
Laboratories surveyed by the Joint Commission or the College of American Pathologists who have earned accreditation have been deemed certifiable under Clinical Laboratory Improvement Amendments of 1988 (CLIA 1988) requirements.

A-41. (**c**) **3 years**
The Joint Commission has been accrediting hospitals for more than 50 years. To earn accreditation, the hospital has to undergo an on-site survey. To maintain their accreditation, hospitals are surveyed every 3 years.

A-42. (**c**) **2006**
Surveys by both the Joint Commission and the College of American Pathologists have been unannounced since the year 2006. The Joint Commission initiated a new survey process that uses patient "tracers," an evaluation process that focuses on service processes and traces patients through the care they have received. The new process has shifted the emphasis from survey preparation to improvement of operational systems. This process enhances safety and reduces medical errors.

A-43. (**b**) **Occupational Safety and Health Administration**
Occupational Safety and Health Administration (OSHA) is a division within the Department of Labor. OSHA's mission is to prevent injuries, illness, and deaths on the job. OSHA conducts inspections in response to reports of high injury rates or imminent danger fatalities or serious accidents and employee complaints. Violation of standards can result in stiff monetary penalties. Of particular relevance to cytology laboratories are OSHA's Bloodborne Pathogens Standard and the OSHA Laboratory Standard, both of which are available on the OSHA website.

A-44. (**e**) **American Society for Cytotechnology**
To bill for and receive Medicare or Medicaid payments, a clinical laboratory must have a CLIA certificate. To obtain a certificate, a laboratory must be accredited by one of two approved organizations, the Joint Commission or CAP. Specialized surveys required by CLIA 1988 are performed by the American Society for Cytotechnology (ASCT) on a small proportion of cytology laboratories with CLIA certificates. The laboratory is either selected at random, or if a complaint has been made against a laboratory with CMS, they may be selected for a survey. The survey team evaluates the laboratories' operations and reviews a minimum of 100 Pap tests.

A-45. (**d**) **The Clinical Laboratory Improvement Advisory Committee**
An advisory committee known as the Clinical Laboratory Improvement Advisory Committee (CLIAC) consists of twenty members including laboratory professionals

and consumer advocates. CLIAC meets at least twice yearly and advises CMS and other governmental agencies on the need for and nature of any revisions to the standards that regulated laboratory testing.

A-46. (a) **DHHS Office of Civil Rights**
HIPAA is a comprehensive law that regulates several unrelated areas of health care, like the protection of healthcare coverage for those who change jobs and the privacy of medical information. A new ruling governs the use of "individually identifiable" healthcare information and is intended to ensure that a patient's health information is used only for health purposes, unless permission is given for other purposes. This information includes a medical record number that could be linked to the cytology diagnosis. The DHHS Office of Civil Rights (OCR) is responsible for implementing the rule and has issued written guidelines for healthcare providers.

A-47. (e) **World Health Organization International Classification of Diseases**
ICD-9 CM, the International Classification of Disease, Clinical Modification, is based on the official version of the World Health Organization (WHO) International Classification of Diseases. ICD-9 classifies morbidity and mortality information for statistical purposes and for indexing of hospital records by disease and operations and for data storage and retrieval. CMS has designated ICD-9 as the coding system physicians must use.

A-48. (e) **ICD-9 code 795.03 (LSIL)**
It is important to assign the correct and most specific ICD-9 code, as this documents medical necessity for the procedure. For pathology, the proper ICD-9 code may be based on the results of the interpretation performed by the pathologist. For example, if a Pap test is submitted for follow-up of a prior Pap test with atypical squamous cells of undetermined significance (ASCUS) (ICD-9 code 795.01) and the finding is low-grade squamous intraepithelial lesion (LSIL), the code for LSIL (ICD-9 code 795.03) should be used.

A-49. (c) **V76.2**
ICD codes are also required as documentation of necessity for screening tests, including the Pap test, which is covered by Medicare every 2 years for average-risk patients and every year for high-risk patients. There are a number of codes that document the clinical exam and pelvic exam that ensure clinician payment. Only four codes are considered acceptable for documentation for payment to laboratories for screening Pap tests. They are V76.2 (routine cervical Pap smear, intact cervix), V76.47 (routine vaginal Pap, status post-hysterectomy for nonmalignant condition), V76.49 (Pap smear, other site, NOS), and V15.89 (other specified personal history representing hazards to health—use for high-risk Pap tests).

A-50. (b) **Baby boomers**
Increased generational diversity challenges today's cytology manager who employ and direct four generations of employees working side by side. Employees of different generations have distinct workplace viewpoints. The three identified generations are Veterans, born before 1945; Baby Boomers, born between 1965 and 1980; and Nexters, also called Generation Y, born after 1980.

A-51. (c) **Equal employment opportunity**
Equal employment opportunity means that all individuals must be treated legally in the hiring process, in training, and in promotion. Each person has the right to be evaluated as an individual on his or her qualifications without discrimination based on stereotypic preconceptions (of race, color, sex, national origin, religion, age, veteran status, and disability) of members of minority groups or any other protected class classifications protected under federal and state equal employment opportunity laws.

A-52. (a) **Needs assessment**
The notice of a vacancy gives the employer an opportunity to conduct a needs assessment. A needs assessment is a process of gathering information to assist in making static-driven decisions and recommendations about staffing levels and staff mix. A thorough review of current laboratory practices, including the use of technologies, should be performed. It is important to include in consideration the strategic goals that will influence future labor needs and decisions about staffing levels and skills.

A-53. (e) **100 ppm**
OSHA provides a summary of the properties of hazardous chemicals, their health effects, and procedures for sampling the levels of exposure. The current OSHA PEL for xylene is 100 parts per million (ppm) for an 8-h time-weighted average. The odor threshold for xylene is 1 ppm. Because the odor threshold is below the current PEL of 100 ppm, xylene is considered to have adequate warning properties.

A-54. (**c**) **Sampling errors**
False-negative Pap tests are largely due to a sampling error (cells are not effectively collected and transferred to the glass slide) and less likely caused by a laboratory error (abnormal cells missed during screening or misinterpreted as benign). False-negative Pap tests are uncommon when the threshold for false negative is set as SIL.

A-55. (**d**) **False negatives ÷ true positives + false negatives**
False-negative rate (FNR) is the proportion of abnormal Pap tests that are falsely negative, false negative ÷ true positive + false negatives. FNRs can be calculated for individual cytotechnologists and used for performance evaluations, especially if the computer system used in the laboratory is programmed to do the calculations. These numbers cannot be used to compare one laboratory to another for the rescreening documentation may vary.

A-56. (**b**) **In a laboratory setting**
Focused review of cases or knowledge that the patient subsequently developed carcinoma biases the objectivity of a review against the laboratory and does not reflect standard practice. The ASC guidelines for review of Pap tests for litigation purposes suggest the Pap tests be reviewed without knowledge or clinical outcome and in an environment that stimulates normal screening practice as closely as possible.

A-57. (**e**) **Cancer**
Retrospective rescreening which targets archived negative Pap tests from women with a new interpretation on Pap tests of HSIL or cancer was introduced in CLIA 1988. The rescreening of all previous negative Pap tests during the 5 years before a new Pap test diagnosis of HSIL or cancer increases the likelihood of detecting an error.

A-58. (**d**) **Referring physician**
On retrospective rescreening or review of Pap tests, if a significant discrepancy is found that will affect patient care, the patient's physician must be notified and an amended report needs to be issued. These situations are rare because the review is prompted by a current abnormality of HSIL or cancer.

A-59. (**c**) **Number of Pap tests that are reclassified as abnormal**
CLIA 1988 requires that cytology laboratories compile statistics. Among these statistics are the total number of cases examined, the number of specimens by specimen type, the volume of cases by diagnosis, the number of unsatisfactory cases, the number of Pap tests with discrepant histologic results, the number of Pap tests that were reclassified as abnormal, and the number of Pap tests reported as HSIL, adenocarcinoma, and other malignant neoplasms with no histologic follow-up.

A-60. (**d**) **795.05**
A screening or routine Pap test is one that is performed in the absence of signs and symptoms and is only payable when billed with certain ICD-9 codes. Confusion may arise over ICD-9 coding when a screening Pap has findings that have a pathologist review. The correct billing would be to document the reason for the Pap screening as the first code with the interpretive results as the second code. The follow-up Pap test will then be billed as a diagnostic Pap billed as the primary ICD-9 code and will not be subject to screening limitations.

A-61. (**c**) **Referring physician**
The laboratory generally relies on the referring physician to obtain the ABN signatures it needs because it almost never has direct contact with the patient in advance of a Pap test. (Medicare states that an ABN is valid—and the patient is financially liable for the service—only if the ABN is signed in advance of the test; post-test ABN signatures are not valid or binding on the beneficiary.) It is advisable, however, not to rely on the referring physician to store ABNs for you. Many laboratories have solved this problem by making the ABN a part of the requisition form itself.

A-62. (**d**) **Multiple sexual partners (five in lifetime)**
Pap tests are divided into three categories. These are (1) screening (routine) Pap test which are defined as having no sign or symptoms, no abnormal Pap smear, and no high-risk factors. (2) The second category is screening (high risk) Pap test which include abnormal Pap smear in the past 3 years (childbearing age women only), daughter of women given diethylstilbestrol during pregnancy, fewer than three negative Pap smear in the previous 7 years, multiple sexual partners, history of STD (sexually transmitted diseases), and early onset of sexual activity. (3) The third category includes diagnostic Pap test which includes previous abnormal Pap smear; previously diagnosed cancer of vagina, cervix or uterus; current abnormal finding of vagina, cervix, uterus, ovaries, or adnexa; significant complaint of referable to the female reproductive system; and any sign or symptom that might be related to gynecological disorder.

A-63. **(e) Both (c) and (d)**
A small percentage of Pap smear is reported unsatisfactory. If the slide is reported unsatisfactory before it was reviewed in scenario like broken beyond repair and insufficient indentifying information, a charge should not be submitted in the case. If however the slide is reviewed and deemed unsatisfactory in scenarios like obscuring blood and insufficient squamous cells, then a charge should be reported.

A-64. **(a) If pathologist interpretation is precipitated by finding of abnormal, atypical, or reactive cells by the cytotechnician**
Pathologist's profession is legitimate when he or she reviews abnormal, atypical, or reactive cells even though he or she ultimately signs out the smear as "normal." The rest of the scenarios are not separately billable professional service. When a pathologist screens a smear in place of a CT and no abnormality or atypia is identified, the test is billable with the regular technical code.

A-65. **(d) When patient has no current sign or symptom of disease or injury**
Health status or V codes are series of codes only employed when a patient received health care in the absence of any current sign or symptom of a disease or an injury.

A-66. **(c) Inefficient transfer of lesional cell from collection device to glass slide**
Screening (i.e., abnormal cells are missed) and interpretation (i.e., abnormal cells are misinterpreted as benign) are mostly laboratory errors. The sampling error occurs if the collection device does not adequately collect lesional cells and transfer them onto the cytology slide.

A-67. **(d) Laboratories with a solo pathologist and no CT**
Laboratories with a solo pathologist and no CT does need to have 10 % rescreen. The rationale for this requirement is to identify CTs whose work is unreliable.

A-68. **(a) 3 years full-time experience in past 10 years**
This must be done by technical supervisor (TS), general supervisor (GS), or cytotechnologist (CT) with 3 years of full-time experience in the past 10 years.

A-69. **(d) SIL**
The PPV of the Pap test is directly proportional to the degree of a Pap abnormality. The PPV for SIL is 82 % whereas for LSIL is 50–86 %. For ASC, the PPV is 44–62 %.

A-70. **(c) Sampling error**
Discrepancies between Pap test and biopsies, in particular, are not uncommon. The majority of discrepancies are the result of the so-called sampling error. Some biopsies are negative because colposcopy has an inherent FNR (i.e., the lesion is simply not detected colposcopically). Even if the lesion is detected colposcopically and biopsied, sometimes the lesion is not embedded properly.

A-71. **(c) Cytocentrifuge preparation**
Non-gynecologic slides in which the cellular material covers one half or less of the slide surface are counted as half slide. Other slides that are counted as half slides are cytocentrifuge preparations, cell block section, ThinPrep, and SurePath slides (non-gynecologic case).

A-72. **(a) 100**
The minimum amount of time spent examining this maximum number of slides (100/24 h) is 8 h (average, 12.5 slides/h). If CT spends less than an 8-h screening, the maximum number of slide is calculated using this formula:

No. hrs examining slides × 100/8.

A-73. **(c) 10**
Each participant must evaluate gynecologic slides in a span of 2 h. Participants are proctored during a 2-h period. Participants must attain an overall score of 90 % or higher to pass.

A-74. **(c) 3**
The participant can take three cytology PTs, the first two comprising 10 gynecytologic studies in 2 h and third comprising 20 gynecological slides in 4 h. After the third notification of failure, the individual must cease examining Pap slides and must obtain at least 35 h of documented, formally structured, continuing education in diagnostic cytopathology.

A-75. **(a) False-negative detected during rescreening of 10 % of negative PAPs**
CT's screening skills are objectively assessed. In addition to FNs detected during rescreening of 10 % of all negative PAP, their screening skills can also be assessed by percentage of cases called abnormal by CT.

A-76. **(b) Abnormal rate**
Abnormal rate of each CT is useful for performance evaluation because it allows comparison with the laboratory average.

A-77. (**b**) **3:1**
This ratio is based on large surveys of laboratories compiled by the CAP.

A-78. (**a**) **Likelihood ratio (LR)**
Sensitivity and specificity can be expressed simultaneously in likelihood ratio (LR). LRs can be expressed at different decision levels (e.g., negative, atypical, suspicious, or positive), when LRs are calculated for a test at several different decision levels.

A-79. (**b**) **CLIA 1988**
Proficiency test of CT is a CLIA 1988 requirement but not implemented until 2006. Per CLIA'1988, the PT testing is required for both CTs and pathologists. Each individual engaged in the examination of gynecological preparations is enrolled in a PT program approved by CMS. Furthermore, each individual engaged in the examination of gynecological preparations must obtain the required level of proficiency 90 % or higher.

A-80. (**b**) **Exposure determination**
Exposure determination also includes tasks and procedures in which exposure occurs.

A-81. (**b**) **2 years**
Onsite surveys by CAP are performed every 2 years, and they have been unannounced since 1906.

A-82. (**d**) **Joint Commission**
Laboratories surveyed by Joint Commission are certifiable for CLIA 1988. To earn accreditation, the laboratory undergoes an on-site survey, and to maintain accreditation, laboratory have unannounced surveys every 2 years. CAP is also an approved body for accrediting laboratories.

A-83. (**c**) **10 years**
Reports must be retained for 10 years. This may be electronic or hard copy format. Cytology (gynecological and non-gynecological) slides must be retained for at least 5 years. FNA slides must be retained for 10 years. Requisitions and worksheets must be kept for 2 years each.

A-84. (**e**) **Narrative, descriptive terminology**
CLIA 1988 specifies that report must use narrative, descriptive terminology. A numerical reporting system (e.g., class IV) is not acceptable. A TS's written or electronic signature must be present on the cytology report.

A-85. (**b**) **CPT codes**
Medical bill submitted to an insurer for payment needs to describe the medical procedure or service that is being billed. The common language that is used in the United States to communicate the vast majority of procedures is called Current Procedural Terminology or CPT, registered trademark of the AMA.

A-86. (**e**) **CMS**
HCPCS are separate set of codes used to describe drugs, supplies, and certain other services not included under CPT codes. HCPCS codes are five-digit alphanumeric codes. The HCPCS codes are administered not by the AMA but by the CMS.

A-87. (**c**) **CPT modifier 26**
In some circumstances, CPT and HCPCS codes require the use of modifiers to avoid filing a false claim and to assure prompt payment by the payers.

A-88. (**b**) **Specimen collection and transportation, accessioning, slide preparation, slide examination, report results, and retention**
The flow of work in cytopathology follows an established pathway, and CLIA 1988 regulations specify certain requirements for the process of quality control purposes.

A-89. (**c**) **Criteria for specimen rejection**
Laboratory procedure manual must include requirement for specimen collection and processing along with criteria for specimen rejection, procedure for microscopic examination, and step-by-step description of the performance procedures.

A-90. (**d**) **2 years**
Each change in procedure must be approved, signed, and dated by director. Records of discontinued procedures must be kept for 2 years.

A-91. (**e**) **National Fire Protection Association**
Of the numerous standards published by NFPA, the two of the greatest relevance to cytology laboratories are the Standard for Health Care Facilities and Standard on Fire Protection for Laboratories using chemicals. Both can be purchased on NFPA website.

A-92. (**d**) **100 Pap tests**
Survey team evaluates the laboratory operations and reviews at least 100 Pap cases. If applicable, a statement

of deficiencies is forwarded to the laboratory via CMS regional office and the laboratory is given the opportunity to respond with plan of correction.

A-93. (**b**) **20 members**
CLIAC consists of 20 members, including laboratories and consumer advocates. CLIAC meets at least twice yearly and advises CMS and other governmental agencies on the need for and nature of any revisions.

A-94. (**e**) **CAAH EP**
CTs are not required under CLIA 1988 to be certified by a certifying agency, so long as they have graduated from an approved school. Approved schools are accredited by the Council for Accreditation of Allied Health Education Programs (CAAHEP).

A-95. (**d**) **Outpatient laboratory**
Outpatient laboratory services are included in Part B of Medicare plan. Other services include outpatient visits and physician services.

A-96. (**b**) **Resource-based value scale**
Physician professional fees are based on the resource-based value scale (RBVS) using formula based on standard expense variables and local expense factors.

A-97. (**e**) **Test ordered is experimental**
Other reasons for billing the patient directly include ordered more frequently than allowed and testing that was not medically necessary or was ordered as a screening test.

A-98. (**c**) **Quality control**
QC is one set of standards for all non-waived testing. All written policies such as specimen requirements, preparation of reagents, calibration, QC and corrective action procedure, QA, result reporting, limitations of methods, expected values, and references should be included in the policy and procedure manual.

A-99. (**c**) **Privacy of medical information**
HIPAA 1996 also determines the protection of healthcare coverage for those who change job. This requires same coding/transactions/identifiers for electronic business.

A-100. (**c**) **Two identifier**
According to national patient safety goals, one must improve the effectiveness of communication among caregivers. Verbal orders should be written and read back to physician who then confirms the information.

Reading List

Cibas ES, Zou KH, Crum CP, Kuo F. Using the rate of positive high-risk HPV test results for ASC-US together with the ASC-US/SIL ratio in evaluating the performance of cytopathologists. Am J Clin Pathol. 2008;129:97–101.

Cibas ES. Cervical and vaginal cytology. In: Cibas ES, Ducatman BS, editors. Cytology diagnostic principles and clinical correlates. Philadelphia: Saunders/Elsevier; 2009. p. 1–66.

DeMay RM. The Pap test. In: DeMay RM, editor. The art and science of cytopathology. 2nd ed. Chicago: ASCP Press; 2012. p. 2–199.

Koss LG. The Papanicolaou test for cervical cancer detection. A triumph and a tragedy. JAMA. 1989;261:737–43.

Pantanowitz L, Hornish M, Goulart RA. Informatics applied to cytology. Cytojournal. 2008;5:16.

Renshaw AA, Elsheikh TM. Predicting screening sensitivity from workload in gynecologic cytology: a review. Diagn Cytopathol. 2011;39:832–6.

Stoler MH. ASC, TBS, and the power of ALTS. Am J Clin Pathol. 2007;127:489–91.

9 Pelvic Washings for Gynecological Lesions

Marilee Means and Walid E. Khalbuss

Contents

M. Means, PhD, SCT(ASCP) (✉)
School of Health Professions,
University of Kansas Medical Center,
3901 Rainbow Blvd., Mail Stop 4048,
Kansas City, KS 66160, USA
e-mail: mmeans@kumc.edu

W.E. Khalbuss, MD, PhD, FIAC
Director of Cytology and Cytopathology Fellowship Program,
University of Pittsburgh Medical Center Shadyside Hospital,
5150 Centre Avenue, 2, Suite 201,
Pittsburgh, PA 15232, USA
e-mail: khalbussw2@upmc.edu

W.E. Khalbuss, M. Means (eds.), *Gynecological and Breast Cytopathology Board Review and Self-Assessment*,
DOI 10.1007/978-1-4614-7270-4_9,

9.1 Tables and Summary

Table 9.1 Benign and malignant conditions in pelvic washing specimens

Condition	Description	Differentials
Normal mesothelial cells	Sheets of mosaic-like cells in flat sheets or clusters or single mesothelial cells with normal or mildly atypical nuclei	Nuclei show little atypia and are well organized DD: well-differentiated adenocarcinoma or mesothelioma with few large clusters
Muscle cells	Pink-to-orange cells with cross striations in the cytoplasm	Cell block may have tissue fragments from abdominal wall
Adipose tissue	Cells with large clear vacuoles and eccentric nuclei	Cell block may have tissue fragments from abdominal wall
Histiocytes	Clusters of cells with pale nuclei and frothy cytoplasm	DD: mesothelial cells – no windows between cells as in mesothelial cells
Collagen balls	Masses of aqua blue collagen surrounded by flattened mesothelial cells	DD: adenocarcinoma with mucin production has highly abnormal nuclei unlike mesothelial cells
Endosalpingiosis and other proliferative conditions	Psammoma bodies, tubal-type epithelial or mesothelial cells, may have cilia, uniform round nuclei	DD: correlate with concurrent histologic material, if possible. Cell block (CB) is useful
Endometriosis	Hemosiderin-laden macrophages, degenerated groups of endometrial cell clusters, usually cannot dx without CB	DD: if CB has glandular endometrial cells surrounding stromal cells, may be able to dx
Ovarian adenocarcinoma	Clusters and isolated cells, large cells, anisonucleosis, hyperchromasia, macronucleoli, from scant to abundant cytoplasm, may have large vacuoles	DD: borderline ovarian tumors – less nuclear atypia
Endometrial adenocarcinoma	Clusters and isolated cells, enlarged nuclei, powdery to coarse chromatin, scant or finely vacuolated cytoplasm	DD: ovarian adenocarcinoma, overlapping criteria depending on subtypes
Cervical squamous cell carcinoma	Keratinized or nonkeratinized cells with sharp-edged squamous-type cytoplasm and dark, coarse chromatin	DD: nonkeratinizing types are harder to differentiate from crowded mesothelial cells

DD differential diagnosis, *CB* cell block

9.2 Text-Based Questions 1–20

Q-1. Indications for performing a pelvic washing include which of the following?
(a) Staging procedure for gynecologic cancers
(b) Treatment for pseudomyxoma peritonei
(c) Diagnostic procedure for CIS of the cervix
(d) Treatment for endometriosis

Q-2. When performing the procedure to collect a pelvic washing for cytology, the surgeon should:
(a) Add EDTA to preserve the specimen.
(b) Aspirate any preexisting fluid and submit it to cytology separately.
(c) Require flow cytometry on the specimen.
(d) Submit all sites of aspiration separately (e.g., right and left gutter) as it makes a significant difference in the diagnostic accuracy.

Q-3. To optimize diagnostic accuracy, the laboratory should:
(a) Require the specimen to be unfixed and stored at −20 °C prior to slide preparation.
(b) Add formalin prior to preparing the cytology slides.
(c) Compare the slides of the pelvic washing with concurrent or previous histology.
(d) Stain all slides with H and E to better correlate with histologic findings.

Q-4. Normal findings in a pelvic washing include mesothelial cells in sheets, histiocytes, and:
(a) Endometriosis
(b) Psammoma bodies
(c) Collagen balls
(d) Mesenchymal tissue from the broad ligament

Q-5. Endometriosis in the pelvic washing may be identified by the presence of endometrial cells as well as cell block evidence of:
(a) Histiocytes
(b) Endometrial glands with stroma
(c) Marked mesothelial proliferation
(d) Serous adenofibroma

Q-6. Endosalpingiosis in a pelvic washing would be morphologically the most similar to:
(a) Serous borderline tumor
(b) Squamous cell carcinoma of the cervix
(c) Leiomyosarcoma
(d) Metastatic pancreatic carcinoma

Q-7. Which of the following is often seen in conjunction with endosalpingiosis and serous adenofibroma of the ovary?
(a) Collagen balls
(b) Sheets of flat uniform mesothelial cells
(c) Hemosiderin-laden macrophages
(d) Psammoma bodies

Q-8. Pale blue staining (Pap stain) masses covered by flattened, benign mesothelial cells are often found in pelvic washings. They are known as:
(a) Psammoma bodies
(b) Adipocytes
(c) Muscle cells
(d) Collagen balls

Q-9. The most common type of ovarian cancer seen in pelvic washings is:
(a) Serous adenocarcinoma
(b) Granulosa cell tumor
(c) Germ cell tumor
(d) Clear cell carcinoma

Q-10. Features of serous adenocarcinoma in a pelvic washing include marked variation in size of the nucleus, scant or abundant vacuolated cytoplasm, and:
(a) Hypochromasia
(b) Tall columnar palisading cells
(c) Metachromatic mucinous background
(d) Macronucleoli

Q-11. On cell block, one can use which of the following features to differentiate an ovarian serous borderline tumor from endosalpingiosis or mesothelial hyperplasia?
(a) Wide fibrovascular cores lined by atypical epithelial cells
(b) Positive staining for chromogranin
(c) Presence of psammoma bodies
(d) Positive staining for SMA

Q-12. Which of the following is the most common subtype of endometrial adenocarcinoma?
(a) Papillary serous
(b) Endometrioid
(c) Clear cell
(d) Mucinous

Q-13. Clamping of the fallopian tubes prior to hysterectomy is done in order to prevent:
(a) The spread of squamous cell carcinoma of the cervix into the abdominal cavity

(b) The dissemination of mixed Mullerian tumors into the abdominal cavity
(c) Retrograde spread of endometrial adenocarcinoma into the abdominal cavity
(d) Retrograde spread of ovarian adenocarcinoma into the abdominal cavity

Q-14. Tumors of the cervix which are the most easily recognized in the pelvic washing are:
(a) Nonkeratinized squamous cell carcinoma
(b) Keratinized squamous cell carcinoma
(c) Endocervical adenocarcinoma
(d) Borderline serous ovarian tumors

Q-15. Malignancies other than those from a gynecologic origin which are searched for in a pelvic washing for staging purposes include:
(a) Breast and lung
(b) Gastric and pancreatic
(c) Esophageal and oral
(d) Leukemia and lymphoma

Q-16. Features of treatment effect useful in the analysis of "second-look" laparoscopic procedures include:
(a) Enlarged, multinucleated mesothelial cells
(b) Hyperchromasia
(c) Scant cytoplasm
(d) Abnormal N/C ratio

Q-17. A positive pelvic washing is significant because it alters the patient's staging in ovarian adenocarcinoma and in:
(a) Uterine corpus cancers
(b) Leukemia
(c) CIS of the cervix
(d) VAIN I

Q-18. Features of endometrioid endometrial adenocarcinoma include which of the following?
(a) Psammoma bodies
(b) Collagen balls
(c) Coarse chromatin
(d) Dense, hyaline cytoplasm

Q-19. Unlike the mesothelial cells found in effusions, the mesothelial cells found in benign pelvic washings often occur:
(a) Singly
(b) In small clusters
(c) In large flat cohesive sheets with a mosaic-appearance
(d) In large papillary groupings

Q-20. In cell block preparations of pelvic washing specimens, benign mesothelial cells often occur:
(a) In three-dimensional papillary formations
(b) As long, thin ribbonlike arrangements
(c) As hyperchromatic crowded groups
(d) In syncytial arrangements

9.3 Image-Based Questions 21–60

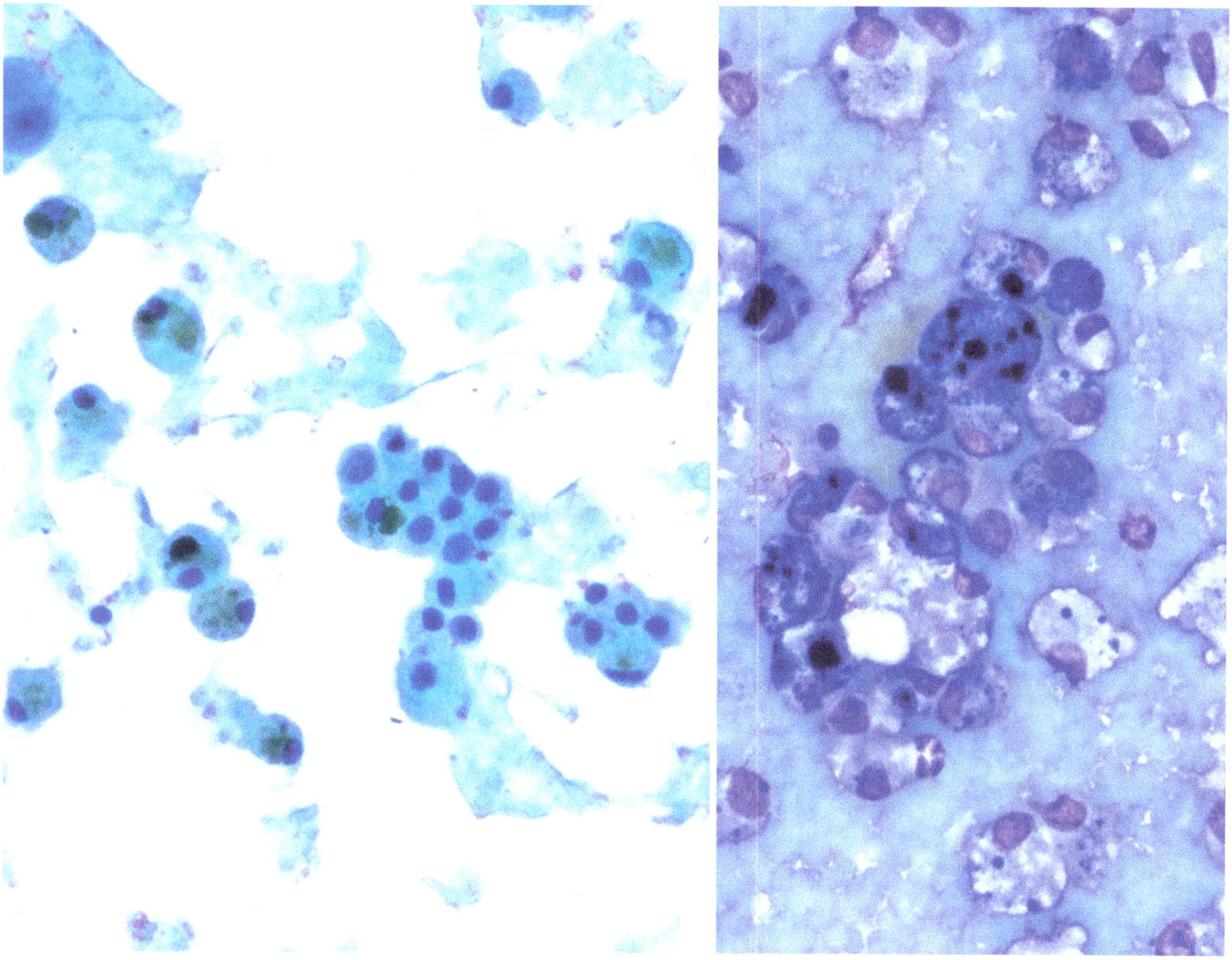

Fig. 9.21

Q-21. Although pelvic washings are not usually performed to diagnose endometriosis, features displayed here (left, SurePath, medium power; right, SurePath, high power) which are the most suggestive of an interpretation of endometriosis in this 28-year-old woman are:

(a) Hemosiderin-laden macrophages and ovarian stromal cells
(b) Psammoma bodies and blood
(c) Granulosa cells and endometrial glandular cells
(d) Hemosiderin-laden macrophages and endometrial cells

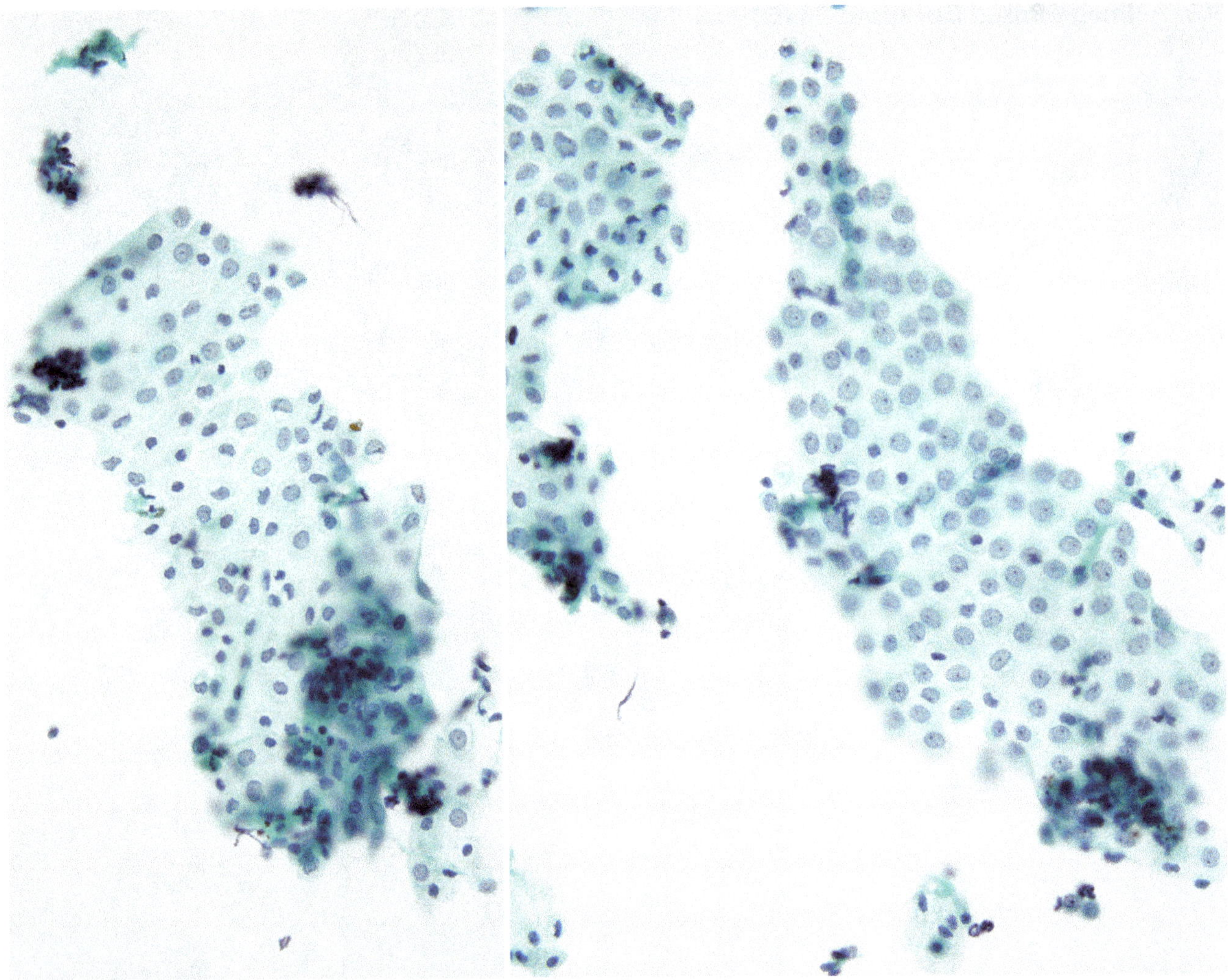

Fig. 9.22

Q-22. These cells were obtained from the pelvic washing of a 36-year-old female (ThinPrep, low power). These cells were found in large flat sheets, with a mosaic-like pattern of polygonal cells. The best interpretation of these groups is:
(a) Histiocytes
(b) Ovarian adenocarcinoma
(c) Endometrial cells suggestive of endometriosis
(d) Benign sheets of mesothelial cells

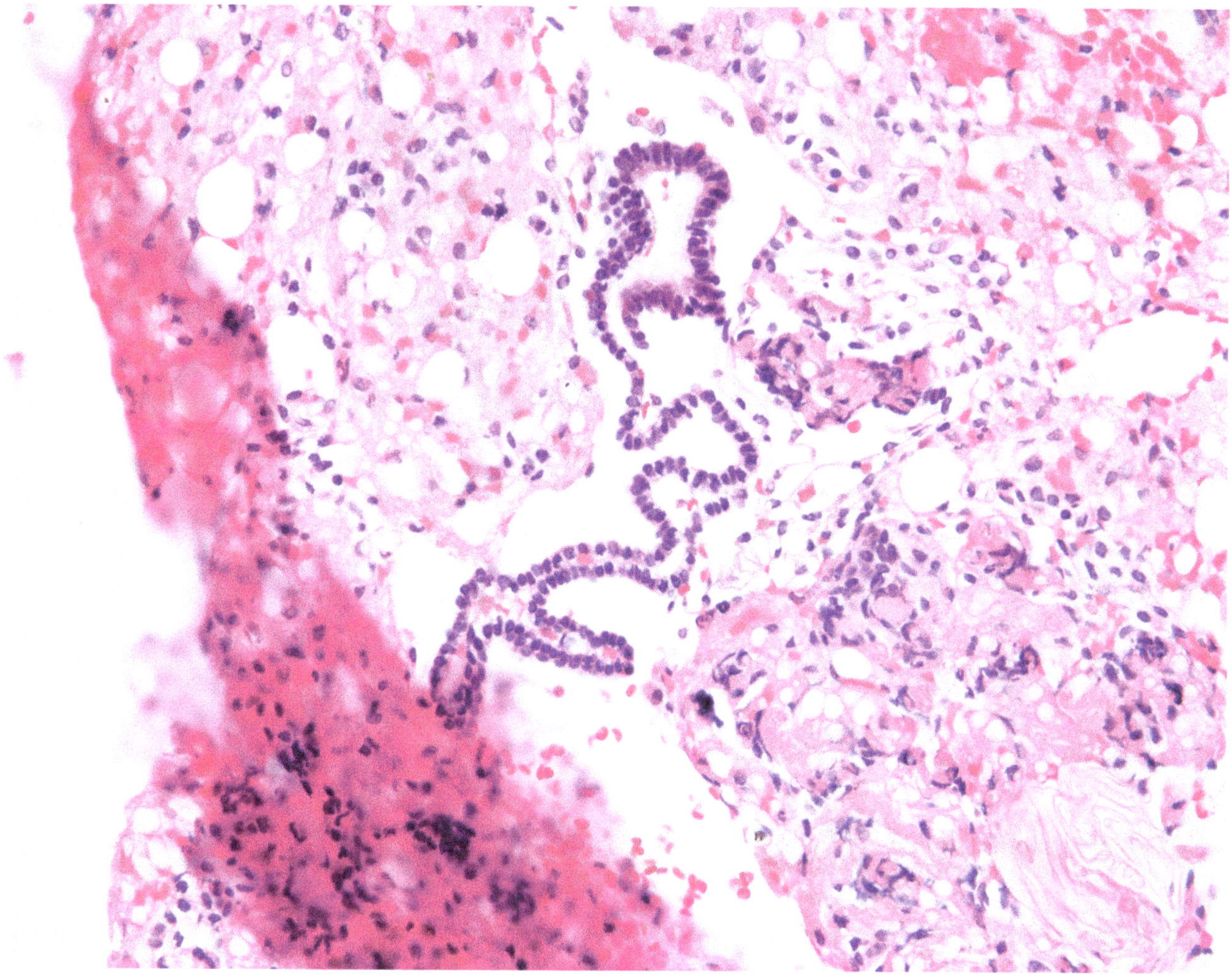

Fig. 9.23

Q-23. This finding in a pelvic washing cell block from a 40-year-old woman (CB, low power) is most consistent with an interpretation of:

(a) Metastatic endometrial adenocarcinoma
(b) Metastatic endocervical adenocarcinoma
(c) Normal sheet of mesothelial cells
(d) Mixed Mullerian tumor
(e) Granulosa cell tumor of the ovary

Fig. 9.24

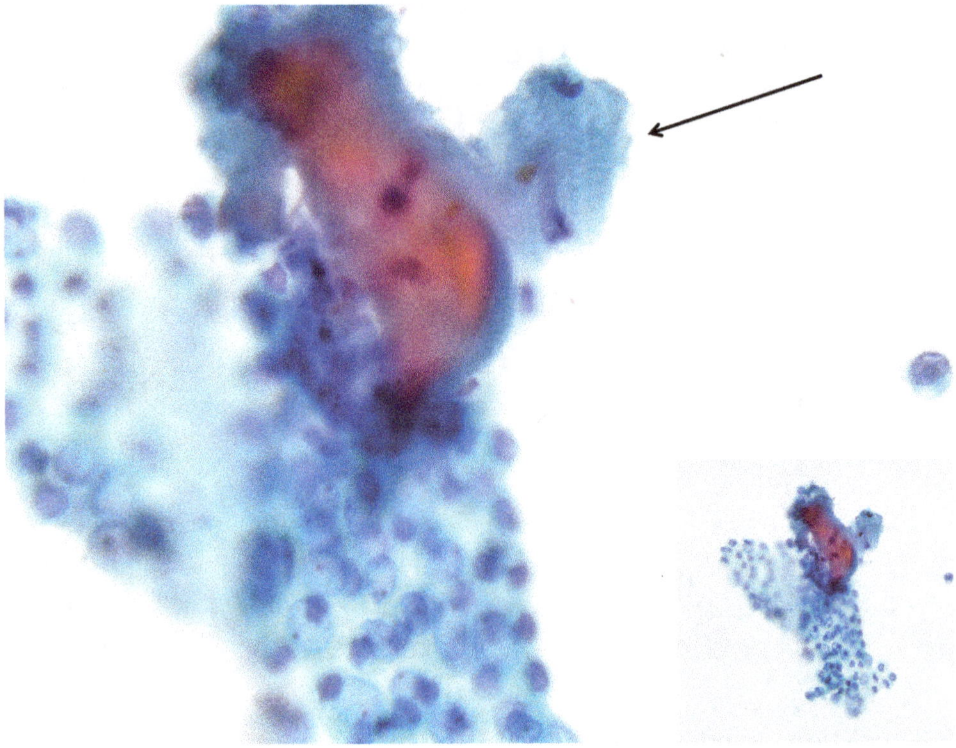

Q-24. This cell fragment was found in the pelvic washing of a 53-year-old woman (ThinPrep, left, high power; inset, low power). The arrow is pointing to a feature which aids in the interpretation of this pink-to-blue staining group of cells as:

(a) Mesothelial cells
(b) Psammoma bodies
(c) Muscle cells
(d) Hemosiderin-laden macrophages

Fig. 9.25

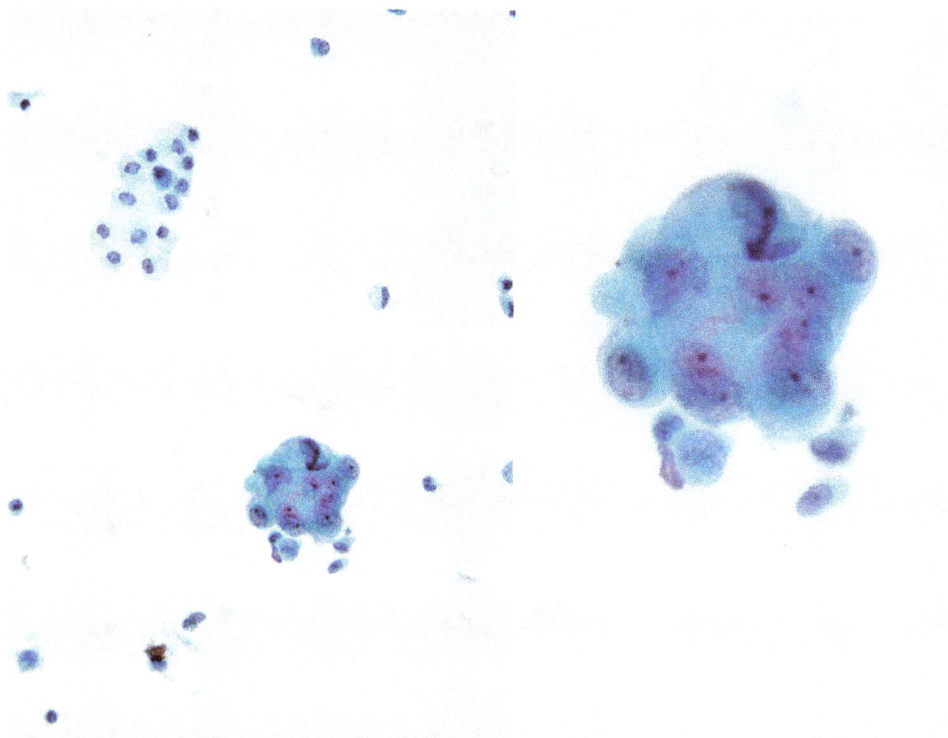

Q-25. These cells were found in the pelvic washing of a 39-year-old woman. The left image shows two cell groups (ThinPrep, low power; right, high power), and the right image shows a high-power image of one of the same groups. The best interpretation of these groups is:

(a) These cell groups represent benign mesothelium and papillary adenocarcinoma of the ovary.
(b) These cell groups are both benign and reactive mesothelial cells.
(c) These cell groups represent metastatic squamous cell carcinoma of the cervix.
(d) These cell groups are consistent with endocervical adenocarcinoma.

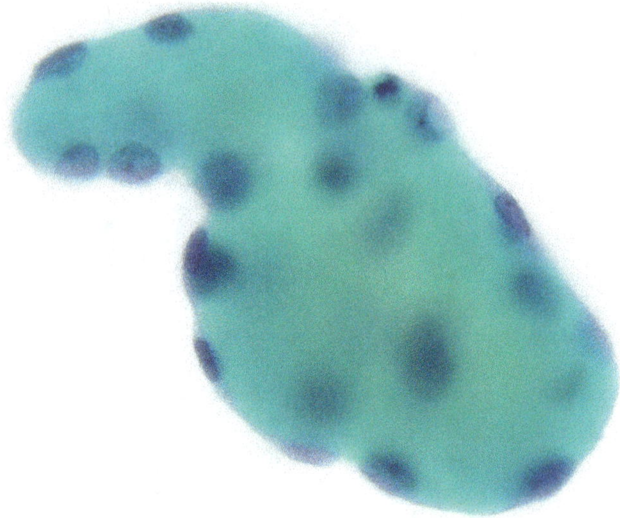

Fig. 9.26

Q-26. This finding is most consistent with (ThinPrep, high power):

(a) Psammoma body
(b) Adipocytes
(c) Collagen ball
(d) Papillary adenocarcinoma

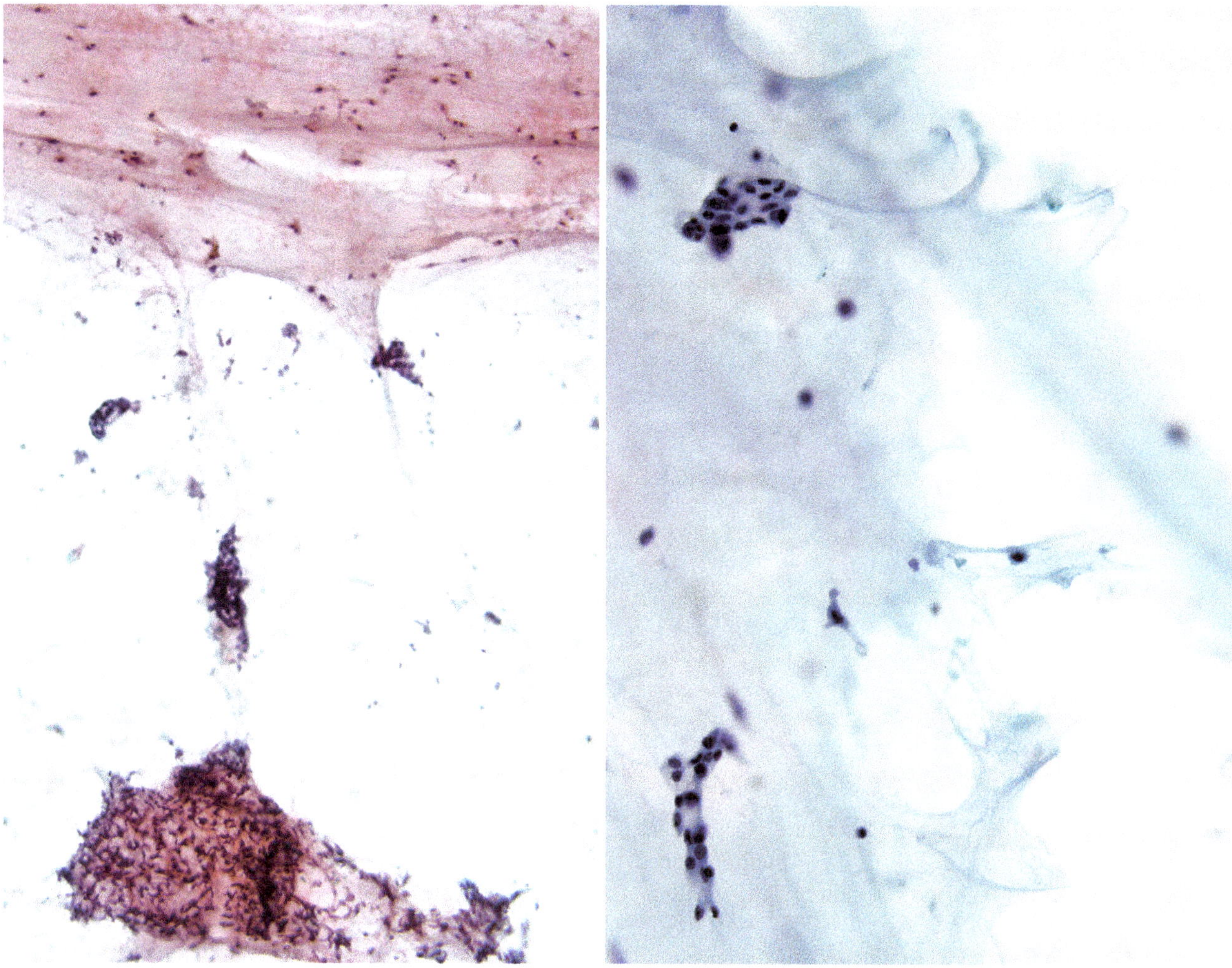

Fig. 9.27

Q-27. This pelvic washing was performed on a patient with a previous history of appendiceal adenocarcinoma (right and left, ThinPrep, low power). Small clusters of cells as seen here were found within large amounts of background pinkish or bluish distinctly edged material. The most likely interpretation of this pattern is:

(a) Recurrent appendiceal adenocarcinoma
(b) Pseudomyxoma peritonei
(c) Endosalpingiosis
(d) Ovarian serous adenocarcinoma

Fig. 9.28

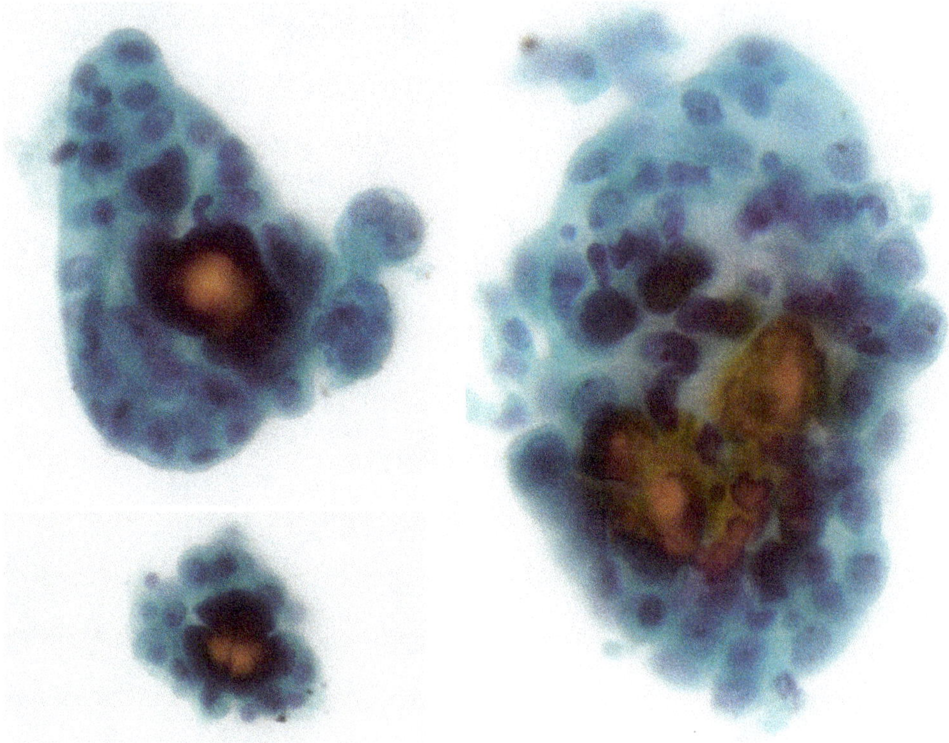

Q-28. The deep red structures noted here are ______, and the case is suggestive of _________ (ThinPrep, upper right and left, high power, lower left, medium power):

(a) Psammoma bodies, papillary serous adenocarcinoma of the ovary
(b) Collagen balls, mucinous adenocarcinoma of the ovary
(c) Staining artifact, keratinized squamous cell carcinoma
(d) *Schistosoma haematobium* ova, metastatic bladder carcinoma

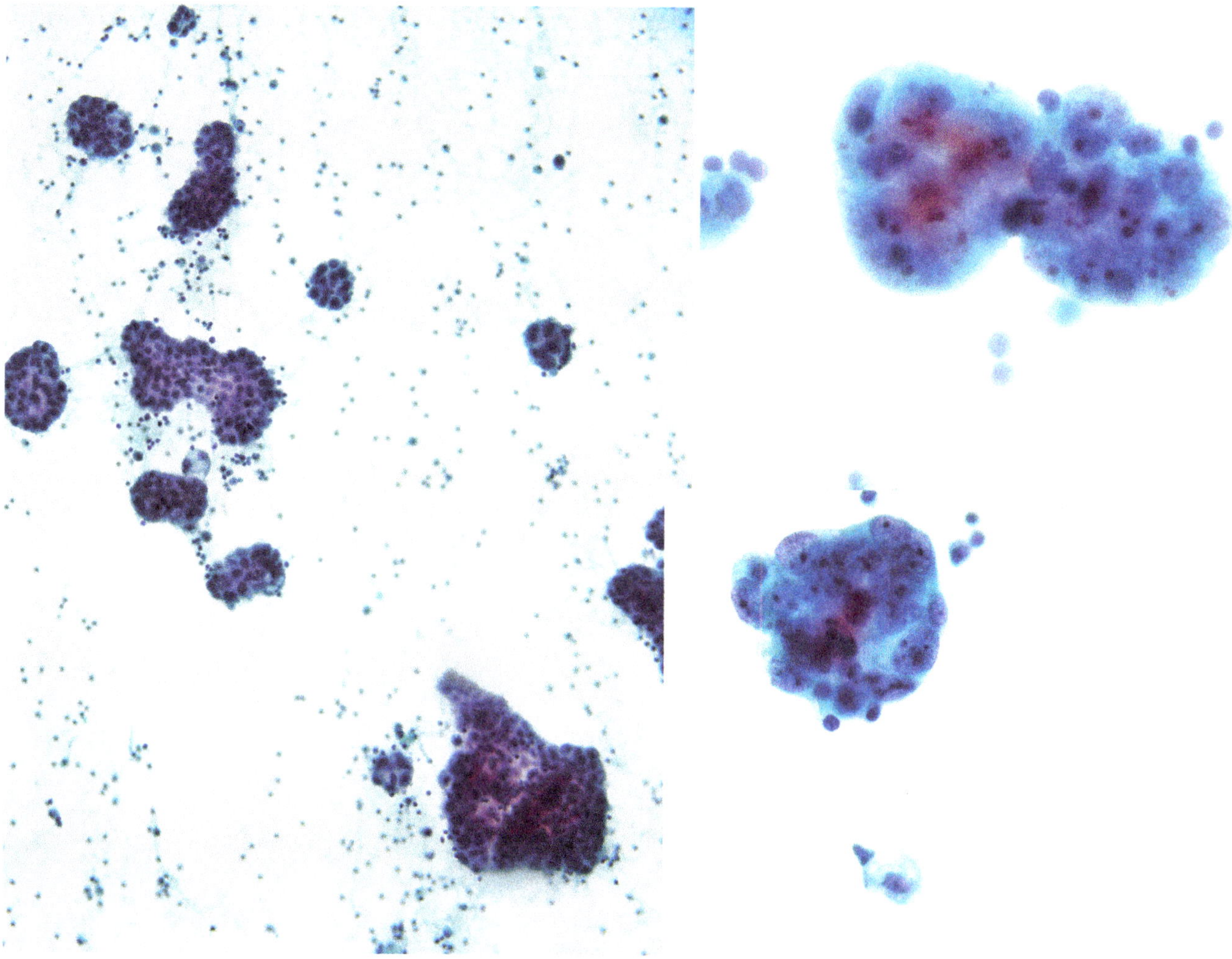

Fig. 9.29

Q-29. This pelvic washing was obtained from a 36-year-old female as a part of a staging procedure (ThinPrep, left, low power; right, upper and lower, high power). Given the appearance of the cells, the most likely interpretation of these groups is:

(a) Normal mesothelial cells
(b) Ovarian adenocarcinoma
(c) Metastatic squamous cell carcinoma
(d) Leukemic infiltrate into the abdominal cavity

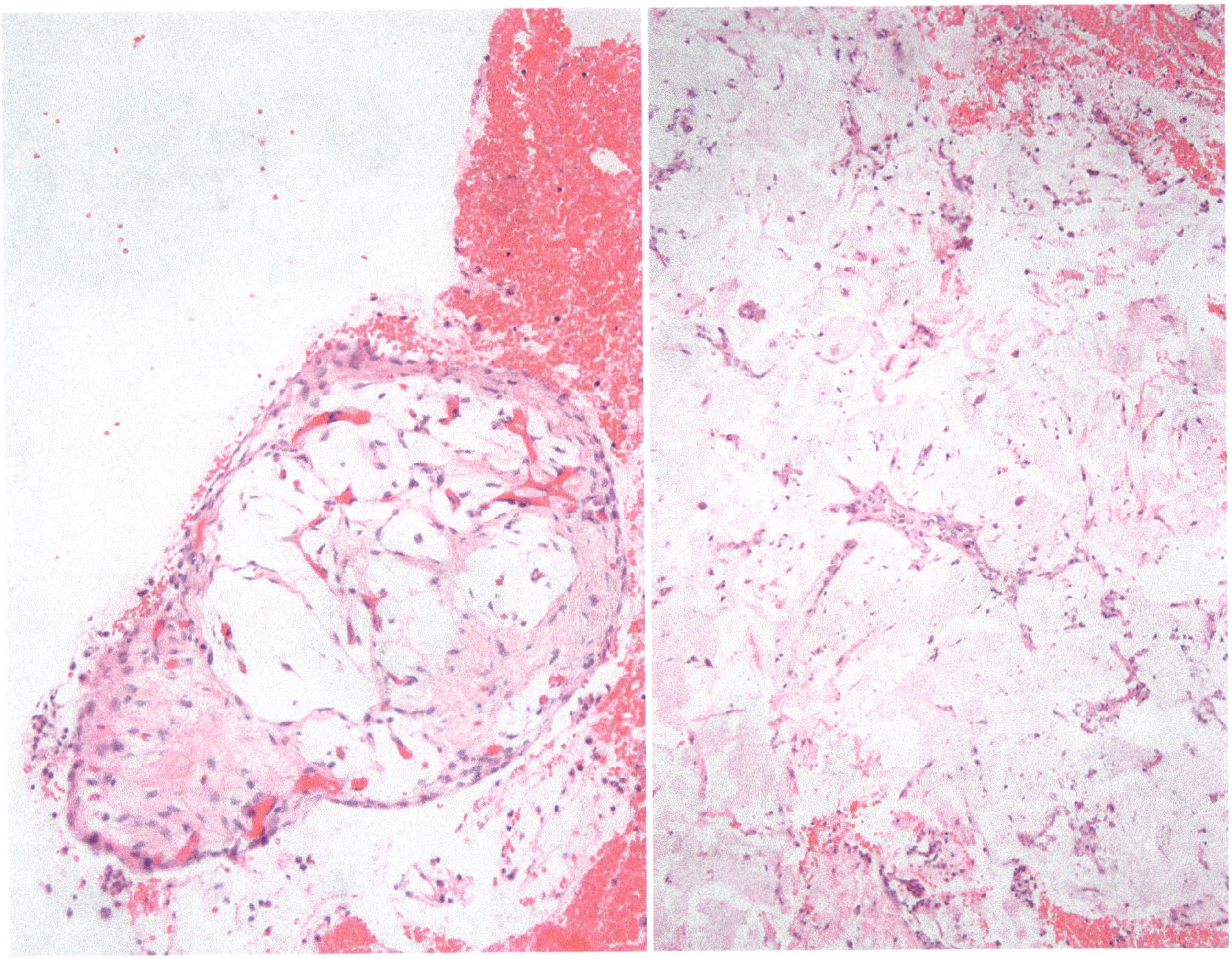

Fig. 9.30

Q-30. These images (cell block, left, low power; right, medium power, H&E) were representative of the pelvic washing from a 42-year-old female. The large amounts of acellular pinkish material seen in the cell block suggest which of the following?

(a) Pseudomyxoma peritonei
(b) Inadequate specimen
(c) Endometriosis
(d) Adenofibroma of the ovary

Fig. 9.31

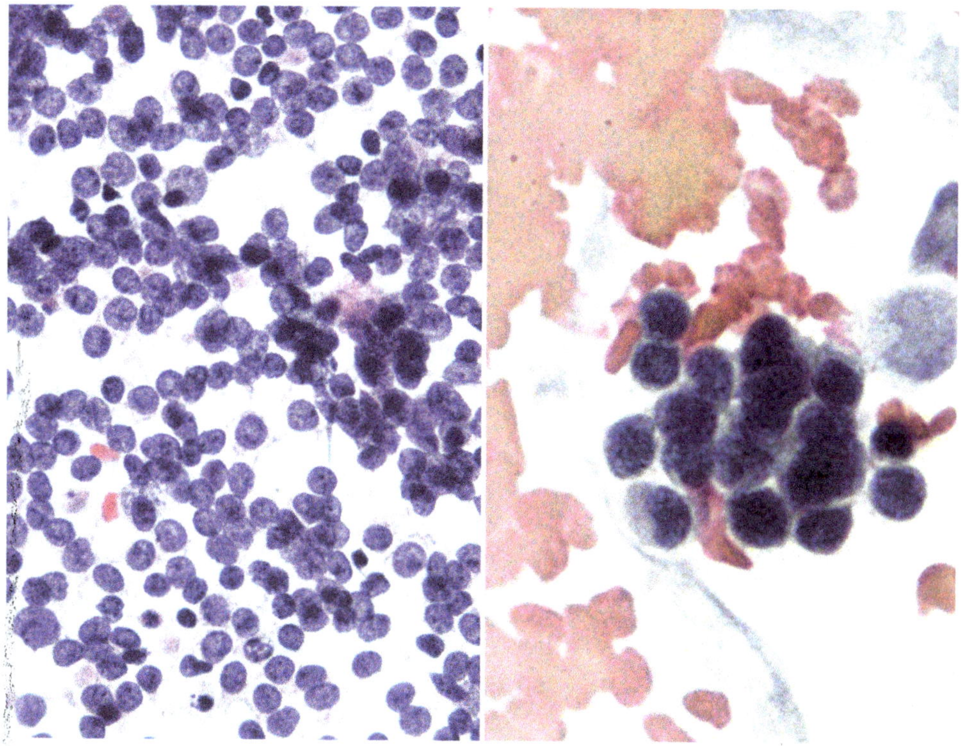

Q-31. These small uniform cells were obtained from the pelvic washing of a 15-year-old female (conventional slide, left, low power; right, high power). Given the appearance of these cells, the most likely interpretation is:

(a) Small cell carcinoma of the lung
(b) Endometrial adenocarcinoma
(c) Small blue cell tumor of childhood
(d) Serous adenocarcinoma of the ovary

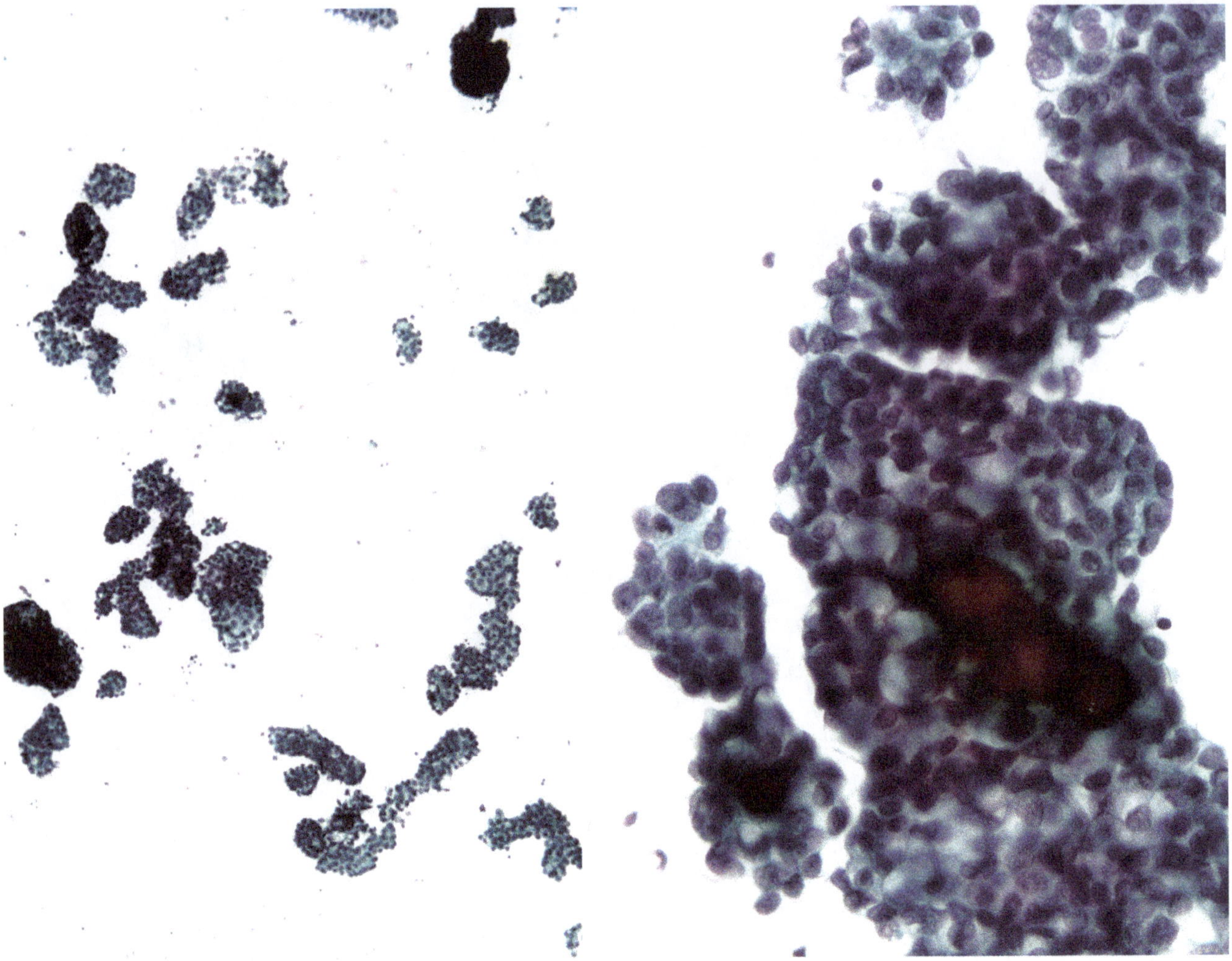

Fig. 9.32

Q-32. The pelvic washing from a 43-year-old woman (ThinPrep, left, low power; right, high power) yielded these cell groups. The most likely interpretation of these cells is:
(a) Serous adenocarcinoma of the ovary
(b) Reactive mesothelial cells
(c) Endometriosis
(d) Squamous cell carcinoma

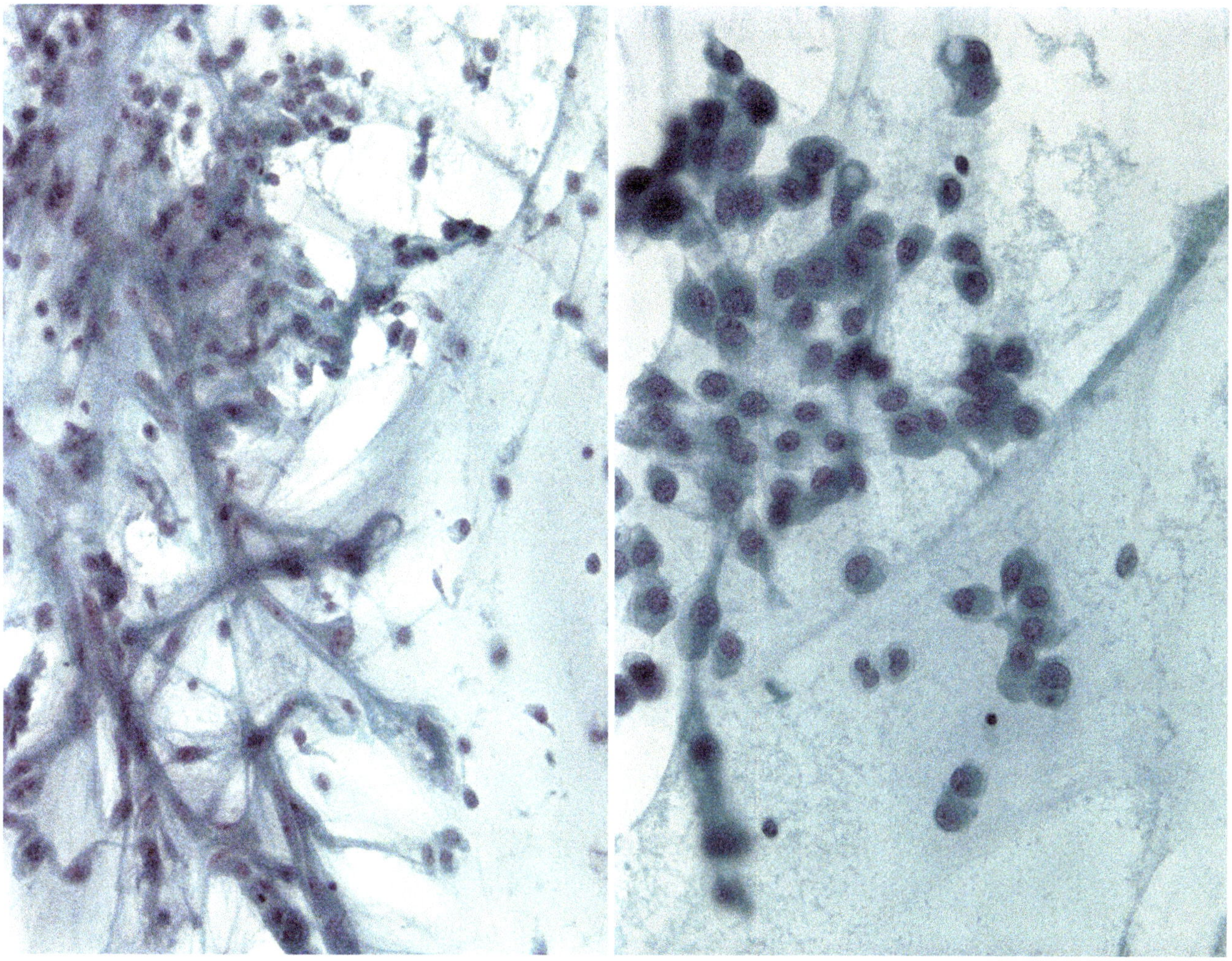

Fig. 9.33

Q-33. (Conventional slide, left, low power; right, high power) This pelvic washing was obtained from a patient with pseudomyxoma peritonei. Which of the following special stains would most likely be positive?

(a) Oil red O
(b) Mucicarmine
(c) Masson-Fontana
(d) GMS

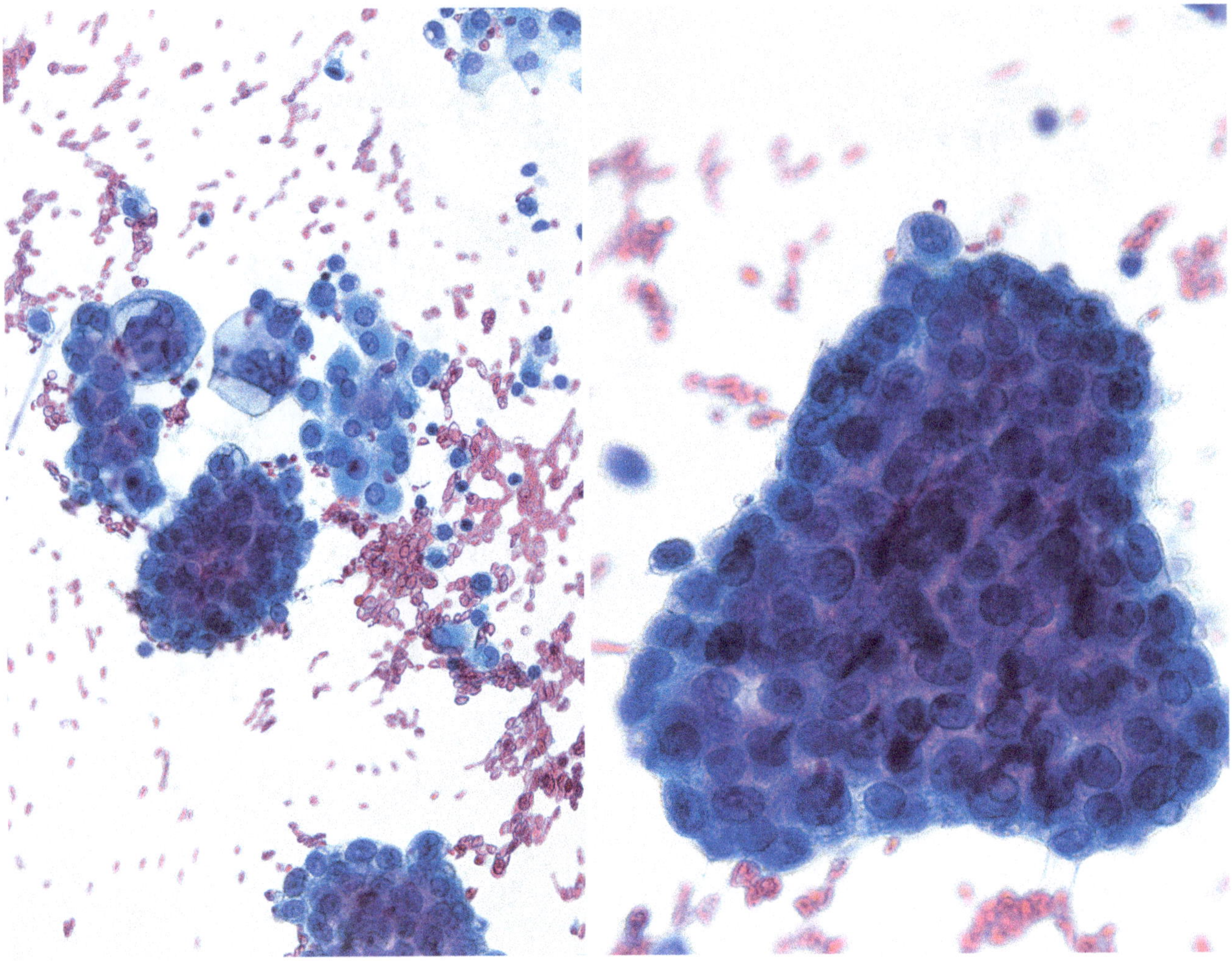

Fig. 9.34

Q-34. Cells such as these (conventional slide, left, low power; right, high power) would be most consistent with an interpretation of:

(a) Normal mesothelial cells
(b) Endometrial cells
(c) Endometrial adenocarcinoma
(d) Ovarian adenocarcinoma

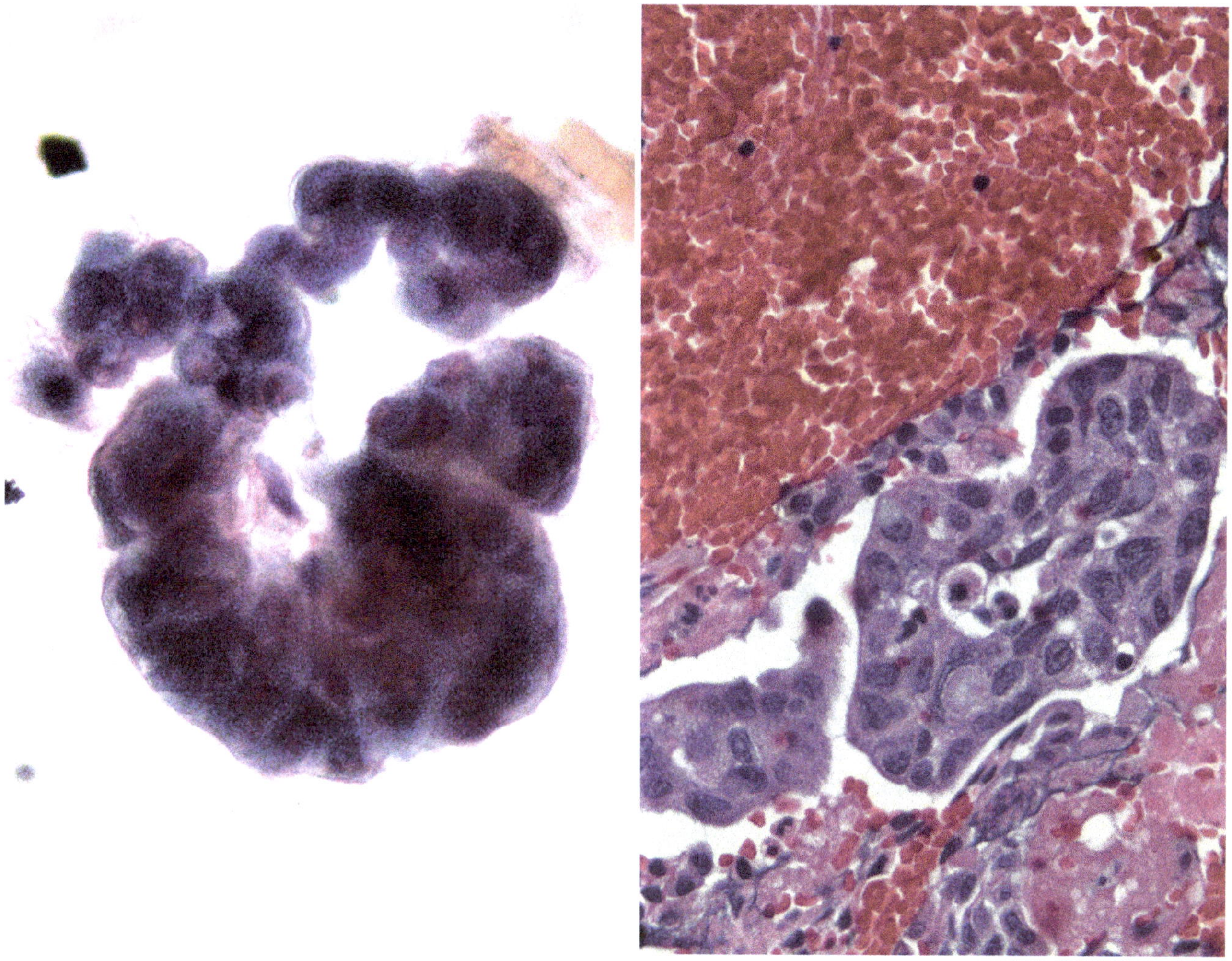

Fig. 9.35

Q-35. These cells were derived from the pelvic washing of a 48-year-old woman with abdominal pain (left, ThinPrep, high power; right, cell block, low power). The specimen was composed of 500 ml of bloody, mucoid fluid. The most likely interpretation of these cells is:

(a) Normal mesothelial cells
(b) Germ cell tumor of the ovary
(c) Mucinous adenocarcinoma of the ovary
(d) Leiomyosarcoma of the uterus

Fig. 9.36

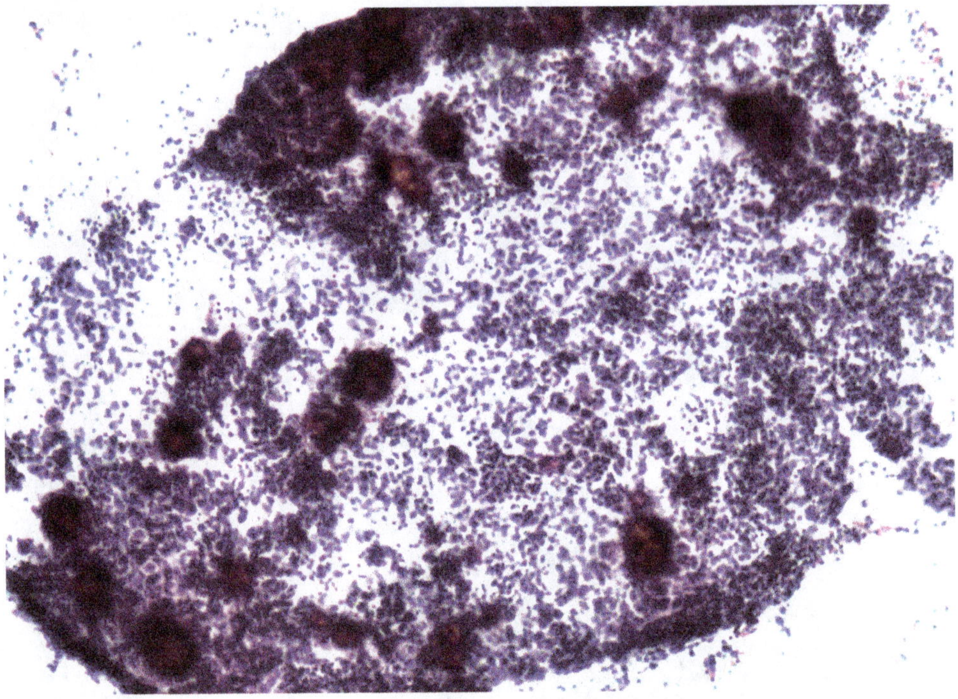

Q-36. A number of red-staining structures are noted in this pelvic washing from a 38-year-old woman (ThinPrep, low power). These structures may be seen in a number of conditions, but the ovarian malignancy which is most likely to display these structures is:

(a) Serous adenocarcinoma
(b) Mucinous adenocarcinoma
(c) Germ cell tumor
(d) Endometrioid carcinoma

Fig. 9.37

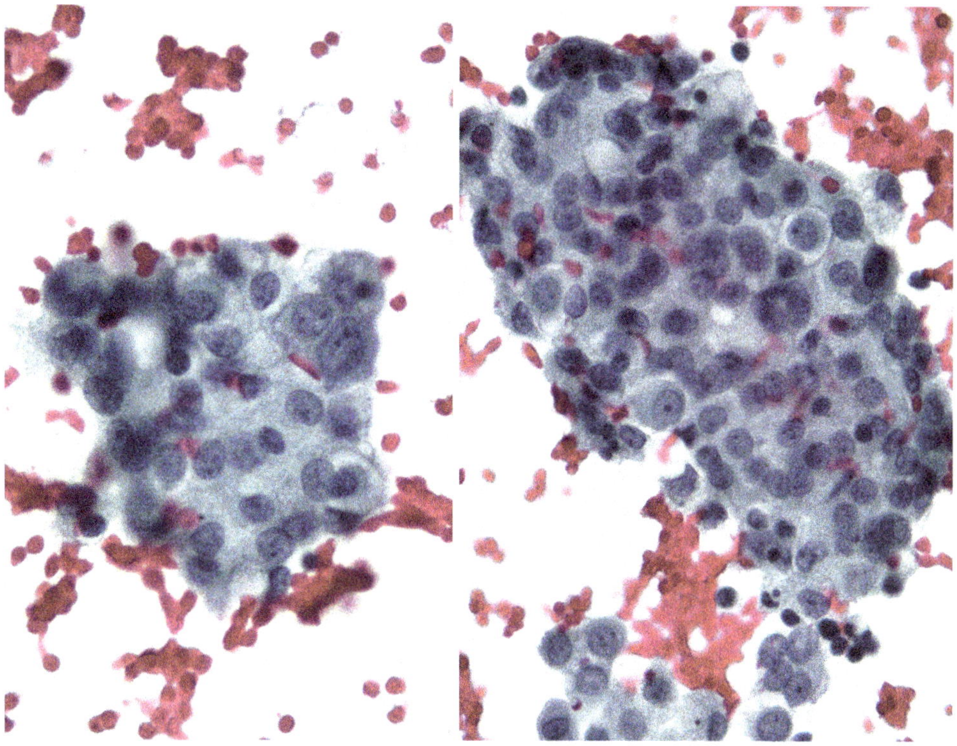

Q-37. Many cells such as these were found in the pelvic washing of a 59-year-old woman (conventional, right and left, high power). The most likely interpretation of these cells is:
(a) Adenocarcinoma of the ovary
(b) Endometrial adenocarcinoma
(c) Endometriosis
(d) Benign mesothelial cells

Fig. 9.38

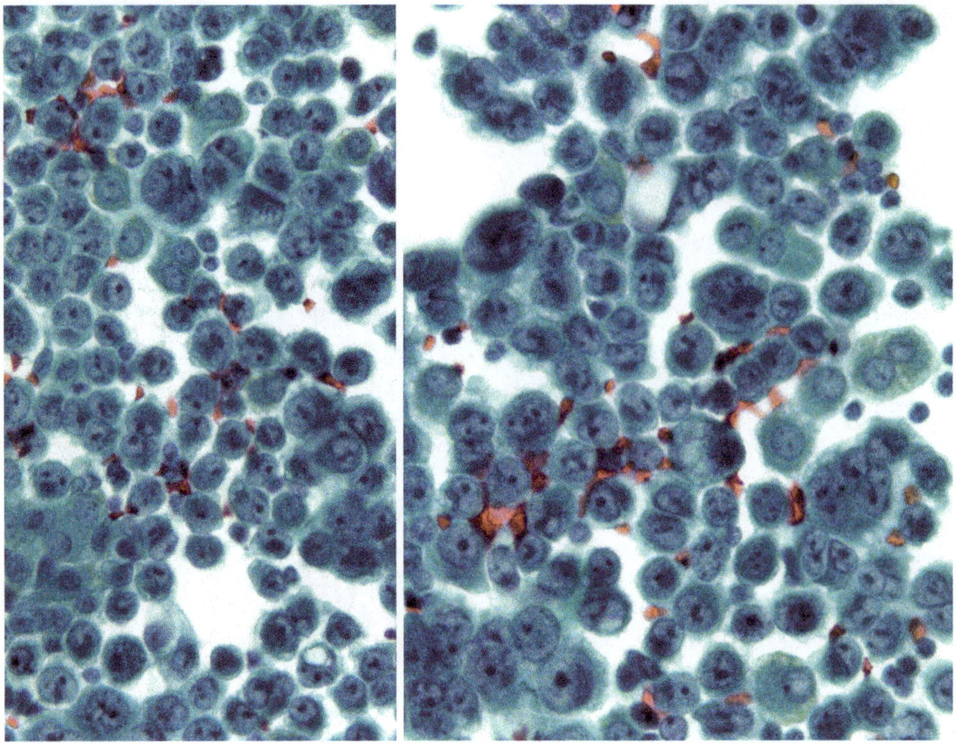

Q-38. These cells were found in the pelvic washing from a patient with a previous history of malignancy (conventional slide, left and right, high power). IHC staining found that the majority of these cells were positive for LCA and CD79a and negative for panCK and S-100. The most likely interpretation of these cells would be:

(a) Ovarian adenocarcinoma
(b) Metastatic melanoma
(c) Acute and chronic inflammation
(d) Lymphoma

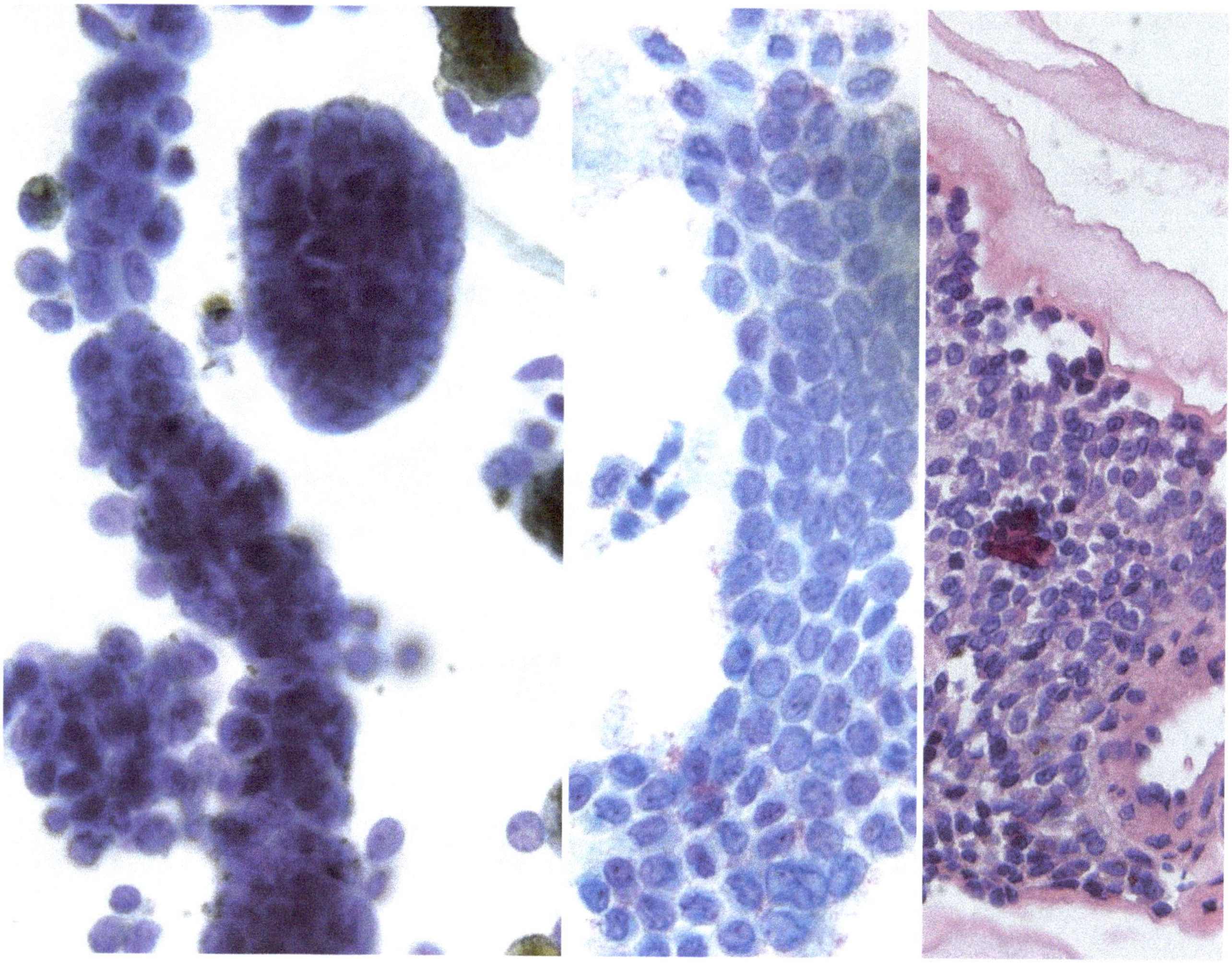

Fig. 9.39

Q-39. These cells were found in the pelvic washing of a 50-year-old woman (ThinPrep, left and center, high power; CB, low power). They were interpreted as consistent with granulosa cell tumor. Common features of this tumor include small round nuclei with scant cytoplasm, loose clusters, and which of the following?

(a) Call-Exner bodies
(b) Psammoma bodies
(c) Collagen balls
(d) CK7 positivity

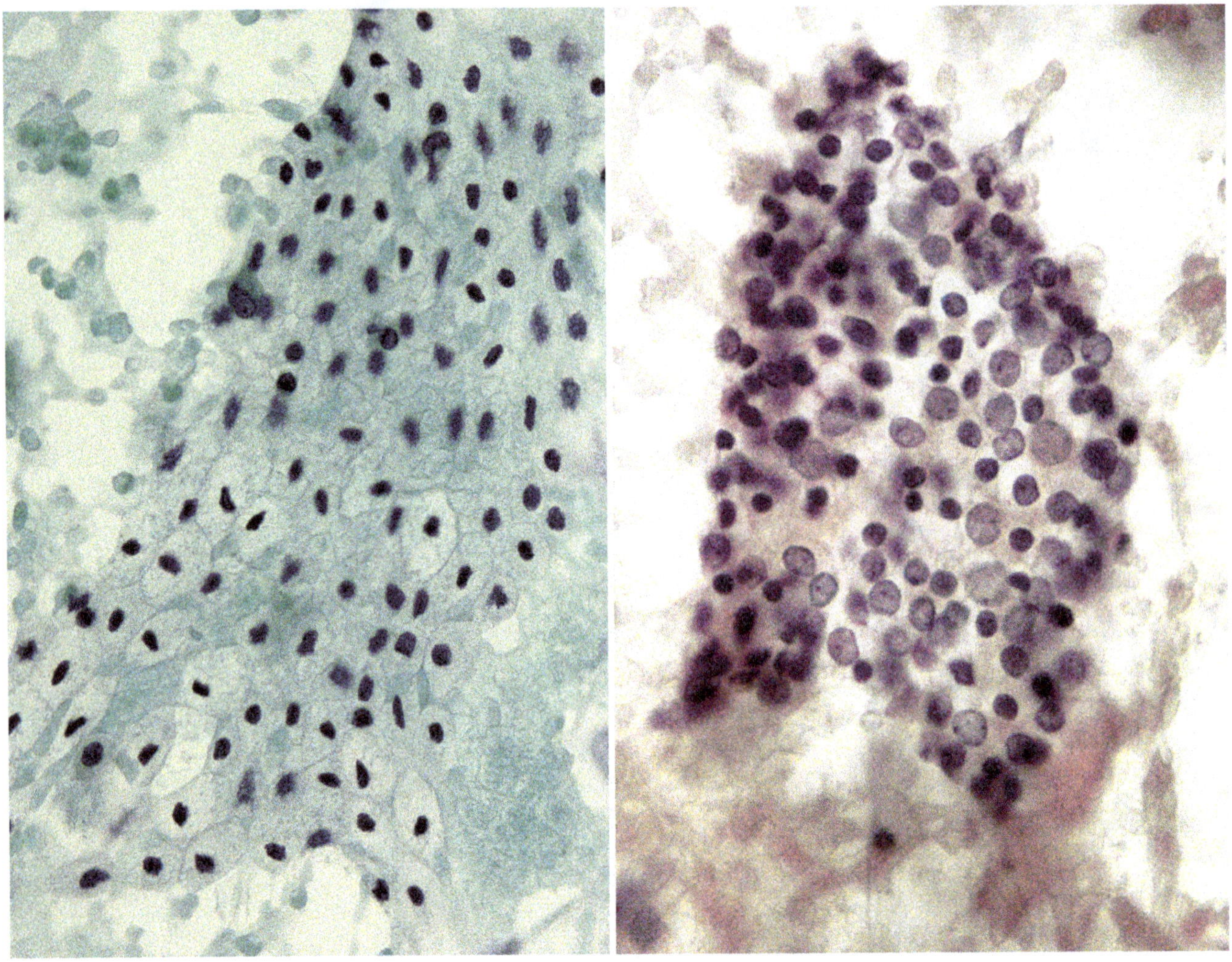

Fig. 9.40

Q-40. These cells illustrate a pattern commonly seen in pelvic washings (conventional slide, right and left, low power). The best interpretation of these cells groups is:
(a) Endometrial cells suggestive of endometriosis
(b) Ovarian adenocarcinoma
(c) Normal mesothelial cells
(d) Histiocytes

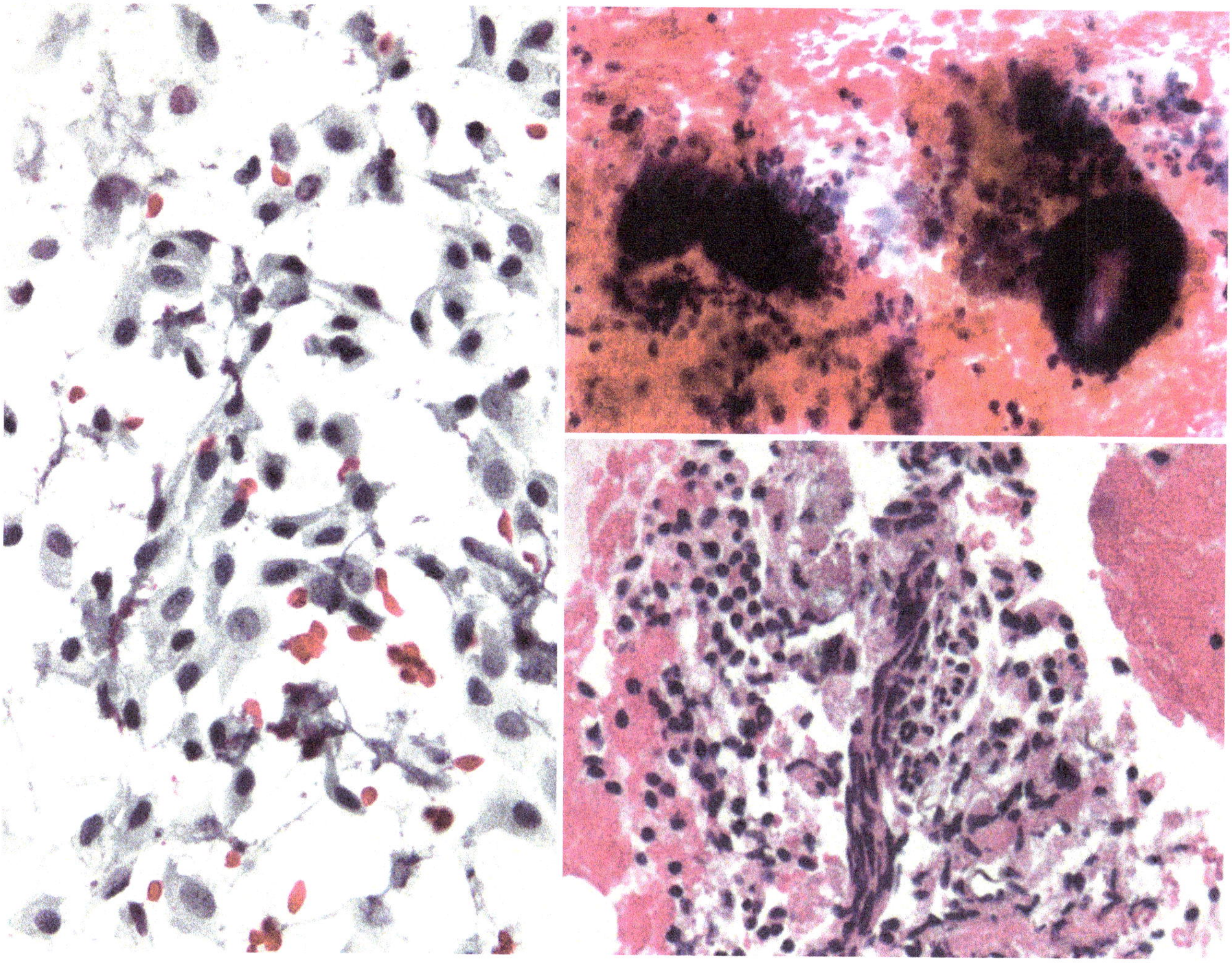

Fig. 9.41

Q-41. In this case of a pelvic washing from a 24-year-old woman (conventional slide, left, high power; upper right, low power; lower right, CB, low power), a consideration of endometriosis would be further strengthened by the finding on the cell block of:

(a) Psammoma bodies
(b) Endometrial glands around endometrial stromal cells
(c) Sheets of benign mesothelial cells
(d) Extracellular mucin

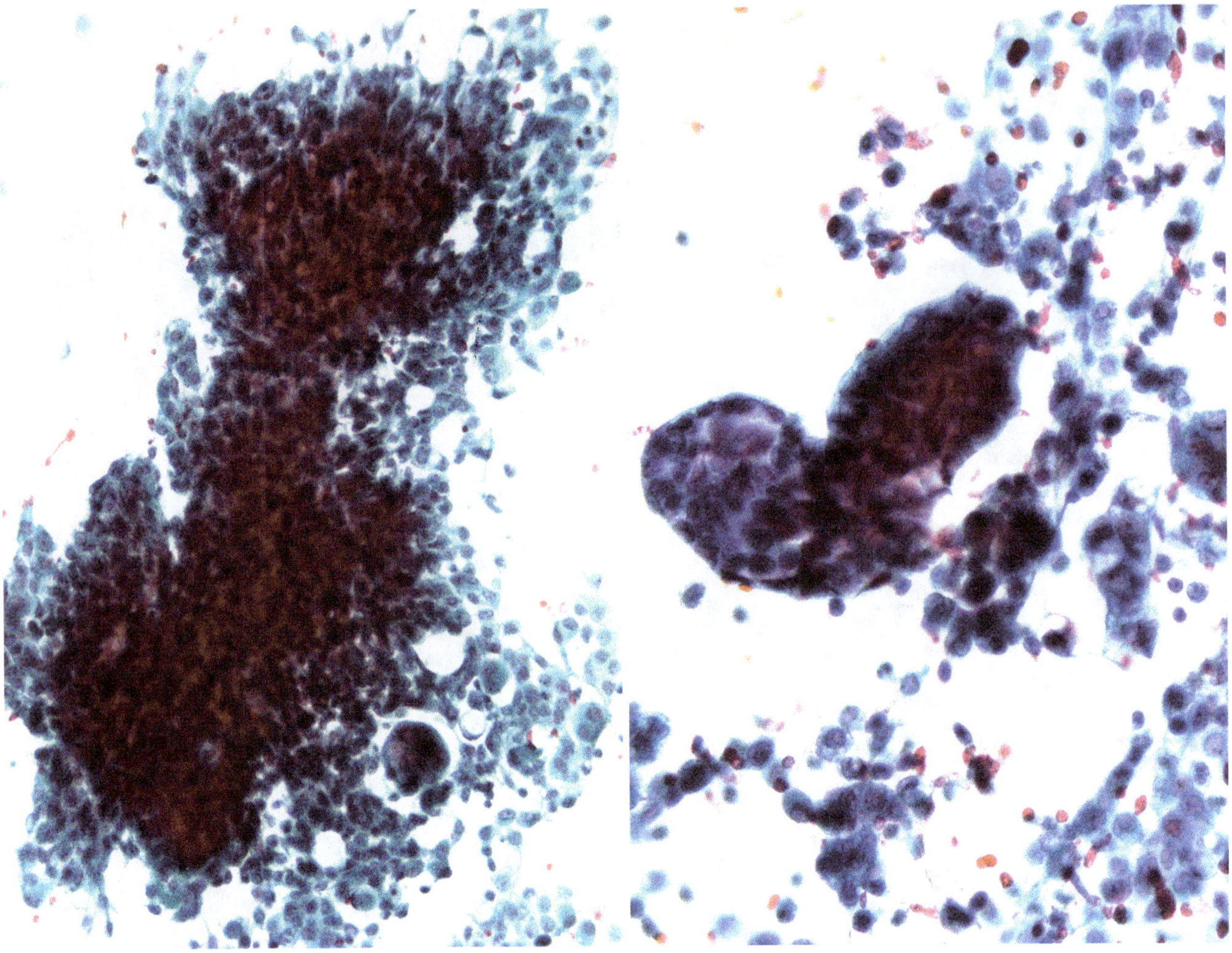

Fig. 9.42

Q-42. Features consistent with ovarian serous adenocarcinoma that may be identified in this pelvic washing from a 52-year-old woman (conventional, left, low power; right, high power) include which of the following?

(a) Smooth-bordered, crowded groups with abnormal nuclei and nucleoli
(b) Flat sheets of cells with centrally placed nuclei
(c) Distorted, hyperchromatic nuclei with single cells and sharp-edged, distinct cytoplasm
(d) Small uniform cells with rare nucleoli, nuclear molding, and coarse chromatin

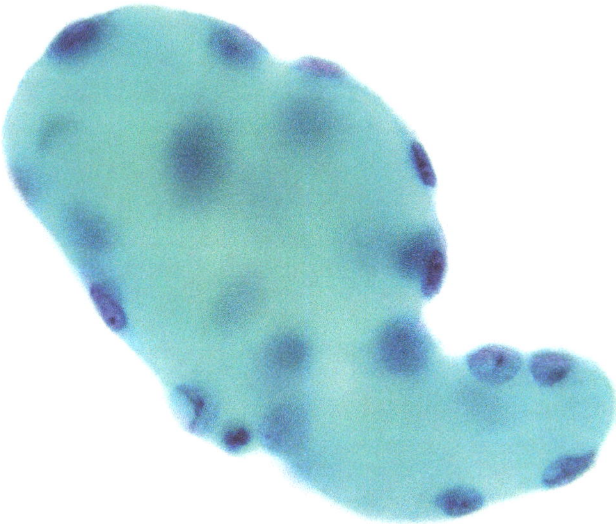

Fig. 9.43

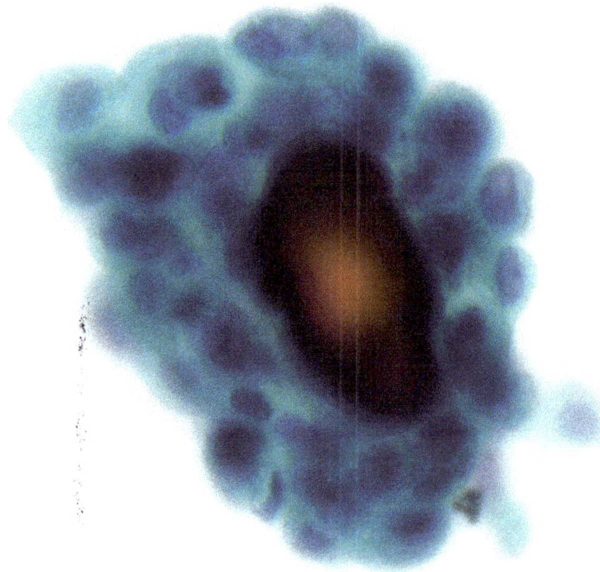

Fig. 9.44

Q-43. This finding (ThinPrep, high power) in the pelvic washing of a 48-year-old patient who is undergoing a "second-look" procedure after treatment for endometrial adenocarcinoma should:

(a) Be suggestive of a second primary
(b) Not be considered in the interpretation
(c) Indicate radiation or chemotherapy effect
(d) Indicate a mucinous component of the original tumor

Q-44. This reddish structure found in the pelvic washing of a 49-year-old woman (ThinPrep, high power):

(a) Is diagnostic of endometrial adenocarcinoma
(b) Is diagnostic of granulosa cell tumor of the ovary
(c) Can be found in benign or malignant conditions
(d) Is diagnostic of fallopian tube adenocarcinoma

Fig. 9.45

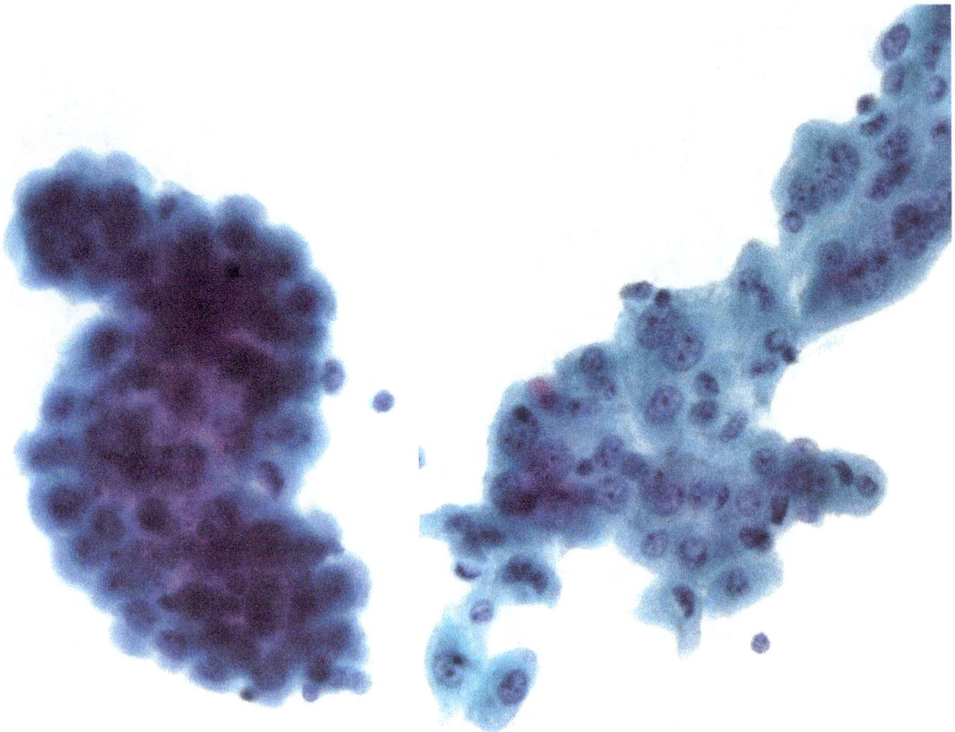

Q-45. This pelvic washing from a 64-year-old female revealed many large three-dimensional clusters and groups of cells with nuclear enlargement, nucleoli, and abundant, dense cytoplasm. Special stains on this case revealed positivity for calretinin and WT1 and negativity for CEA and B72.3. The most likely interpretation is:

(a) Reactive mesothelial cells
(b) Colonic adenocarcinoma
(c) Mesothelioma
(d) Breast carcinoma

Fig. 9.46

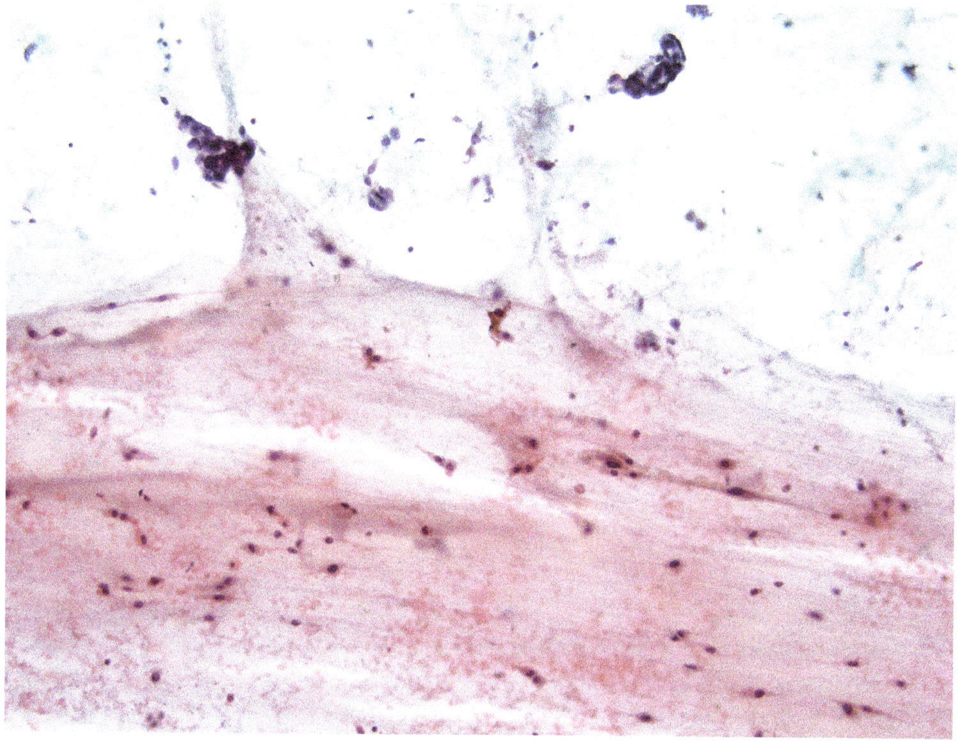

Q-46. This specimen (conventional slide, low power) was created with pelvic washing fluid from a patient with a long history of recurrent abnormal abdominal fluid accumulations. The most likely interpretation of this case is:

(a) Pseudomyxoma peritonei
(b) Endosalpingiosis
(c) Gastric adenocarcinoma
(d) Fallopian tube adenocarcinoma of the ovary

Fig. 9.47

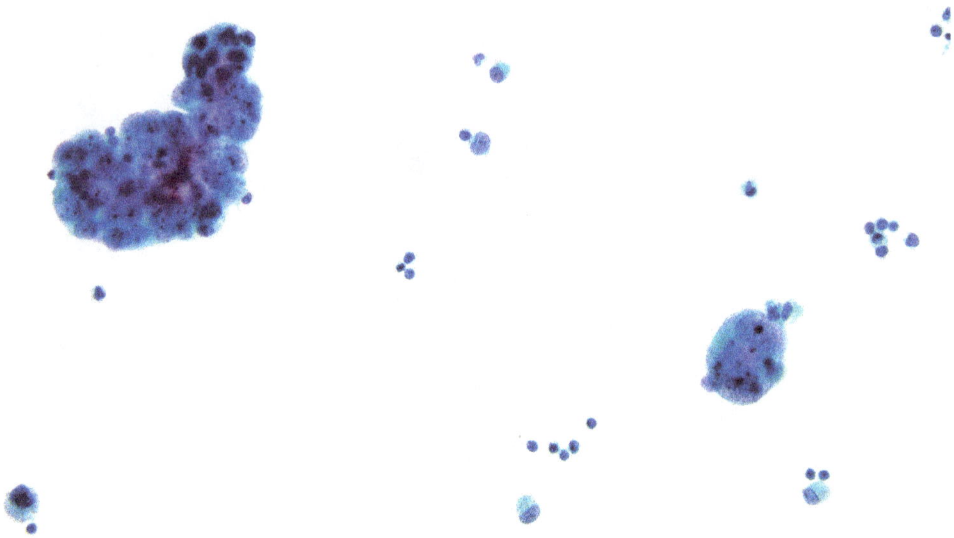

Q-47. Many clusters of cells such as these were seen in the pelvic washing from a 29-year-old woman (ThinPrep, low). Features suggestive of malignancy are cellularity, high N/C ratio, and:
(a) Nucleoli
(b) Psammoma bodies
(c) Collagen balls
(d) Single cells with terminal bars

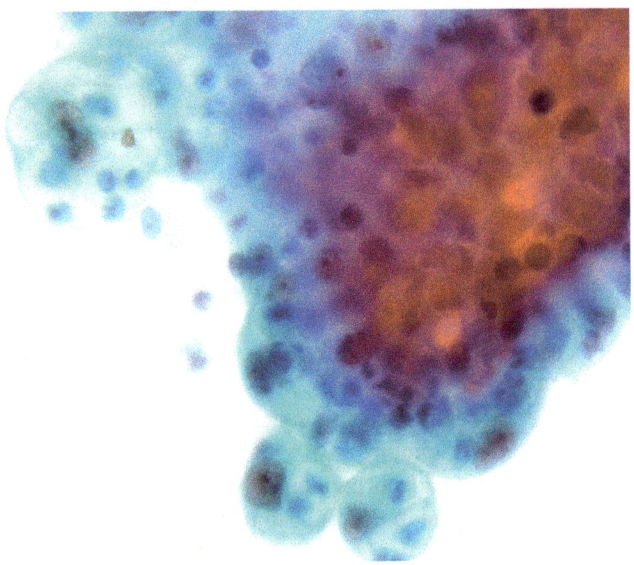

Fig. 9.48

Q-48. Many clusters of cells such as these were seen in the pelvic washing of a 61-year-old woman (ThinPrep, high power). The cells in the fluid were numerous, and many had abundant cytoplasm with vacuolization, enlarged nuclei with nucleoli, and hyperchromasia. The best interpretation of these cells is:
(a) Benign mesothelial cells
(b) Endometrial cell clusters
(c) Ovarian adenocarcinoma
(d) Endometrial leiomyosarcoma

Fig. 9.49

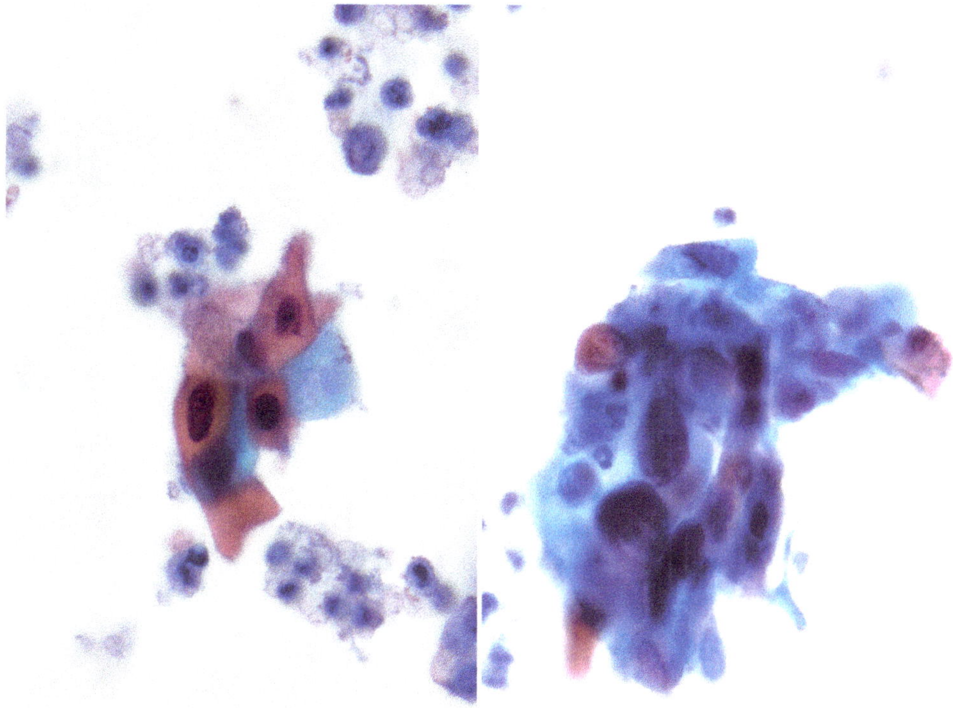

Q-49. This pelvic washing from a 63-year-old woman displayed a number of cells consistent with these images (ThinPrep, right and left, low power). The patient had a previous history of malignancy. Which of the following is the most likely diagnosis?

(a) Adenocarcinoma of the ovary
(b) Adenocarcinoma of the breast
(c) Endometrial adenocarcinoma
(d) Cervical squamous cell carcinoma

Fig. 9.50

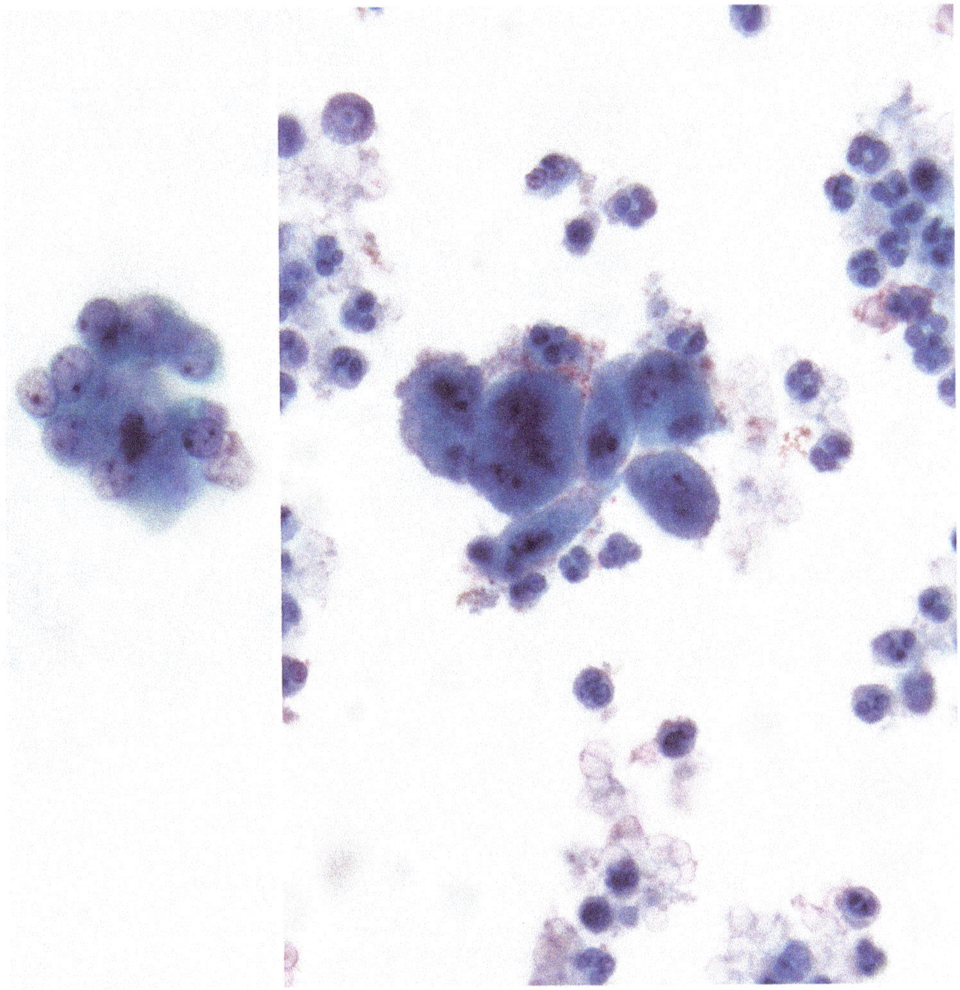

Q-50. Three-dimensional clusters of cells such as these (ThinPrep, right and left, high power) were found in the pelvic washing of a woman undergoing staging for endometrial adenocarcinoma. The best interpretation of these cells would be:

(a) Endometriosis, negative for malignant cells
(b) Reactive mesothelial cells, negative for malignant cells
(c) Adenocarcinoma, favor endometrial origin
(d) Adenocarcinoma, favor endocervical origin

Fig. 9.51

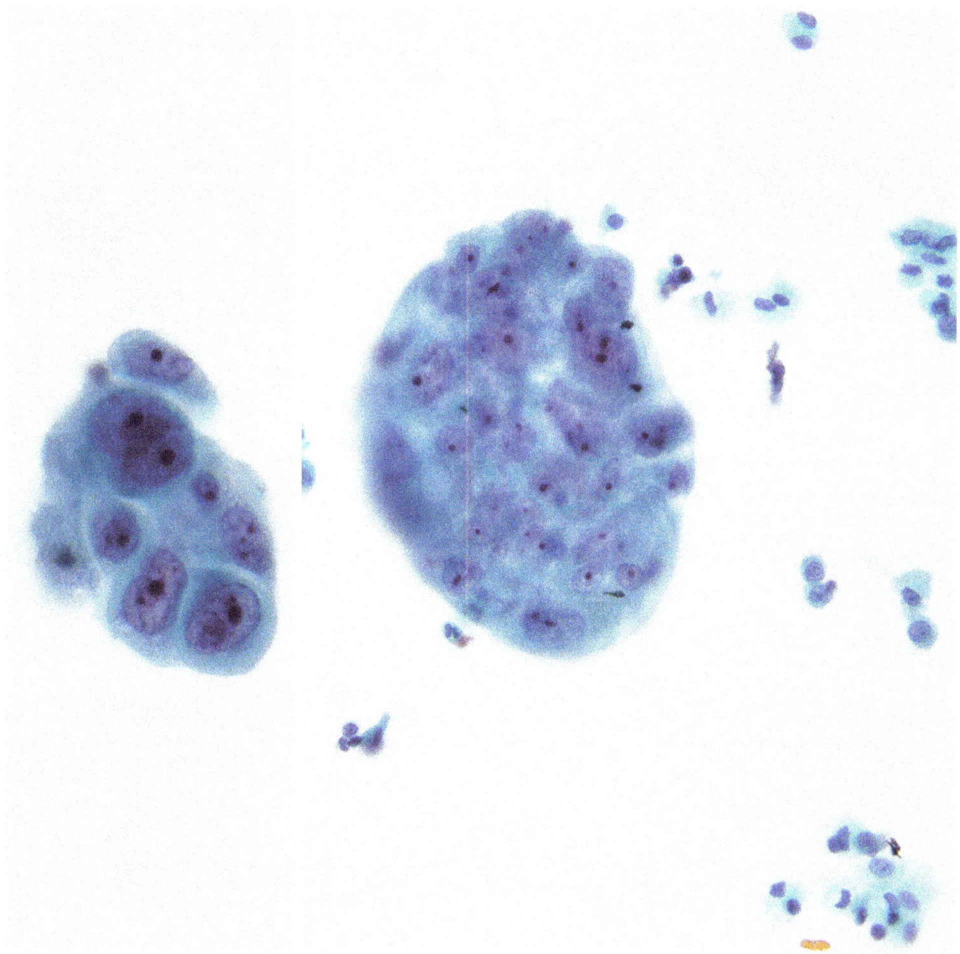

Q-51. These three-dimensional cell groups (ThinPrep, left, high power; right, low power) were found in a pelvic washing from a patient suspected to have a gynecologic malignancy. The cervical/vaginal sample on a ThinPrep done concurrently showed similar three-dimensional cell groups, scant finely vacuolated cytoplasm, prominent nucleoli, finely granular chromatin, and enlargement of the nuclei. The background had a watery diathesis. The most likely interpretation of the pelvic washing is:

(a) Endometrial adenocarcinoma
(b) Endocervical adenocarcinoma
(c) Ovarian adenocarcinoma
(d) Squamous cell carcinoma of the cervix

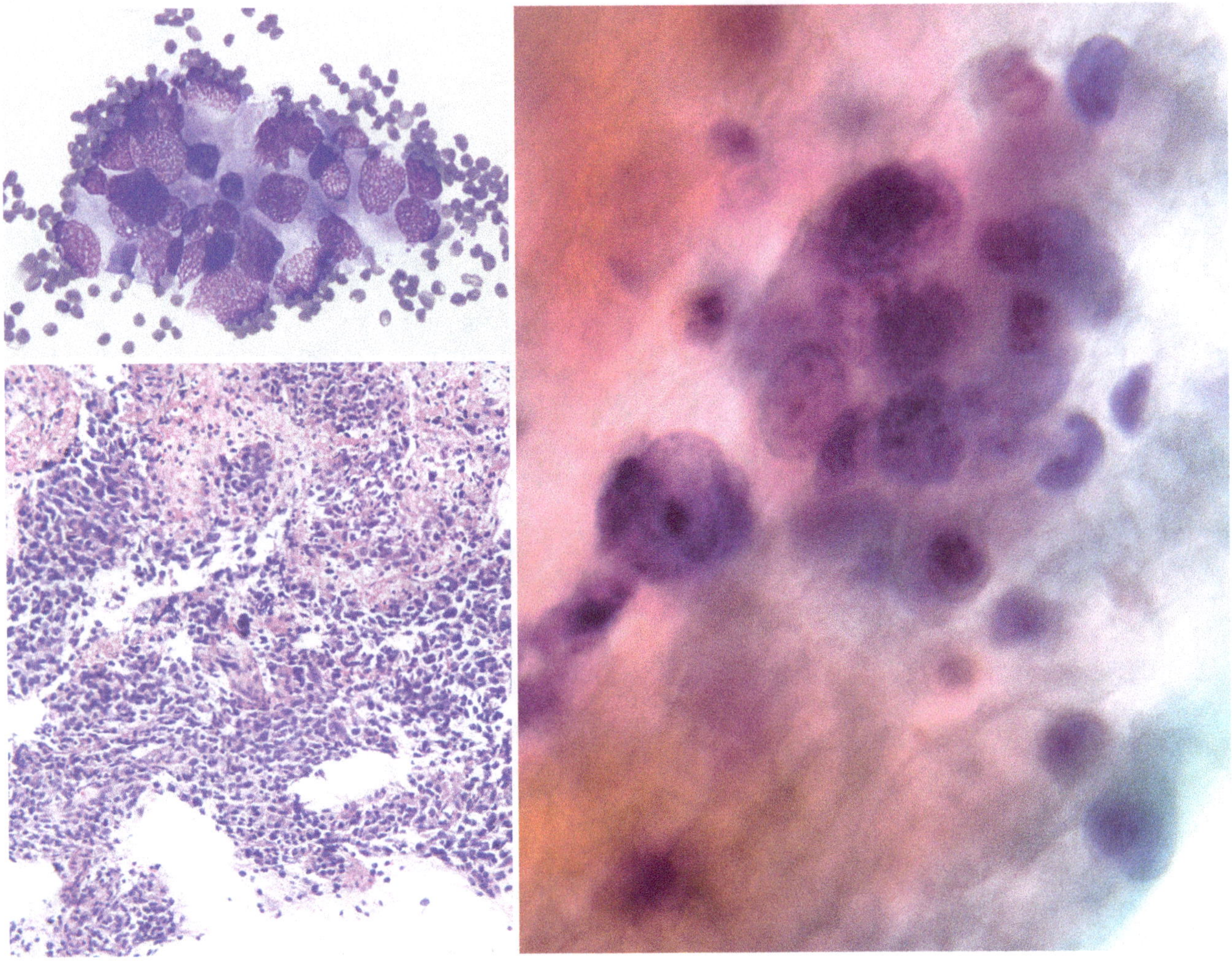

Fig. 9.52

Q-52. A pelvic washing was done for a patient with a previous history of breast carcinoma 5 years earlier. Cell clusters such as these were found in the washing (DQ, upper left, low power; ThinPrep, right, high power). A cell block on this specimen is shown on the lower left (H&E, CB, low power). The CB was sent for special staining and was found to be positive for CA-125 and WT1. Given these findings, the most likely interpretation of these cells is:

(a) Recurrent breast adenocarcinoma
(b) Reactive mesothelial cells
(c) Ovarian adenocarcinoma
(d) GI primary tumor of unknown origin

Fig. 9.53

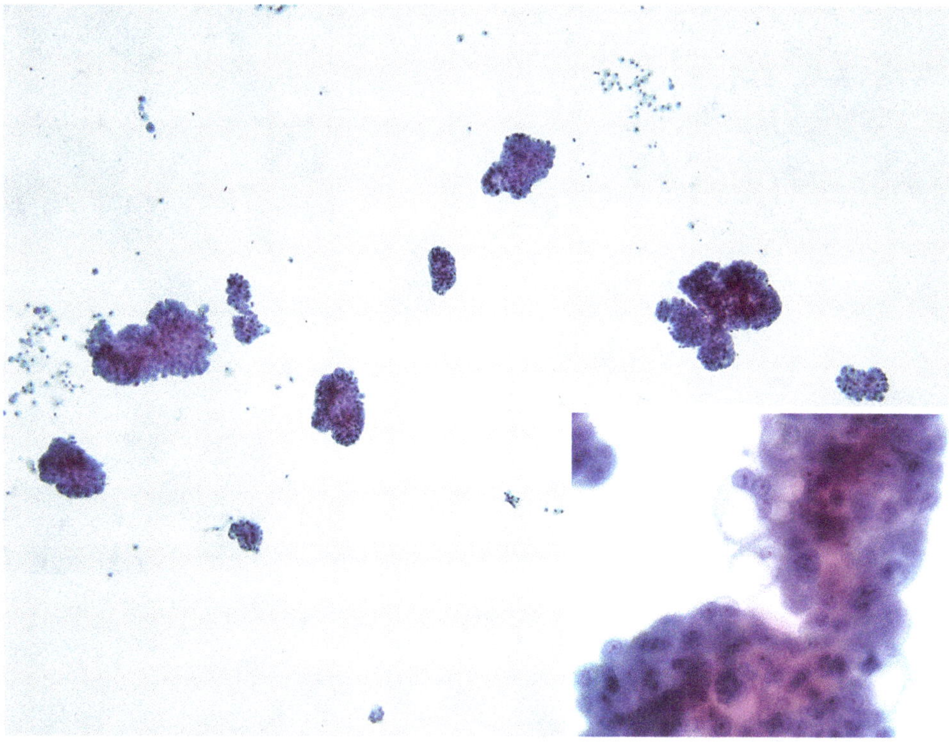

Q-53. This pelvic washing of a 49-year-old woman reveals several characteristics of malignancy in a pelvic wash (ThinPrep, left, low power; right inset, high power). Two features which are seen here include:

(a) Psammoma bodies and collagen balls
(b) Abundant crowded cell groups and nucleoli
(c) Coarse chromatin and lack of cohesion
(d) Cytoplasmic ribboning and preserved polarity

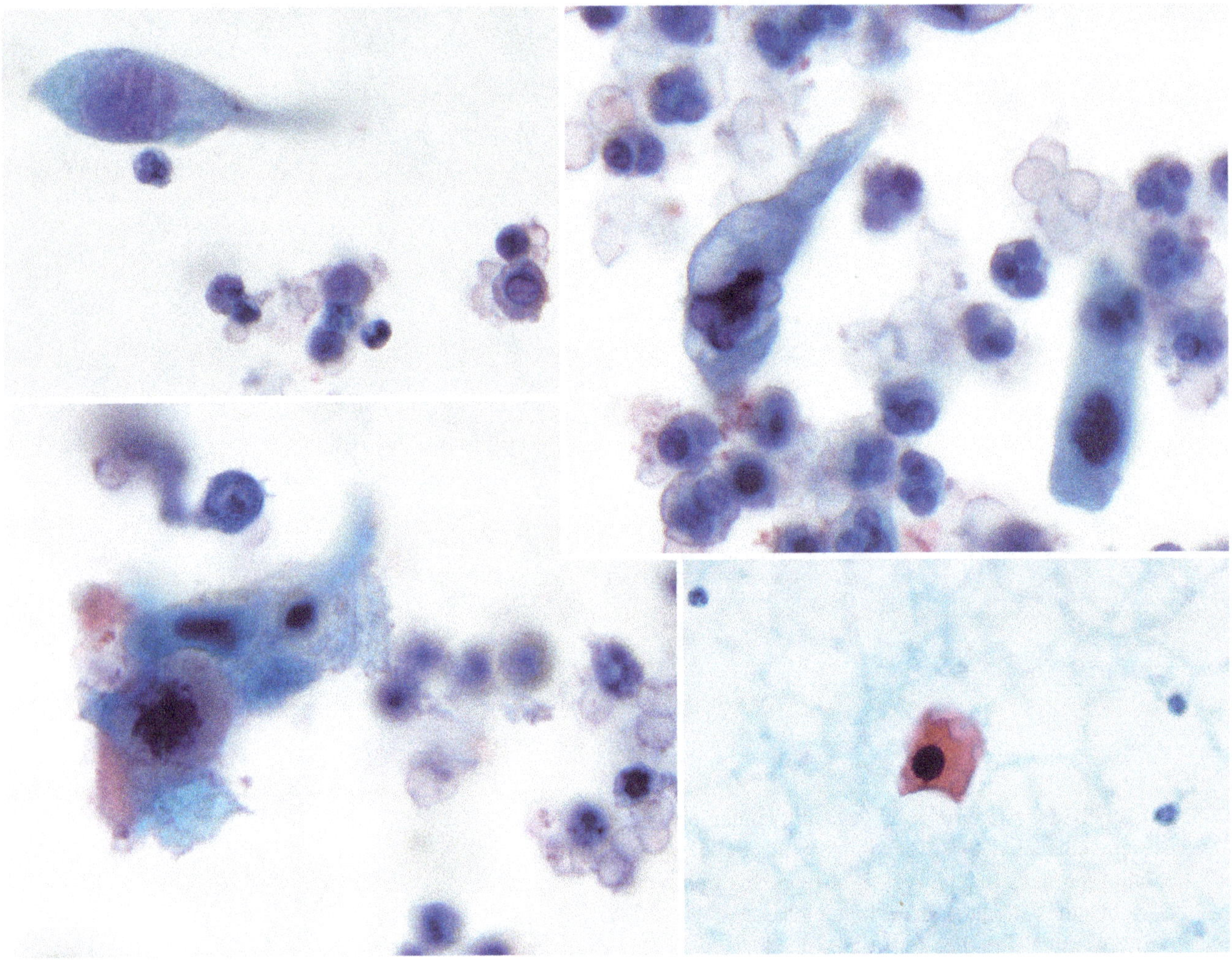

Fig. 9.54

Q-54. This composite slide shows a variety of cells from a patient undergoing pelvic washing for a staging work-up of a known gynecologic malignancy (ThinPrep, upper and lower left, right upper, high power; right lower, low power). The most likely interpretation for this malignancy is:

(a) Metastatic ovarian adenocarcinoma
(b) Squamous cell carcinoma of the cervix
(c) Metastatic endometrial adenocarcinoma
(d) Metastatic breast carcinoma

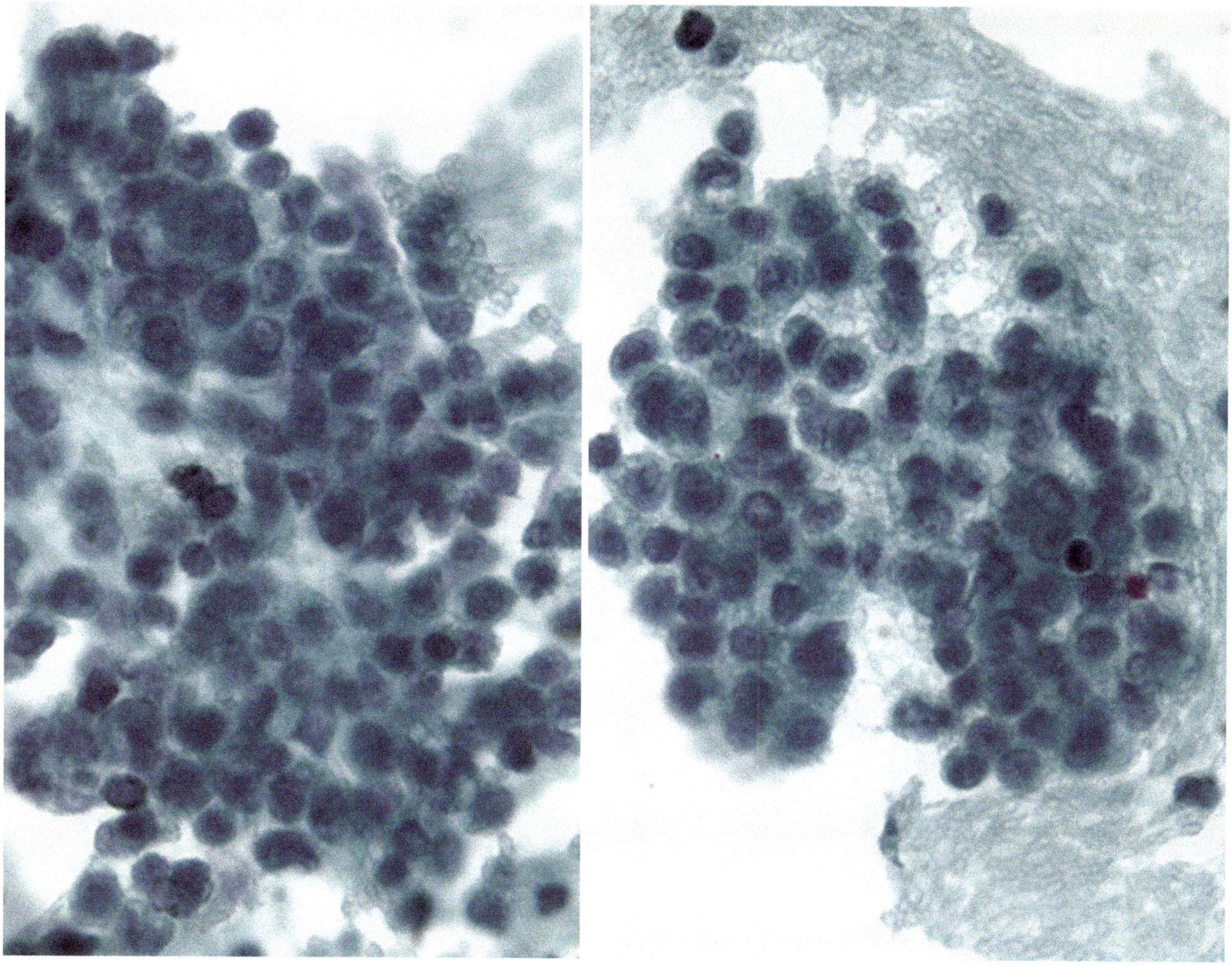

Fig. 9.55

Q-55. A pelvic washing was done as a second-look procedure on a 42-year-old woman with a previous history of ovarian serous adenocarcinoma. The best interpretation of these cells (conventional, right and left, low power) is:
(a) Negative for malignant cells
(b) Squamous cell carcinoma of the cervix
(c) Mesothelioma
(d) Ovarian serous adenocarcinoma

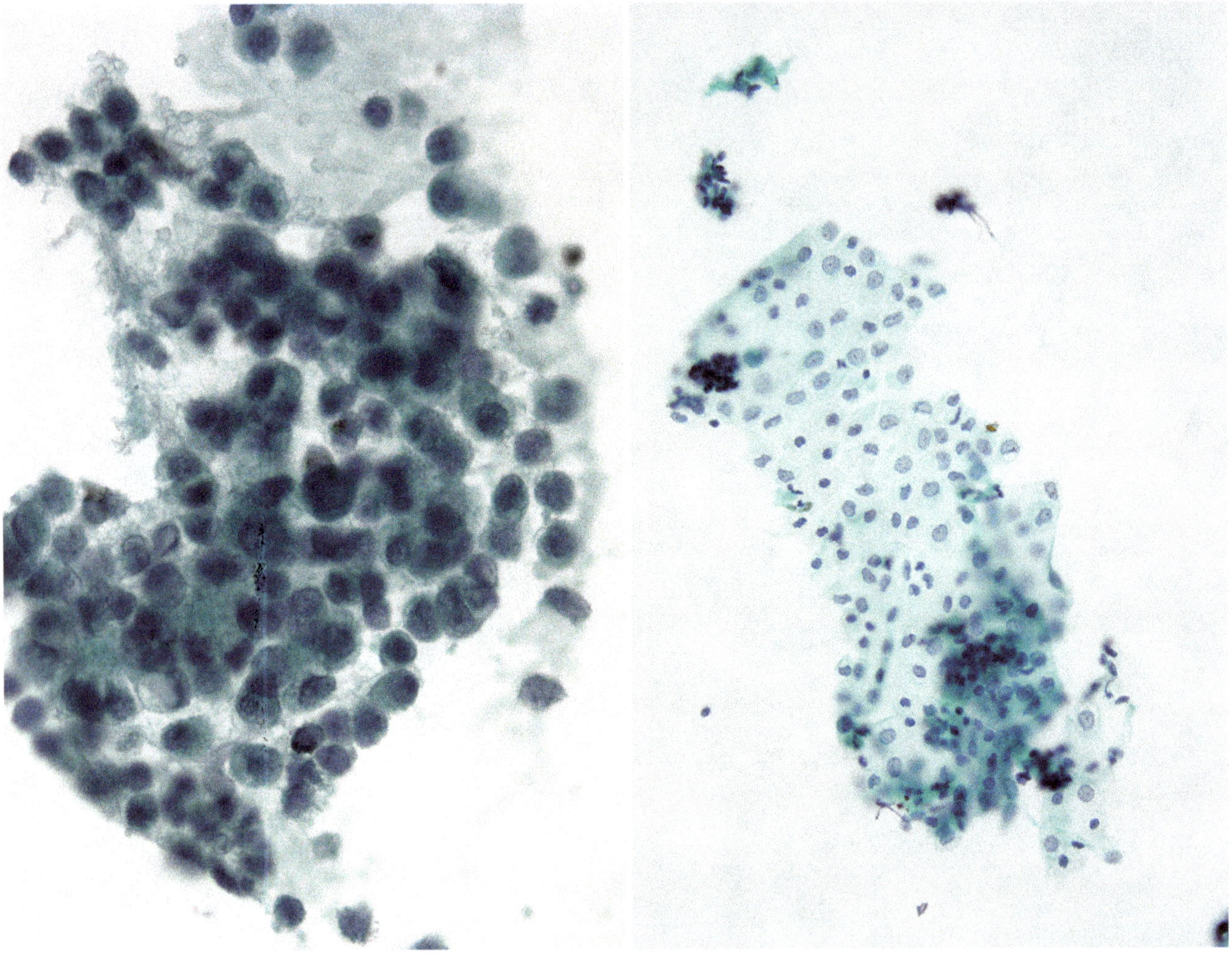

Fig. 9.56

Q-56. These cells were found in the pelvic washing of a 36-year-old woman with abdominal pain and no previous history (ThinPrep, left, high power; right, low power). The most likely interpretation of these cells is:

(a) Endometriosis
(b) Endometrial adenocarcinoma
(c) Mesothelial cells, negative for malignancy
(d) Ovarian adenocarcinoma

Fig. 9.57

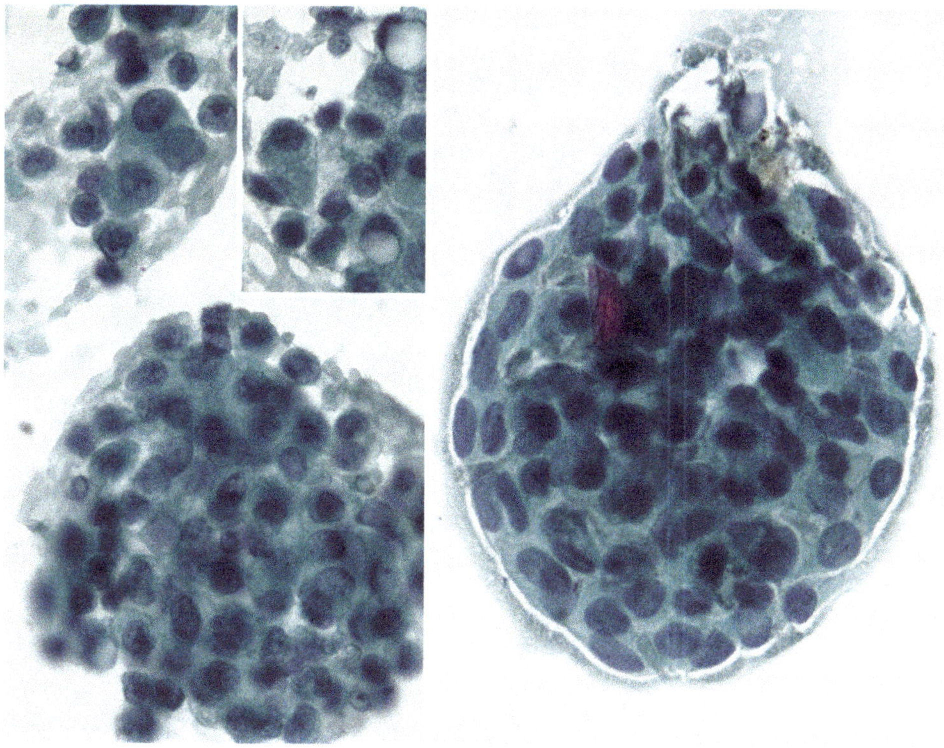

Q-57. A feature of this benign pelvic washing (ThinPrep, left, right, and inset, high power) that helps to identify the cells as derived from normal mesothelium is:

(a) Visible "windows" between the cells
(b) Vacuoles
(c) Nucleoli
(d) Coarse chromatin pattern

Fig. 9.58

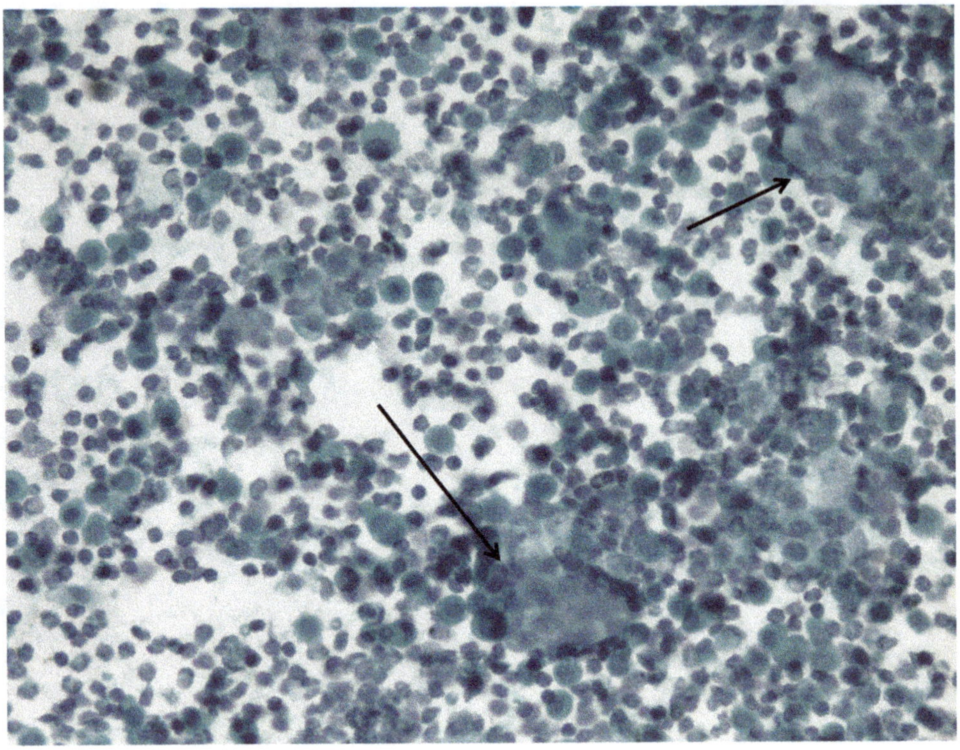

Q-58. This pelvic washing from a 29-year-old woman illustrates at the arrows a common finding in pelvic washings (ThinPrep, low power). The best interpretation of these structures is:

(a) Collagen balls
(b) Psammoma bodies
(c) Glandular epithelium suggestive of metastatic colon adenocarcinoma
(d) Mucinous adenocarcinoma

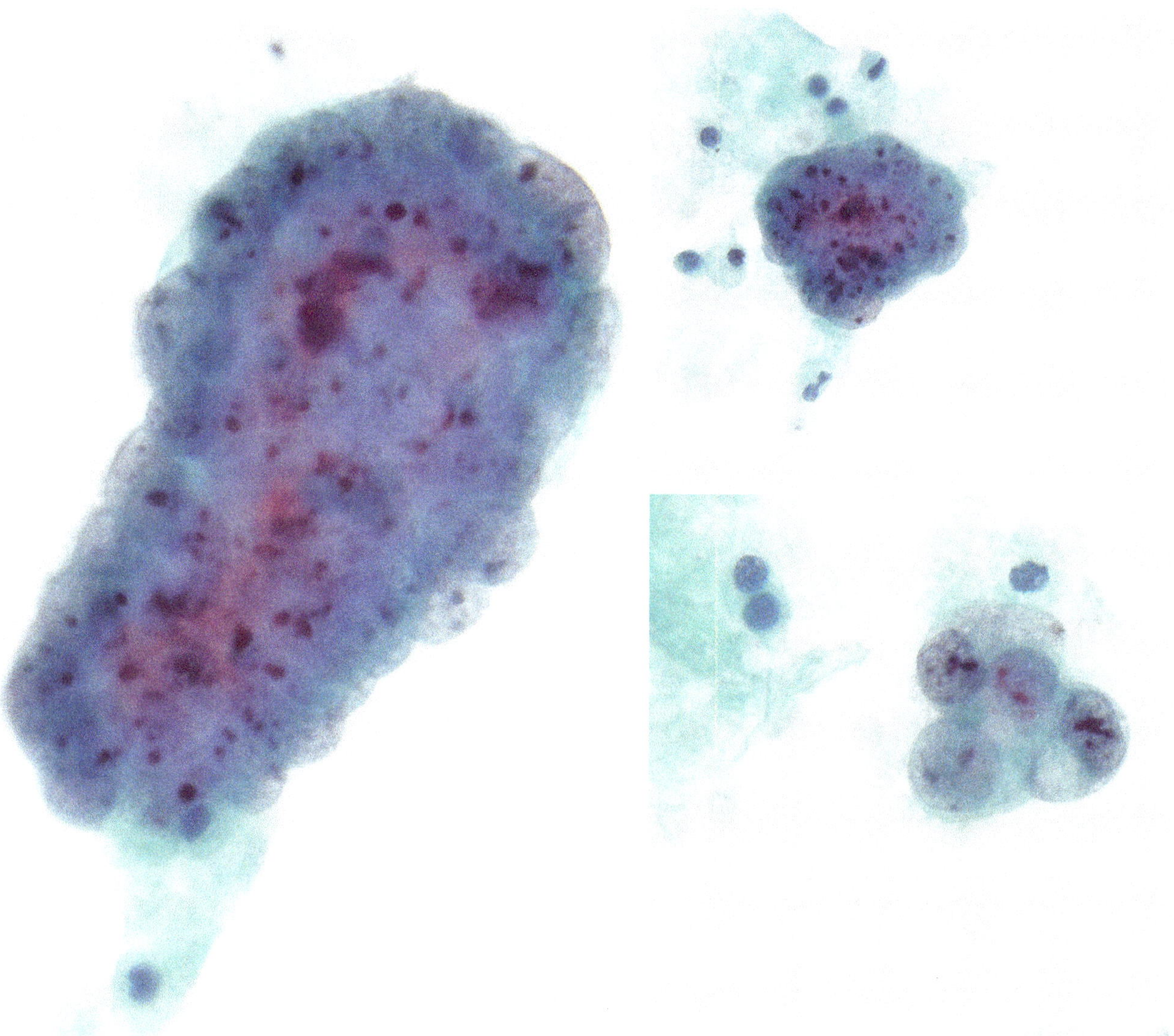

Fig. 9.59

Q-59. Many clusters of cells such as these were found in the pelvic washing of a woman with an abnormal endometrial biopsy. The hysterectomy specimen was found to have a mixed type of tumor with some areas positive for endometrial adenocarcinoma and other areas which stained positive for CD10 and vimentin. Given this information, this case most likely represents:

(a) Breast adenocarcinoma
(b) Serous borderline tumor
(c) Mixed Mullerian tumor
(d) Germ cell tumor

Fig. 9.60

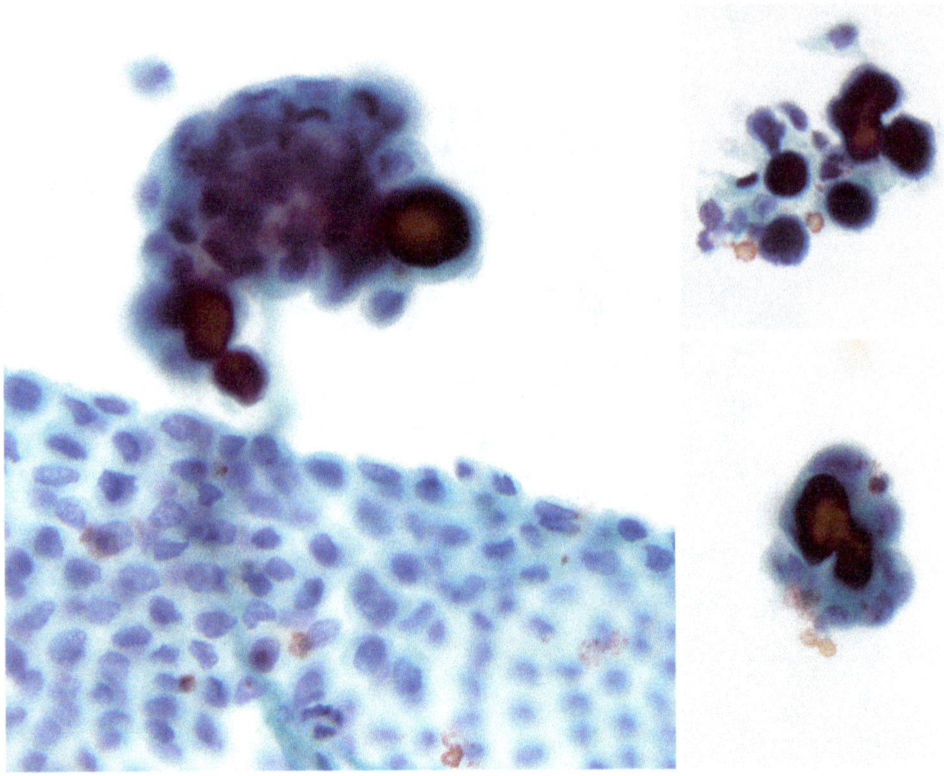

Q-60. These structures in a pelvic washing (ThinPrep, left, high power; right upper and lower, high power):

(a) Are pathognomonic for serous adenocarcinoma of the ovary
(b) May be found in benign or malignant conditions
(c) Are not significant and should not be reported
(d) Are made up of collagen with surrounding flattened mesothelial cells

9.4 Answers and Discussion of Text-Based Questions 1–20

A-1. **(a) Staging procedure for gynecologic cancers**
One of the most common reasons for performing a pelvic washing is to determine the staging of gynecologic cancers from the ovary or endometrium, for example. If the specimen is positive, it changes the staging and affects the further course of treatment the patient will receive. Pseudomyxoma peritonei is the abnormal collection of mucinous material in the abdomen and may be caused by either a benign or malignant condition. A pelvic washing would not be a useful treatment for this condition. CIS of the cervix is, by definition, confined to the cervix, and abnormal cells would not be expected in the abdominal cavity. Endometriosis is not treated by pelvic washing, although it may rarely be diagnosed by cytologic examination of the fluid.

A-2. **(b) Aspirate any preexisting fluid and submit it to cytology separately**.
Any preexisting fluid in the abdominal cavity is a spontaneously accumulated effusion. It should be labeled as an abdominal fluid and treated as a separate specimen by the laboratory. It should not be combined with the subsequent pelvic washing. Heparin, not EDTA, should be added to prevent clotting of the specimen. Flow cytometry would not normally be ordered by the surgeon for pelvic washing specimens. It has been shown that submitting the pelvic washing separately by each site is not advantageous over submitting a combined single specimen.

A-3. **(c) Compare the slides of the pelvic washing with concurrent or previous histology**.
Having the concurrent or previous histologic slides to compare with the washing can be very useful in resolving difficult cases. Comparison can be made with the oophorectomy or endometrial biopsy specimen to assist in detecting similar cells in the fluid. Although the fluid should ideally not be fixed, storage at −20 °C would freeze the cells and result in artifactual changes. Cytology slides should be routinely stained with Papanicolaou stain and not H&E.

A-4. **(c) Collagen balls**
Collagen balls are found in as many as 50 % of pelvic washings but are nondiagnostic and do not need to be mentioned in the report. Endometriosis can only rarely be diagnosed by pelvic washings alone and is an abnormal condition is any case. Psammoma bodies are not a normal finding in pelvic washings but can be noted in either benign or malignant conditions. Mesenchymal tissue from the broad ligament would not be expected to normally exfoliate into the abdominal cavity.

A-5. **(b) Endometrial glands with stroma**
The presence of benign ectopic endometrial glands and stroma in a pelvic washing can be quite difficult to distinguish from normal mesothelial cells, but the cell block material may be diagnostic if tissue fragments with cores of stromal cells surrounded by endometrial glandular cells are identified. Histiocytes are a normal component of pelvic washings. Marked mesothelial proliferation is not associated with endometriosis. A serous adenofibroma contains benign fallopian tube-like cells with or without cilia and may contain psammoma bodies. It may also contain elements of the fibrous stromal component that are not present in endosalpingiosis. It is not an expected finding in endometriosis.

A-6. **(a) Serous borderline tumor**
Serous borderline tumor would be the most likely differential with endosalpingiosis in that there are clusters of mesothelial-appearing cells, psammoma bodies or other calcifications, and nuclei with mild atypia and pale nuclear staining. Cell block material may provide the best differential clue: serous borderline tumors may have papillary fragments with stromal cores, unlike endosalpingiosis. The other conditions would be expected to have hyperchromatic, highly abnormal nuclei which would be easier to differentiate from endosalpingiosis.

A-7. **(d) Psammoma bodies**
Psammoma bodies are often seen in both endosalpingiosis and adenofibroma. Collagen balls are nonspecific and can occur in any pelvic washing. Sheets of flat mesothelial cells are a normal finding in pelvic washings. Hemosiderin-laden macrophages may be seen in cases of endometriosis but are not specific.

A-8. **(d) Collagen balls**
Collagen balls are often seen in pelvic washings but are nonspecific and do not need to be mentioned in the report. Psammoma bodies are concentrically laminated calcified bodies and usually stain deep red to orange. Adipocytes are empty-appearing fat cells with a single, compressed nucleus. Muscle cells stain deep pink and have cross striations.

A-9. **(a) Serous adenocarcinoma**
Serous adenocarcinoma is the most common ovarian carcinoma, and it is also the most common ovarian tumor seen in pelvic washings. Granulosa cell tumor,

germ cell tumor, and clear cell carcinoma occur more rarely in pelvic washings than serous adenocarcinoma of the ovary.

A-10. (**d**) **Macronucleoli**

Macronucleoli are commonly present in the cells of serous adenocarcinoma. The cells of serous adenocarcinoma are usually hyperchromatic, with coarse chromatin, nuclear irregularities, and enlarged nuclei. The cells are not tall columnar, but are more commonly round cells in large or small clusters with either scant or abundant vacuolated cytoplasm. A mucinous background is more common in mucinous tumors of the ovary.

A-11. (**a**) **Wide fibrovascular cores lined by atypical epithelial cells**

The best feature to differentiate ovarian serous borderline tumor from endosalpingiosis is found on cell block specimens in which one can find the typical broad fibrovascular cores of tissue lined by atypical epithelial cells. Chromogranin or SMA positivity is not useful in this differential. The presence of psammoma bodies alone in a pelvic washing should not be the basis for a diagnosis of borderline tumor because they can occur in endosalpingiosis or mesothelial hyperplasia as well.

A-12. (**b**) **Endometrioid**

Endometrioid endometrial adenocarcinoma makes up about 85 % of the various histologic subtypes and is the most common subtype seen in pelvic washings. The morphology of the cells may range from well differentiated with little nuclear atypia to poorly differentiated with marked pleomorphism. However, subdividing the various subtypes is not reliable on pelvic washings and is not usually necessary as histologic samples can be obtained.

A-13. (**c**) **Retrograde spread of endometrial adenocarcinoma into the abdominal cavity**

The most likely scenario that would be prevented by the clamping of the fallopian tubes prior to the removal of the uterus is the retrograde spread of endometrial adenocarcinoma into the abdominal cavity. Squamous cell carcinoma of the cervix would not be as likely to spread in this fashion. MMT also would be unlikely to disseminate in this manner. The ovaries are already in contact with the abdominal cavity so that clamping the tubes would not prevent dissemination of ovarian carcinoma into the cavity.

A-14. (**b**) **Keratinized squamous cell carcinoma**

Keratinized squamous cell carcinoma of the cervix has the more easily recognized keratinized cells with sharp-edged, dense orange cytoplasm, bizarre tadpole and pleomorphic cells, and extremely hyperchromatic densely staining nuclei. Nonkeratinizing squamous cell carcinoma may be more difficult to correctly classify as the cells may look similar to groups of mesothelial cells. Endocervical adenocarcinoma may resemble other malignant adenocarcinomas, depending on its appearance. Borderline serous ovarian tumors are perhaps the most difficult to correctly classify, and differentials would include well-differentiated serous adenocarcinoma or even benign proliferations such as endosalpingiosis.

A-15. (**b**) **Gastric and pancreatic**

Pelvic washings for staging purposes are most commonly performed for gastric and pancreatic malignancies of the non-gynecologic choices given. The other choices mentioned are not often considered for the performance of the pelvic washing procedure in the search for possible metastatic disease. Interestingly, even in patients with biopsy-proven metastases to the abdominal cavity, positivity of pelvic washings is seen in only 23–52 % of patients.

A-16. (**a**) **Enlarged, multinucleated mesothelial cells**

Enlarged multinucleated mesothelial cells with a relatively normal N/C ratio are typical for either radiation or chemotherapy effect. These cells are usually normochromatic and have increased amounts of cytoplasm while maintaining their normal N/C ratio. Thus, "a" is the best answer.

A-17. (**a**) **Uterine corpus cancers**

The two types of cancers in which the staging procedures include pelvic washings are ovarian adenocarcinoma and endometrial adenocarcinomas. Pelvic washing is not utilized for staging purposes in the other tumor types listed.

A-18. (**c**) **Coarse chromatin**

Coarse chromatin is the best of these features to indicate an endometrioid endometrial adenocarcinoma. Psammoma bodies or collagen balls may be found in any washing, benign or malignant. Dense, hyaline cytoplasm is more usually a feature of squamous cell carcinomas. Endometrial lesions usually have finely vacuolated wispy cytoplasm.

A-19. (**c**) **In large flat cohesive sheets with a mosaic appearance**

One of the most striking features differentiating pelvic washings from abdominal fluids which spontaneously accumulate in the abdominal cavity is the flat,

mosaic-like sheets of uniform mesothelial cells which have probably been traumatically exfoliated during the procedure. Mesothelial cells in effusions tend to round up, occur in scalloped clusters, and do not occur in sheets. These sheets may fold over on themselves, but the cells can be seen to be more polygonal than those usually seen in effusions. Both types of specimens may have single cells or small clusters of cells. Large papillary groups more often occur in effusions from the abdominal cavity than in benign pelvic washings.

A-20. **(b) As long, thin ribbonlike arrangements**
Cell block specimens most often reveal benign mesothelial cells as long, thin ribbons of cells, reflecting their sheetlike arrangement in the washing. Three-dimensional papillary formations, hyperchromatic crowded groups, and syncytial arrangements would be more likely to be found in malignancy.

9.5 Answers and Discussion of Image-Based Questions 21–60

A-21. (**d**) **Hemosiderin-laden macrophages and endometrial cells**

The presence of hemosiderin-laden macrophages indicates only that bleeding has taken place in the abdominal cavity. However, their presence is suggestive of endometriosis in a young woman. Another finding suggestive of endometriosis in these images is the presence of endometrial clusters, similar to those shed during menses. The best diagnostic feature is the finding of tissue fragments in a cell block representing intact endometrial glands and stromal cells. However, this is a rare finding. Ovarian stromal cells would not be a feature of endometriosis. Psammoma bodies are found in many types of conditions, both benign and malignant, and their presence does not specifically indicate endometriosis. Granulosa cells would be derived from the ovary and would not suggest endometriosis.

A-22. (**d**) **Benign sheets of mesothelial cells**

Benign mesothelial cells in a pelvic washing can appear in large sheets with a mosaic-like pattern, as seen here. The cells have distinct borders, appear polygonal, and have small centrally placed nuclei. This appearance is probably a result of the traumatic exfoliation of cells during the pelvic washing procedure. These cells can appear quite different than the clusters of mesothelial cells commonly seen in spontaneous effusions. The mesothelial cells seen in effusions often occur in three-dimensional clusters and may show a clear "window" between cells, indicating the presence of microvilli. Both of these cellular patterns can be seen in pelvic washings and should be properly identified. Histiocytes have less distinct cell borders and have finely vacuolated cytoplasm. They may occur singly or in clusters but do not have the clear windows seen in mesothelial cell clusters. Ovarian adenocarcinoma would have enlarged nuclei with nucleoli and irregular chromatin and would usually occur in three-dimensional clusters. These cells have too much cytoplasm and are not showing the loose three-dimension clusters usually seen in endometrial cells.

A-23. (**c**) **Normal sheet of mesothelial cells**

The cell block appearance of a normal sheet of mesothelial cells from a pelvic washing resembles beads on a string. This ribbonlike form may twist back on itself as seen here and should be differentiated from a glandular tissue fragment. Thus, this is not endometrial or endocervical adenocarcinoma. Also the cells are very uniform and thus are unlikely to be derived from a malignancy. Mixed Mullerian tumor is also not indicated in the cell block. Germ cell tumor of the ovary rarely causes malignant effusions, and the cells would likely have more cytoplasm than seen here.

A-24. (**c**) **Muscle cells**

The arrow is pointing to cross striations of striated muscle, probably from the abdominal wall, that may be normally found in pelvic washings. Adipose tissue can also be found from the same source. These are most often found in cell block tissue fragments but may also be seen in the washing preparation itself. Mesothelial cells would not have this feature. Although psammoma bodies may stain orange to red, this image lacks the characteristic concentric calcification structure of psammoma bodies. Hemosiderin-laden macrophages would show pink-to-orange pigmentation in cells with abundant finely vacuolated cytoplasm.

A-25. (**b**) **These cell groups are both benign and reactive mesothelial cells**.

The flat sheet in the upper left image is typical of mesothelial cells traumatically removed from the abdominal cavity during the pelvic washing procedure. However, the lower group is also benign or reactive mesothelial cells and can be more difficult to distinguish as benign because it gives an initial impression of two cell types in the fluid, suggestive of malignancy. Careful examination of the higher-power image reveals, however, that these cells have smooth nuclear membranes with even, finely granular chromatin and small nucleoli. Some faint clearing between the borders of the cells (windows) also suggests their mesothelial origin. Papillary adenocarcinoma of the ovary would have more anisonucleosis, larger more irregular nuclei, and larger nucleoli. Metastatic squamous cell carcinoma of the cervix would have irregular, sharp-edged cytoplasm, hyperchromatic nuclei, and might also feature keratinization. Endocervical adenocarcinoma would also have more irregular chromatin, larger nucleoli, more anisonucleosis, and often a more two-dimensional appearance.

A-26. (**c**) **Collagen ball**

Collagen balls such as represented in this image are a quite frequent finding in pelvic washings. They are bluish in color on Pap stain and have compressed, flat mesothelial cells surrounding the central core of collagen. Found in as many as half of all pelvic washings, they have no significance and should not be reported. Psammoma bodies usually stain orange to

red and display concentric layers of calcification. Unlike collagen balls, psammoma bodies are associated with ovarian adenocarcinomas as well as other malignant and benign conditions and are usually mentioned in the report. Adipocytes might be found in a normal pelvic washing but would display an eccentric compressed nucleus and a large clear vacuole containing lipid. Although the general formation of this cell cluster might resemble a cluster of adenocarcinoma cells, the nuclei are not sufficiently abnormal and the central core does not display cell borders as it would in a papillary adenocarcinoma.

A-27. (**b**) **Pseudomyxoma peritonei**
Pseudomyxoma peritonei is the accumulation of mucinous material in the abdominal cavity, and it may be caused by a mucinous adenocarcinoma, especially of the appendix, or even from benign conditions such as a ruptured appendix. The mucin-producing cells proliferate in the fluid and may grow on peritoneal surfaces. The fluid from such a case is often gelatinous and is mostly made up of acellular mucin with rare or absent epithelial cells present. Muciphages may also be present. This case shows the distinctly edged light blue-to-pink homogenous background of mucin, along with some rare cells which cannot be interpreted as malignant. A recurrent appendiceal adenocarcinoma cannot be diagnosed from the appearance of this case. Endosalpingiosis is a benign condition of the pelvic cavity in which there is a proliferation of glands made up of ciliated tubal-type epithelium. It may be diagnosed by the presence of cuboidal mesothelial-like cells, with or without psammoma bodies. Cilia are an aid to correct diagnosis but may not always be identifiable. Ovarian serous adenocarcinoma would likely have large, smooth-bordered clusters of abnormal cells with enlarged nuclei and macronucleoli and lack of mucinous background.

A-28. (**a**) **Psammoma bodies, papillary serous adenocarcinoma of the ovary**
Serous adenocarcinoma of the ovary is commonly associated with the presence of psammoma bodies, as seen here. A case should never be called malignant based only on the presence of psammoma bodies since psammoma bodies may occur in benign as well as malignant conditions. However, the large papillary clusters with hyperchromatic nuclei, crowded arrangements, and moderately sized nucleoli lead one to the correct interpretation. Note the fragmented appearance in the lower left image with pie-shaped sections missing from the usual rounded calcification. The red staining and the concentric calcified structure lead to the correct identification of the psammoma bodies. Collagen balls are usually blue staining in Pap stain with flattened mesothelial cells edging the core of collagen. Metastatic squamous cell carcinoma of the cervix would have single cells or sheets of cells with opaque, hyperchromatic chromatin, sharply defined squamous-type cytoplasm, and pleomorphic cell shapes. Keratinization is not observed in these images. Parasite ova would be much larger and would tend to stain orange rather than the reddish calcified structures seen here. Also, ova would lack the concentric laminations seen here.

A-29. (**b**) **Ovarian adenocarcinoma**
The left low-power view of this pelvic washing shows the high cellularity of the fluid and the rounded, smooth-bordered malignant groups. In the high-power view, a careful examination of the cells reveals anisonucleosis, macronucleoli, and irregular chromatin patterns consistent with an ovarian adenocarcinoma. Normal mesothelial cells would not show this degree of anisonucleosis and irregularity of the chromatin. Metastatic squamous cell carcinoma would have more single cells with opaque, hyperchromatic chromatin, pleomorphic cell shapes and may have evidence of keratinization. These clustered groups would be incompatible with a diagnosis of leukemia since leukemic cells occur singly.

A-30. (**a**) **Pseudomyxoma peritonei**
This cell block from a case of pseudomyxoma peritonei displays the typical finding of large amounts of mucin from the abdominal cavity. The mucin-producing cells may be scant or absent in the fluid, and so a presumptive interpretation of pseudomyxoma peritonei rather than a conclusive diagnosis may be the most specific interpretation available. The specimen is not inadequate, however, since the finding of the mucin is significant. Endometriosis cannot usually be diagnosed on pelvic washing alone, but one would expect clusters of endometrial cells and hemosiderin-laden macrophages which are not in evidence here. Adenofibroma of the ovary would have benign tubal-type epithelium with mild atypia as well as a fibrous stromal component. It often cannot be differentiated from endosalpingiosis or other benign proliferations of the pelvic cavity.

A-31. (**c**) **Small blue cell tumor of childhood**
This case is from a patient with a history of Ewing's sarcoma (ES/PNET). The interpretation as a small blue cell tumor of childhood is appropriate without further information since the case displays small,

uniform cells with very scant cytoplasm. The other choices, small cell carcinoma of the lung, endometrial adenocarcinoma, and serous adenocarcinoma of the ovary, are all inappropriate for a patient of this age. Additionally, only the small cell carcinoma of the lung might morphologically resemble this case, and it would usually display more molding than is seen here.

A-32. (**a**) **Serous adenocarcinoma of the ovary**
This case is consistent with a diagnosis of malignancy based on the numerous hyperchromatic, crowded groups seen in the low-power view. The higher-power view shows a glandular configuration of cells which have anisonucleosis, small vacuoles, and nucleoli consistent with an adenocarcinoma. Serous adenocarcinoma is the most common of the ovarian tumors to shed cells into the pelvic cavity. Thus, these cells are morphologically inconsistent with a benign condition such as reactive mesothelial cells or endometriosis. Squamous cell carcinoma would show more single cells; a more hyperchromatic, irregular chromatin pattern; and more sharp-edged squamous appearing cytoplasm.

A-33. (**b**) **Mucicarmine**
This pattern of distinctly edged, bluish background material and scanty cellular material in a pelvic washing is consistent with pseudomyxoma peritonei. This background material is mucicarmine positive and is secreted into the abdominal cavity by mucin-producing cells of malignant or even benign origin. This can be easily seen in a Romanowsky-type stain as metachromatic abundant background material. Oil red O stains positive if lipid is present which is not the case here. Masson-Fontana stain is used to detect melanin and would be negative here. GMS is used to detect fungal organisms or *Pneumocystis jiroveci* and would be negative in this case.

A-34. (**d**) **Ovarian adenocarcinoma**
These cells would be most consistent with a diagnosis of ovarian adenocarcinoma. Note the large crowded groups with hyperchromatic nuclei (compare with the group of mesothelial cells in the center of the left image). The enlarged nuclei, nucleoli, and hypercellularity all indicate a malignant process. Normal mesothelial cells would have less variation in nuclear size, smaller nucleoli, and more uniformity. Endometrial cells would be quite uniform in their size (no larger than an intermediate cell nucleus) and should not have nucleoli. An endometrial adenocarcinoma would have enlarged nuclei and larger nucleoli, but would not be as hyperchromatic as seen here, usually showing powdery fine chromatin.

A-35. (**c**) **Mucinous adenocarcinoma of the ovary**
These images show a three-dimensional glandular cell group with malignant-appearing nuclei. The cell block clearly shows the angularity and anisonucleosis of the nuclei. Thus, normal mesothelial cells are not a consideration. Germ cell tumors of the ovary usually do not shed into the peritoneal cavity until after widespread dissemination in the body. They are usually large with pale, finely granular chromatin. Leiomyosarcoma of the uterus also does not often shed cells into the abdomen and would not occur in the three-dimensional group shown here but would tend to be more single. Additionally, neither germ cell tumors nor leiomyosarcoma would show the pale blue-tinged intracytoplasmic mucin vacuoles seen here in the cell block preparation. Thus, the best answer is mucinous adenocarcinoma of the ovary which would be morphologically consistent with the images seen here.

A-36. (**a**) **Serous adenocarcinoma**
This highly cellular pelvic washing is displaying many psammoma bodies among the malignant cells. These red-staining, concentrically calcified structures are most often found in serous adenocarcinoma of the ovary. However, their presence alone should not trigger a malignant diagnosis as they may also occur in benign conditions as well as in other malignancies. The ability to focus up and down on the psammoma bodies would assist in their correct interpretation. The other malignancies of the ovary are not as highly associated with psammoma bodies as serous adenocarcinoma.

A-37. (**d**) **Benign mesothelial cells**
A careful examination of the cells seen here will reveal that the nuclei are relatively uniform, smooth bordered, and have regular finely granular chromatin. Additionally, the cell borders are more distinct than would be expected in an adenocarcinoma. Small, clear "windows" between the cells can also be identified and may assist in the correct interpretation as benign mesothelial cells. Adenocarcinoma of the ovary would be expected to have more anisonucleosis, irregularity of the chromatin, and three-dimensional glandular groups. Endometrial adenocarcinoma usually has more powdery chromatin, loose three-dimensional groups, and increase in the size of the nucleus with nucleoli. One would expect to find endometrial cells in a pelvic washing of endometriosis, although their

differentiation from mesothelial cells can be difficult. However, the cells in these images have too much cytoplasm to be considered as endometrial cells.

A-38. **(d) Lymphoma**
This highly cellular case was found to be positive for LCA and CD79a, highly suggestive of a high-grade B-cell lymphoma. The cells are single lying, show variation in the enlarged nuclei, contain nucleoli, and morphologically are most consistent with a lymphoma. Ovarian adenocarcinoma would show more cohesive groups with more abundant cytoplasm. Metastatic melanoma might be a consideration, but the negative S-100 stain argues against that interpretation. Acute and chronic inflammation would show cells which are positive for LCA. But the morphology argues against that interpretation. Also, few polymorphonuclear leukocytes are present and the lymphoid cells are immature and quite variable.

A-39. **(a) Call-Exner bodies**
Call-Exner bodies occur in the most common pattern of granulosa cell tumors, the microfollicular pattern. They consist of tumor cells surrounding eosinophilic fluid, as seen in the cell block material. This feature is seen in about 40 % of cases. The oval, uniform nuclei have pale finely granular chromatin. A minority of cases (20 %) may have "coffee-bean nuclei" with grooves in the nucleus (center image). Psammoma bodies are not associated with granulosa cell tumor. Collagen balls occur in about one half of pelvic washings but are of no significance. CK7 is negative in granulosa cell tumors.

A-40. **(c) Normal mesothelial cells**
Pelvic washings can remove sheets of mesothelial cells with polygonal cells, centrally placed nuclei, and distinct cell borders. There may be some slight variation in the size of the nuclei, possibly related to fixation artifacts. These mesothelial cells occur in a different arrangement than the rounded clusters of cells usually seen in abdominal effusions. The lack of hyperchromasia, irregular nuclei, macronucleoli, anisonucleosis, and irregular architecture help to rule out malignancies such as endometrial adenocarcinoma or ovarian adenocarcinoma. Histiocytes would have more abundant cytoplasm and would occur in clusters, not sheets. They would also have the typical finely vacuolated cytoplasm and micronucleoli seen in histiocytes.

A-41. **(b) Endometrial glands around endometrial stromal cells**
The diagnosis of endometriosis is not usually the reason for a pelvic washing to be performed. However, if cell block material contains evidence of glandular endometrial cells surrounding a central core of degenerating stromal cells, then the fluid may be able to be diagnosed. Other findings in endometriosis which commonly occur include hemosiderin-laden macrophages and degenerated clusters of endometrial cells. Psammoma bodies may occur with endometriosis but are nonspecific. Sheets of benign mesothelial cells would be expected and would not assist in this diagnosis. Extracellular mucin also would not be a useful feature in this diagnosis.

A-42. **(a) Smooth-bordered, crowded groups with abnormal nuclei and nucleoli**
A serous adenocarcinoma of the ovary often shows smooth-bordered, crowded groups with enlarged hyperchromatic nuclei and nucleoli. Flat sheets of cells with centrally placed nuclei would be consistent with normal mesothelial cells. Hyperchromatic nuclei with pleomorphic single cells and sharp-edged, distinct cytoplasm would be most consistent with a squamous cell carcinoma. Small uniform cells with molding and coarse chromatin would be more consistent with a metastatic small cell carcinoma of some type.

A-43. **(b) Not be considered in the interpretation**
This aqua staining structure with flattened mesothelial cells surrounding it is a collagen ball, and it is found in about half of all pelvic washings. It has no significance and does not need to be included in the report. It is not indicative of a malignancy. It does not suggest either chemotherapy or radiation effect. Large multinucleated mesothelial cells with normal chromatin patterns, prominent nucleoli, abundant cytoplasm, and normal N/C ratios would be more consistent with that interpretation. Also, the central portion of the structure is collagen, not mucin which would stain much more lightly and would not be surrounded by normal mesothelial cells.

A-44. **(c) Can be found in benign or malignant conditions**
The central reddish structure is a psammoma body which is often associated with serous adenocarcinoma of the ovary. However, it can occur in several other malignancies as well as in any benign condition. Therefore, its presence alone should not trigger an interpretation of adenocarcinoma in a pelvic washing. Granulosa cell tumor is not associated with psammoma bodies. Focusing up and down will usually reveal the concentric layers of this calcified structure.

A-45. **(c) Mesothelioma**
This interpretation might be quite difficult without the appropriate special stains. Calretinin and WT1 will stain positive in most cases of mesothelioma. Calretinin

will show a strongly positive nuclear and cytoplasmic staining pattern, while most adenocarcinomas will be negative. Of those few that are positive, the staining pattern is cytoplasmic. WT1 also shows strong positivity in the nuclei of most mesotheliomas. Most adenocarcinomas except serous carcinoma are negative for WT1. CEA and B72.3 are usually negative in cases of mesothelioma but positive for adenocarcinomas. All special staining should be evaluated in conjunction with the morphology of the case and knowledge of the technical and biologic pitfalls which may give unexpected results. This case was described as having high cellularity, three-dimensional clusters, nucleoli, and abundant, dense cytoplasm. Thus, the morphology is consistent with a mesothelioma, an extremely rare entity in a pelvic washing. As discussed above, adenocarcinomas do not fit the reported staining pattern. Reactive mesothelial cells will not have a staining differentiation from mesothelioma. The morphologic difference is the usual appearance of many large morulae in most mesothelioma cases, whereas these very large clusters are not usually present in reactive mesothelial cells.

A-46. (a) **Pseudomyxoma peritonei**
This case shows the distinctly edged pink mucinous background consistent with a diagnosis of pseudomyxoma peritonei in the proper clinical setting. Note that the material is not highly cellular and this is often true whether the condition is caused by a mucin-producing adenocarcinoma or by a benign condition such as peritoneal seeding of normal mucin-producing cells after a ruptured appendix. Endosalpingiosis is one of a number of benign conditions that may be found in the pelvic washing. It usually contains cuboidal cells, with or without cilia, mildly atypical nuclei, and psammoma bodies. Gastric adenocarcinoma would usually contain signet ring cells with macronucleoli and eccentric vacuoles. Fallopian tube adenocarcinoma usually resembles ovarian adenocarcinoma and features consistent with that diagnosis are not seen here.

A-47. (a) **Nucleoli**
The only feature listed that would assist in a diagnosis of malignancy is nucleoli. Both psammoma bodies and collagen balls may be found in either benign or malignant conditions so they are not good differentiating features. Single cells with terminal bars are in fact a feature of benignity. Thus, the best answer is nucleoli.

A-48. (c) **Ovarian adenocarcinoma**
This cell group shows a large cluster of cells with abundant, vacuolated cytoplasm and irregular large nucleoli. The anisonucleosis, variation in nuclear size and shape, and appearance of the cytoplasm are most consistent with ovarian adenocarcinoma. The nuclear changes and large size of the cell clusters are beyond the appearance of benign or reactive mesothelial cells. The cells are also inconsistent with an appearance of endometrial cells which would have smaller nuclei and no nucleoli. Endometrial leiomyosarcoma would generally not shed into the pelvic washing fluid and would have elongated, highly abnormal nuclei which would be less cohesive than the cell cluster depicted here.

A-49. (d) **Cervical squamous cell carcinoma**
These sharp-edged cells with keratinization and opaque, hyperchromatic nuclei are most consistent with the appearance of metastatic squamous cell carcinoma of the cervix. The other choices of ovarian, breast, or endometrial adenocarcinomas would not display keratinization or the opaque, hyperchromatic appearance of the nuclei seen here.

A-50. (c) **Adenocarcinoma, favor endometrial origin**
These cells show enlargement and anisonucleosis, pale, finely granular, powdery chromatin, and occurrence as loose three-dimensional clusters. These features are most consistent with an endometrial adenocarcinoma. While the cells do appear to be of endometrial origin, the variation in nuclear size, especially evident in the right image, removes a benign process from consideration. Similarly, benign mesothelial cells would have more abundant cytoplasm and less anisonucleosis. Finally, endocervical adenocarcinoma usually has a more hyperchromatic, coarse chromatin pattern than is seen here.

A-51. (a) **Endometrial adenocarcinoma**
These nuclei are quite large with nucleoli and finely granular chromatin and would best coincide with an interpretation of endometrial adenocarcinoma. The finding of a watery tumor diathesis in the concurrent Pap also helps to strengthen this impression. Note also the considerable anisonucleosis present in both images. Endocervical adenocarcinoma would most likely have a very bloody background rather than a watery tumor diathesis. Also, usually the nuclei are more hyperchromatic, the cell groups are more two dimensional than three dimensional, and the chromatin pattern is more coarse than is seen here. Ovarian adenocarcinoma would also usually have larger macronucleoli; more irregular, coarse chromatin pattern; and more abundant vacuolated cytoplasm. These cell groups are clearly glandular, and the nuclear features are not consistent with a squamous cell carcinoma.

A-52. (c) **Ovarian adenocarcinoma**
These cells are consistent with an adenocarcinoma, given their glandular appearance, macronucleoli, and anisonucleosis. Although the history of a previous breast adenocarcinoma is concerning, the positive results on immunostaining for CA-125 and WT1 make ovarian adenocarcinoma a likely choice. The cells are too anaplastic to be considered for reactive mesothelial cells. GI tumors are also unlikely to be positive for both CA-125 and WT1.

A-53. (b) **Abundant crowded cell groups and nucleoli**
The low-power view of this pelvic washing reveals a quite cellular fluid with many clusters of crowded cells. The higher-power view shows some cytoplasmic vacuolization and the presence of nucleoli. Psammoma bodies and collagen balls may occur in either benign or malignant fluids and are not useful differentiating features by themselves. These cells are not displaying particularly coarse chromatin, and they are certainly not showing lack of cohesion. Thus, "c" is not the best choice. Cytoplasmic ribboning and preserved polarity are traditionally characteristics of reparative cells. Thus, the best answer is "b."

A-54. (b) **Squamous cell carcinoma of the cervix**
The pleomorphic shapes of these singly occurring cells as well as the evidence of keratinization help to lead one to an interpretation of squamous cell carcinoma of the cervix. Ovarian adenocarcinoma would not usually occur as single cells but as clusters of glandular-appearing cells. Endometrial adenocarcinoma would also likely occur as groups of glandular cells, although usually with less cytoplasm, more powdery chromatin, and less hyperchromasia than ovarian adenocarcinoma. Certainly the nuclei in these images are much more hyperchromatic than one would expect for an endometrial adenocarcinoma. Breast carcinoma also would usually occur in clusters and would show less cytoplasmic pleomorphism.

A-55. (a) **Negative for malignant cells**
These cells are too uniform in their size, shape, and arrangement to be consistent with a serous adenocarcinoma of the ovary. Benign mesothelial cells can occur in these uniform sheets with a mosaic-like pattern of the flat mesothelial cells with moderate amounts of cytoplasm. It is important to be able to differentiate these from a recurrent malignancy. The cells are too uniform for squamous cell carcinoma of the cervix which would have more single, pleomorphic cells. Mesothelioma would have abundant, large morulae with nucleoli and abundant cytoplasm. Thus, the best answer is negative for malignant cells.

A-56. (c) **Mesothelial cells, negative for malignancy**
These two images show the flat sheets of normal mesothelial cells typically seen in pelvic washings. The cells are in orderly arrangements and have more distinct cytoplasmic borders than in most adenocarcinomas. Endometriosis would usually have degenerated endometrial cells with three-dimensional arrangements. Endometrial adenocarcinomas would have anisonucleosis, fine powdery chromatin, and nucleoli, as well as three-dimensional clusters. Ovarian adenocarcinomas would also occur in glandular groups with coarser chromatin patterns and larger abnormal nuclei.

A-57. (a) **Visible "windows" between the cells**
Normal mesothelial cells often display the so-called windows or small clear spaces between adjoining cells. The microvilli of the cells are nearly submicroscopic, but they prevent the close adhesion of neighboring cells. Vacuolization is nonspecific for benign mesothelial cells. Small nucleoli may be present in benign or reactive mesothelial cells, and larger ones are in malignant cells so this is not a useful criterion. Coarse chromatin patterns are more usually found in malignancy than in benign mesothelial cells. Thus, the best answer is "a."

A-58. (a) **Collagen balls**
Although this image is quite crowded with cells, one can distinguish at the arrows evidence of collagen balls with flattened mesothelial cells surrounding spherical or oval collagen masses. These are of no clinical significance and are usually not included on the report. As many as 50 % of pelvic washings contain these structures. Psammoma bodies would be calcified with concentric rings. Colonic adenocarcinoma would have abnormal nuclei, macronucleoli, and glandular arrangements. Mucinous adenocarcinoma would also have glandular-appearing cells with malignant features.

A-59. (c) **Mixed Mullerian tumor**
It is uncommon for the sarcomatous portion of an MMT to shed cells into the pelvic cavity; therefore, often, the only malignant cells seen are from the carcinomatous portion of the tumor. Endometrial adenocarcinoma is the most common carcinoma found in MMTs. The fact that the other portion of the tumor was positive for CD10 and vimentin helps to more accurately classify the tumor. None of the other tumors would be positive for both of these stains.

A-60. **(b) May be found in benign or malignant conditions** These dense reddish structures are psammoma bodies and may be found often in association with serous adenocarcinoma of the ovary. However, any benign or malignant conditions can give rise to these structures. They are usually reported due to their possible association with adenocarcinomas. The "d" choice is a description of collagen balls which are commonly found in pelvic washings, but they have no clinical significance.

Reading List

Bibbo M, Wood MD, Fitzpatrick BT. Peritoneal washings and ovary. In: Bibbo M, Wilbur D, editors. Comprehensive cytopathology. 3rd ed. Philadelphia: Saunders/Elsevier; 2008.

Cibas ES. Peritoneal washings. In: Cibas ES, Ducatman BS, editors. Cytology: diagnostic principles and clinical correlates. Philadelphia: Saunders/Elsevier; 2009.

DeMay RM. The art and science of cytopathology, Exfoliative cytology, vol. 1. 2nd ed. Chicago: ASCP Press; 2012.

Breast FNA: Cytomorphology and Diagnostic Pitfalls

10

Reda S. Saad, Walid E. Khalbuss, and Marilee Means

Contents

R.S. Saad, MD, PhD, FRCPC (✉)
Department of Pathology, Hotel Dieu Grace Hospital,
Windsor, ON, Canada

137 Brian Drive, Toronto, ON M2J 3Y8, Canada
e-mail: reda.saad@hdgh.org

W.E. Khalbuss, MD, PhD, FIAC
Director of Cytology and Cytopathology Fellowship Program,
University of Pittsburgh Medical Center Shadyside Hospital,
5150 Centre Avenue, 2, Suite 201,
Pittsburgh, PA 15232, USA
e-mail: khalbussw2@upmc.edu

M. Means, PhD, SCT(ASCP)
School of Health Professions,
University of Kansas Medical Center,
3901 Rainbow Blvd., Mail Stop 4048,
Kansas City, KS 66160, USA
e-mail: mmeans@kumc.edu

10.1 Tables and Summary

Table 10.1 Indication of FNA/core needle biopsy: palpable versus nonpalpable

In palpable breast lesions
Palpable masses of clinical/patient concern
Young patients with palpable persistent/suspicious masses
Patients with family history regardless of imaging findings
In nonpalpable breast lesions
Lesions suspicious for malignancy by imaging study
Lesions with discordance between clinical and radiologic findings

Table 10.2 Limitations of breast FNA

Lack of ability to distinguish between in situ and invasive carcinoma
Lack of ability to distinguish between atypical ductal hyperplasia and low-grade in situ carcinoma
Lack of ability to distinguish between low-grade carcinomas and benign proliferative changes need to biopsy all lesions with atypical "gray zone" diagnoses
Lack of specific diagnosis for most benign lesions

Table 10.3 Advantages of breast FNA

Economical/cost-effective outpatient procedure
Minimally traumatic (physically and psychologically) with high acceptance rate and minimal or no morbidity
Rapid and accurate diagnosis stress relief of anxiety for the patient for benign diagnosis and more time for pretreatment planning for malignant diagnosis
Permit involvement of the patient in the decision-making process when malignancy is identified
Offers evaluation of multiple nodules/lesions
Sampling tumor for biomarkers and molecular studies
Diagnosis of cystic/inflammatory lesions with therapeutic evacuation
Offers rapid diagnosis of locally advanced cancer, axillary lymph node metastases, or recurrence for better tumor staging and treatment decision

W.E. Khalbuss, M. Means (eds.), *Gynecological and Breast Cytopathology Board Review and Self-Assessment*,
DOI 10.1007/978-1-4614-7270-4_10,

Table 10.4 Complications of breast FNA

Bleeding/hematoma
Infection
Pneumothorax/vasovagal reaction
Epithelial displacement/tumor seeding
Post-FNA changes may interfere with images studies

Table 10.5 Reporting terminology for breast FNA

Negative for malignant cells (no malignant cells seen)
Atypical/indeterminate
Suspicious for malignancy
Positive for malignant cells
Nondiagnostic (inadequate or unsatisfactory)

Table 10.6 Lesions associated with architectural patterns

Sheets
Fibrocystic changes
Fibroadenomas
Tightly cohesive three-dimensional aggregates
Fibroadenomas and phyllodes tumors
Intraductal papilloma
Ductal proliferative lesions from intraductal hyperplasia to ductal carcinoma in situ
Well-differentiated ductal carcinomas
Mucinous carcinomas
Loosely cohesive three-dimensional clusters
Phyllodes tumor
Ductal carcinoma in situ
Branching papillary clusters
Fibroadenoma
Intraductal papilloma
Papillary carcinoma
Numerous single cells
Carcinoma
Pregnancy or lactation

Table 10.7 Breast lesions diagnosed as "papillary" on FNA

Intraductal papilloma
Papillomatosis
Fibroadenoma
Fibrocystic changes with papillary hyperplasia
Malignant on follow-up: ductal carcinoma and phyllodes tumor

Table 10.8 Nipple discharge cytology

Uncommon specimen
The second most common sign of breast lesion after a breast lump
Can be physiologic or pathologic causes
Physiological causes: drugs, metabolic conditions, pituitary adenoma with high prolactin levels, and hormonal fluctuation resulting from pregnancy or lactation
Pathological: 3 % of breast malignancies are associated with nipple discharge (bloody, unilateral, accompanied by a lump, a positive mammogram, or patient is over 50 years old)
Cytological examination should only be performed on bloody discharges, although others have cautioned that carcinoma can also be associated with a non-bloody discharge

Table 10.9 Diagnostic pitfalls in breast FNAs

Causes of false-negative diagnoses
Small focus of carcinoma
Carcinoma arising in a complex proliferative lesion
Well-differentiated carcinomas (low grade)
Specific histologic subtypes (such as tubular carcinoma, colloid carcinoma)
Rare tumor types (such as metaplastic carcinoma, apocrine carcinoma)
Large tumors with extensive necrosis or cystic changes
Sampling errors (in lesions that are small, deep, or have densely fibrotic stroma)
Causes of false-positive diagnoses
Fibroadenoma
Papilloma/papillary lesions
Atypical ductal hyperplasia
Pregnancy associated or lactational changes
Skin adnexal tumors
Other lesions (fat necrosis, collagenous spherulosis)

10.2 Text-Based Questions 1–5

Q-1. The advantages of breast fine-needle aspiration include:
- (a) Economical/cost-effective outpatient procedure
- (b) Minimally invasive procedure
- (c) Therapeutic for benign cysts
- (d) Rapid and accurate diagnosis and rare morbidity
- (e) All of the above

Q-2. Which of the following is true about breast FNA?
- (a) Ability to distinguish between in situ and invasive carcinoma.
- (b) Ability to distinguish between atypical ductal hyperplasia and low-grade in situ carcinoma.
- (c) Ability to distinguish between low-grade carcinomas and benign proliferative changes.
- (d) It offers rapid diagnosis of locally advanced cancer or recurrence for better tumor staging and treatment decision.

Q-3. What is the least possible complication of breast fine-needle aspiration?
- (a) Pain and bleeding/hematoma
- (b) Pneumothorax
- (c) Infection
- (d) Needle tract seeding of tumor and epithelial displacement of tumor cells

Q-4. Which of the following is least accurate about primary neuroendocrine carcinoma in breast FNA?
- (a) Smears are highly cellular.
- (b) Cells may be arranged in a single cell discohesive pattern.
- (c) There is nuclear molding, hyperchromasia, "salt-and-pepper" chromatin, and inconspicuous nucleoli.
- (d) The differential diagnosis includes metastatic carcinoid or small cell carcinoma from the lung.
- (e) Immunohistochemical staining for ER, PR, and GCDFP-15 is helpful.

Q-5. A breast FNA from a 23-year-old woman who presented with mammogram suspicious for malignancy showed abundant vacuolated cytoplasm with lipid-laden-like and hemosiderin-laden-like morphology, granular necrotic-like debris, and inflammatory cells including neutrophils, plasma cells, and lymphocytes. Few multinucleated foreign-body-type giant cells and spindle-shaped cells are also seen. The patient recalled a traumatic blow to her breast. Which of the following is the most likely diagnosis?
- (a) Invasive ductal carcinoma
- (b) Invasive secretor carcinoma
- (c) Fat necrosis
- (d) Fibroadenoma
- (e) Basal-like breast carcinoma

10.3 Image-Based Questions 6–65

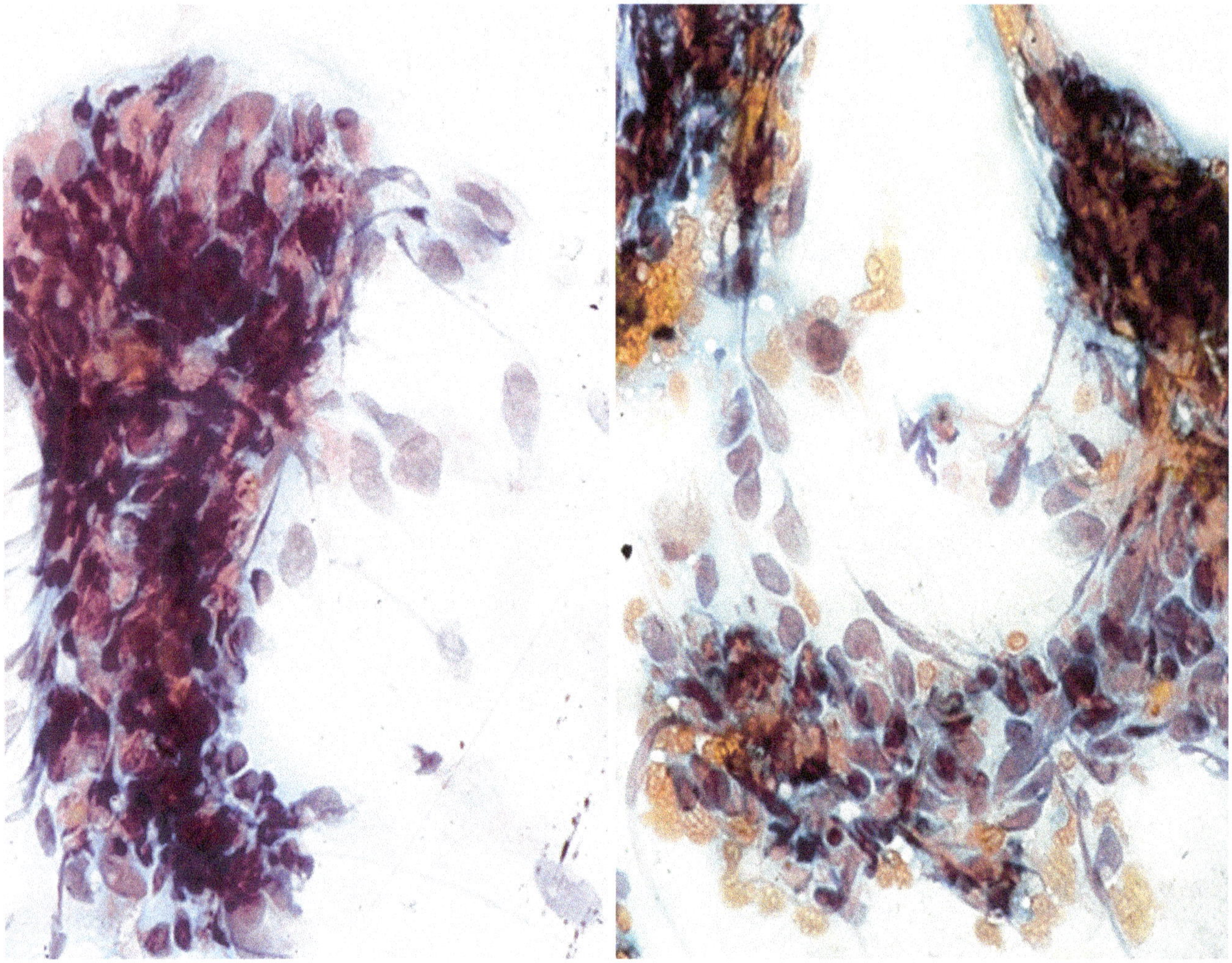

Fig. 10.6

Q-6. This aspirate is from a 56-year-old woman who has noticed a mass in her left breast. On physical examination, a large vague mass was identified. Mammogram shows an ill-defined breast lesion with microcalcifications, indeterminate for malignancy. FNA was performed. Which of the following is the most likely diagnosis?

(a) Unsatisfactory for evaluation
(b) Fibroadenoma
(c) Benign breast cyst
(d) Granulomatous mastitis
(e) Negative for malignancy

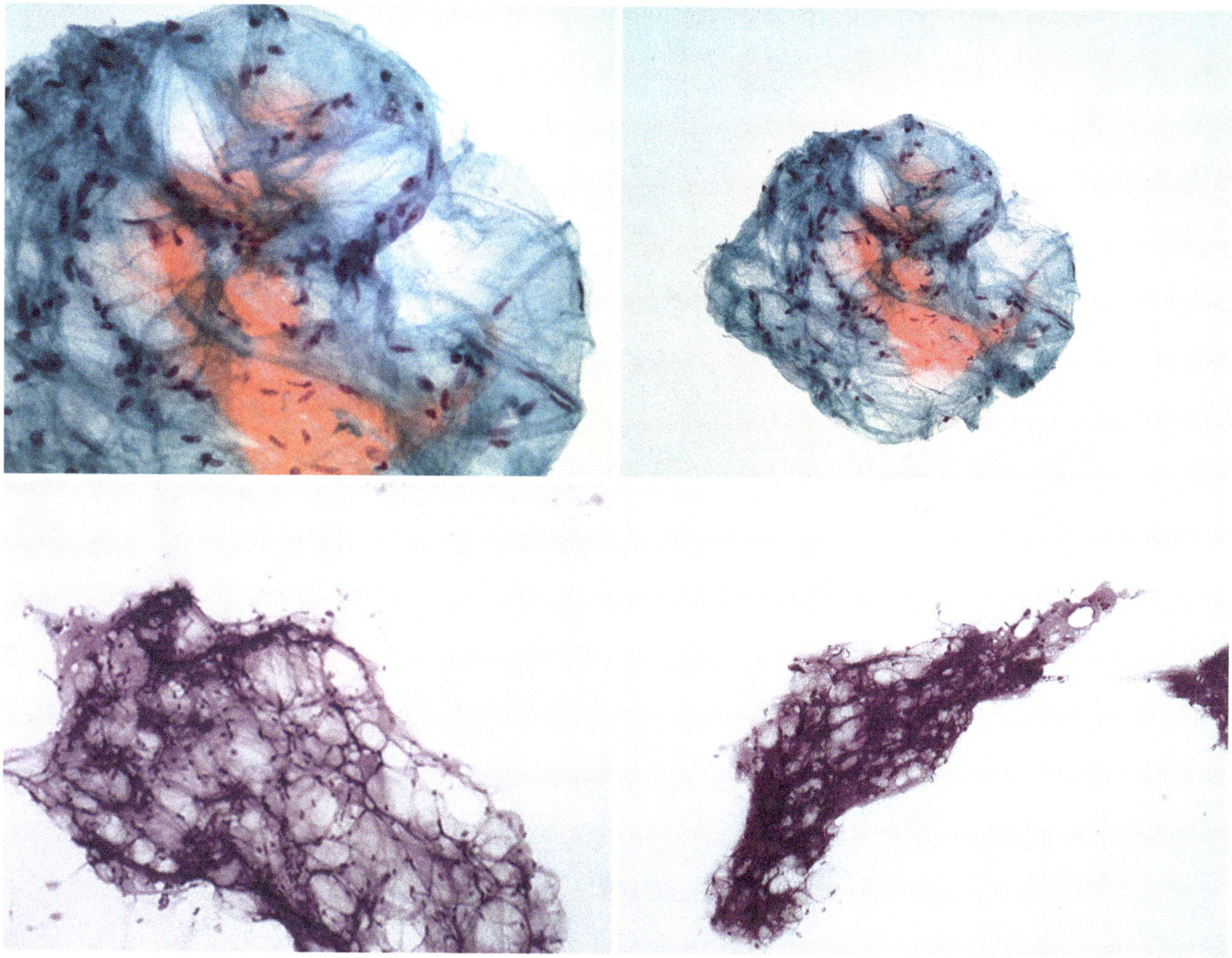

Fig. 10.7

Q-7. This aspirate is from a 43-year-old woman who presents with a well-defined mass. Mammogram demonstrates a well-defined mass with benign features located in the subcutaneous area of the breast. FNA was performed. Which of the following is the most likely diagnosis?
(a) Fibroadenoma
(b) Phyllodes tumor
(c) Lipoma
(d) Chronic mastitis
(e) Fat necrosis

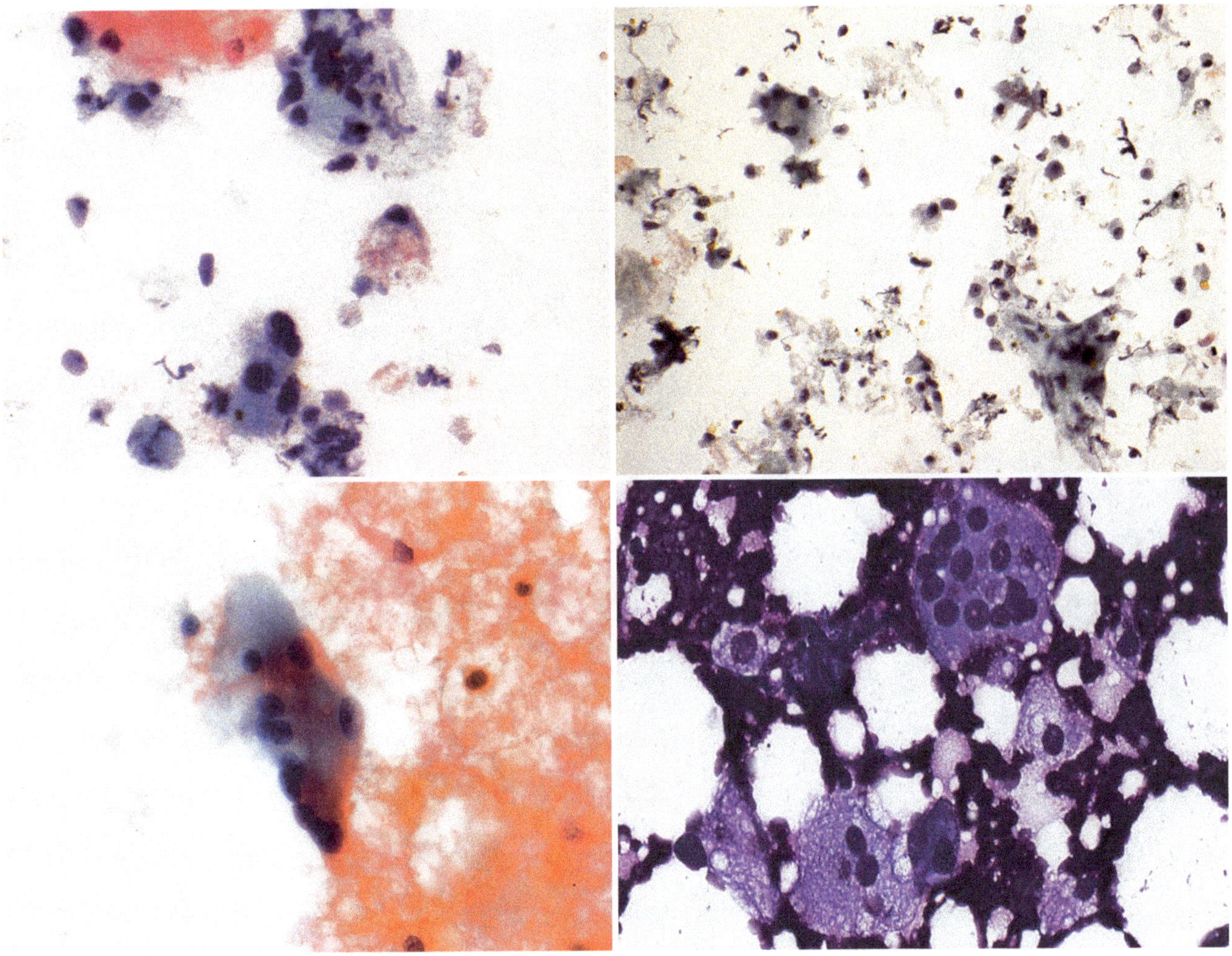

Fig. 10.8

Q-8. This aspirate is from a 30-year-old woman who suffered a traumatic blow to her right breast. Initially, there was a 3-cm contusion that resolved within a few weeks. After a while she developed a breast mass. On physical examination, a 2.5-cm firm and irregular lump was identified. Mammogram was suspicious for malignancy. FNA was performed. Which of the following is the most likely diagnosis?

(a) Invasive ductal carcinoma
(b) Sclerosing adenosis
(c) Fat necrosis
(d) Fibroadenoma
(e) Mammary duct ectasia

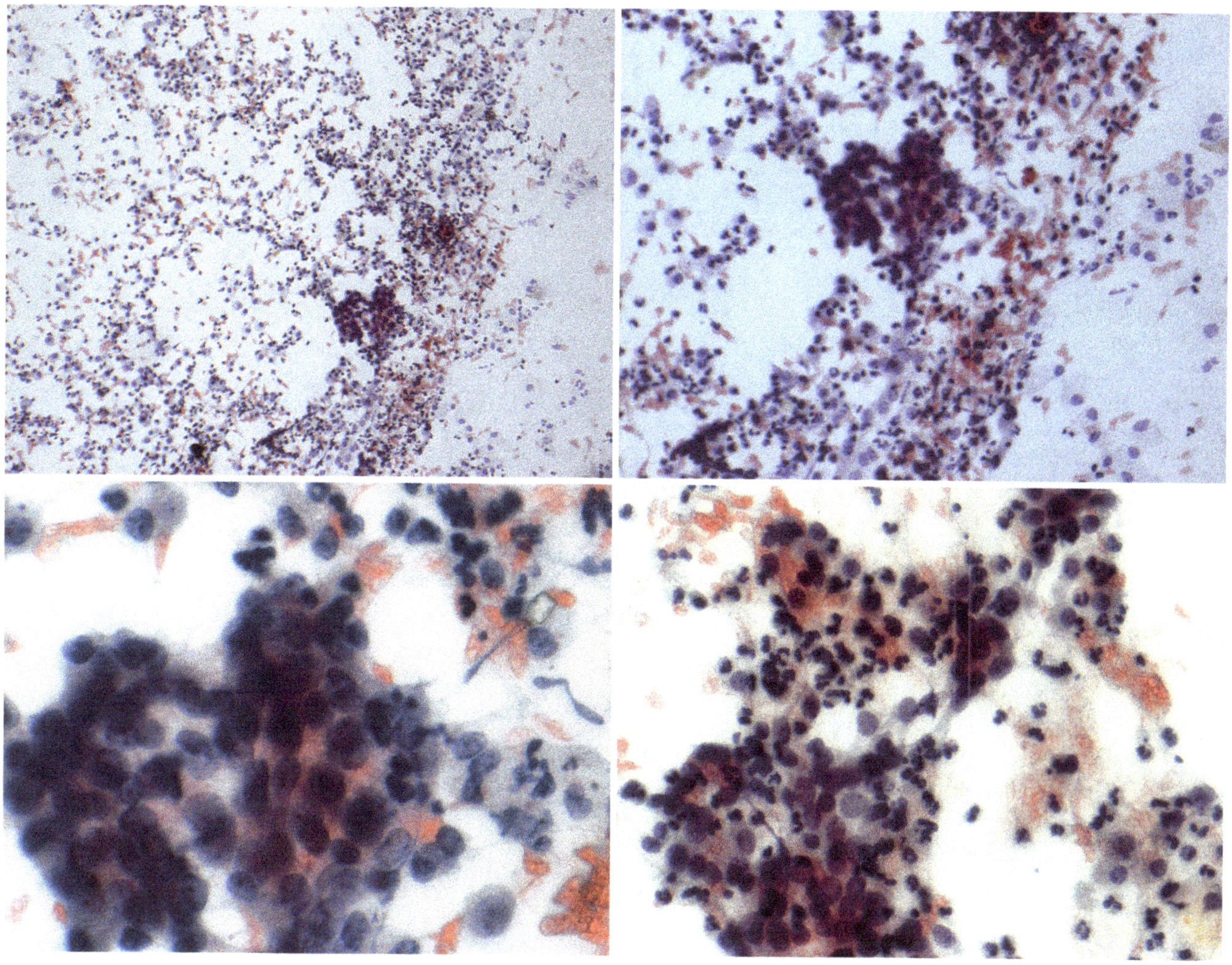

Fig. 10.9

Q-9. This aspirate is from a 30-year-old lactating woman who has noticed redness and pain in the nipple of her left breast. On physical examination, an area of hotness and redness was identified. Palpation showed an ill-defined and tender mass. FNA was performed. Which of the following is the most likely diagnosis?

(a) Fibroadenoma
(b) Inflammatory carcinoma
(c) Fat necrosis
(d) Acute mastitis/breast abscess
(e) Lymphoma

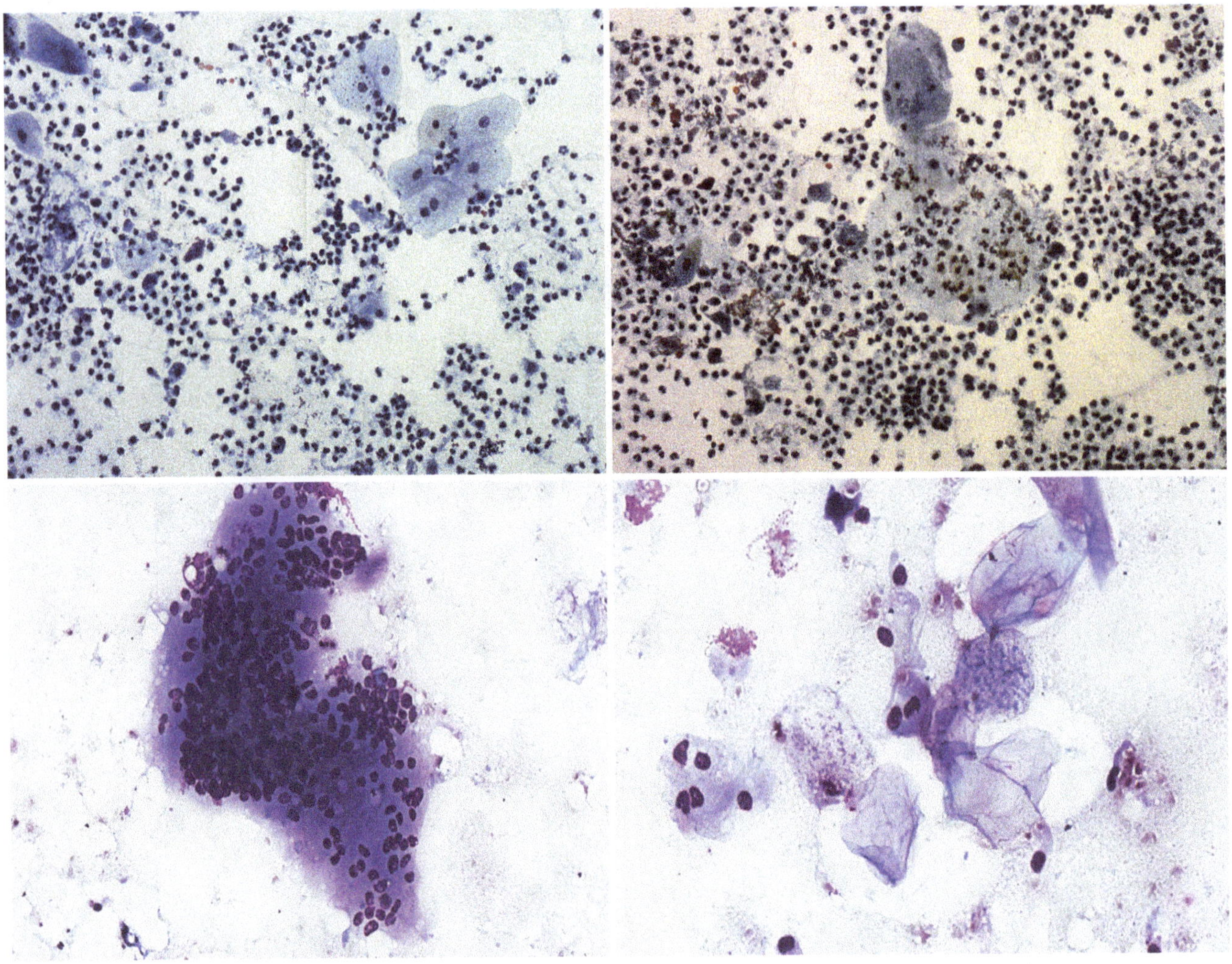

Fig. 10.10

Q-10. This aspirate is from a 37-year-old woman who has noticed pain in the nipple of her left breast. There is a tender nodule seen in the areola of her left breast. On physical examination, a tender 2.0-cm mass was identified. Mammogram shows an ill-defined mass in the areolar area, suspicious for malignancy. FNA was performed. Which of the following is the most likely diagnosis?

(a) Inflammatory carcinoma
(b) Fibroadenoma
(c) Fat necrosis
(d) Subareolar abscess
(e) Granulomatous mastitis

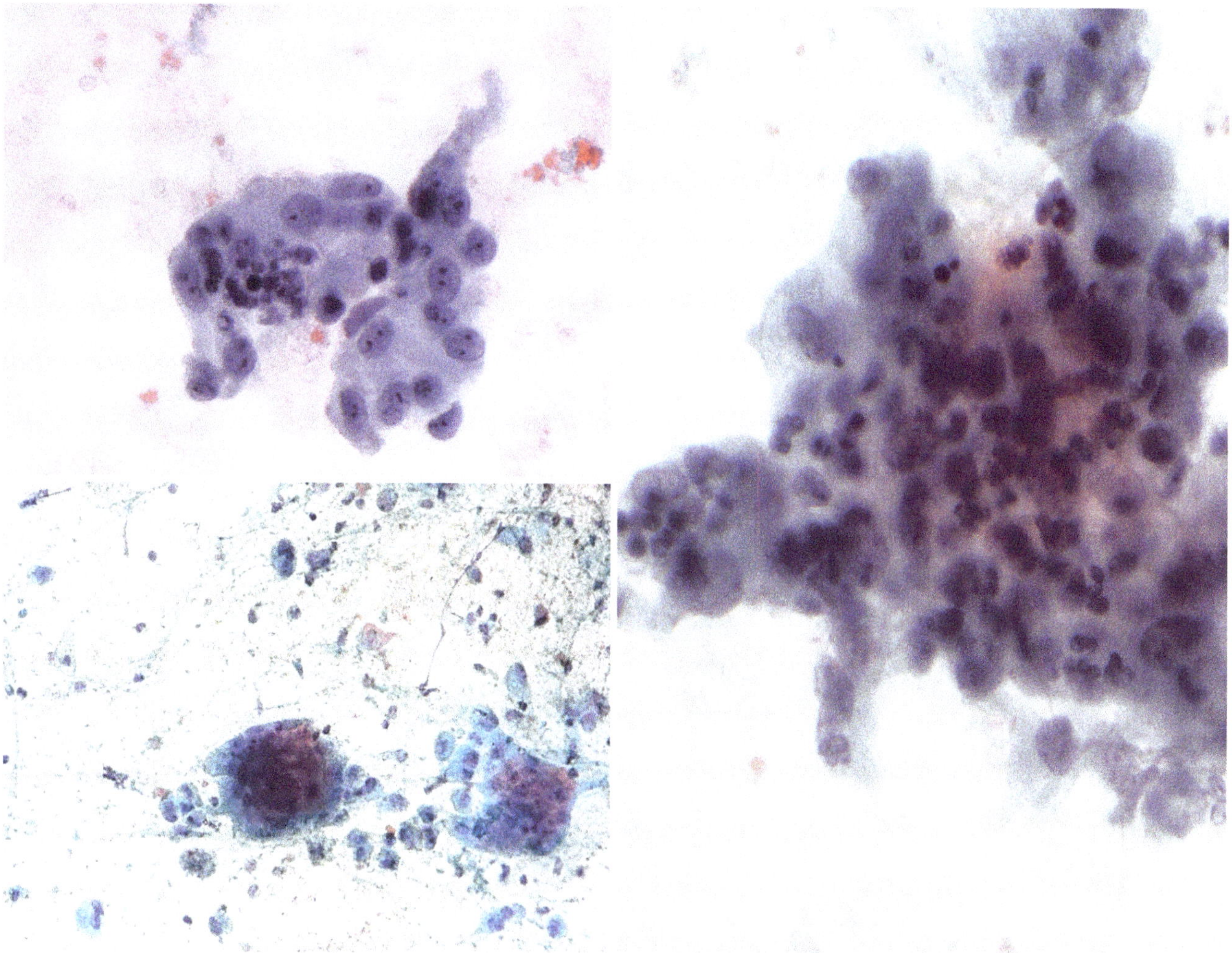

Fig. 10.11

Q-11. This aspirate is from a 40-year-old woman who has noticed pain in the nipple of her left breast. There is a small painful nodule. On physical examination, a small tender mass, without hotness and redness, was identified. FNA was performed. The aspirate showed a creamy, thick secretion. Which of the following is the most likely diagnosis?

(a) Fibroadenoma
(b) Inflammatory carcinoma
(c) Plasma cell mastitis
(d) Granulomatous mastitis
(e) Lymphoma

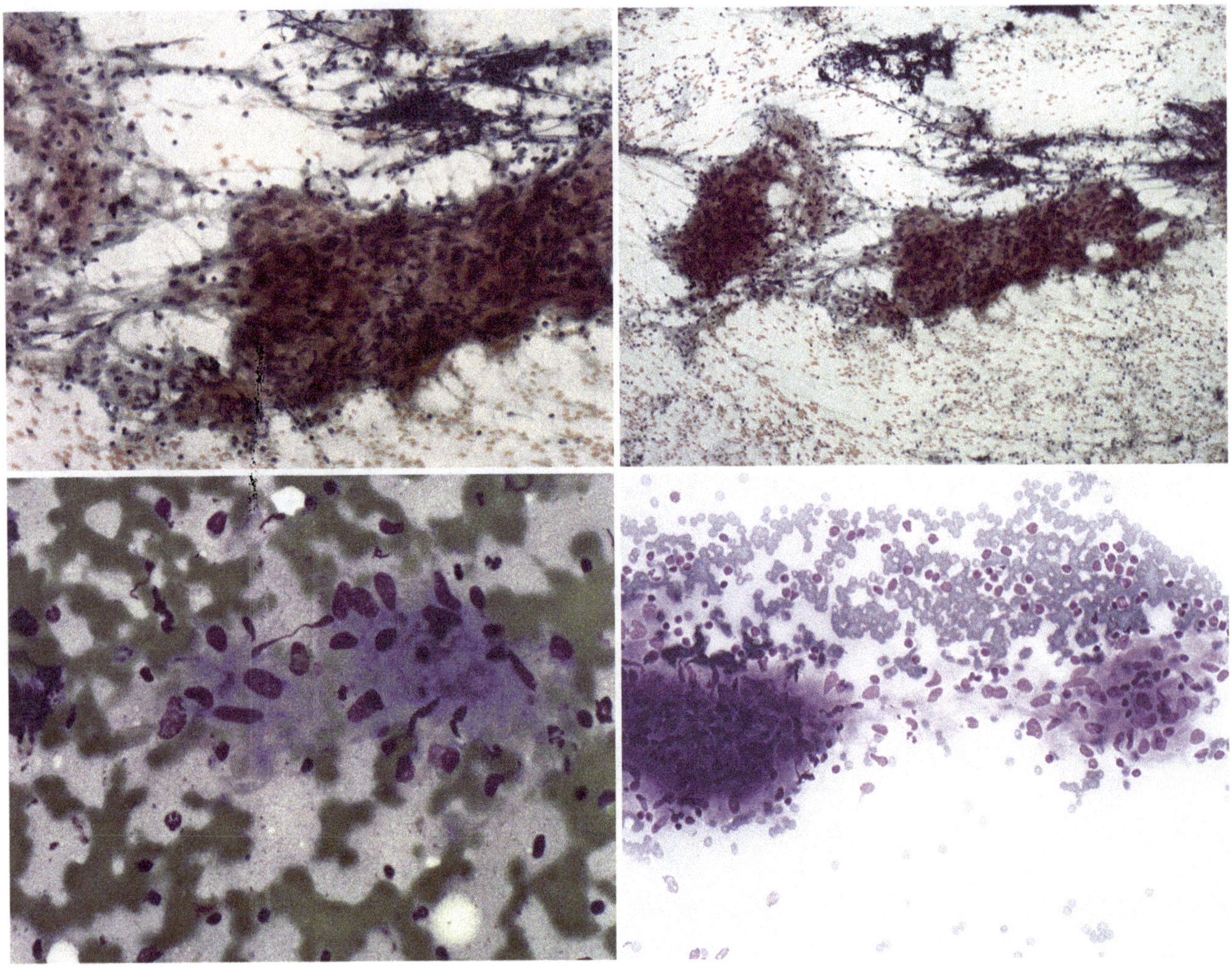

Fig. 10.12

Q-12. This aspirate is from a 45-year-old woman who has noticed pain in her left breast. On physical examination, a large vague tender mass was identified. Mammogram shows an ill-defined breast lesion with microcalcifications, indeterminate for malignancy. FNA was performed. Which of the following is the most likely diagnosis?

(a) Ductal carcinoma
(b) Fibroadenoma
(c) Benign breast cyst
(d) Granulomatous mastitis
(e) Intraductal papilloma

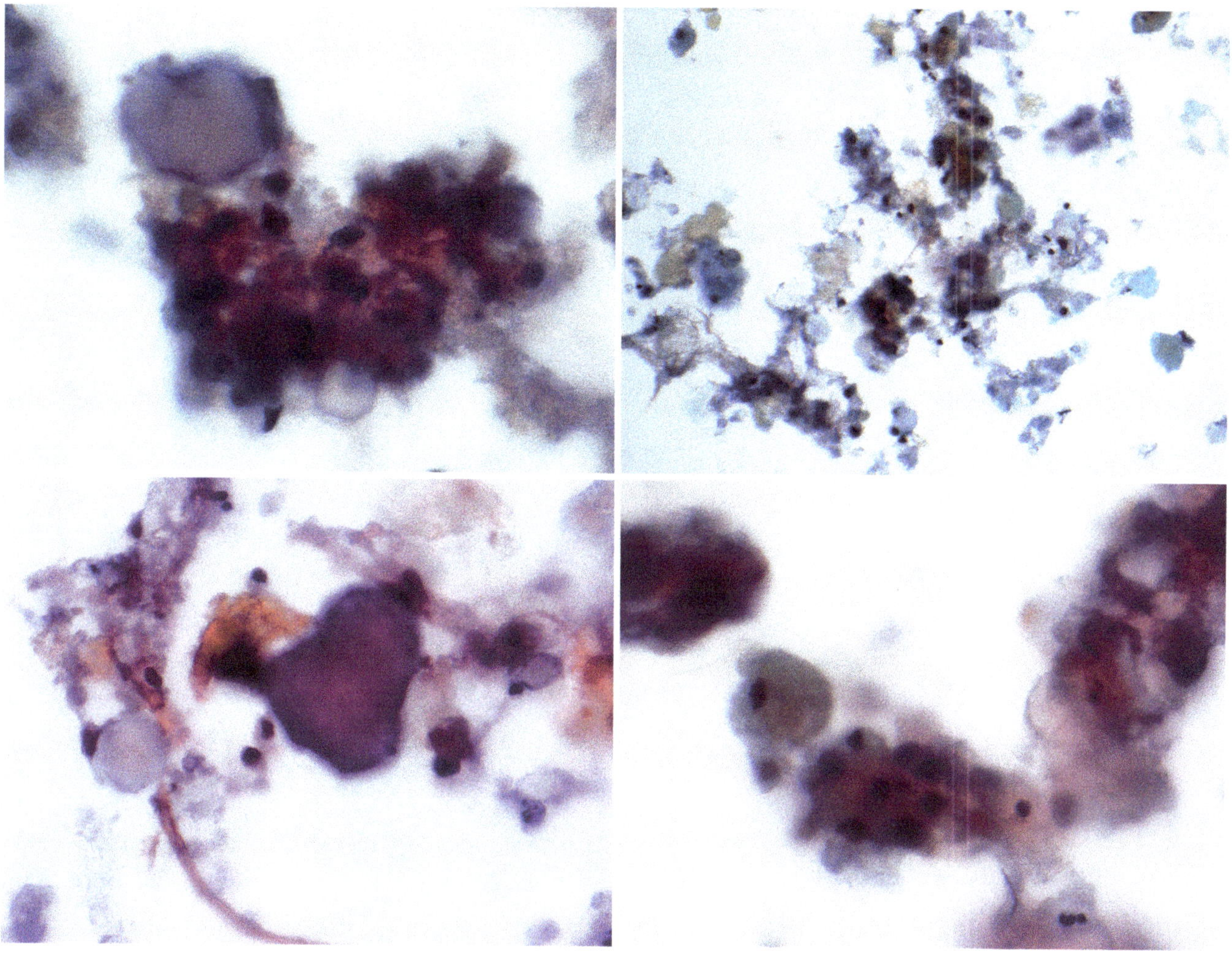

Fig. 10.13

Q-13. This aspirate is from a 45-year-old woman who has noticed pain in her left breast. The patient has a history of silicone implant. On physical examination, there are multiple vague tender nodules, without hotness or redness. Mammogram shows ill-defined breast lesions around the silicone implant with microcalcifications. FNA was performed. Which of the following is the most likely diagnosis?

(a) Ductal carcinoma
(b) Fibroadenoma
(c) Silicone granuloma
(d) Intraductal papilloma
(e) Acute mastitis

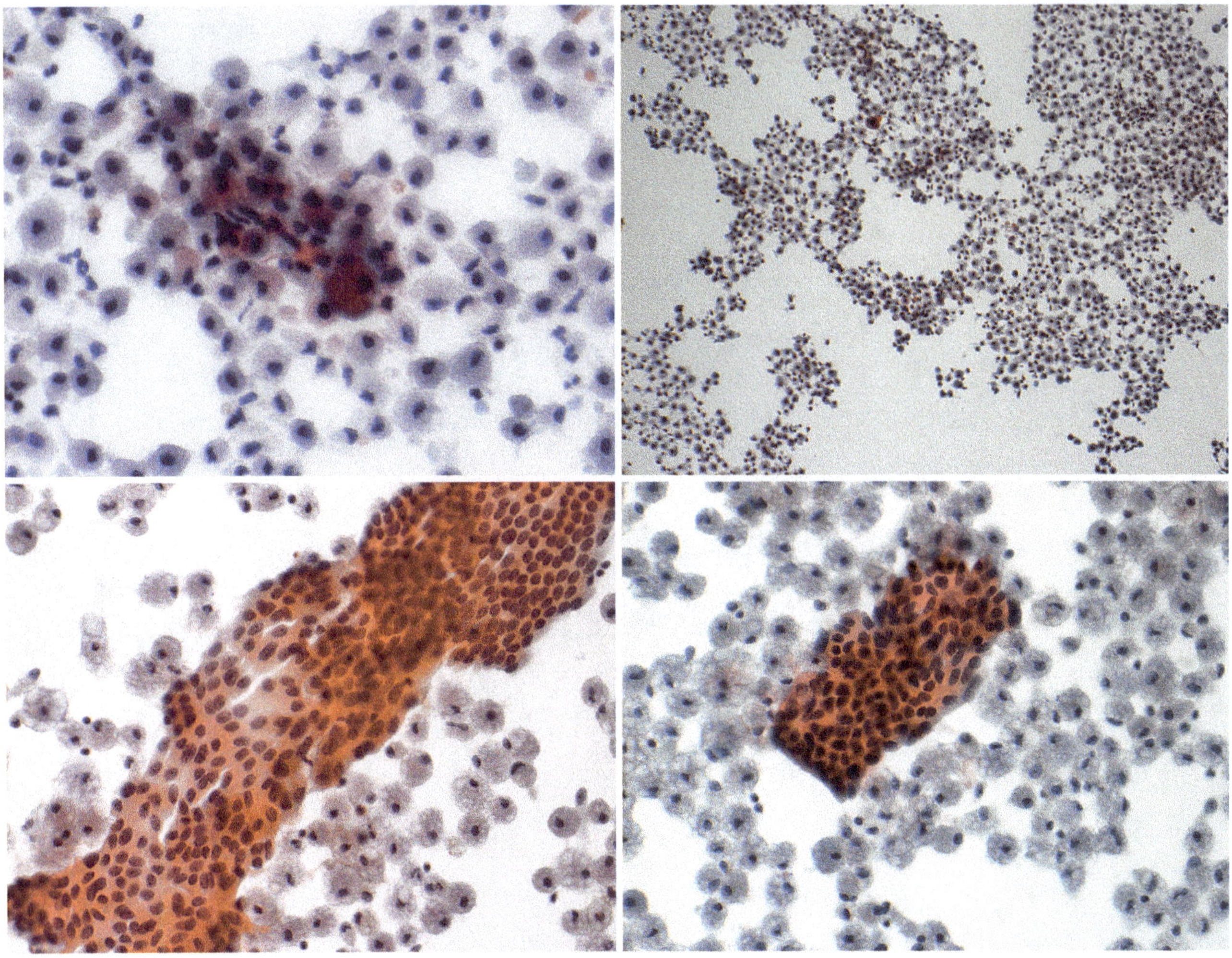

Fig. 10.14

Q-14. This aspirate is from a 40-year-old nulliparous woman who complains that her breasts are swollen and nodular upon palpation. Patient complains of an increase in the fullness and tenderness of her breast in the premenstrual period. A mammogram discloses benign changes with multiple cysts, ranging from 0.5 to 1.0 cm. No calcification was identified. FNA was performed to yield 3.0 mL of clear cyst fluid. What is the appropriate diagnosis?

(a) Ductal carcinoma
(b) Fibroadenoma
(c) Granulomatous mastitis
(d) Benign breast cyst
(e) Intraductal papilloma

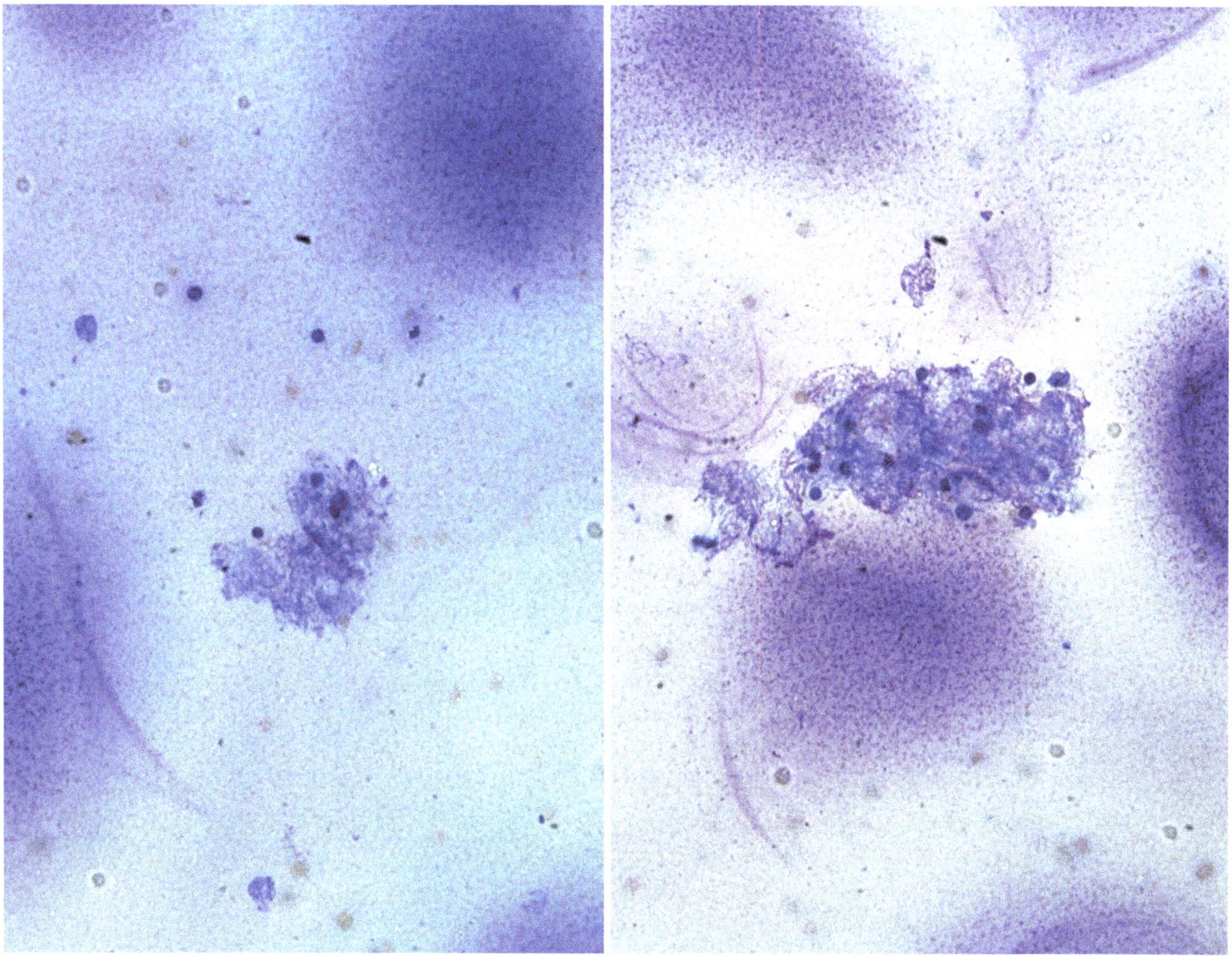

Fig. 10.15

Q-15. This aspirate is from a 50-year-old woman with a past history of breast cancer. Lumpectomy was performed and patient later developed a hard mass in the scar tissue area. Physical examination demonstrates a well-circumscribed, hard mass, measuring 1.5 cm and arising in the previous operation site. Patient has a history of breast radiation to the surgery bed. FNA was performed and yielded 10-mL clear fluid. The aspirate was centrifuged and smears were prepared. Which of the following is the most likely diagnosis?

(a) Ductal carcinoma
(b) Lobular carcinoma
(c) Fibrocystic changes
(d) Postsurgical seroma
(e) Fibroadenoma

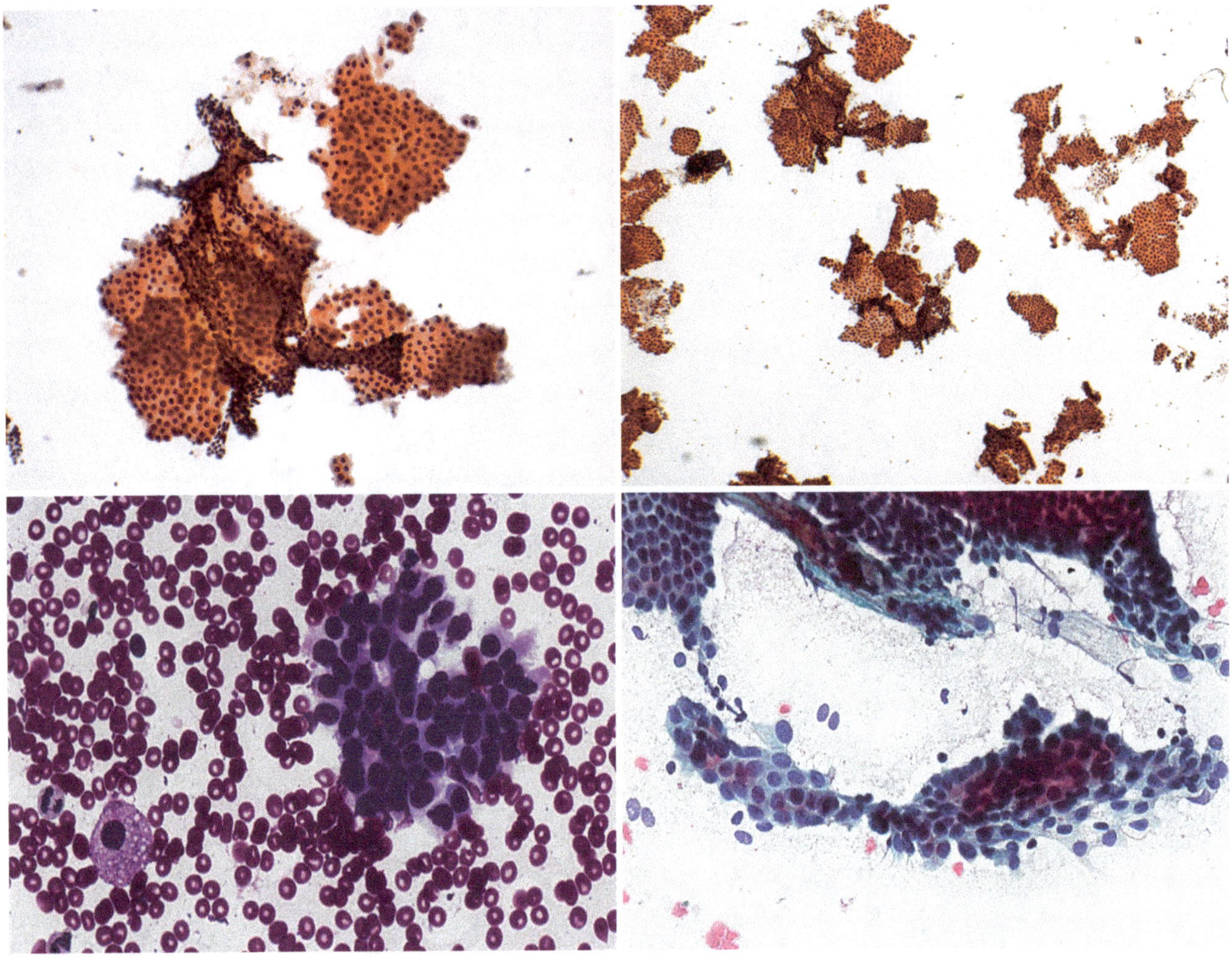

Fig. 10.16

Q-16. This aspirate is from a 35-year-old nulliparous woman who complains that her breasts are swollen and nodular upon palpation. The patient complains of an increase in the fullness and tenderness of her breasts in the premenstrual period. Physical examination shows bilateral nodularity but with no definitive breast mass. A mammogram discloses foci of calcifications in both breasts and was reported as benign. FNA was performed and smears were prepared. What is the most likely diagnosis?

(a) Ductal carcinoma in situ
(b) Fibroadenoma
(c) Granulomatous mastitis
(d) Intraductal papilloma
(e) Nonproliferative fibrocystic changes

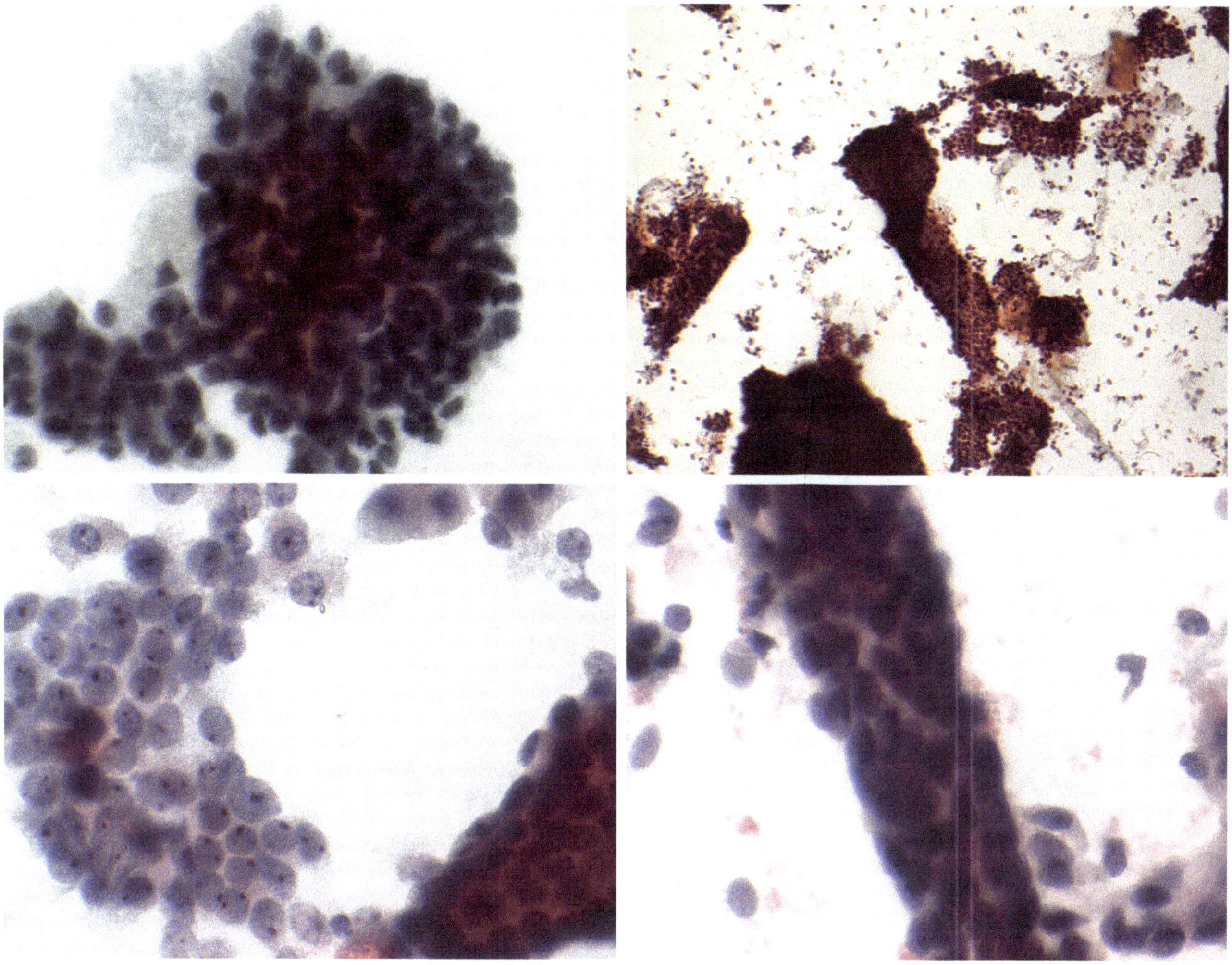

Fig. 10.17

Q-17. This aspirate is from a 45-year-old woman who has noticed several lumps in her right breast 2 months ago with some breast pain during the premenstrual period. A mammogram shows several foci of irregular density in both breasts; the densities measure from 0.5 to 1.0 cm in diameter, without calcifications. FNA of the most prominent lesion was performed. Which of the following is the most likely diagnosis?

(a) Infiltrating ductal carcinoma
(b) Phyllodes tumor
(c) Fibrocystic changes, proliferative type
(d) Fibroadenoma
(e) Fibrocystic changes, nonproliferative type

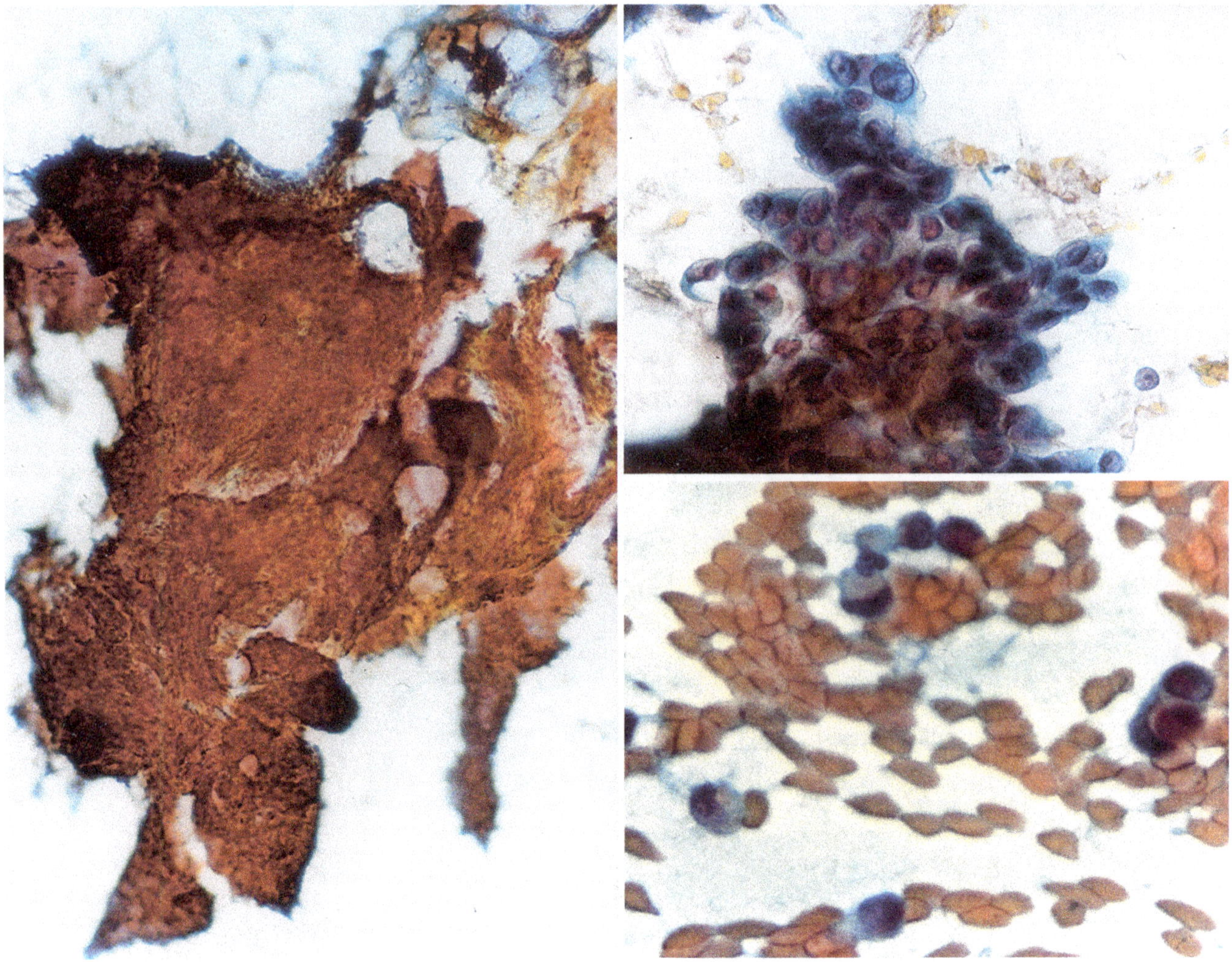

Fig. 10.18

Q-18. This aspirate is from a 35-year-old woman who discovered a lump in her left breast. Physical examination confirms a mass in the lower outer quadrant of the left breast. Mammography demonstrates an ill-defined, stellate lesion, measuring 1.5 cm. Needle aspiration reveals hypercellular smears with mild atypical cells with occasional cytoplasmic vacuoles. No individual cells with intact cytoplasm were identified. Which of the following is the most likely pathologic diagnosis?

(a) Ductal carcinoma
(b) Lactating adenoma
(c) Phyllodes tumor
(d) Galactocele
(e) Radial scar and complex sclerosing lesion

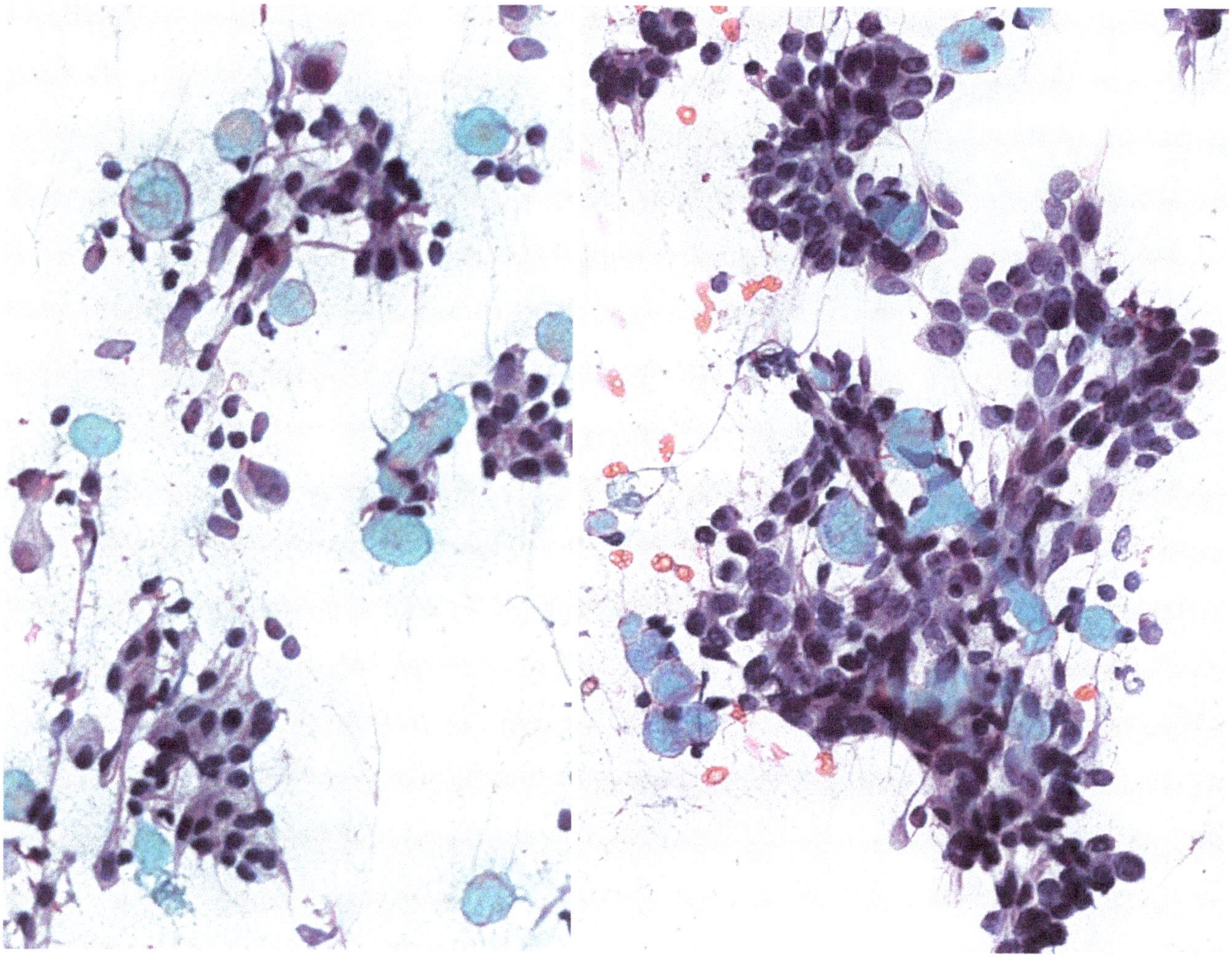

Fig. 10.19

Q-19. This aspirate is from a 52-year-old woman who noticed one lump in her right breast 2 weeks ago with breast tenderness and fullness in the premenstrual period. A mammogram shows several foci of irregular densities measuring 0.5–1.0 cm in diameter in both breasts. FNA was performed. Which of the following is the most likely diagnosis?

(a) Collagenous spherulosis
(b) Ductal carcinoma
(c) Adenoid cystic carcinoma
(d) Fibroadenoma
(e) Fibrocystic changes, nonproliferative

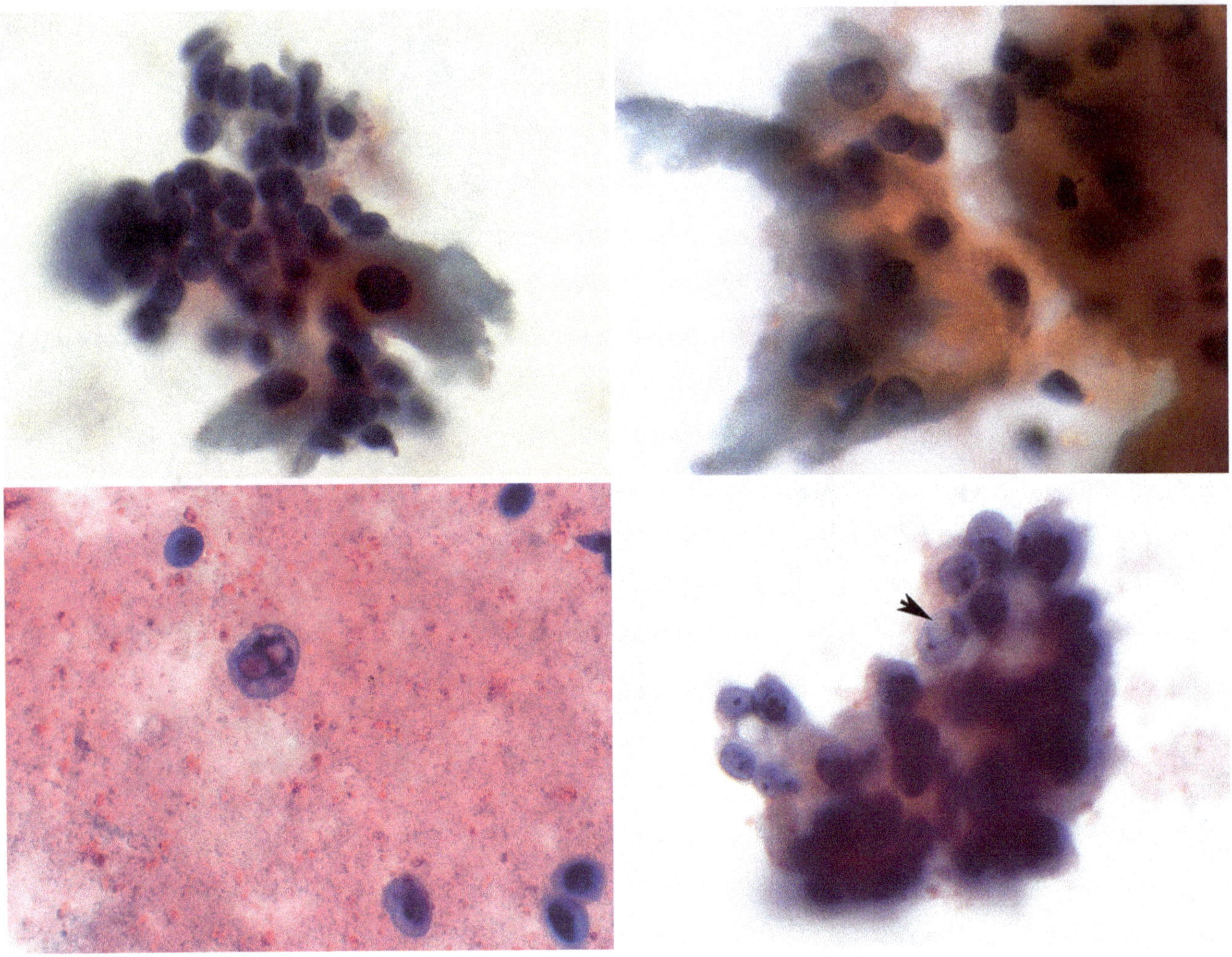

Fig. 10.20

Q-20. This aspirate is from a 36-year-old woman who presents with a breast mass that was detected on self-examination 2 weeks earlier. Mammography reveals a round, sharply demarcated 1.5-cm nodule in the right breast. The mammographic finding is consistent with benign breast lesion. FNA was performed. Which of the following is the most likely diagnosis?

(a) Adenomyoepithelioma
(b) Metastasis to regional lymph node
(c) Invasive ductal carcinoma
(d) Intraductal papilloma
(e) Phyllodes tumor

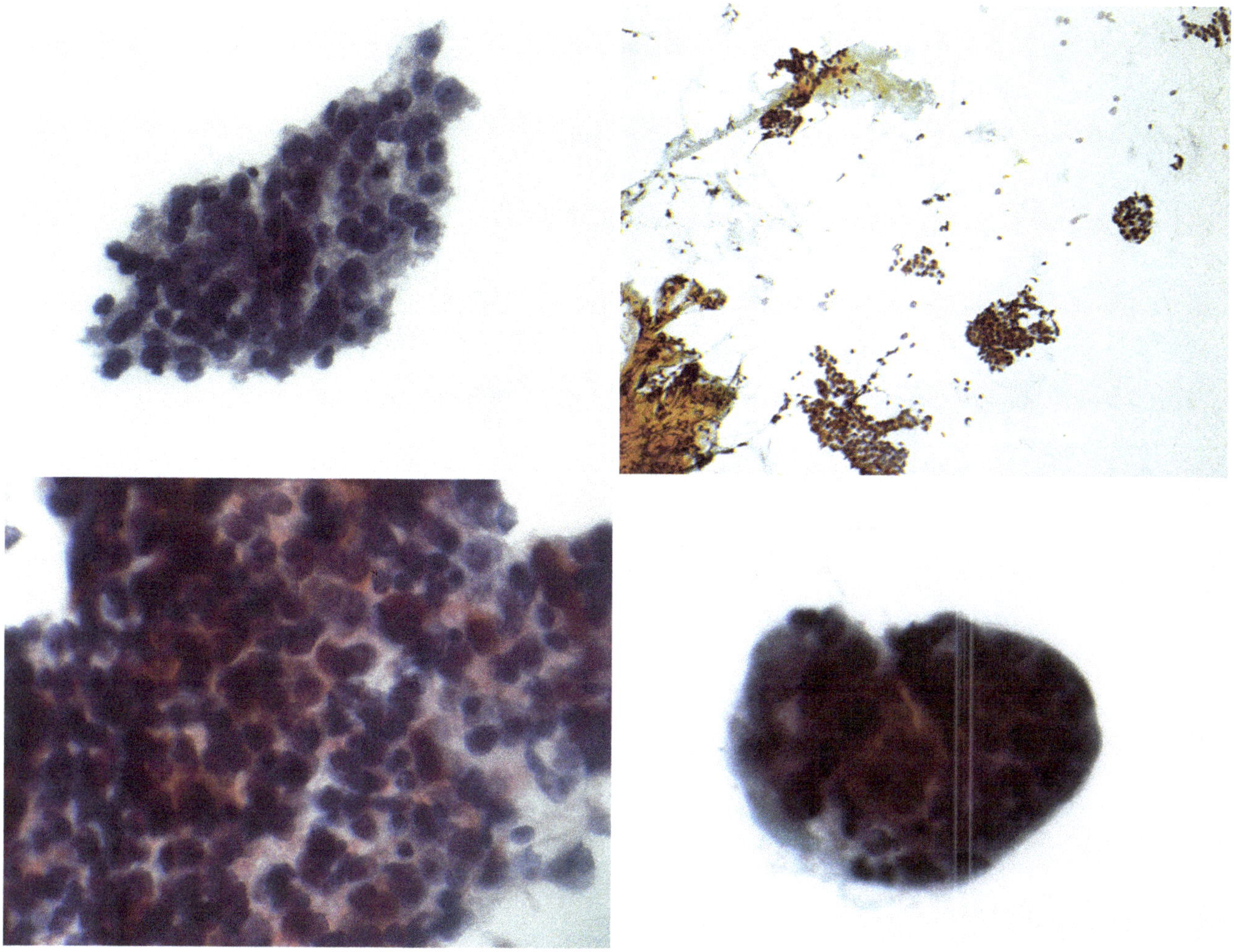

Fig. 10.21

Q-21. This aspirate is from a 52-year-old woman who comes for her routine mammogram. The mammogram demonstrates calcifications in her left breast. No axillary lymph node enlargement is detected on physical examination. Needle aspiration of the lesion was performed. Which of the following is the most likely diagnosis?

(a) Intraductal papilloma
(b) Phyllodes tumor
(c) Proliferative fibrocystic changes with atypia
(d) Fibroadenoma
(e) Fibrocystic changes, nonproliferative

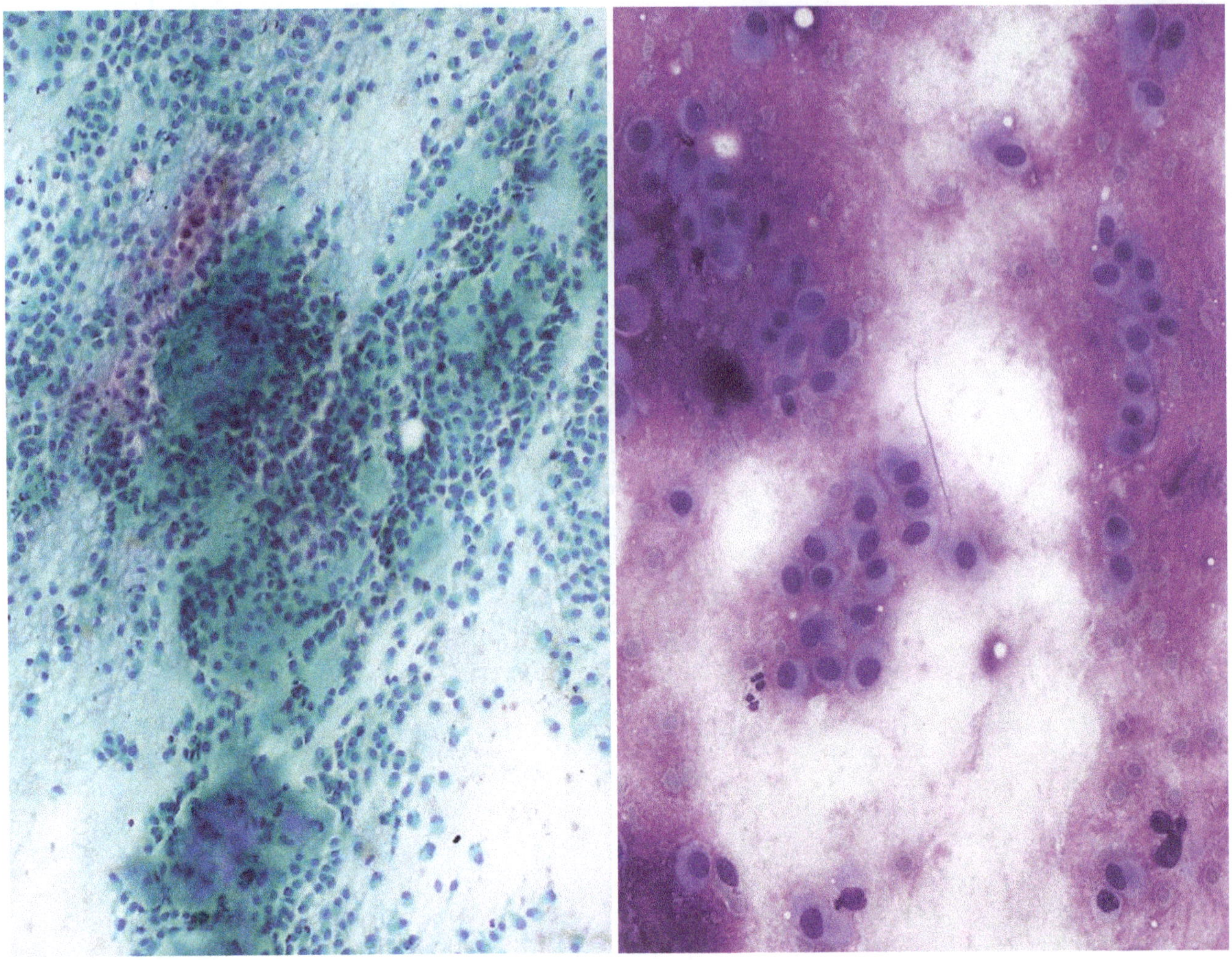

Fig. 10.22

Q-22. This aspirate is from a 35-year-old woman who presents with a breast mass that was detected on self-examination 4 weeks earlier. The lesion is slowly growing. Mammogram reveals a round, sharply demarcated 2-cm nodule in the left breast located under the skin. The mammographic finding is consistent with benign breast lesion. FNA was performed. Which of the following is the most likely diagnosis?

(a) Adenomyoepithelioma
(b) Metastasis to regional lymph node
(c) Invasive ductal carcinoma
(d) Intraductal papilloma
(e) Pleomorphic adenoma

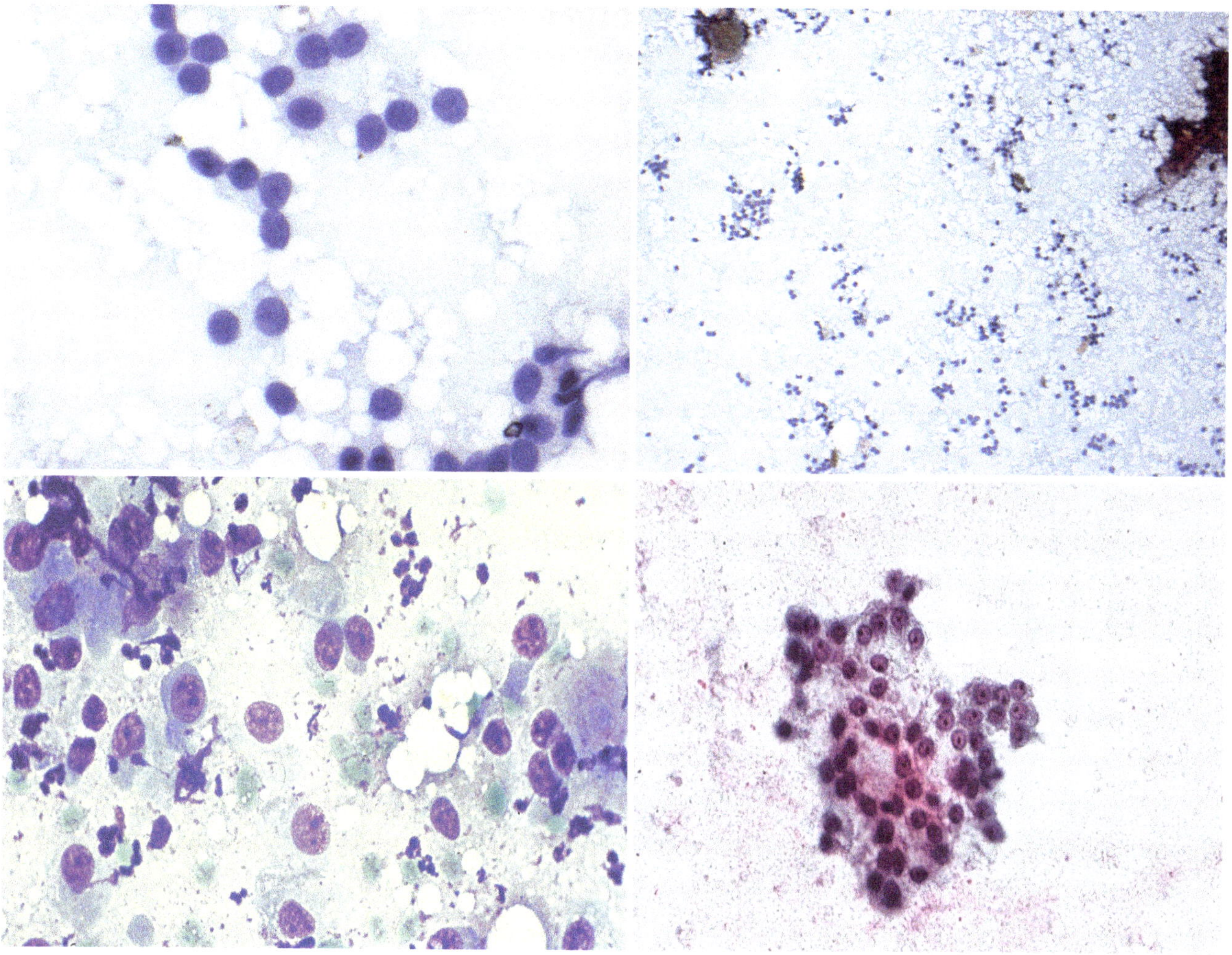

Fig. 10.23

Q-23. This aspirate is from a 24-year-old woman who noticed a breast lump in the upper inner quadrant of her left breast 1 month after giving birth to a normal full-term infant. She is breast-feeding without any significant history. On physical examination, the lump is well circumscribed and movable. The nipple shows a few fissures in the skin around the nipple. Mammogram shows a well-defined mass and reported as benign breast lesion, favor fibroadenoma. FNA was performed. What is the mostly likely diagnosis?

(a) Inflammatory carcinoma
(b) Lactating adenoma
(c) Phyllodes tumor
(d) Galactocele
(e) Fibroadenoma with lactating changes

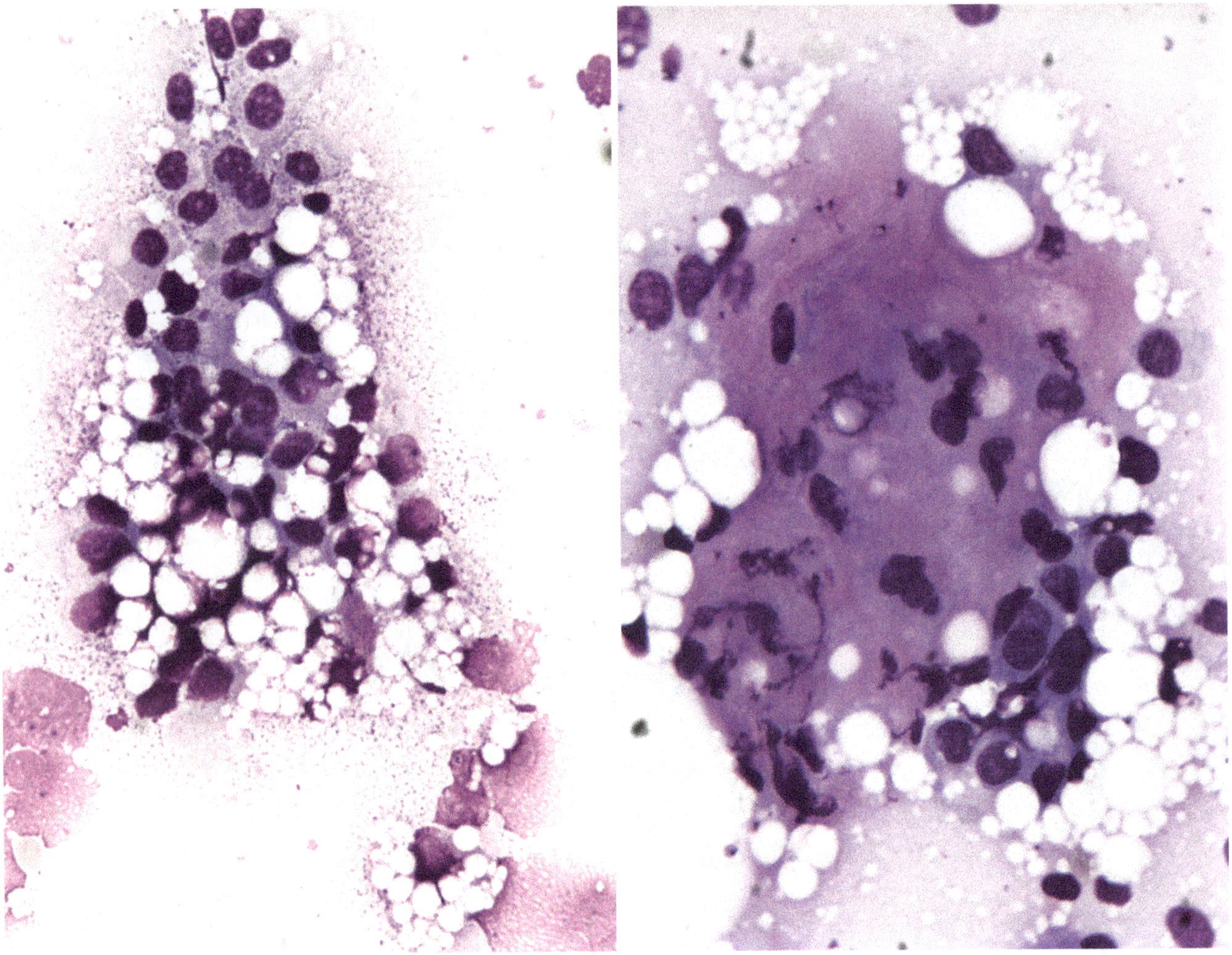

Fig. 10.24

Q-24. This aspirate is from a 24-year-old woman who noticed an increase in the size of a breast lump in the upper inner quadrant of her left breast during pregnancy. On physical examination, the lump is well circumscribed and movable. Previous mammogram shows a well-defined mass and was reported as benign breast lesion, favor fibroadenoma. FNA was performed. What is the most likely diagnosis?

(a) Inflammatory carcinoma
(b) Lactating adenoma
(c) Phyllodes tumor
(d) Galactocele
(e) Fibroadenoma with lactational changes

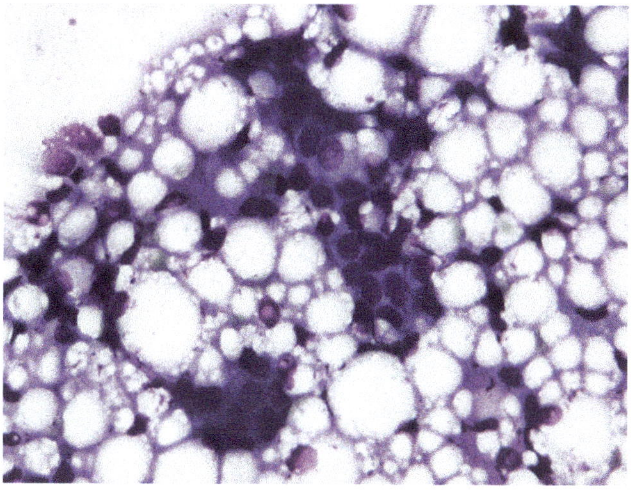

Fig. 10.25

Q-25. This aspirate is from a 26-year-old woman who noticed a breast lump in her left breast, 2 months after giving birth to a normal full term infant. She is breast-feeding without any significant history. On physical examination, the lump is well circumscribed and movable. The nipple shows a few fissures in the skin. The mammogram shows a well-defined mass and reported as benign breast cystic lesion. FNA was performed. What is the mostly likely your diagnosis?

(a) Inflammatory carcinoma
(b) Lactating adenoma
(c) Fibroadenoma
(d) Galactocele
(e) Paget's disease of the breast

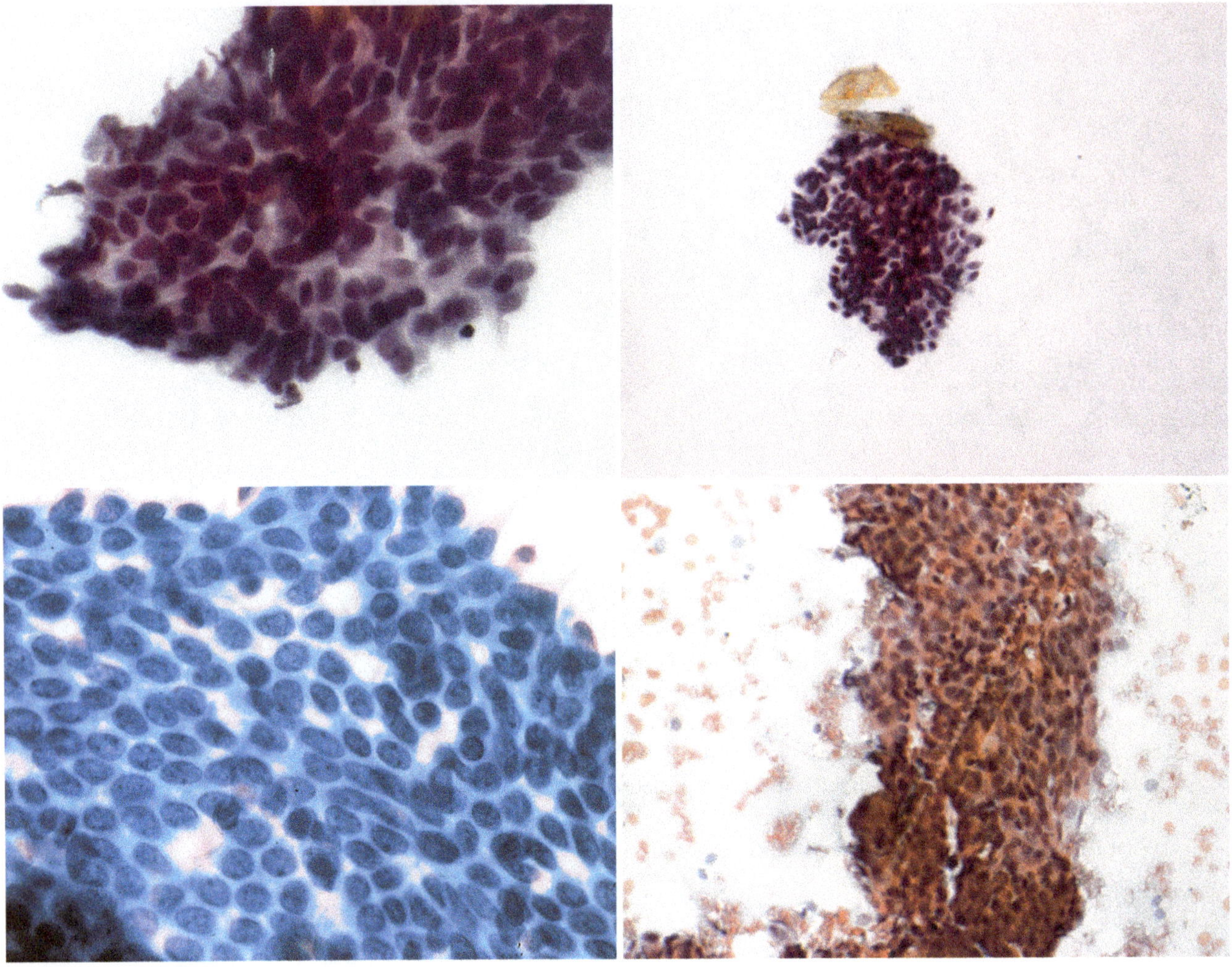

Fig. 10.26

Q-26. This aspirate is from a 17-year-old man who has developed bilateral breast enlargement over the past year. On physical examination, the enlargement is symmetric and is not painful to palpation. A vague left breast lump was identified. The patient is not obese and is not taking any medication. Which of the following is the most likely diagnosis?

(a) Fibroadenoma
(b) Phyllodes tumor
(c) Ductal carcinoma
(d) Gynecomastia
(e) Fat necrosis

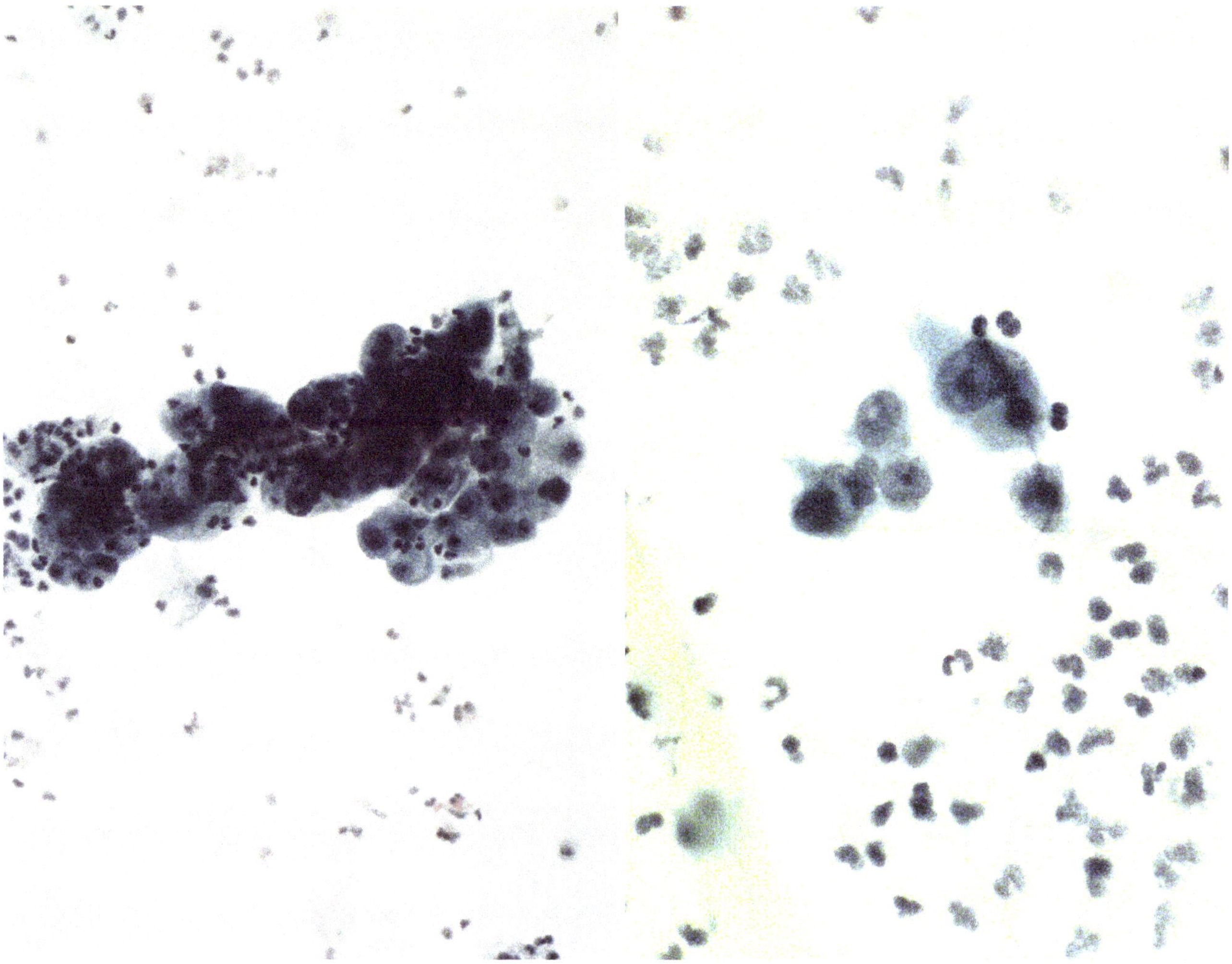

Fig. 10.27

Q-27. This aspirate is from a 45-year-old woman who has a past history of lumpectomy in her left breast. The pathologic examination of the lumpectomy specimen showed ductal carcinoma in situ with negative, but close resection margins. She received postoperative radiation in the lumpectomy bed. One month ago, she started to feel an ill-defined breast lesion at the lumpectomy site. FNA was performed. Which of the following is the most likely diagnosis?

(a) Recurrent ductal carcinoma in situ
(b) Radiation effect
(c) Invasive ductal carcinoma
(d) Fibrocystic changes
(e) Fibroepithelial lesion

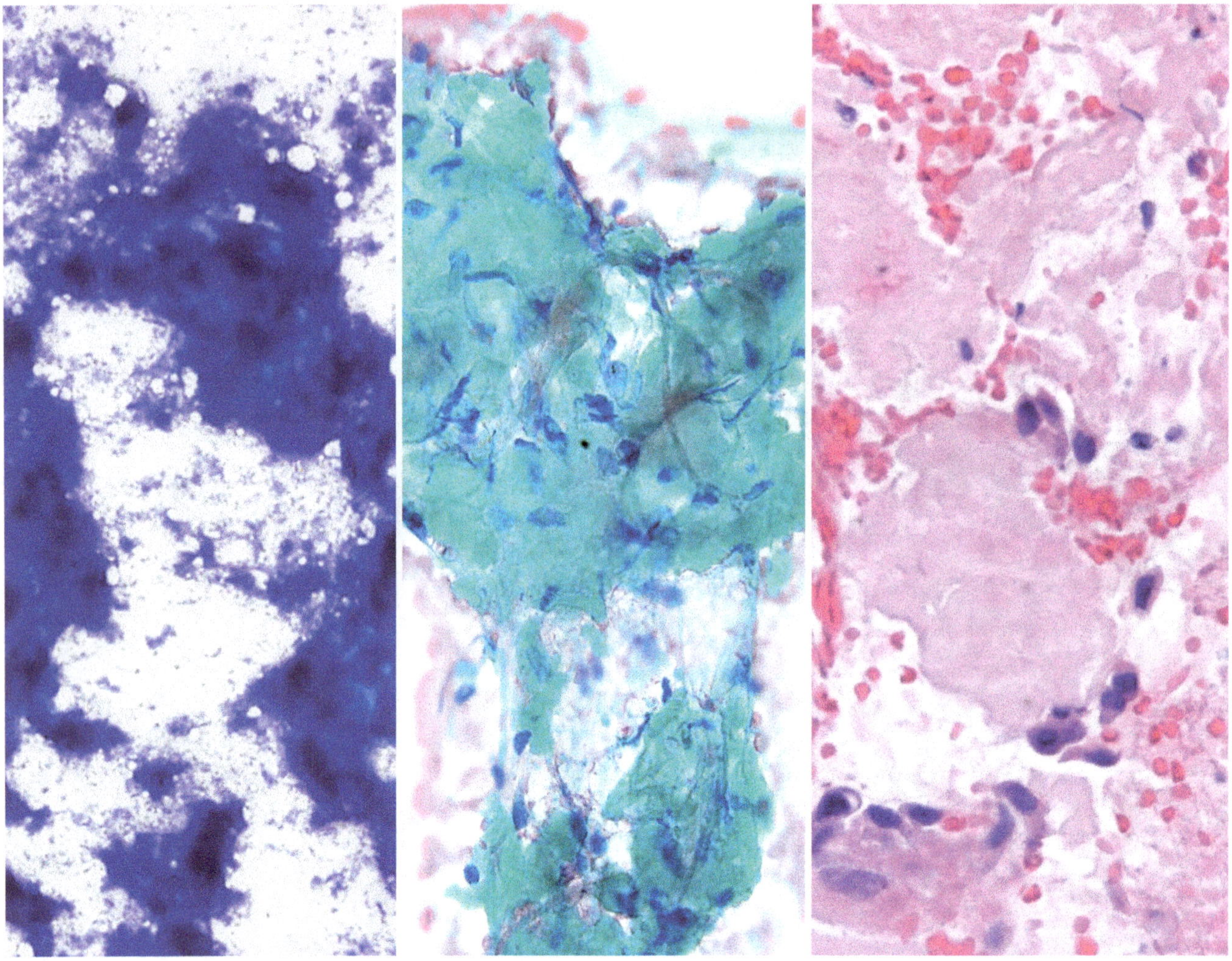

Fig. 10.28

Q-28. This aspirate is from a 54-year-old woman who presents with a breast mass in right side. Past history was unremarkable. Clinical examination shows a well-defined breast lesion, measuring 2.5 cm. Axillary lymph nodes are not clinically palpable. Mammogram is indeterminate. FNA was performed. Which of the following is the most likely interpretation?

(a) Invasive ductal carcinoma
(b) Plasmacytoma
(c) Invasive lobular carcinoma
(d) Amyloid tumor
(e) Papillary lesion

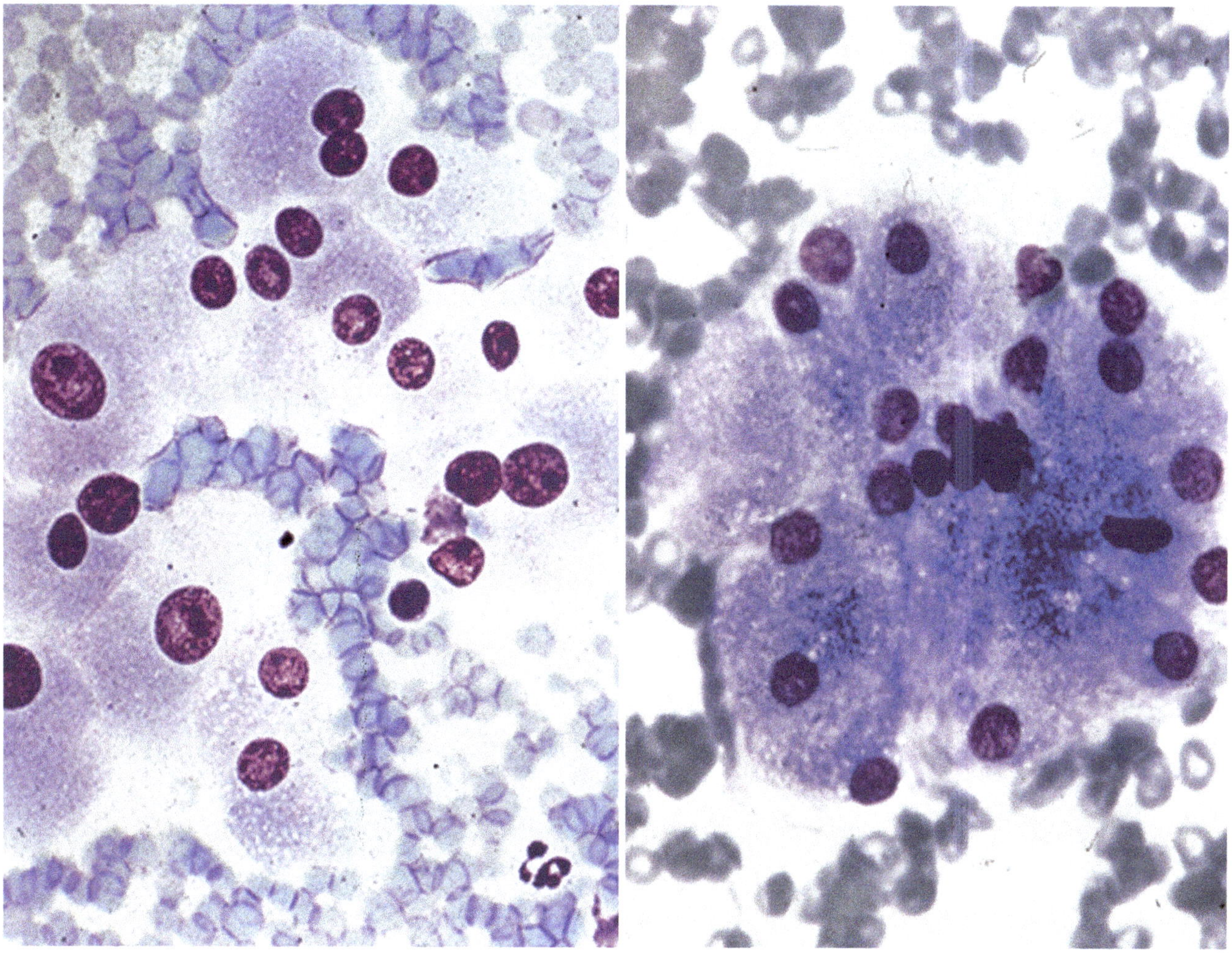

Fig. 10.29

Q-29. This aspirate is from a 43-year-old woman who presents with an ill-defined infiltrative mass. Mammogram demonstrates an infiltrating breast lesion with suspicious features of malignancy, located in the subcutaneous area of the breast. FNA was performed. Which of the following is the most likely diagnosis?

(a) Fibrocystic changes with apocrine metaplasia
(b) Phyllodes tumor
(c) Apocrine carcinoma
(d) Granular cell tumor of the breast
(e) Fat necrosis

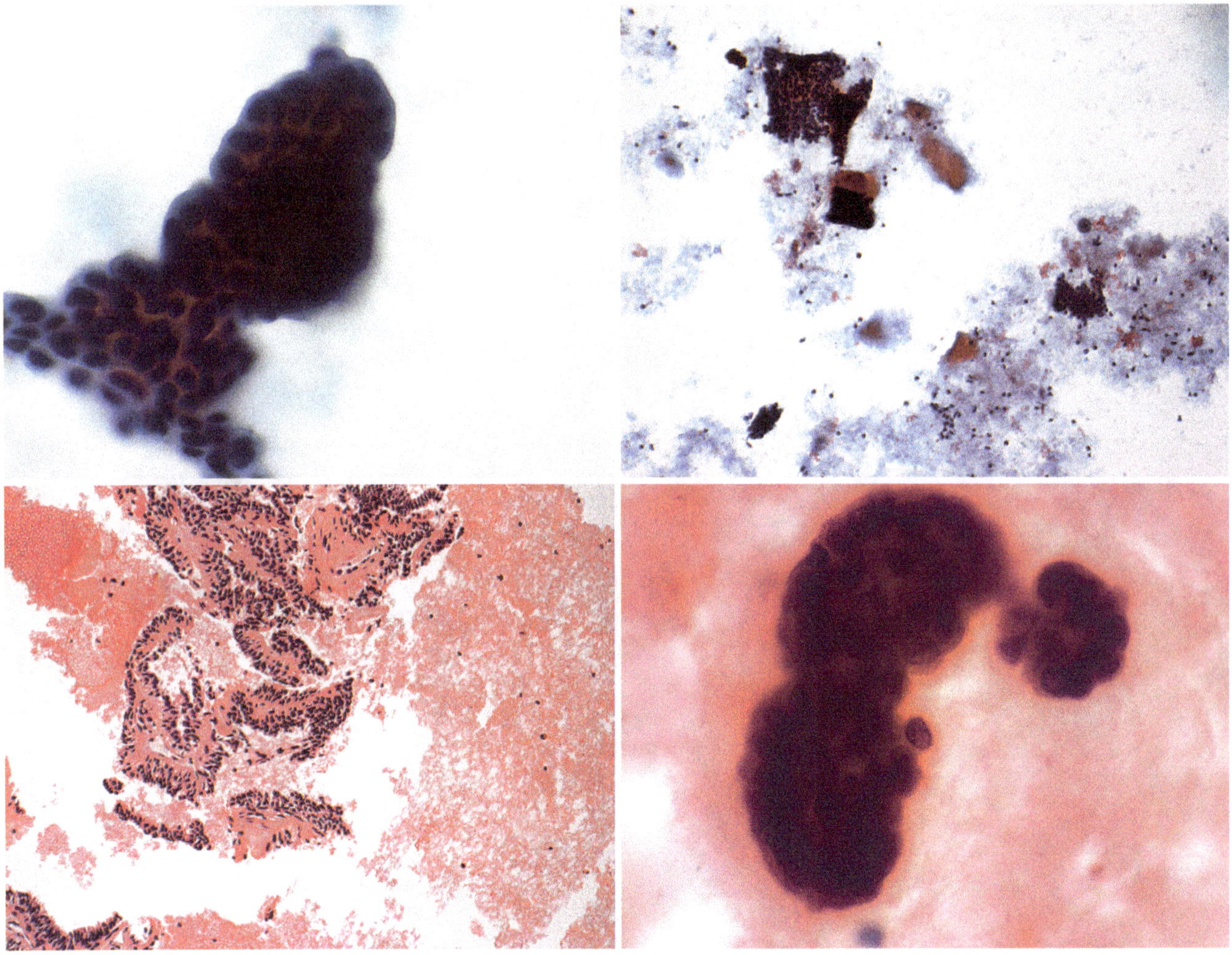

Fig. 10.30

Q-30. This aspirate is from a 34-year-old woman who has noticed a bloody discharge from the nipple associated with a small mass of her right breast for the past week. On physical examination, the skin is normal, and a small mass in the retro-areolar area is palpated. There is no axillary lymphadenopathy. The patient has regular menstrual cycles and is using oral contraceptives. There is scant nipple discharge history. FNA was performed. Which of the following is the most likely diagnosis?

(a) Ductal carcinoma
(b) Fat necrosis
(c) Fibrocystic changes
(d) Fibroadenoma
(e) Intraductal papilloma

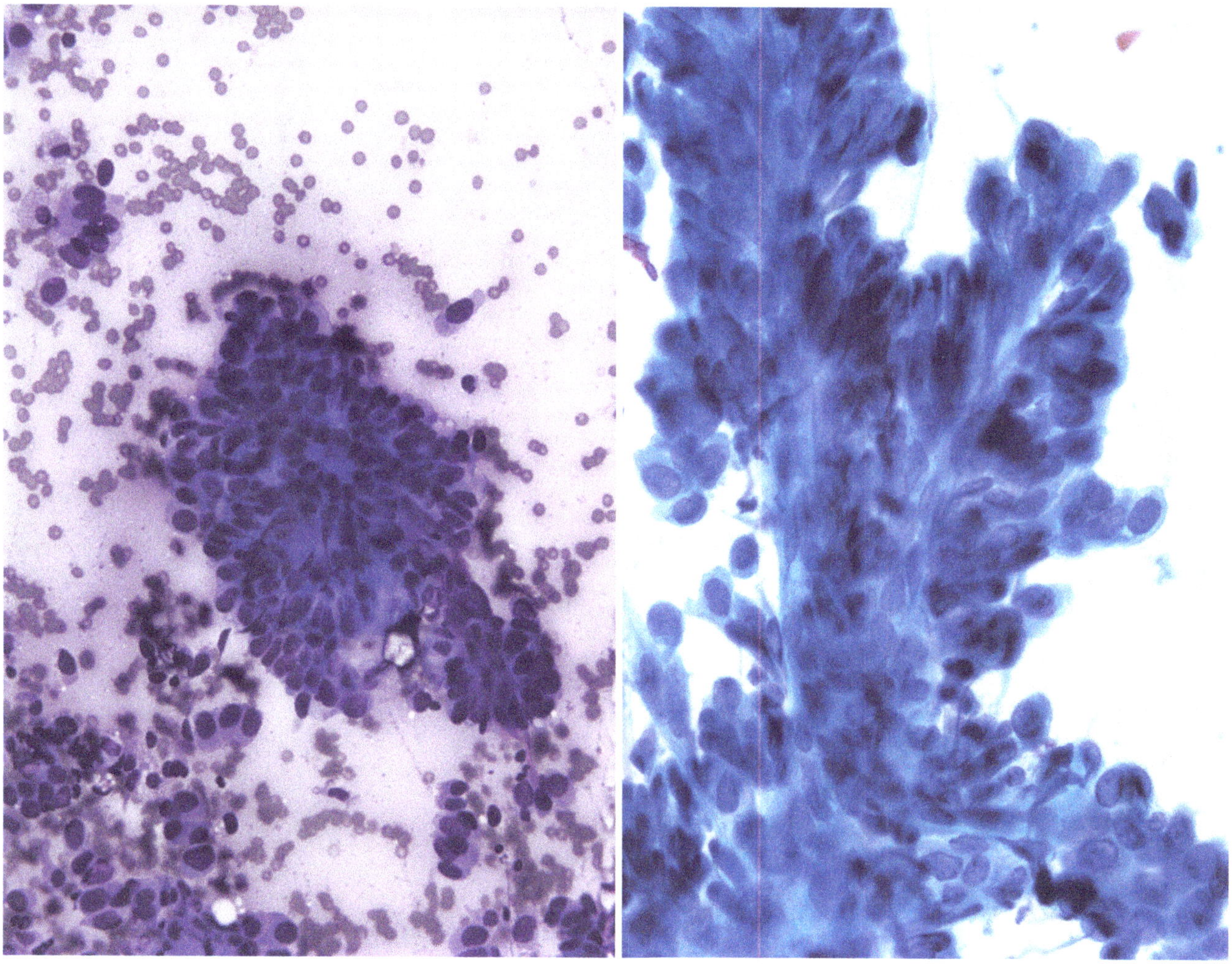

Fig. 10.31

Q-31. This aspirate is from a 54-year-old lady who has noticed a breast mass in the periareolar area of her right breast. On physical examination, a well-defined circumscribed subareolar mass was identified on palpation, with normal overlying skin. There is no axillary lymphadenopathy. FNA was performed. What is the most likely diagnosis of this lesion?

(a) Intraductal papilloma
(b) Fibrocystic changes
(c) Lobular carcinoma in situ
(d) Medullary carcinoma
(e) Papillary carcinoma

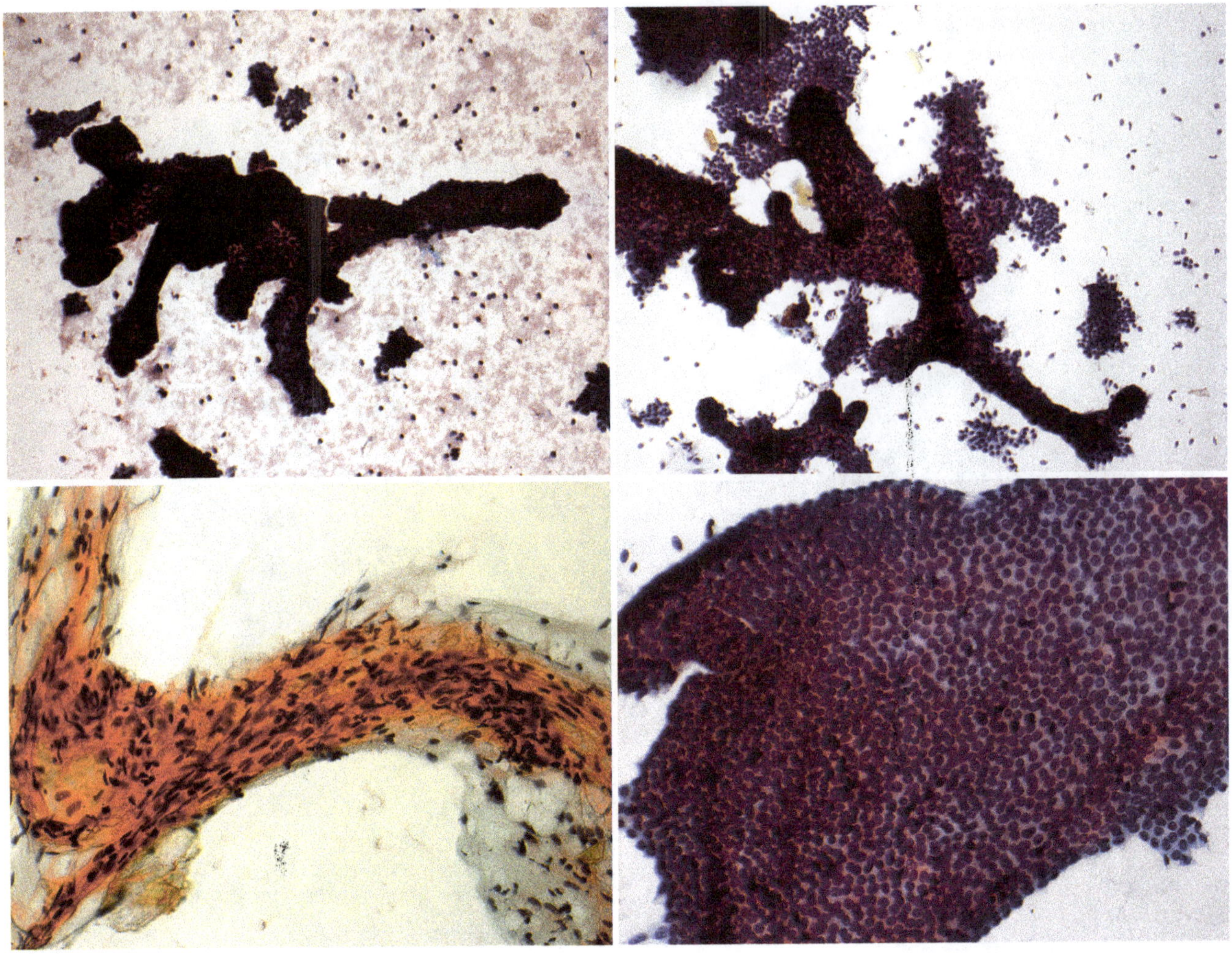

Fig. 10.32

Q-32. This aspirate is from a 20-year-old woman who visited her physician because of a lump in her left breast. On physical examination, there is a 3.0-cm firm, well-circumscribed mass in the lower outer quadrant of her left breast. Mammogram was performed and interpreted as BIRAD 2, consistent with benign breast lesion. To confirm this conclusion, the physician decides to perform FNA of the mass. Which of the following is the most likely diagnosis?

(a) Phyllodes tumor
(b) Fibrocystic changes
(c) Fat necrosis
(d) Fibroadenoma
(e) Infiltrating ductal carcinoma

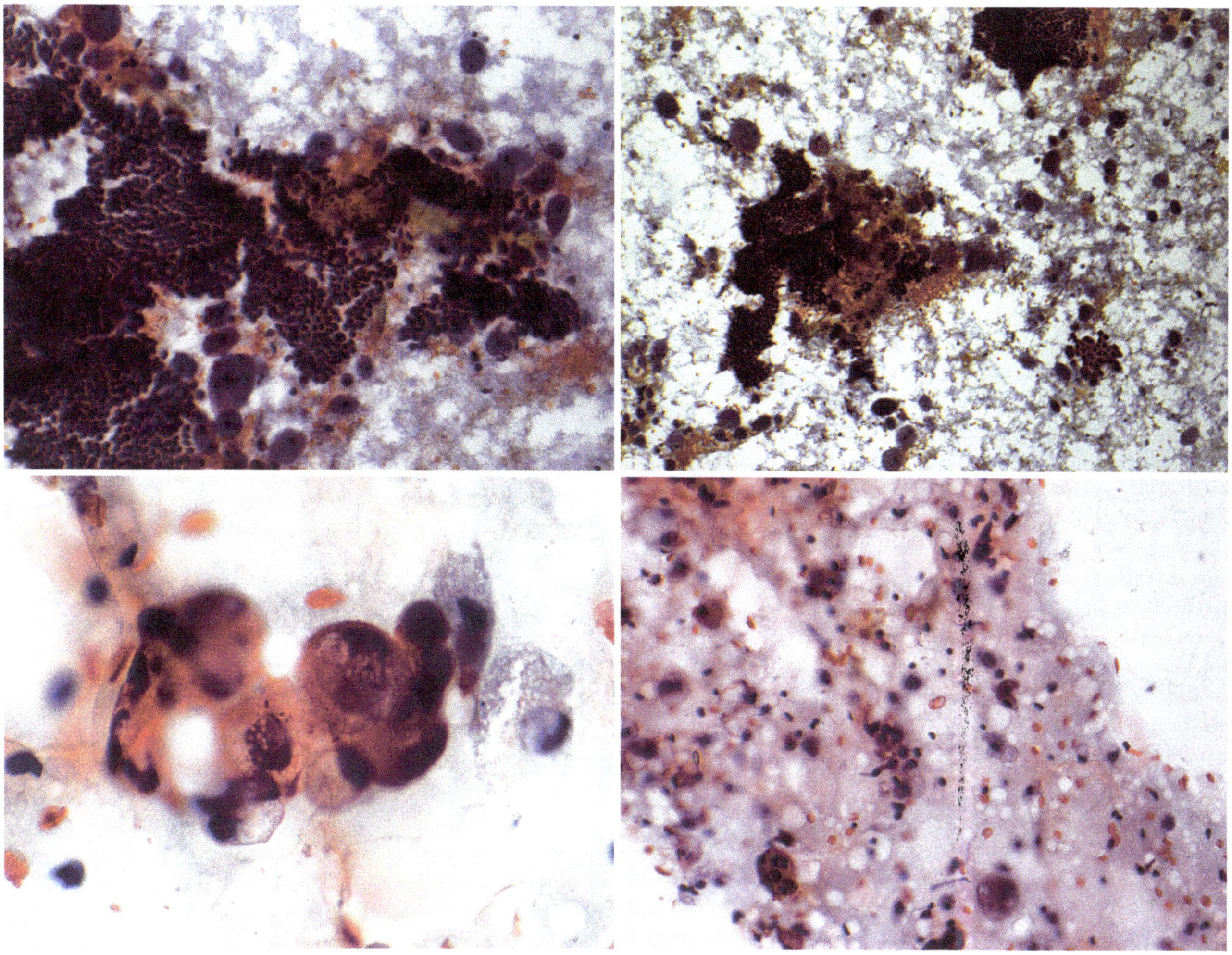

Fig. 10.33

Q-33. This aspirate is from a 37-year-old woman who presents with a lump in her right breast. On physical examination, a 3.0-cm, firm, circumscribed mass in the upper outer quadrant of her breast was identified. Mammogram was performed and interpreted as suspicious. To confirm this conclusion, the physician decides to perform FNA of the mass. Which of the following is the most likely diagnosis?

(a) Fibroadenoma
(b) Sarcoma
(c) Medullary carcinoma
(d) Fat necrosis
(e) Ductal carcinoma

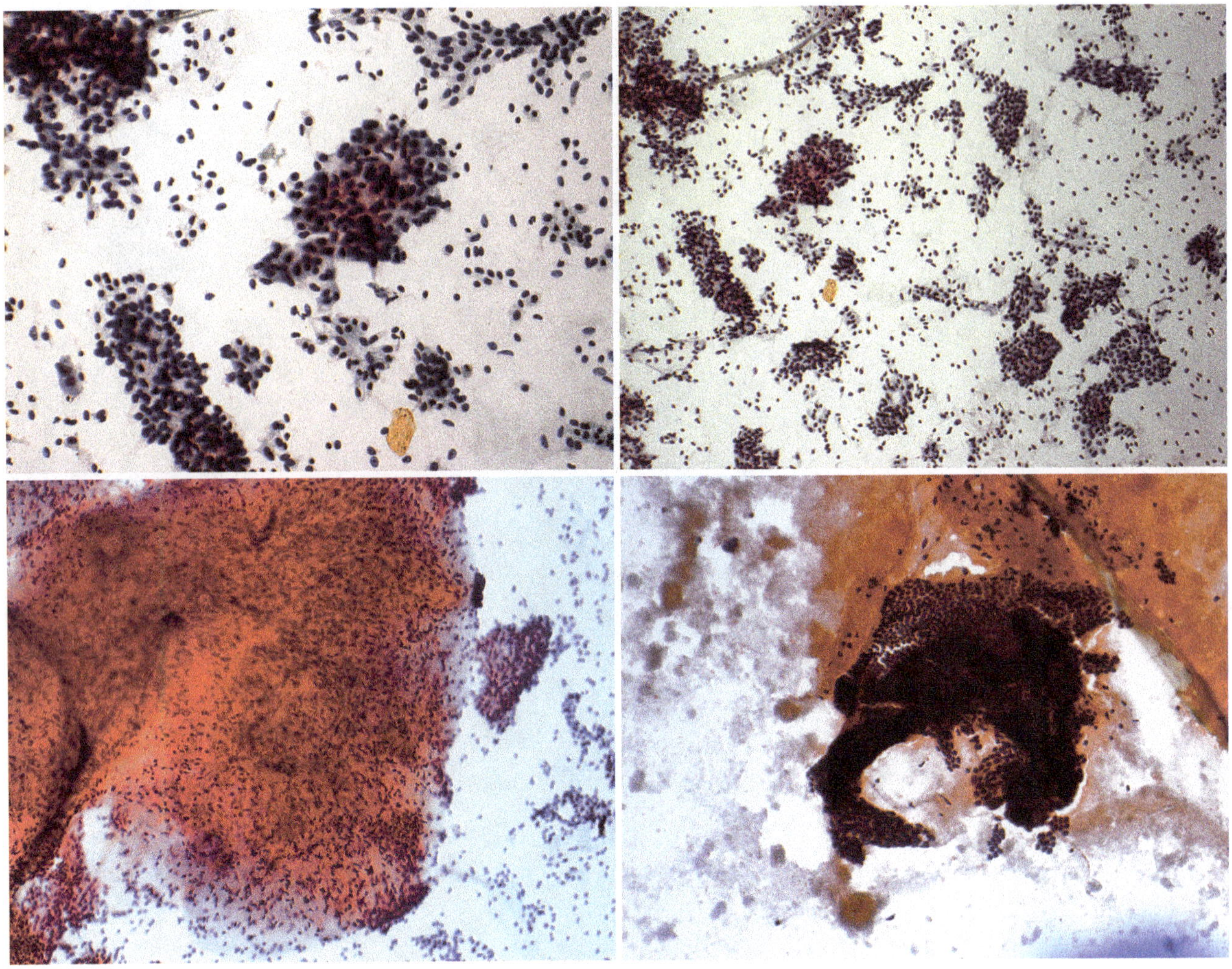

Fig. 10.34

Q-34. This aspirate is from a 50-year-old woman who presents with a painless mass in the lower outer quadrant of the right breast. The mass is slowly growing and has been present for the last 5 months. Recently, the mass is increasing in size, reaching 8.0 cm in greatest diameter. The mass appears to be sharply demarcated from the surrounding parenchyma and firm. A mammogram demonstrates a well-circumscribed, homogenous density. FNA was performed and is shown in these images. Which of the following is the most likely diagnosis?

(a) Phyllodes tumor
(b) Fibrocystic changes
(c) Fat necrosis
(d) Fibroadenoma
(e) Ductal carcinoma

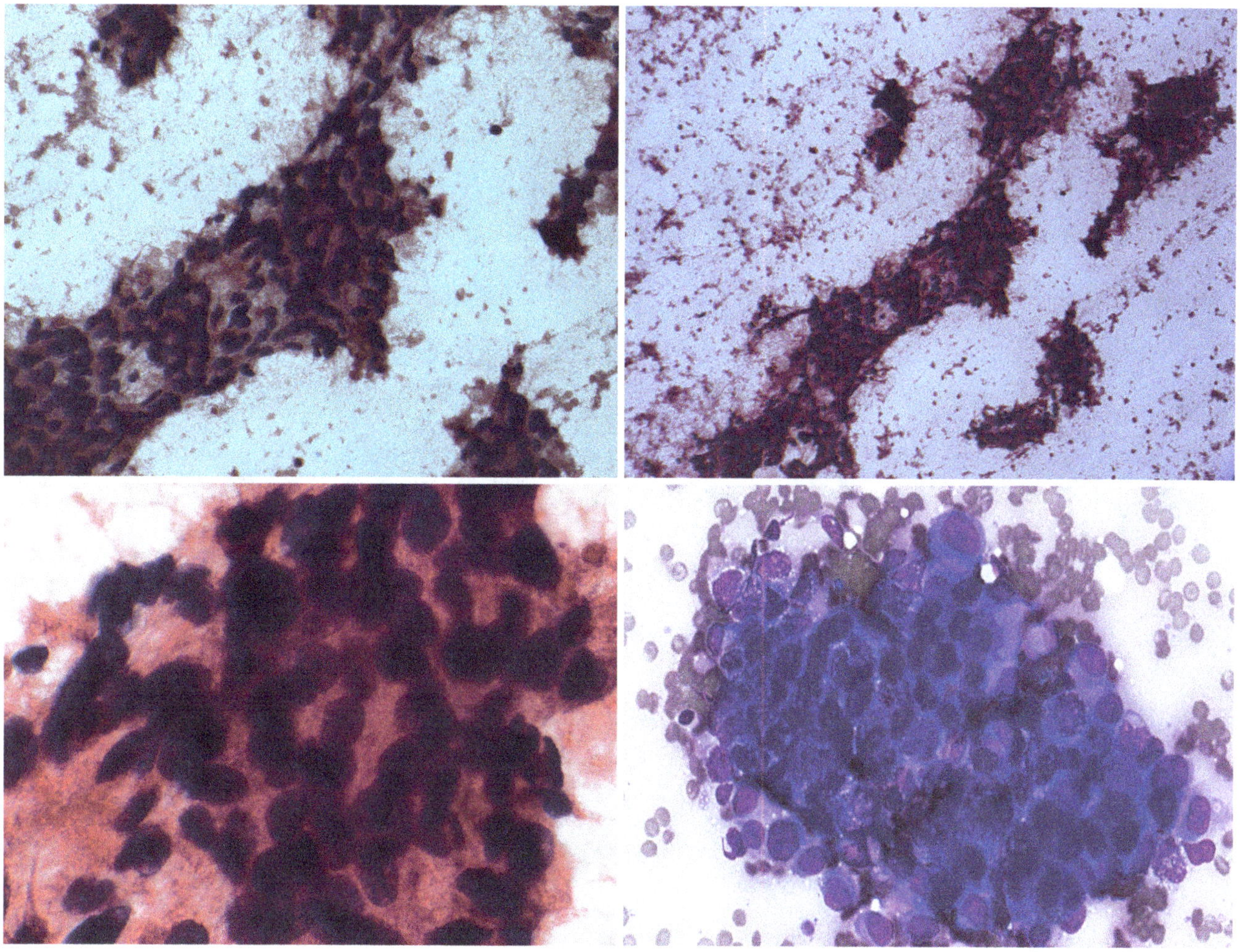

Fig. 10.35

Q-35. This aspirate is from a 55-year-old woman who discovers an ill-defined breast mass on self-examination. Mammogram demonstrates clusters of fine calcifications and the lesion was interpreted as suspicious for carcinoma (BIRADS 4). FNA was performed. Which of the following is the most likely diagnosis?

(a) Ductal carcinoma
(b) Lobular carcinoma
(c) Fibrocystic changes
(d) Fibroadenoma
(e) Chronic mastitis

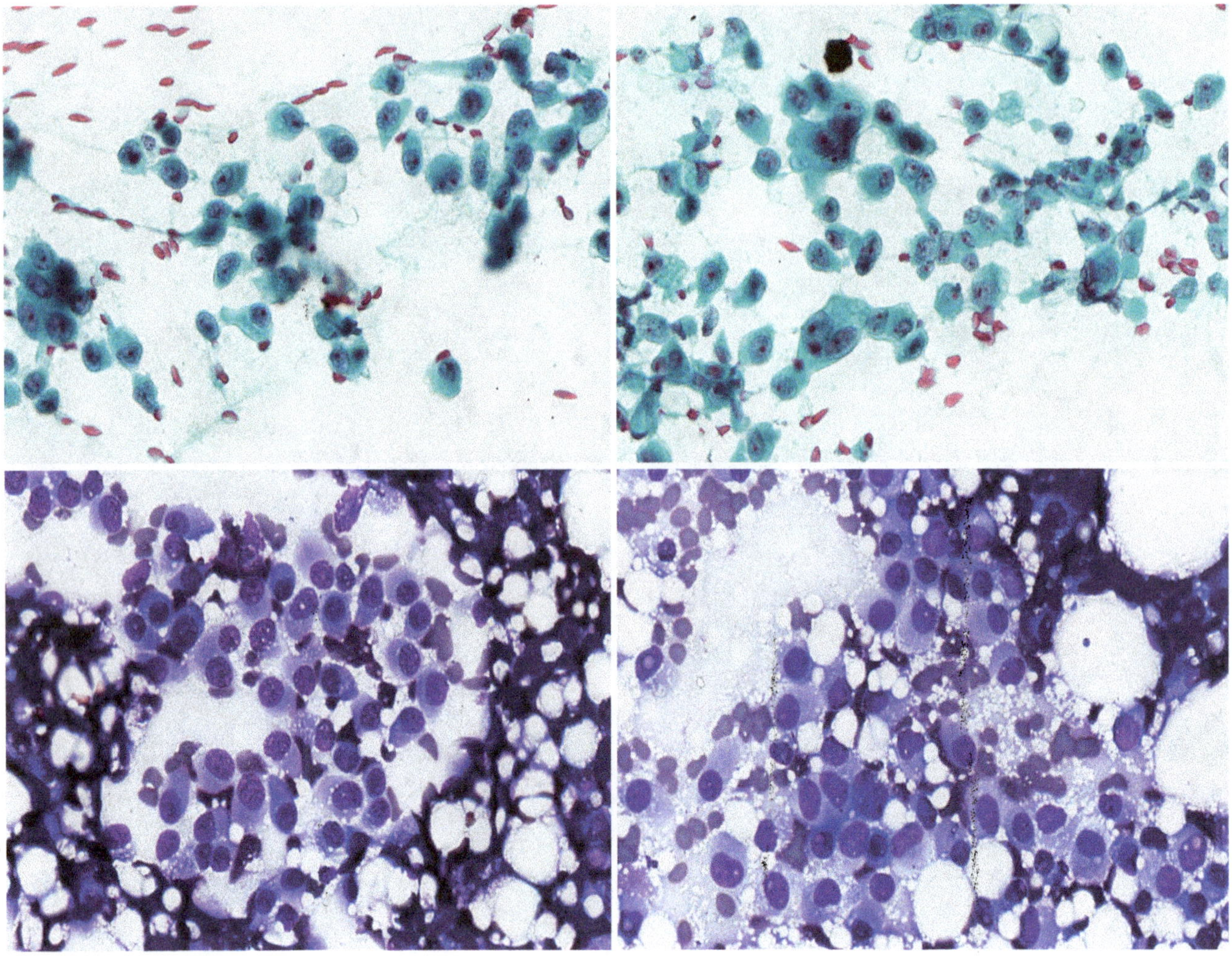

Fig. 10.36

Q-36. This aspirate is from a 48-year-old woman who sees her physician because she felt a lump in her right breast. On palpation, there is a firm, irregular lump in the lower outer quadrant of the right breast. There is overlying skin retraction. Mammogram shows a suspicious mass (BIRADS 4). There is no axillary lymphadenopathy. FNA was performed. Which of the following is the most likely diagnosis?

(a) Fat necrosis
(b) Ductal carcinoma
(c) Fibroadenoma
(d) Proliferative fibrocystic changes
(e) Chronic mastitis

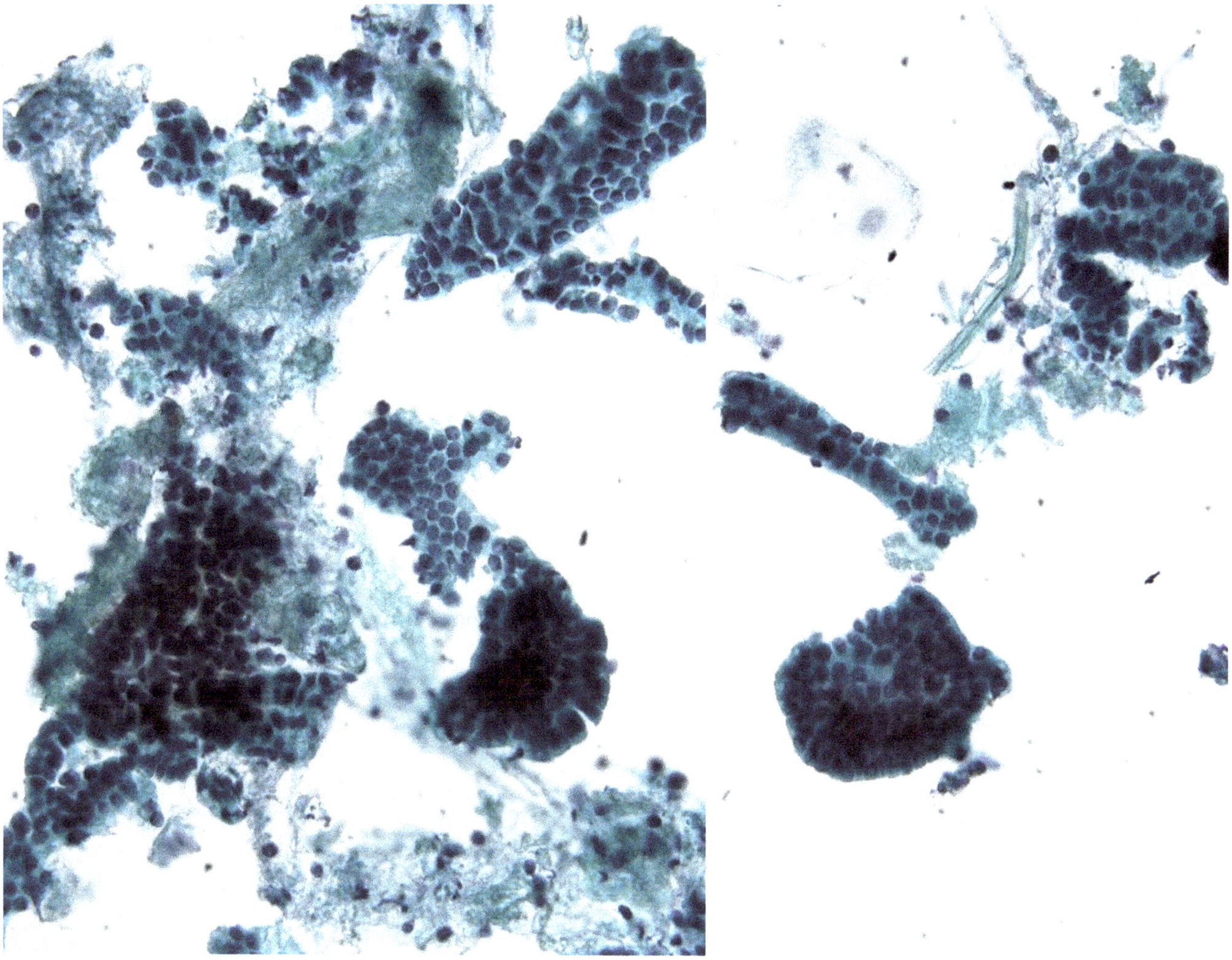

Fig. 10.37

Q-37. This aspirate is from a 48-year-old woman who sees her physician because she felt a lump in her right breast. On palpation, there is a small firm, irregular mass in the upper outer quadrant of the right breast. Mammogram shows a stellate lesion, measuring 1.5 cm. No skin retraction was identified. There is no axillary lymphadenopathy. FNA was performed. Which is the most likely diagnosis?

(a) Ductal carcinoma
(b) Fat necrosis
(c) Fibroadenoma
(d) Proliferative fibrocystic changes
(e) Tubular carcinoma

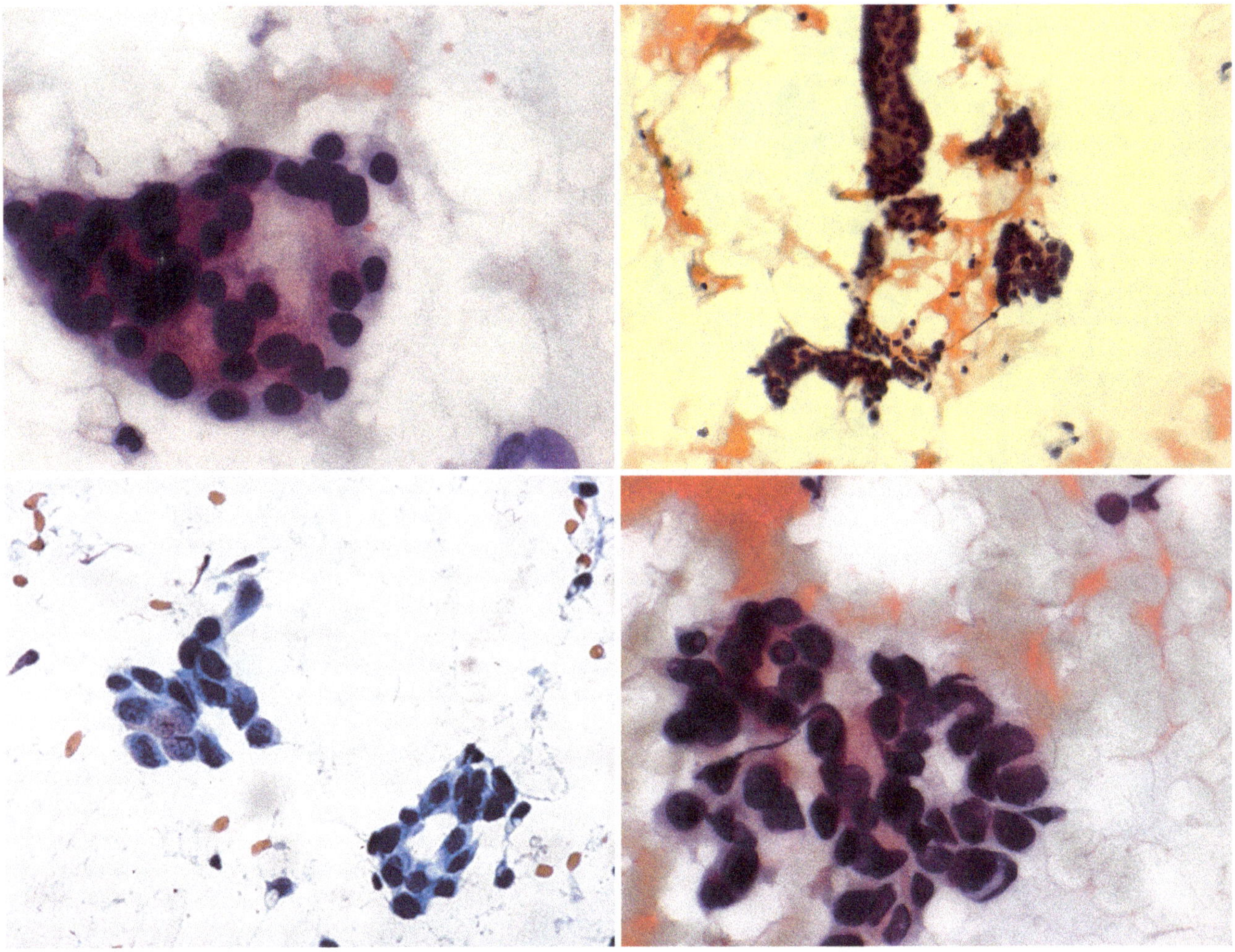

Fig. 10.38

Q-38. This aspirate is from a 52-year-old woman who presents with a 3-month history of an ill-defined breast mass. Physical examination demonstrates an area of firmness in the upper outer quadrant of the right breast. Mammogram shows a diffuse ill-defined mass, BIRADS 4. FNA was performed. Which of the following is the most likely diagnosis?

(a) Ductal carcinoma
(b) Invasive lobular carcinoma
(c) Proliferative fibrocystic changes
(d) Tubular carcinoma
(e) Fibroadenoma

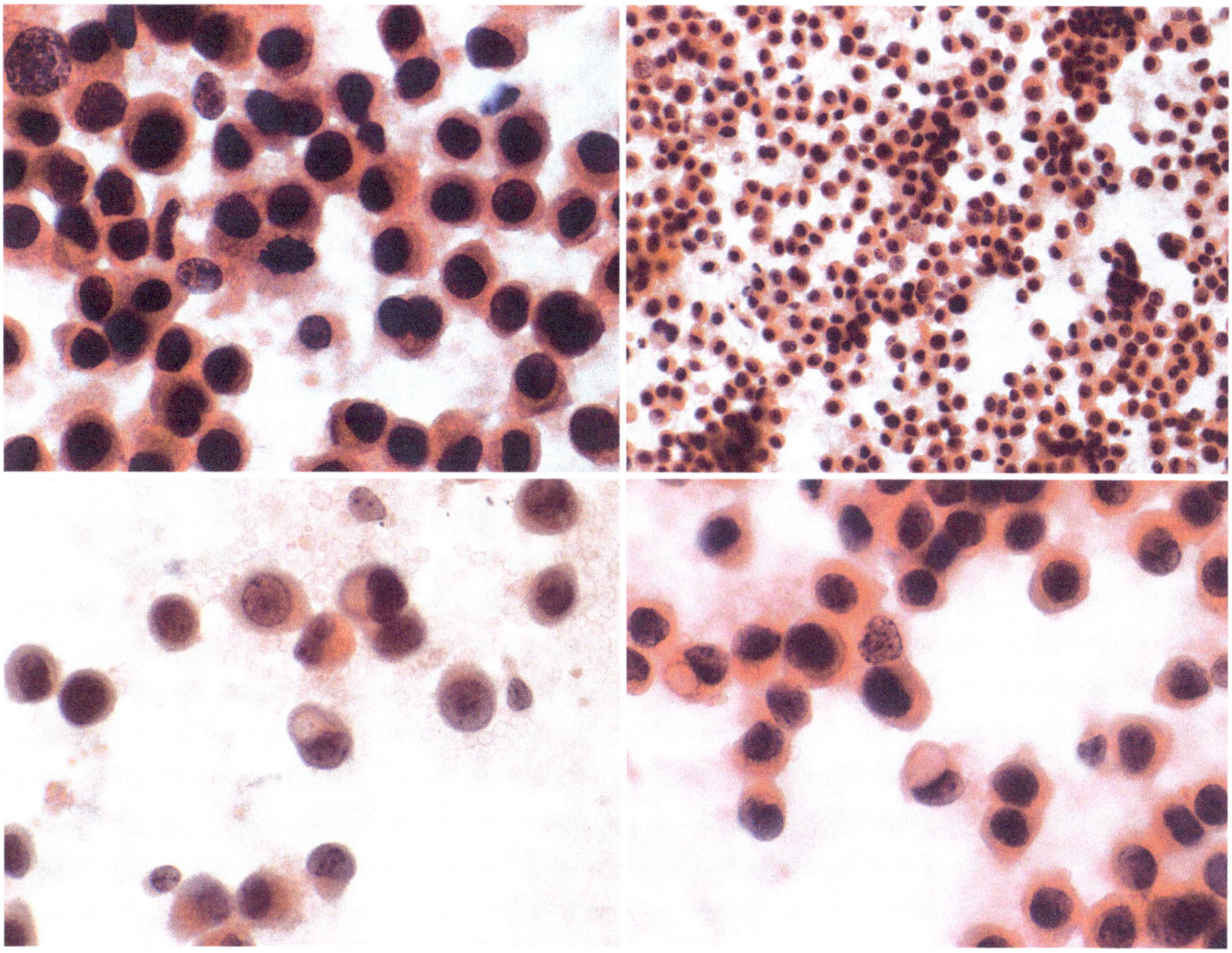

Fig. 10.39

Q-39. This aspirate is from a 62-year-old woman who presents with a 5-month history of an ill-defined breast mass. Physical examination demonstrates an area of firmness in the upper outer quadrant of the right breast. Mammogram shows a diffuse ill-defined mass. FNA was performed. Which of the following is the most likely diagnosis?

(a) Ductal carcinoma
(b) Proliferative fibrocystic changes
(c) Tubular carcinoma
(d) Fibroadenoma
(e) Invasive lobular carcinoma, pleomorphic type

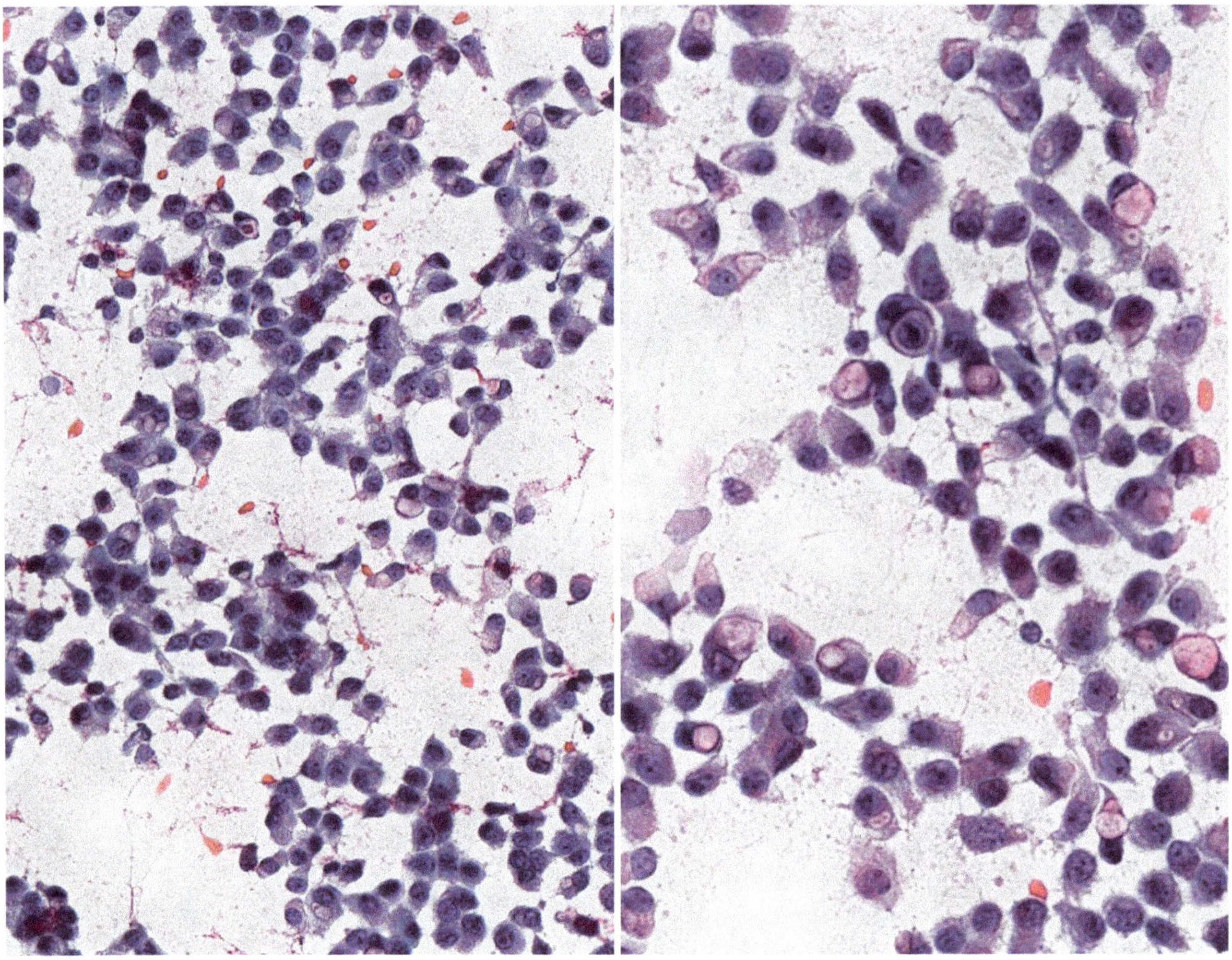

Fig. 10.40

Q-40. This aspirate is from a 62-year-old woman who presents with a 5-month history of an ill-defined breast mass. Physical examination demonstrates an area of diffuse infiltration involving her right breast tissue. Mammogram shows a diffuse ill-defined mass suspicious for malignancy. FNA was performed. Which of the following is the most likely diagnosis?

(a) Signet ring carcinoma
(b) Invasive lobular carcinoma, classic type
(c) Proliferative fibrocystic changes
(d) Radial scar
(e) Fibroadenoma

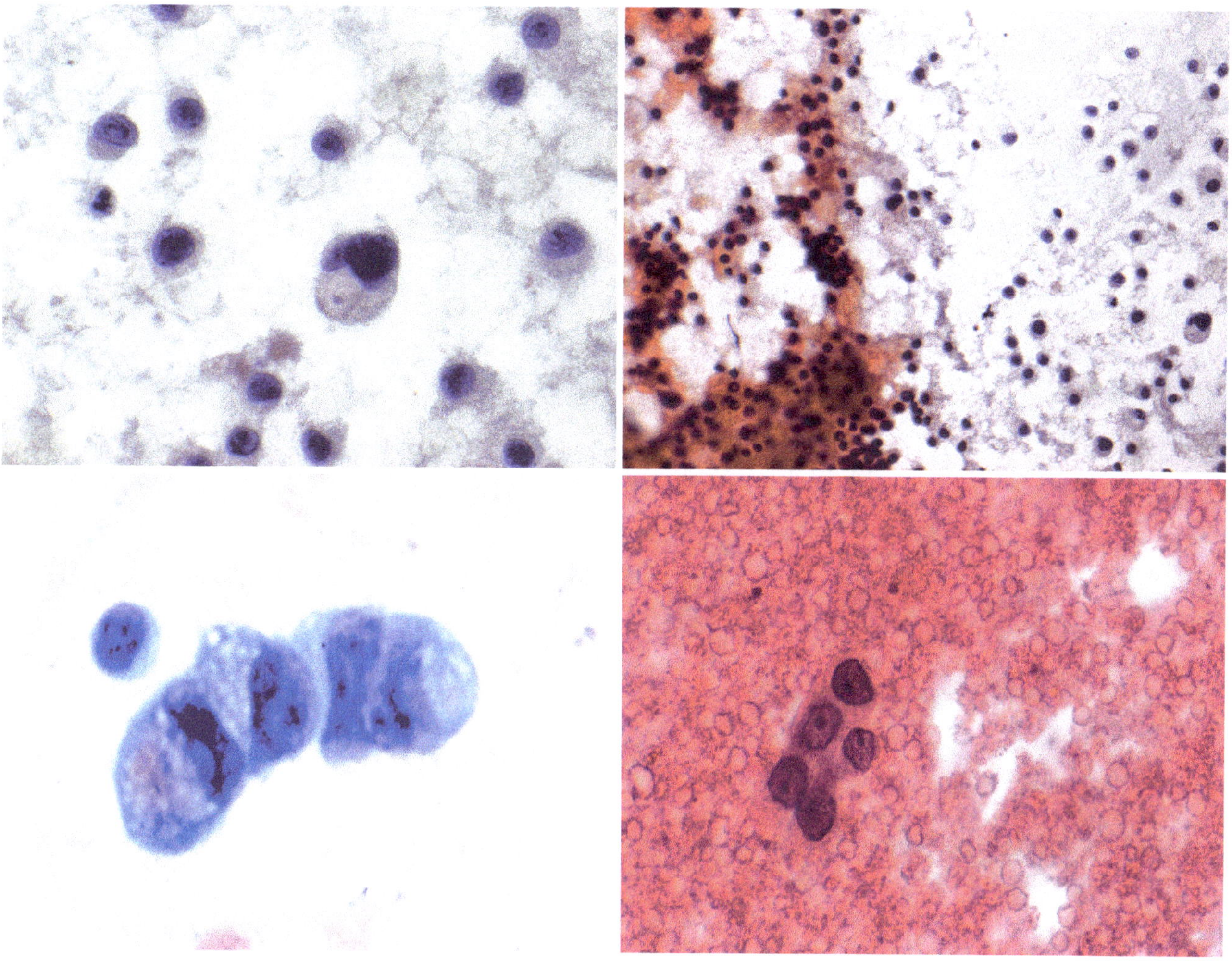

Fig. 10.41

Q-41. This aspirate is from a 32-year-old woman who noticed diffuse left breast hotness and redness 1 month after giving birth to a normal term infant. She is breast-feeding without any significant history. She visited her family physician who has prescribed her antibiotics without any significant improvement. On physical examination, the breast shows a diffuse area of redness with an ill-defined lesion and skin edema. Diffuse breast edema with peau d'orange skin architecture was seen. Axillary palpation reveals a few enlarged lymph nodes. FNA was performed. What is the mostly likely diagnosis?

(a) Inflammatory carcinoma
(b) Lactating adenoma
(c) Phyllodes tumor
(d) Acute mastitis
(e) Paget's disease of the breast

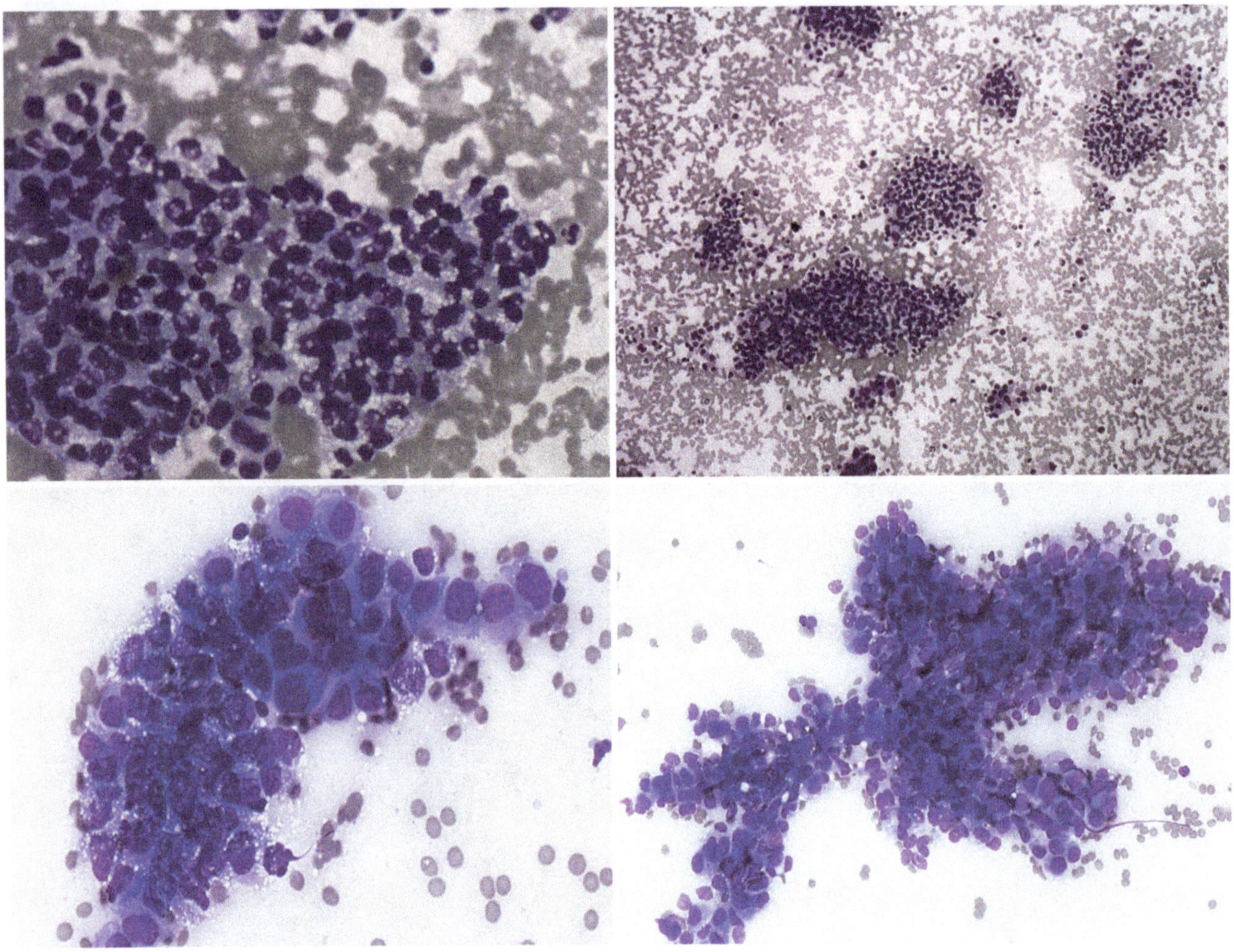

Fig. 10.42

Q-42. This aspirate is from a 52-year-old woman who presents with a breast lump in the upper outer quadrant of her left breast. There is no family history of breast cancer. On physical examination, the breast shows an ill-defined mass, measuring 2.5 cm. The overlying skin is unremarkable. Axillary palpation reveals a few enlarged lymph nodes. The mammogram was suspicious. FNA was performed. What is the mostly likely diagnosis?

(a) Inflammatory carcinoma
(b) Lactating adenoma
(c) Fibroadenoma with lactational changes
(d) Acute mastitis
(e) Glycogen-rich ductal carcinoma

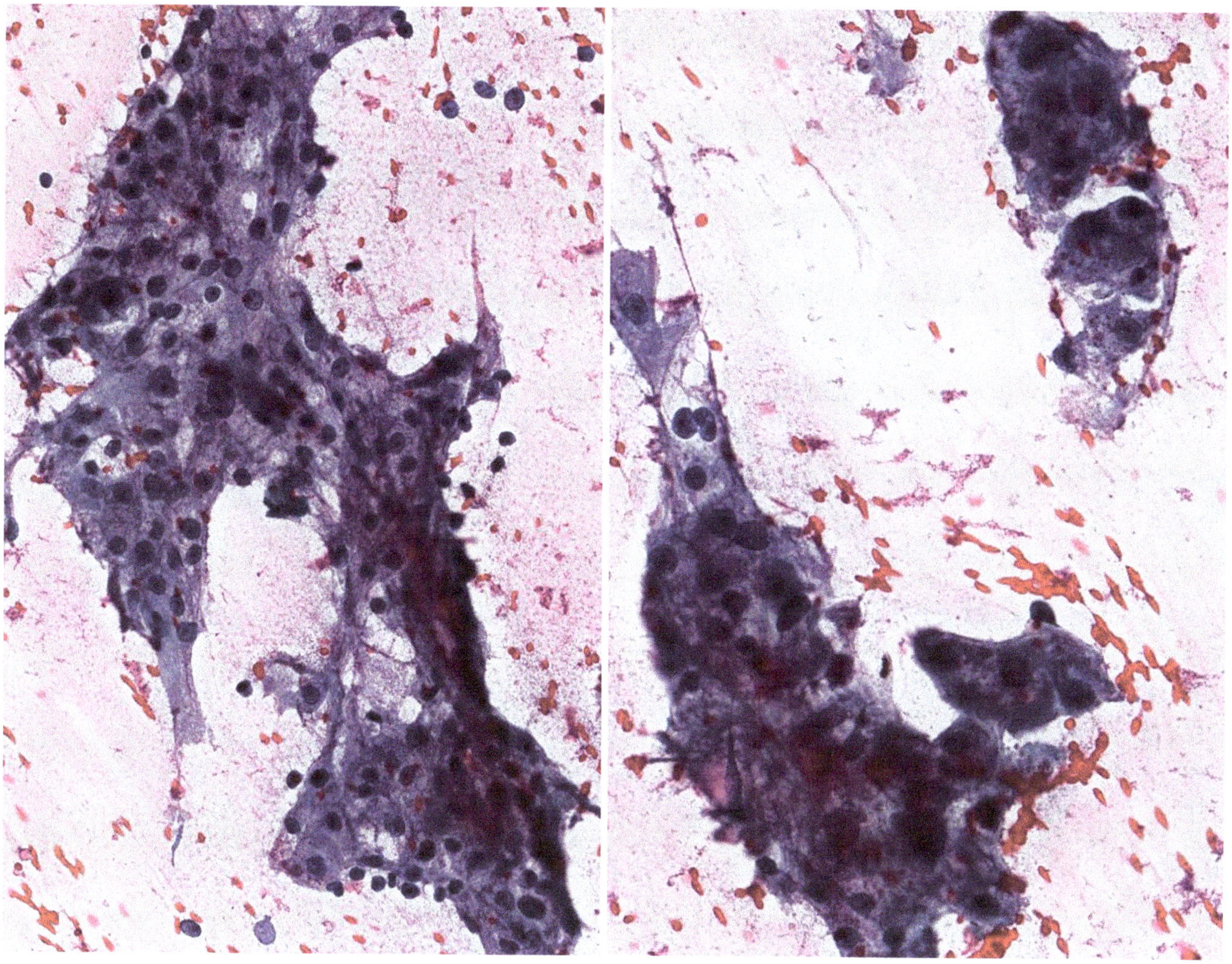

Fig. 10.43

Q-43. This aspirate is from a 44-year-old woman who presents with an ill-defined breast mass. Physical examination confirms a 2.2-cm mass in the upper outer quadrant of the left breast. Mammogram shows an infiltrating breast mass, suspicious for malignancy. FNA was performed. Which of the following is the most likely diagnosis?

(a) Ductal carcinoma
(b) Mucinous carcinoma
(c) Lobular carcinoma
(d) Metaplastic carcinoma
(e) Secretory carcinoma

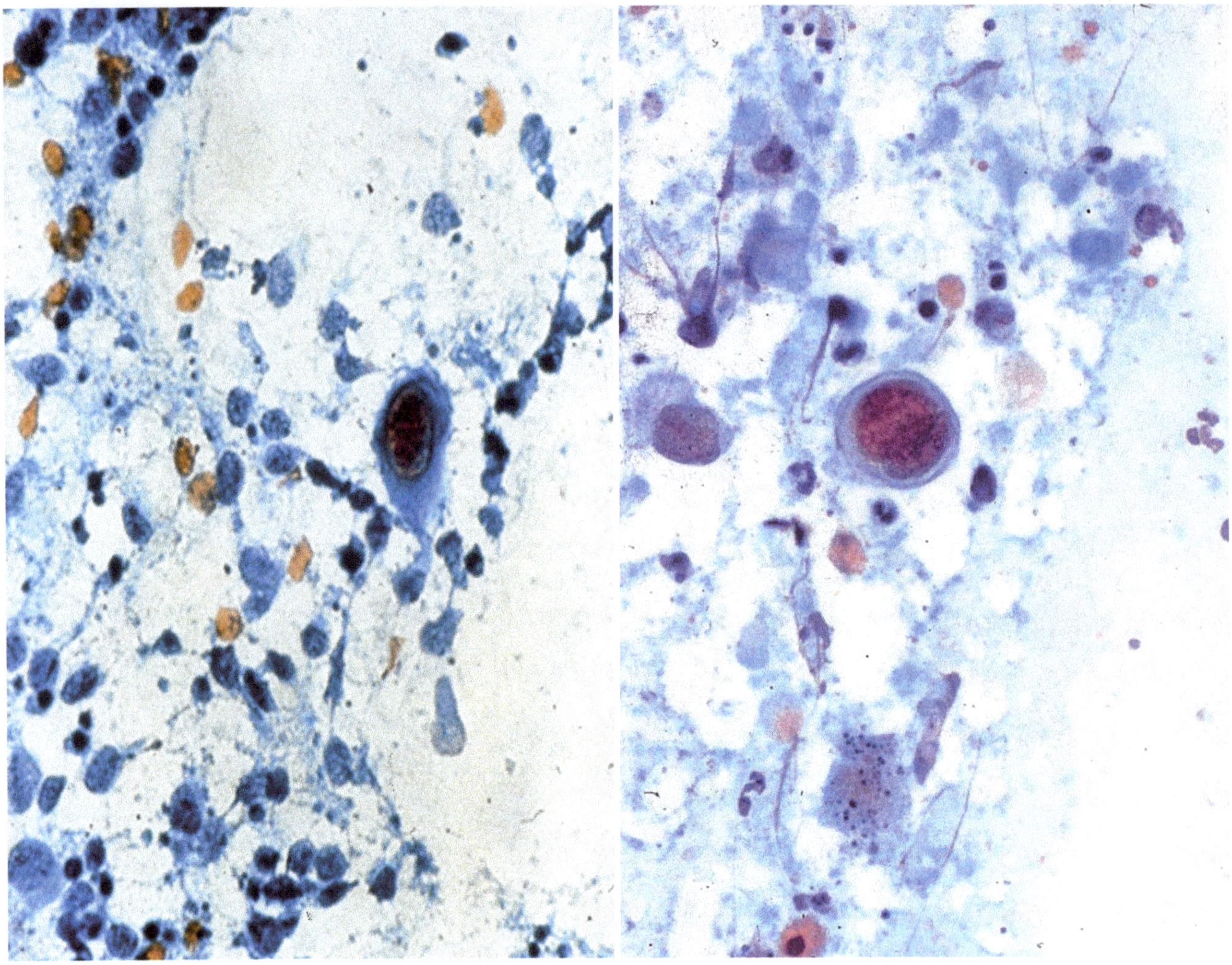

Fig. 10.44

Q-44. This aspirate is from a 43-year-old woman who has noticed a red, scaly area of skin on her left breast that has grown slightly larger over the past 4 months. On physical examination, there is a 1-cm area of eczematous skin just lateral to the areola. Scrape smears were performed and are shown in the figures. Which of the following is the most likely diagnosis?

(a) Apocrine metaplasia
(b) Melanoma
(c) Inflammatory carcinoma
(d) Fat necrosis
(e) Paget's disease of the nipple

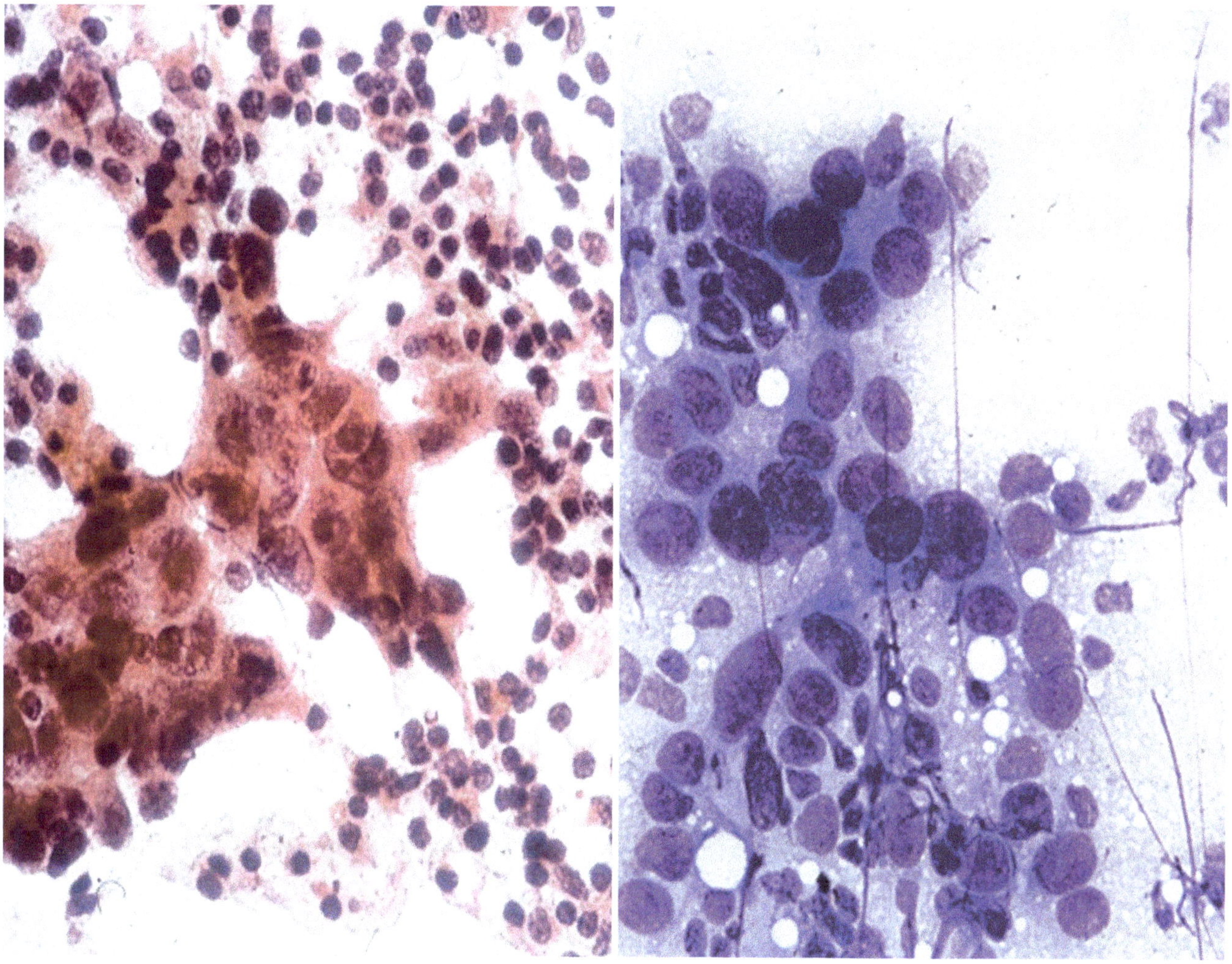

Fig. 10.45

Q-45. This aspirate is from a 34-year-old woman who has noticed an enlarging mass in her left breast for the past 2 years. On physical examination, a well-circumscribed firm mass, measuring 4 cm, is identified. The mammogram shows a well-circumscribed mass that is indeterminate (BIRADS 3). The patient has a family history of breast cancer. FNA was performed. What is the most likely diagnosis?

(a) Lobular carcinoma
(b) Medullary carcinoma
(c) Mucinous carcinoma
(d) Breast lymphoma
(e) Chronic mastitis

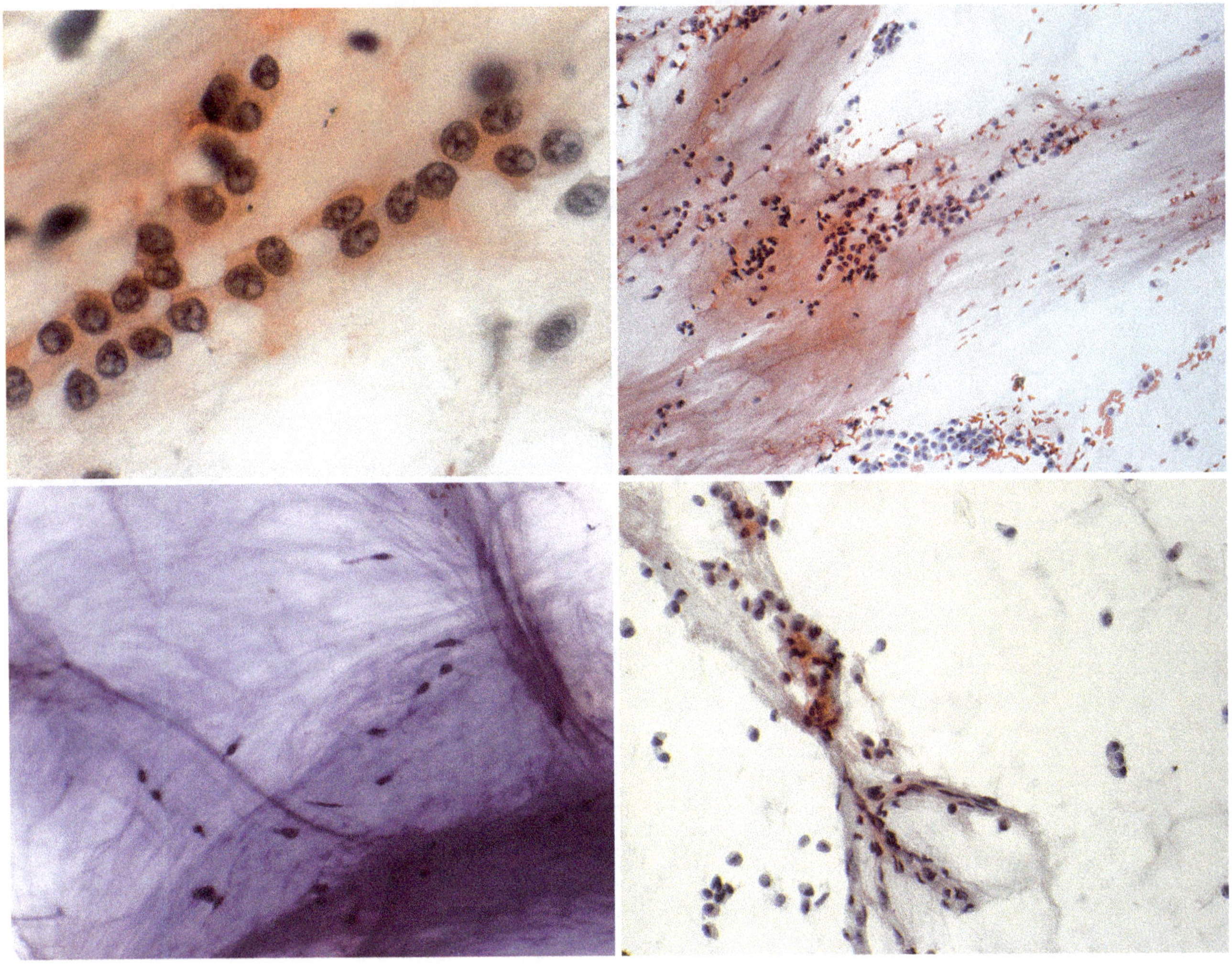

Fig. 10.46

Q-46. This aspirate is from a 50-year-old woman who presents with a palpable breast mass that she noticed on self-examination 1 month earlier. The mammogram shows a circumscribed mass and was interpreted as a benign breast lesion – BIRADS 2 (?fibroadenoma). Physical examination reveals a soft tumor measuring 5.0 cm in diameter. FNA was performed. Which of the following is the appropriate diagnosis?

(a) Tubular carcinoma
(b) Medullary carcinoma
(c) Mucinous carcinoma
(d) Lobular carcinoma
(e) Chronic mastitis

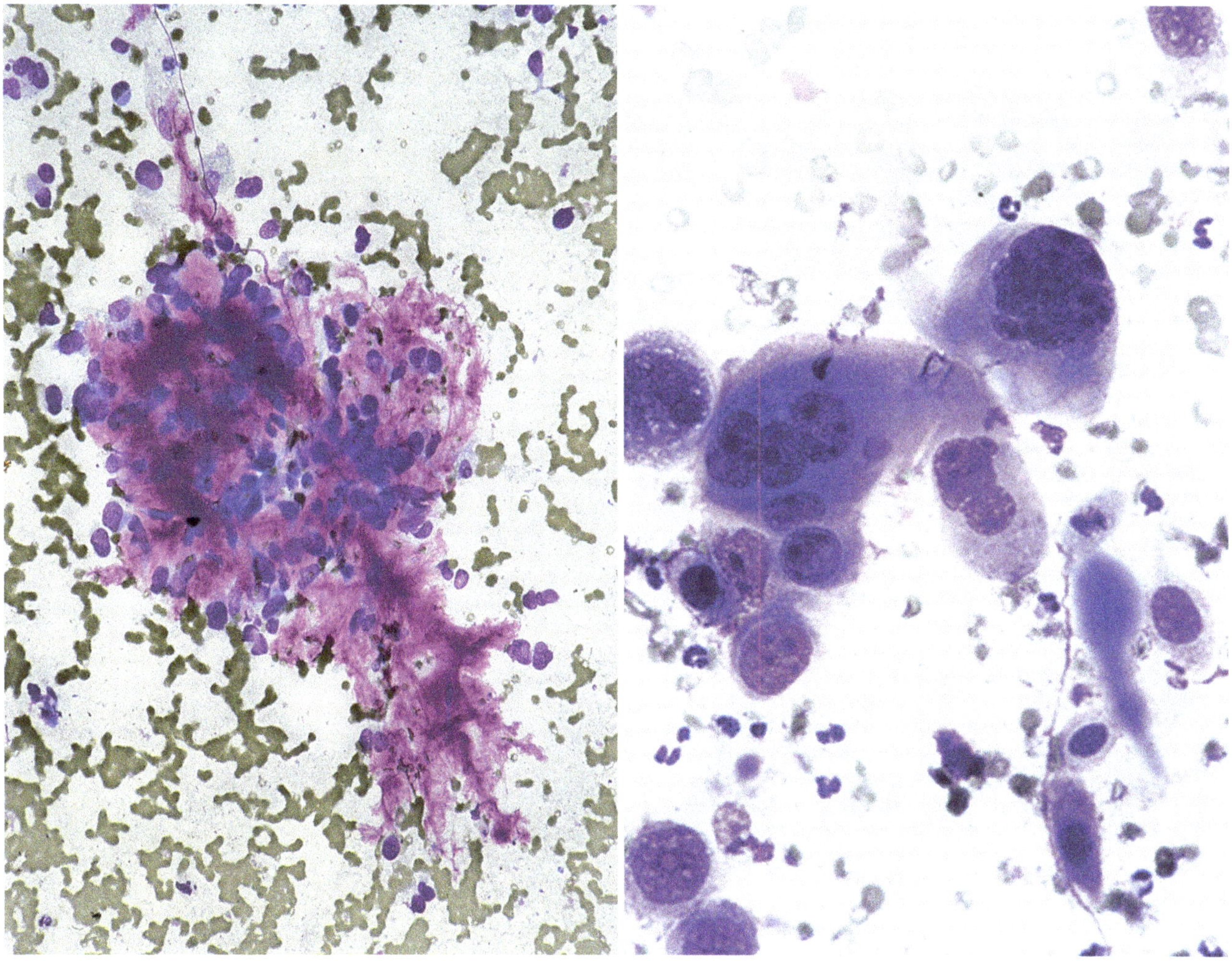

Fig. 10.47

Q-47. This aspirate is from a 54-year-old woman who discovered an ill-defined breast mass on self-examination. Mammogram shows an infiltrating breast mass, suspicious for malignancy. Physical examination confirms a 3-cm mass in the lower outer quadrant of the left breast. FNA was performed. Which of the following is the most likely diagnosis?

(a) Ductal carcinoma
(b) Mucinous carcinoma
(c) Lobular carcinoma
(d) Metaplastic carcinoma
(e) Paget's disease

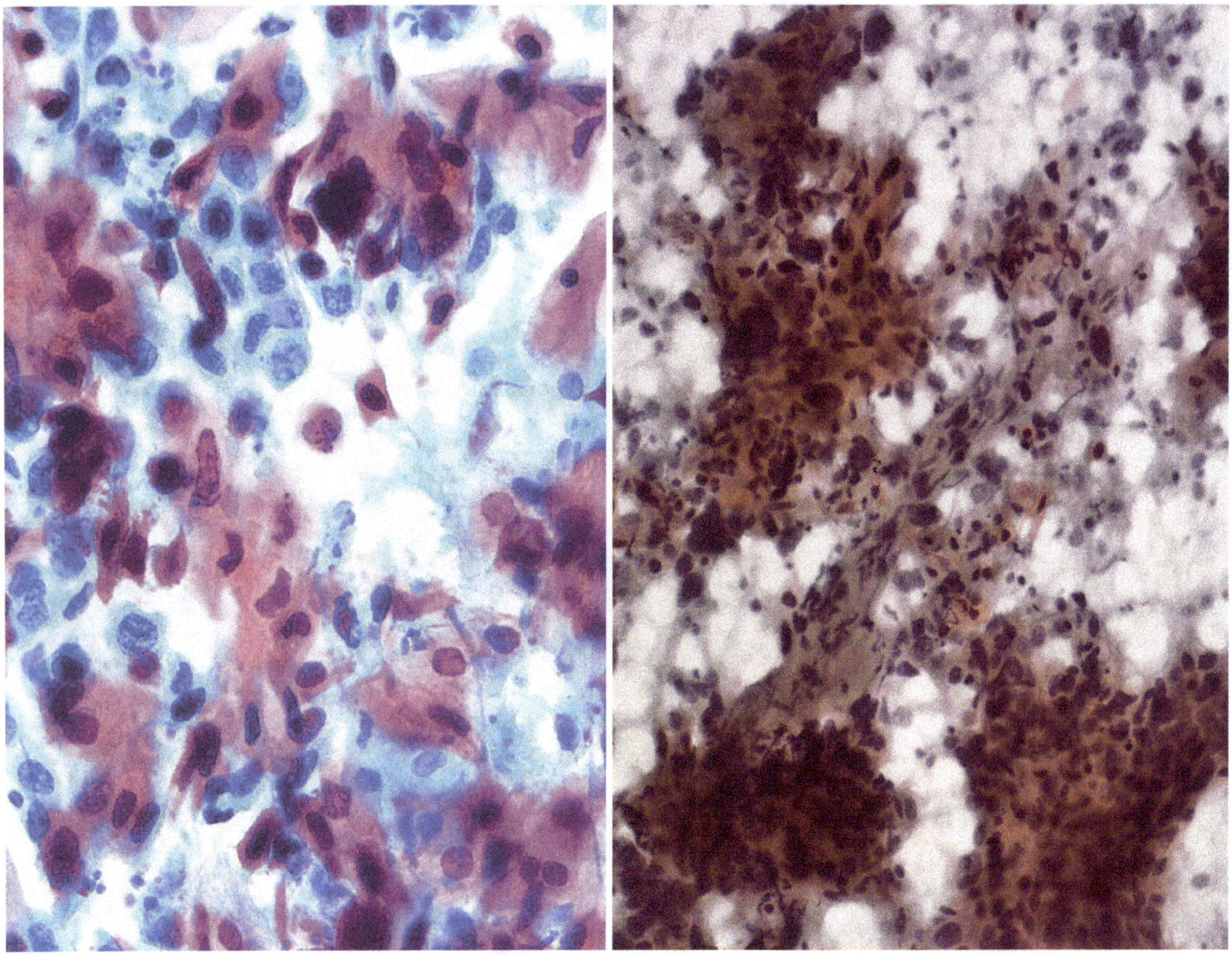

Fig. 10.48

Q-48. This aspirate is from a 54-year-old woman who presents with an ill-defined breast mass in her left breast. Physical examination confirms a 2.5-cm mass in the lower outer quadrant of the left breast, located mainly in the underlying subcutaneous tissue. Mammogram shows an infiltrating breast mass, suspicious for malignancy. FNA was performed. Which of the following is the most likely diagnosis?

(a) Lobular carcinoma
(b) Medullary carcinoma
(c) Mucinous carcinoma
(d) Metaplastic carcinoma
(e) Chronic mastitis

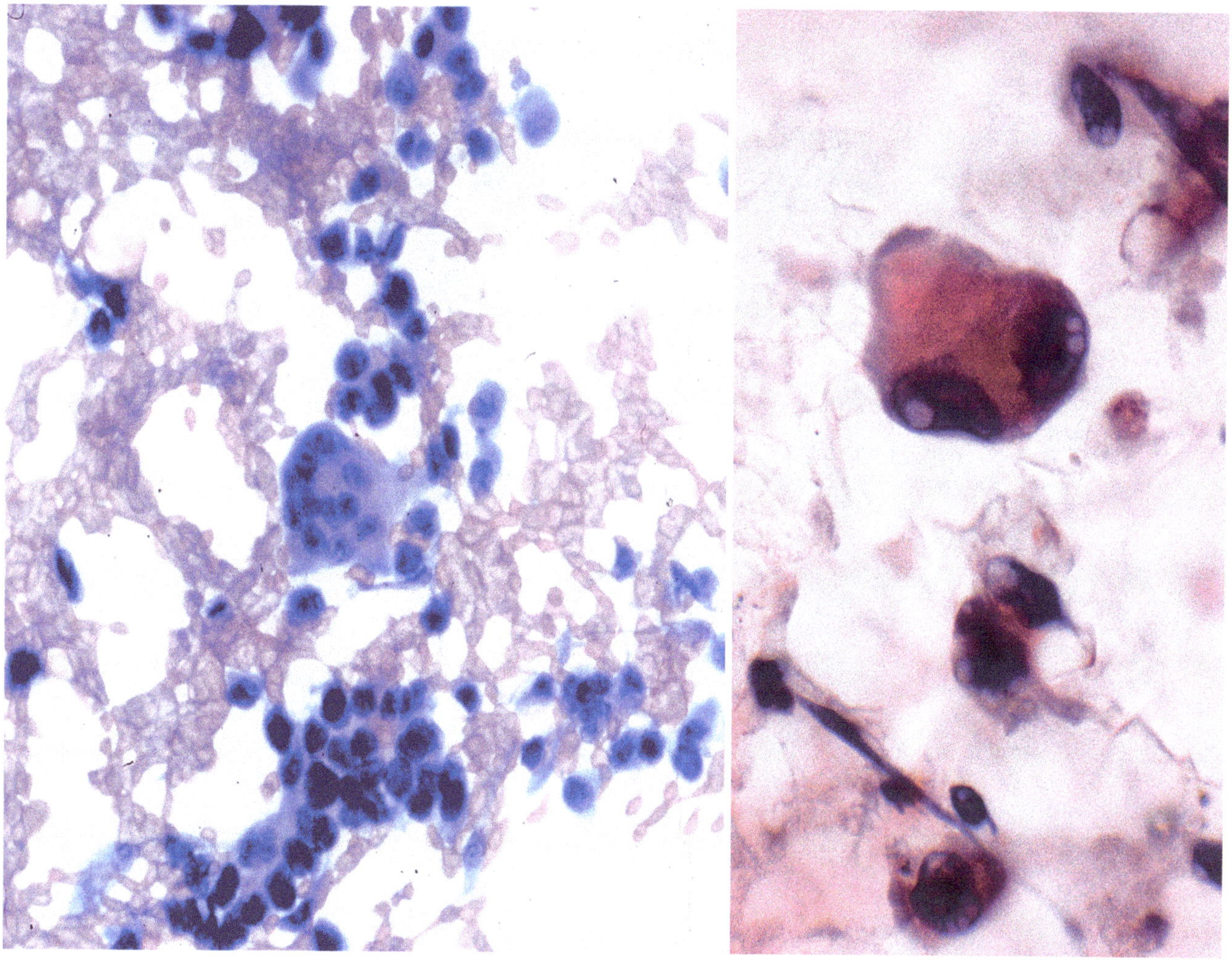

Fig. 10.49

Q-49. This aspirate is from a 64-year-old woman who presents with a breast mass in her right breast. Mammogram shows an ill-defined mass, suspicious for malignancy. Physical examination confirms a 2.0-cm mass in the lower outer quadrant of the left breast, located mainly in the underlying subcutaneous tissue. FNA was performed. Which of the following is the most likely diagnosis?

(a) Lobular carcinoma
(b) Medullary carcinoma
(c) Osteoclastic-type giant cell carcinoma
(d) Metaplastic carcinoma
(e) Chronic mastitis

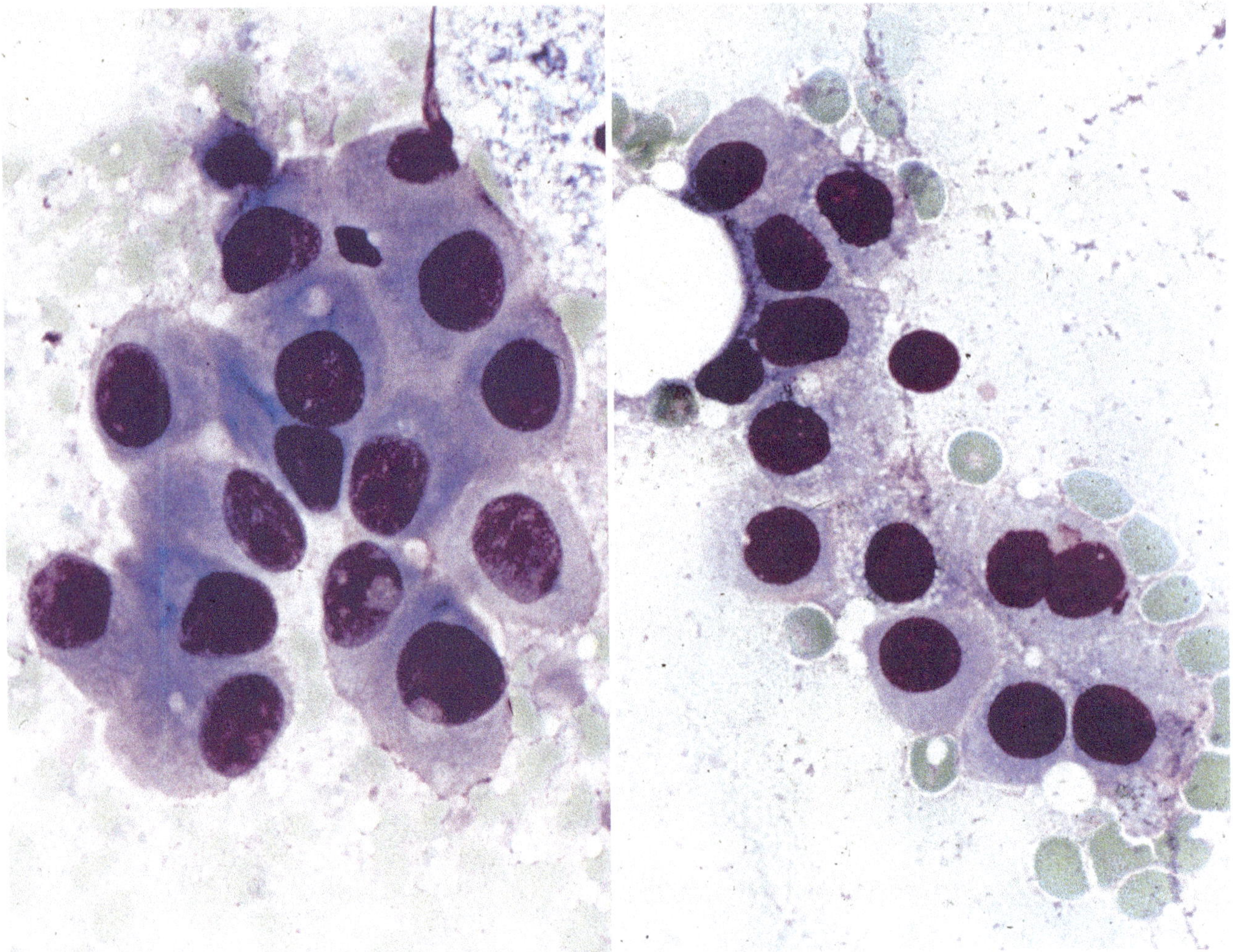

Fig. 10.50

Q-50. This aspirate is from a 64-year-old woman who presents to her family doctor with an ill-defined breast mass fixed to her chest wall. Mammogram shows an infiltrating breast mass with malignant features. Physical examination confirms a 3-cm mass in the upper outer quadrant of the left breast. Axillary palpatin reveals a few enlarged lymph nodes. FNA was performed. Which of the following is the most likely diagnosis?

(a) Ductal carcinoma
(b) Mucinous carcinoma
(c) Lobular carcinoma
(d) Metaplastic carcinoma
(e) Apocrine carcinoma

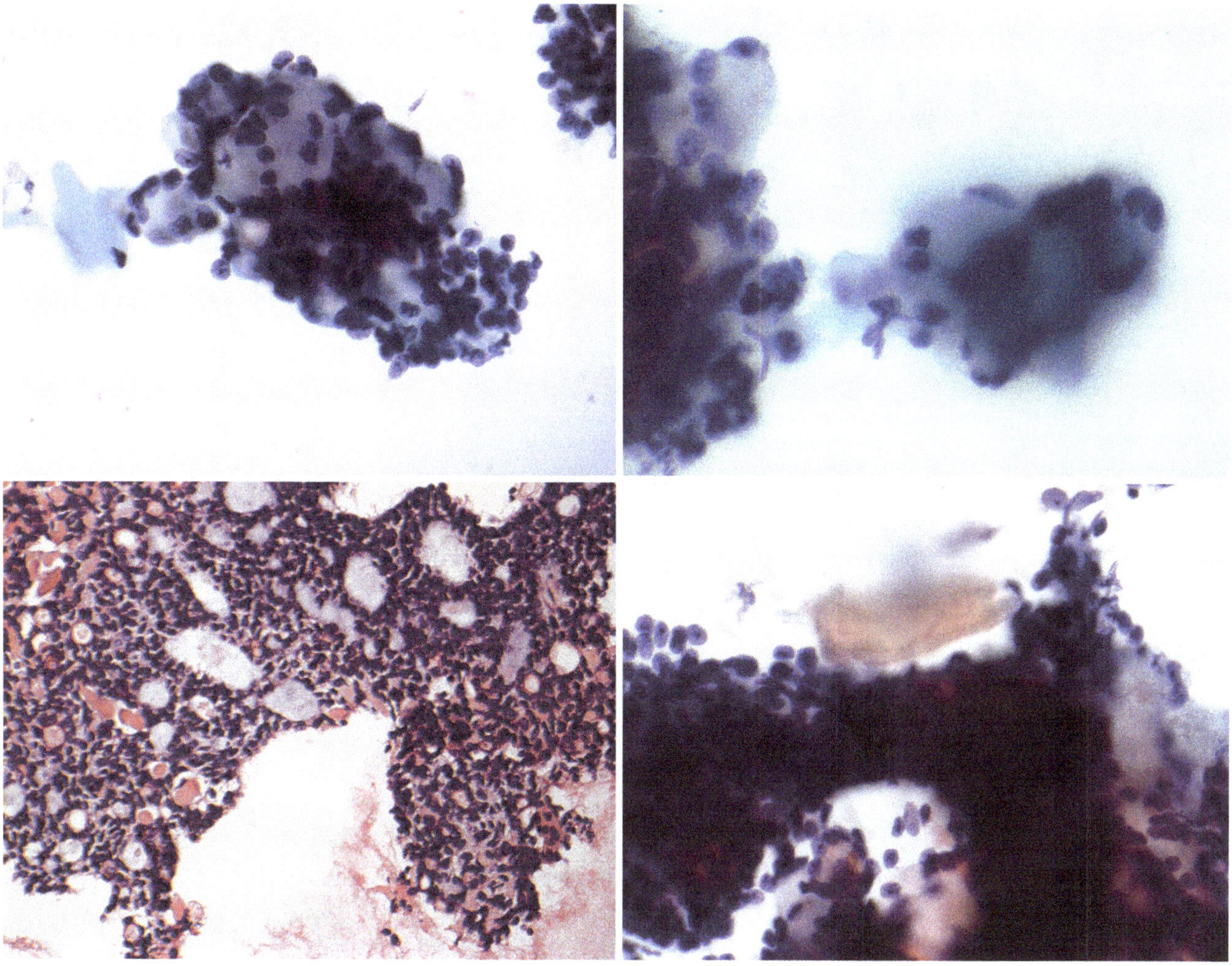

Fig. 10.51

Q-51. This aspirate is from a 56-year-old woman who presents with an ill-defined breast mass on self-examination. Physical examination confirms a 3-cm mass in the lower outer quadrant of the left breast. The mammogram shows an infiltrating breast mass, suspicious for malignancy. Which of the following is the most likely diagnosis?

(a) Ductal carcinoma
(b) Adenoid cystic carcinoma
(c) Mucinous carcinoma
(d) Lobular carcinoma
(e) Metaplastic carcinoma

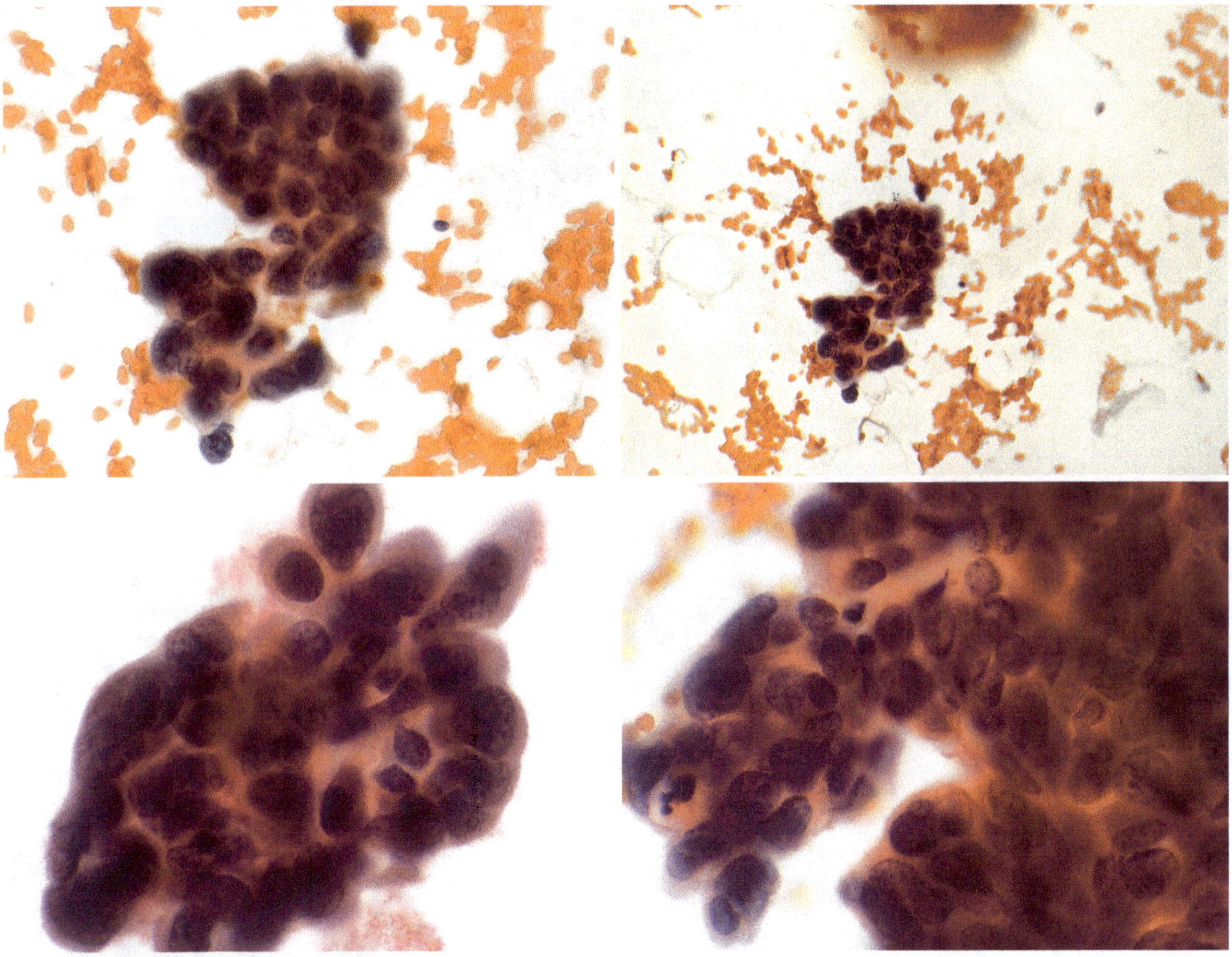

Fig. 10.52

Q-52. This aspirate is from a 50-year-old woman who has been aware of a mass in her left breast for the past 6 months. A 4-cm mass is palpated on examination. The mass is hard, tender, and fixed to the overlying skin. Mammogram shows malignant features. Axillary palpatin reveals a few enlarged lymph nodes. FNA was performed. Which of the following is the most likely diagnosis?

(a) Mucinous carcinoma
(b) Lobular carcinoma
(c) Micropapillary carcinoma
(d) Apocrine carcinoma
(e) Tubular carcinoma

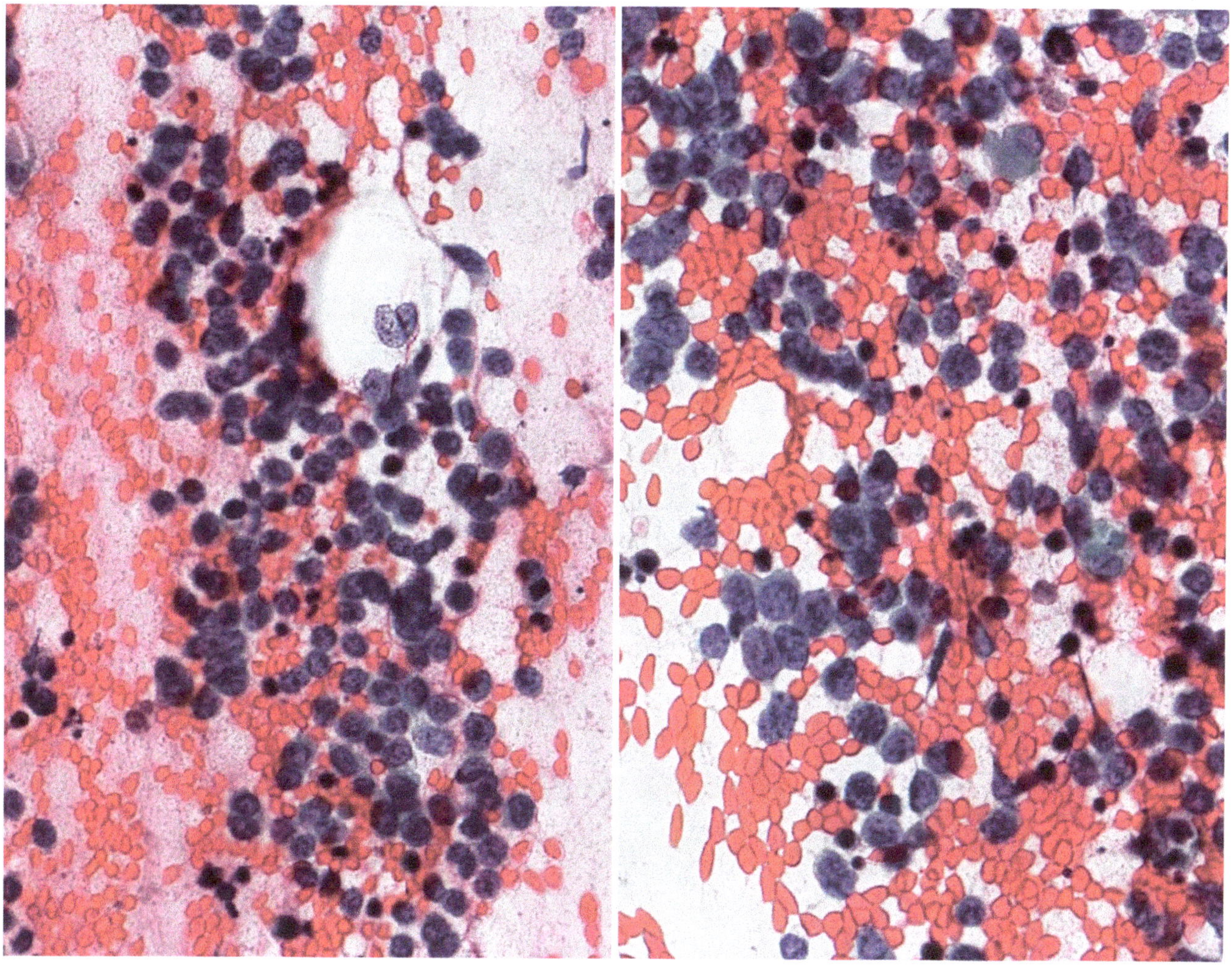

Fig. 10.53

Q-53. This aspirate is from a 74-year-old woman who presents with a well-defined circumscribed breast mass. Physical examination confirms a 3-cm mass in the upper outer quadrant of the left breast. Mammogram shows a well-circumscribed breast mass with indeterminate features. FNA was performed. Which of the following is the most likely diagnosis?

(a) Ductal carcinoma
(b) Mucinous carcinoma
(c) Lobular carcinoma
(d) Metaplastic carcinoma
(e) Neuroendocrine carcinoma

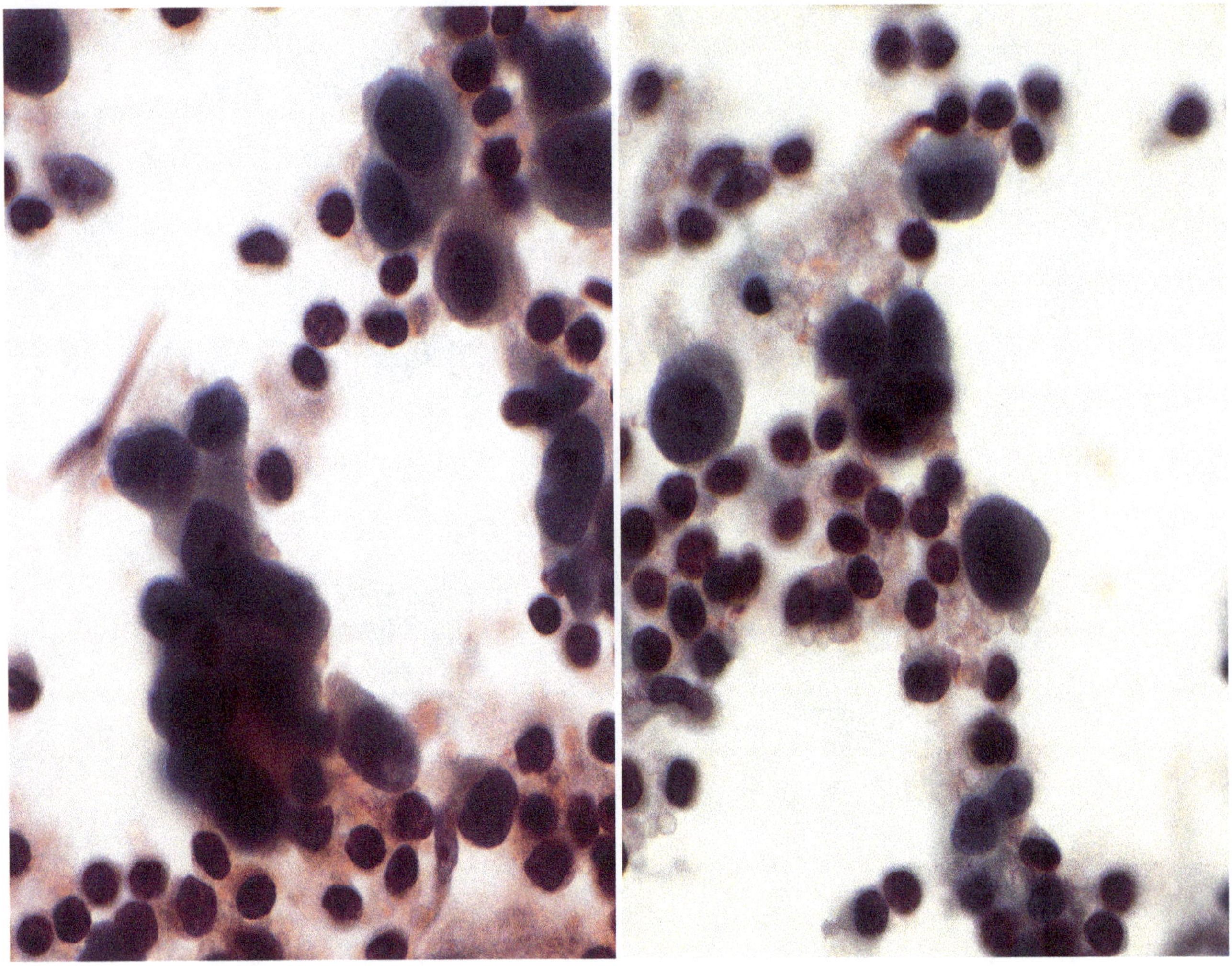

Fig. 10.54

Q-54. This aspirate is from a 74-year-old woman who presents with an ill-defined breast mass. Physical examination confirms a 3-cm mass in the upper outer quadrant of the left breast. Mammogram shows an infiltrating breast mass, with malignant features. FNA was performed. Which of the following is the most likely diagnosis?

(a) Ductal carcinoma, high grade
(b) Mucinous carcinoma
(c) Lobular carcinoma
(d) Metaplastic carcinoma
(e) Ductal carcinoma, low grade

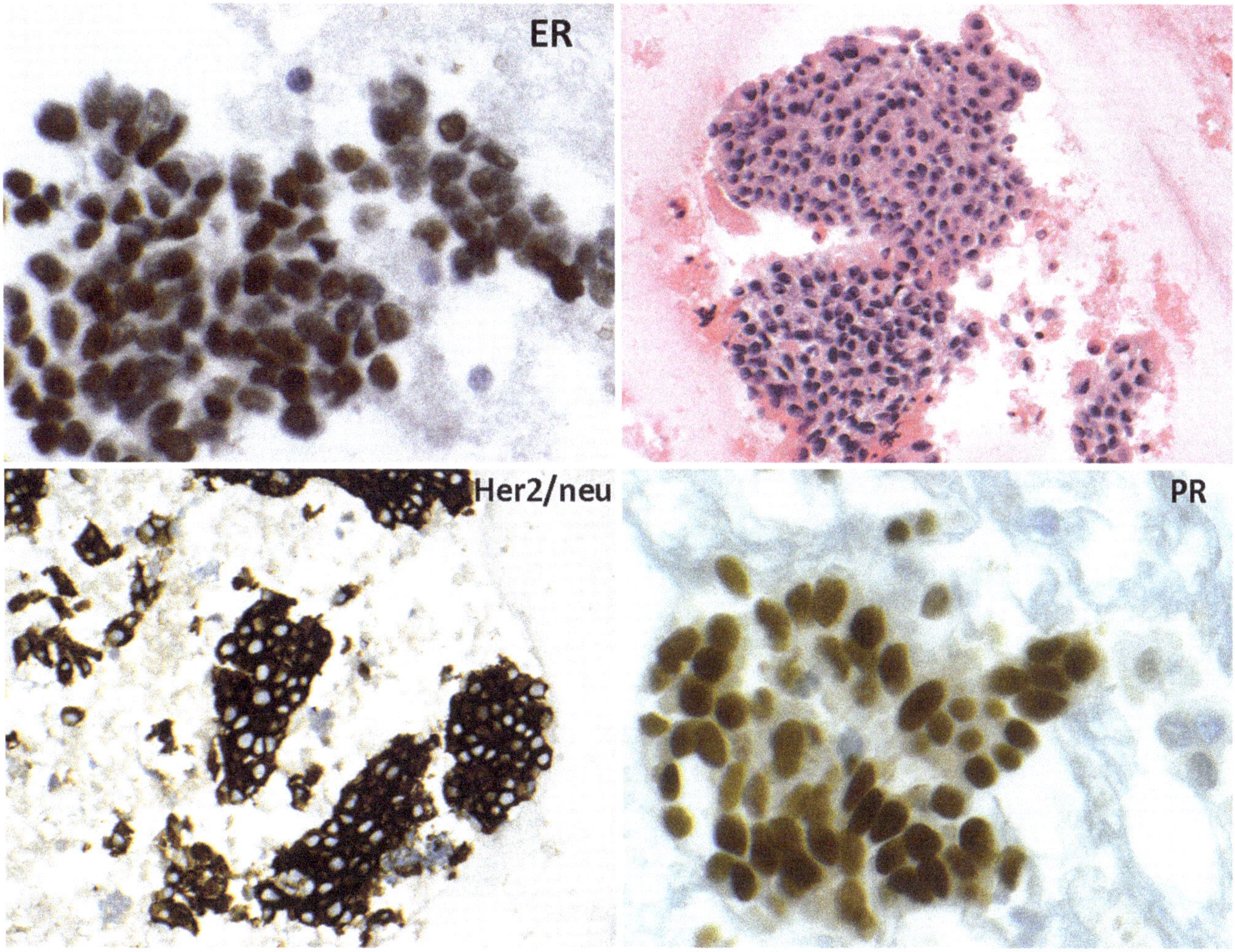

Fig. 10.55

Q-55. This aspirate is from a 54-year-old woman who presents with a breast mass on the right side. She first palpated the lesion 5 days ago while taking a shower. Axillary lymph nodes are large and can be clinically palpated. FNA was performed and hormonal receptor analysis was performed on the cell block. Which of the following is the most likely interpretation?

(a) Positive for hormonal receptors
(b) Negative for hormonal receptors
(c) Equivocal for hormonal receptors
(d) Cannot be assessed in the specimen
(e) Positive internal control

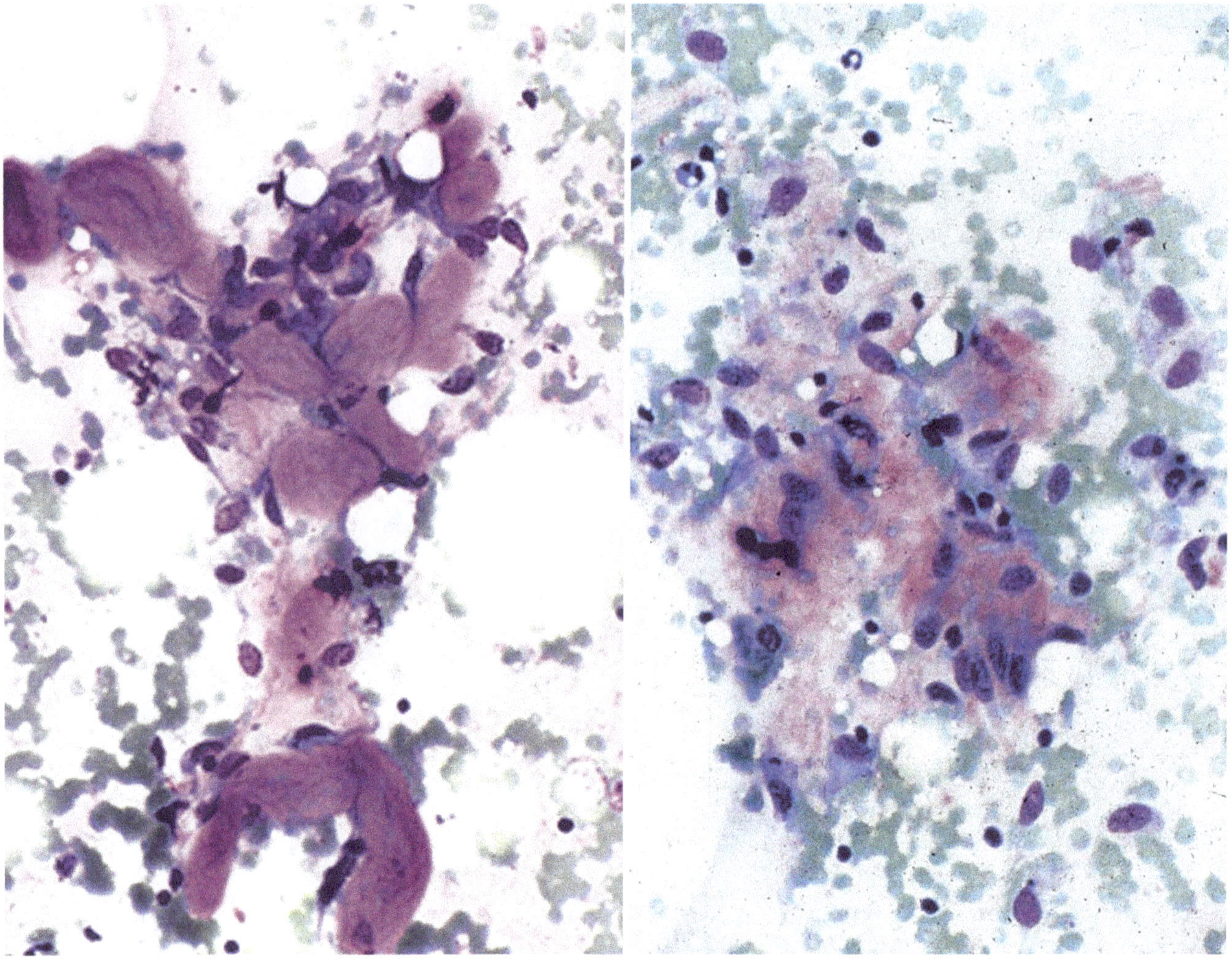

Fig. 10.56

Q-56. This aspirate is from a 58-year-old woman who presents with a breast mass on the right side. On physical examination, there is a deep-seated lesion in the right breast. Axillary lymph nodes are normal in size. FNA was performed. Which of the following is the most likely diagnosis?

(a) Ductal carcinoma
(b) Lobular carcinoma
(c) Fibroadenoma
(d) Spindle cell lesion
(e) Angiosarcoma

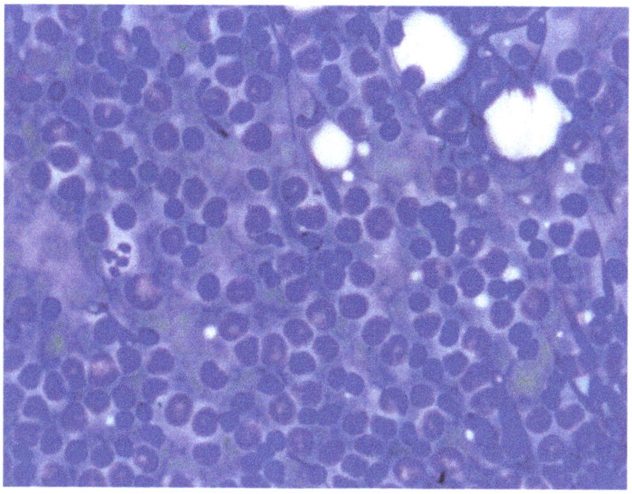

Fig. 10.57

Q-57. This aspirate is from a 54-year-old woman who presents with a well-defined breast mass. Physical examination shows a well-defined, movable 2.0-cm mass in the upper inner quadrant. The overlying skin is unremarkable. There is no axillary lymph node enlargement. The mammogram shows a well-demarcated mass, with a differential diagnosis of fibroadenoma versus intramammary lymph node. The needle aspiration is shown in the images below. Which is the most likely appropriate diagnosis?
(a) Ductal carcinoma
(b) Mucinous carcinoma
(c) Lobular carcinoma
(d) Non-Hodgkin lymphoma
(e) Paget's disease

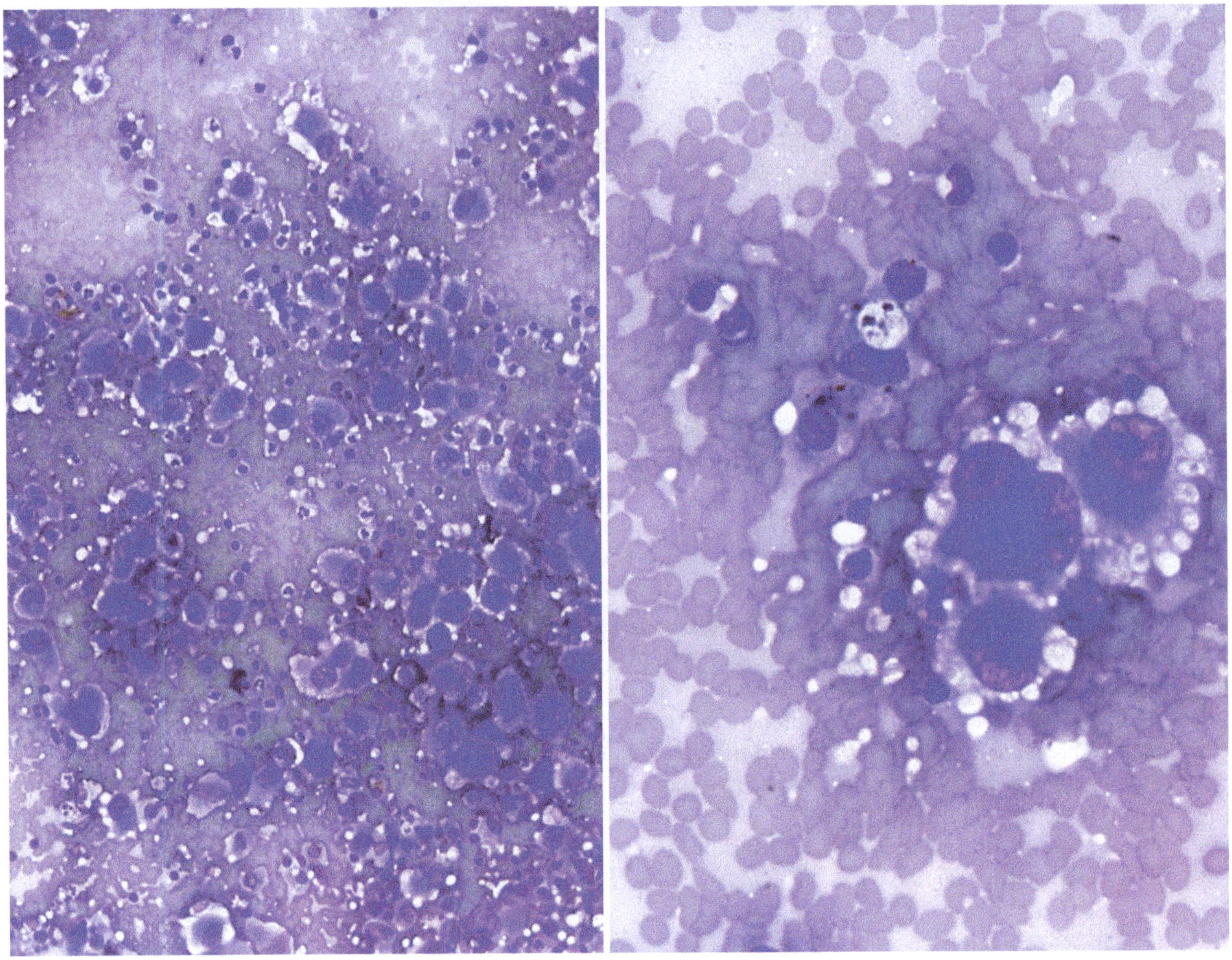

Fig. 10.58

Q-58. This aspirate is from a 54-year-old woman who has a history of breast cancer with lumpectomy 10 years ago. The patient had received radiation as adjuvant therapy. A few months ago she developed a small breast nodule which grew rapidly and reached a size of 5 cm. Physical examination shows a well-defined mass in the upper inner quadrant at the lumpectomy site. The overlying skin is red and hot. There is no axillary lymph node enlargement. Mammogram shows a suspicious vascular lesion. FNA was performed. Which of the following is the most likely diagnosis?

(a) Recurrent ductal carcinoma
(b) Fibroadenoma
(c) Seroma
(d) Angiosarcoma
(e) Lymphoma

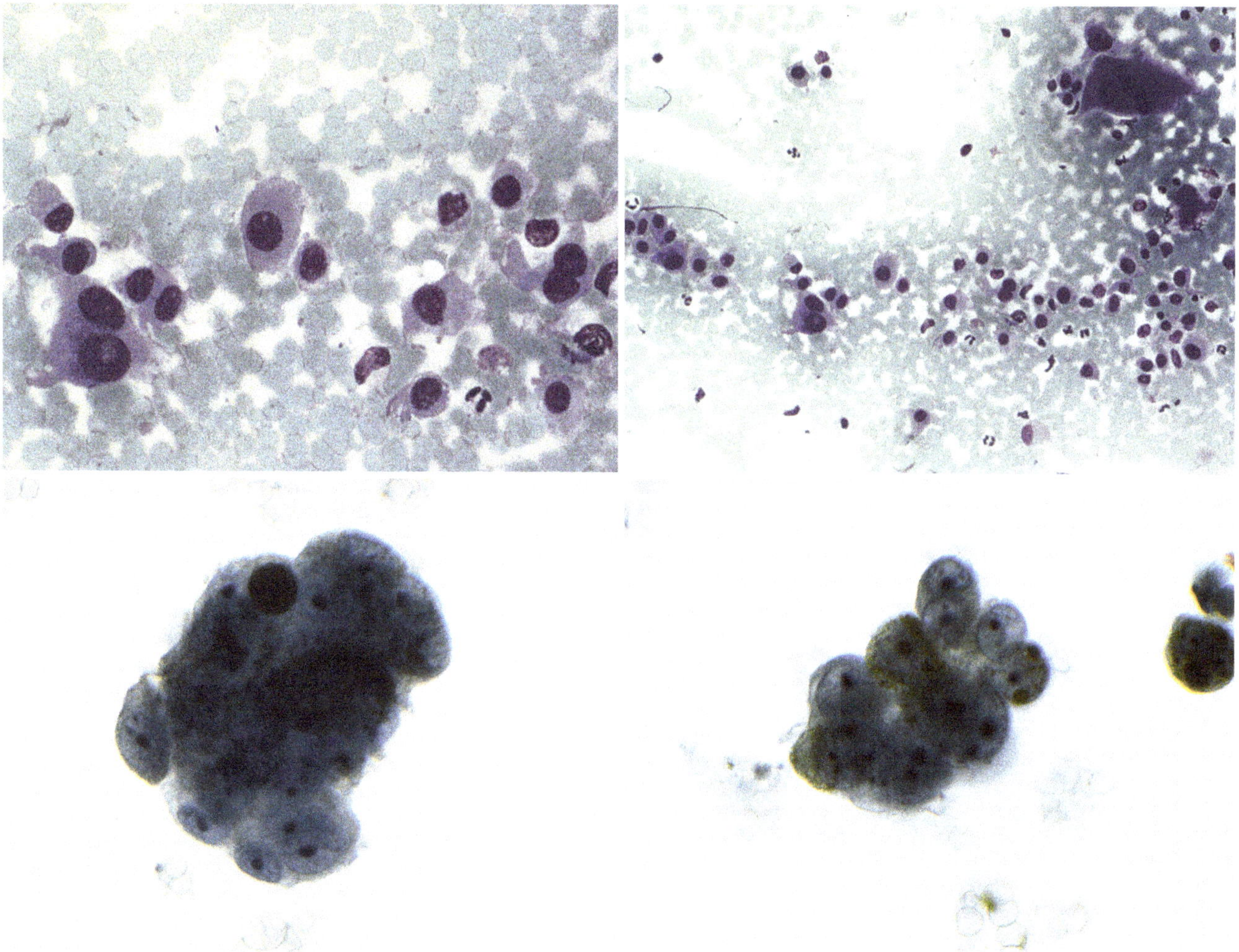

Fig. 10.59

Q-59. This aspirate is from a 59-year-old woman who presents with two well-defined breast masses. Physical examination shows a well-defined, movable lesion, located in the lower inner and outer quadrants. The overlying skin is unremarkable. There is axillary lymph node enlargement. Mammogram shows well-demarcated masses, with a differential diagnosis of benign breast lesions. The patient has a past history of a pigmented lesion which was excised 7 years ago. She does not recall the diagnosis of the pigmented lesion. FNA was performed. Which of the following is the most likely diagnosis?

(a) Fibroadenoma
(b) Mucinous carcinoma
(c) Metastatic malignant melanoma
(d) Non-Hodgkin lymphoma
(e) Metastatic small cell carcinoma

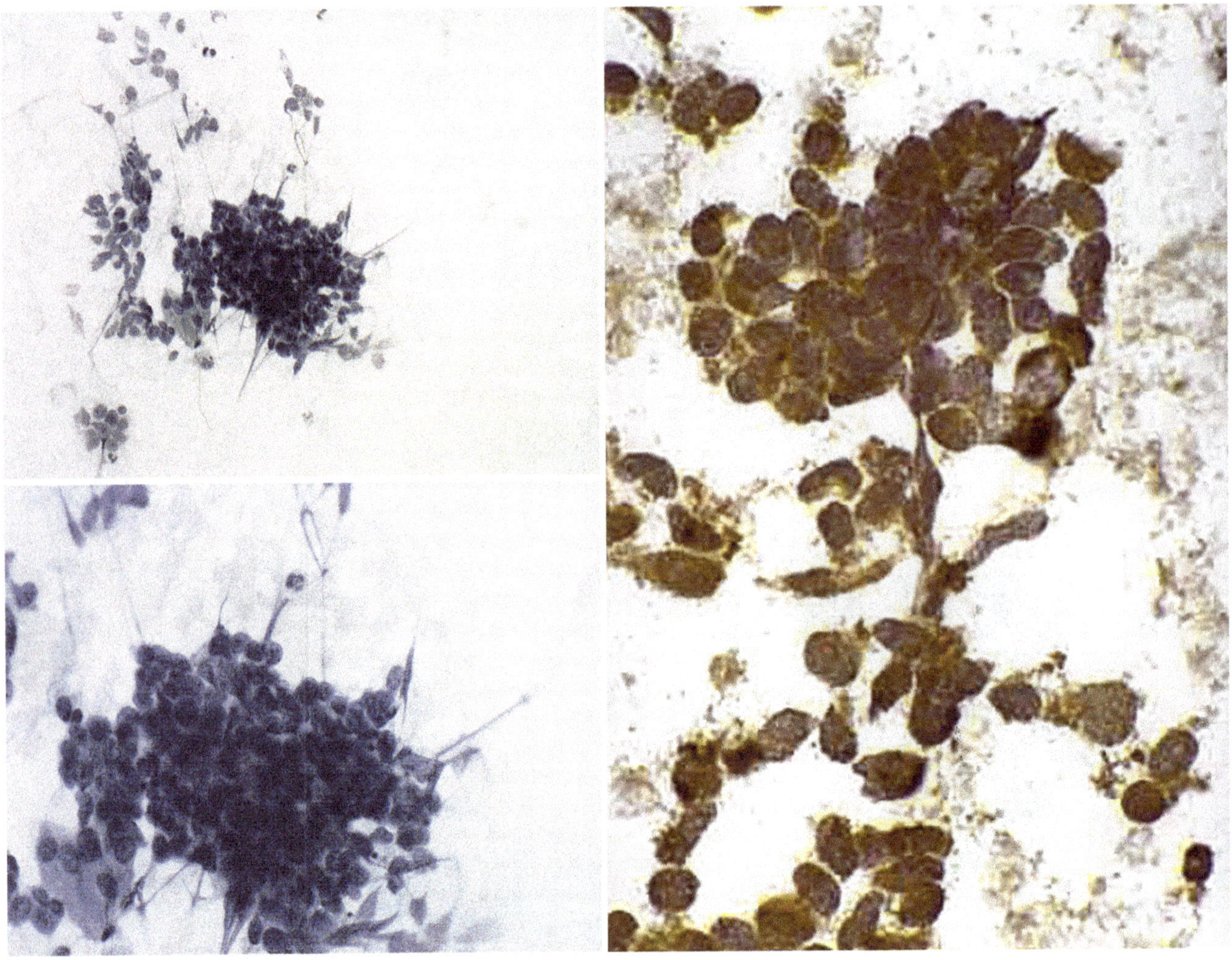

Fig. 10.60

Q-60. This aspirate is from a 54-year-old woman who presents with two well-defined breast masses. Physical examination shows well-defined, movable lesions, located in the upper inner and outer quadrants. The overlying skin is unremarkable. There is no axillary lymph node enlargement. The mammogram shows well-demarcated masses, with a differential diagnosis of benign breast lesions. However, ultrasound examination shows vascularity of the lesions, and metastatic carcinoma cannot be totally excluded. The patient has a past history of heavy smoking with 3 packs/day for 25 years. CT examination shows hilar lymphadenopathy with a possible mediastinal mass. FNA was performed. Which of the following is the most likely diagnosis?

(a) Fibroadenoma
(b) Mucinous carcinoma
(c) Medullary carcinoma
(d) Non-Hodgkin lymphoma
(e) Metastatic small cell carcinoma

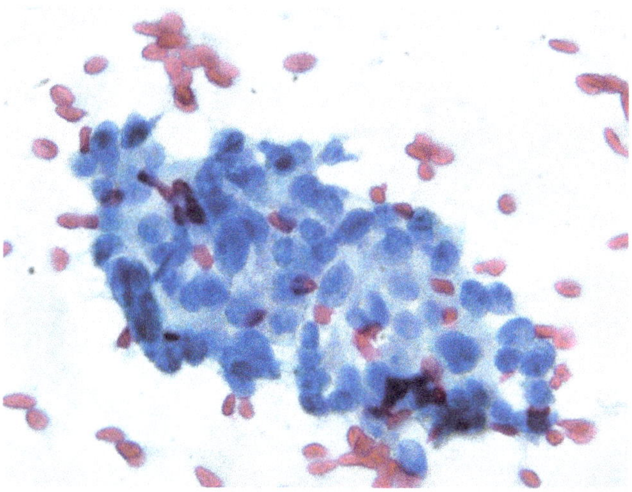

Fig. 10.61

Q-61. This aspirate is from a 72-year-old man who presents with a well-defined breast mass. Physical examination shows a well-defined breast mass infiltrating the underlying tissue. The overlying skin is unremarkable. There is no axillary lymph node enlargement. The mammogram shows a well-demarcated mass. However, ultrasound examination shows tumor vascularity, and a metastatic carcinoma cannot be totally excluded. An FNA was performed. Which of the following is the most likely diagnosis?

(a) Fibroadenoma
(b) Metastatic small cell carcinoma
(c) Medullary carcinoma
(d) Metastatic prostatic adenocarcinoma
(e) Papillary lesion

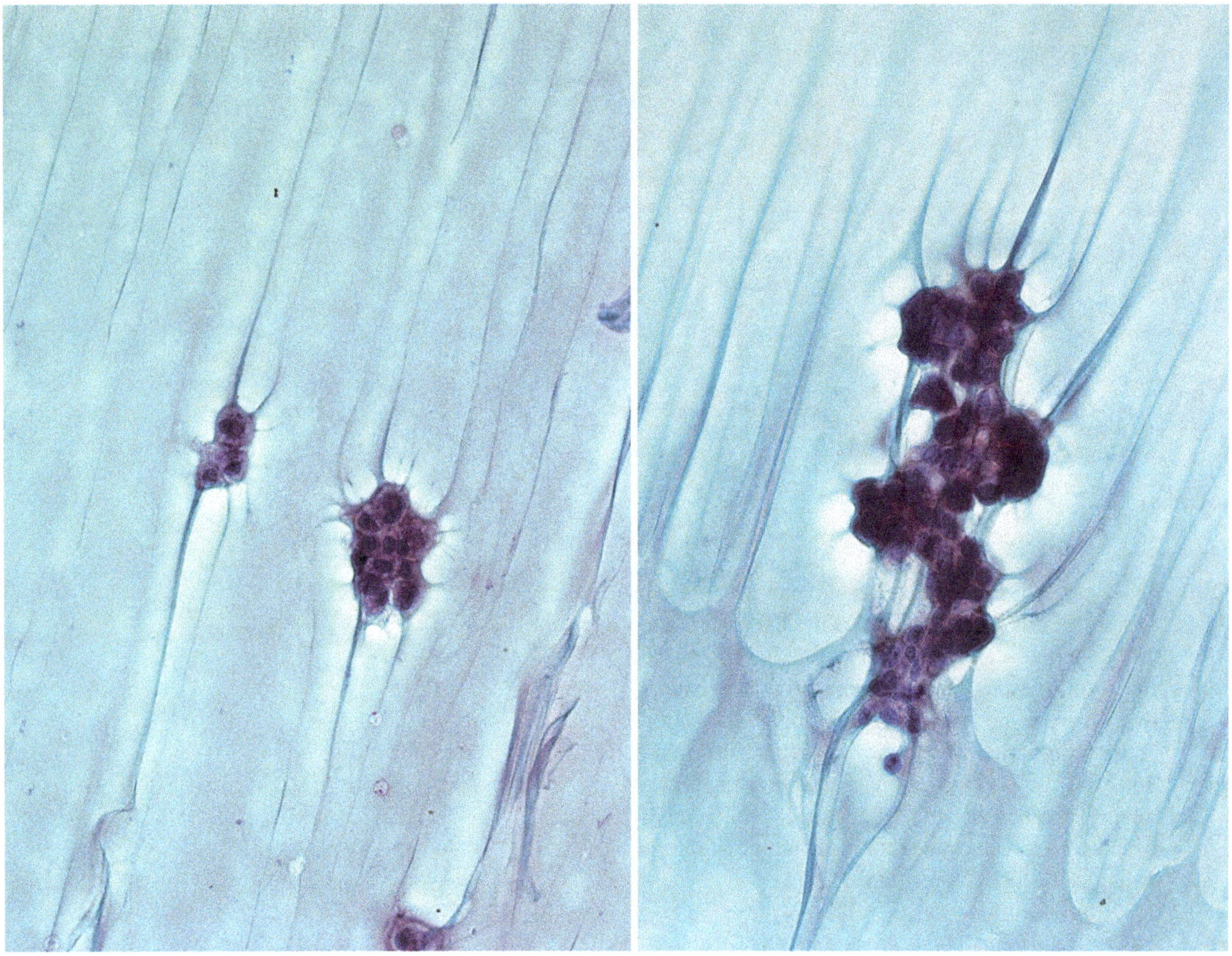

Fig. 10.62

Q-62. This nipple discharge smear is from a 34-year-old who noticed a colorless discharge from the nipple of both her breasts for the past week. On physical examination, the skin was normal, and no mass was palpated. There is no axillary lymphadenopathy. The patient has regular menstrual cycles and is using oral contraceptives. There is colorless nipple discharge which was smeared. Which of the following is the most likely interpretation?

(a) Ductal carcinoma
(b) Physiologic nipple discharge
(c) Fibrocystic changes
(d) Fibroadenoma
(e) Intraductal papilloma

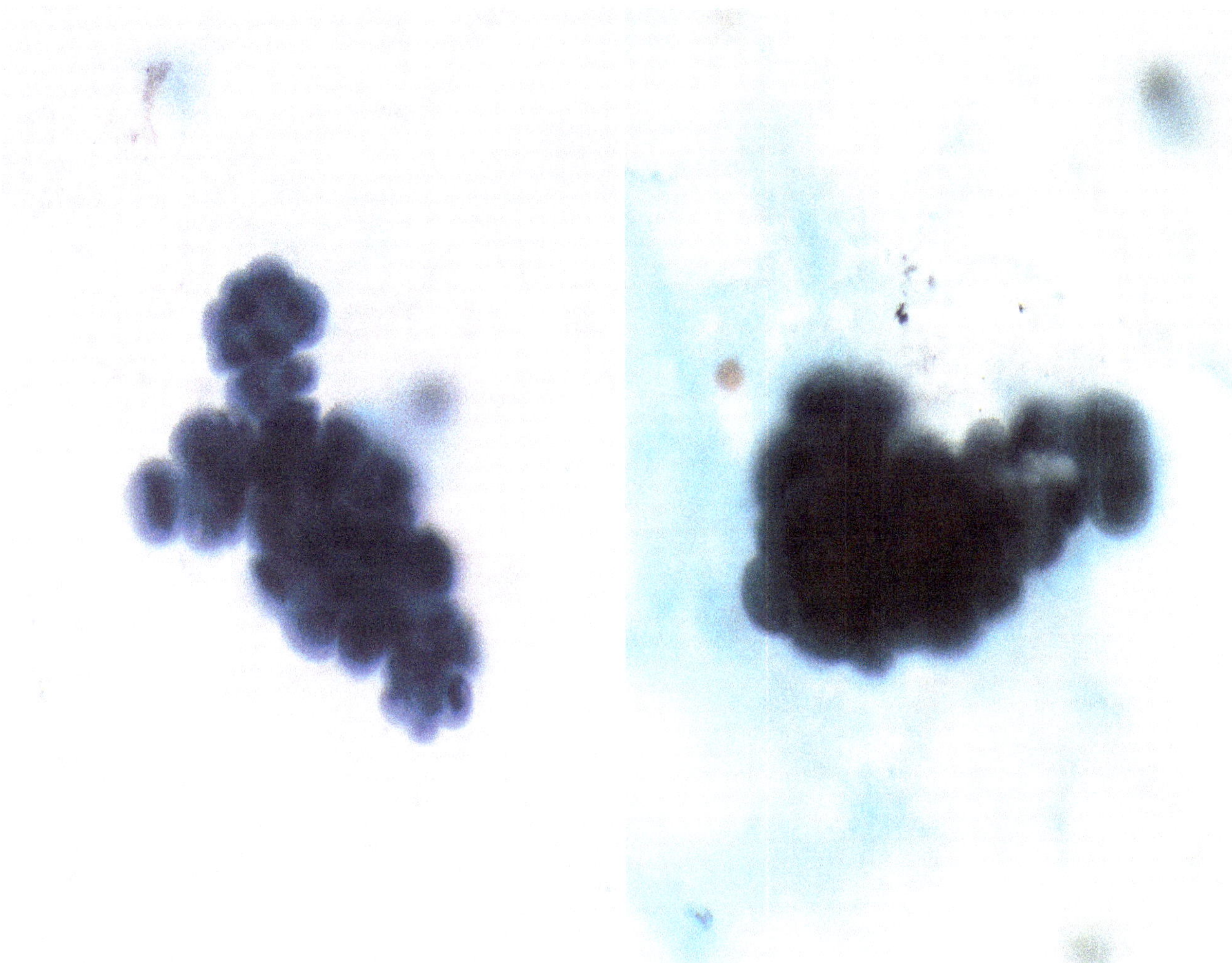

Fig. 10.63

Q-63. This nipple discharge smear is from a 49-year-old who has noticed a bloody discharge from the nipple of her right breast for the past week. On physical examination, the skin is normal, and a small mass in the retro-areolar area was palpated. There is no axillary lymphadenopathy. The nipple discharge was smeared. Excisional biopsy is most likely to show which of the following lesions?

(a) Ductal carcinoma
(b) Fat necrosis
(c) Fibrocystic changes
(d) Fibroadenoma
(e) Intraductal papilloma

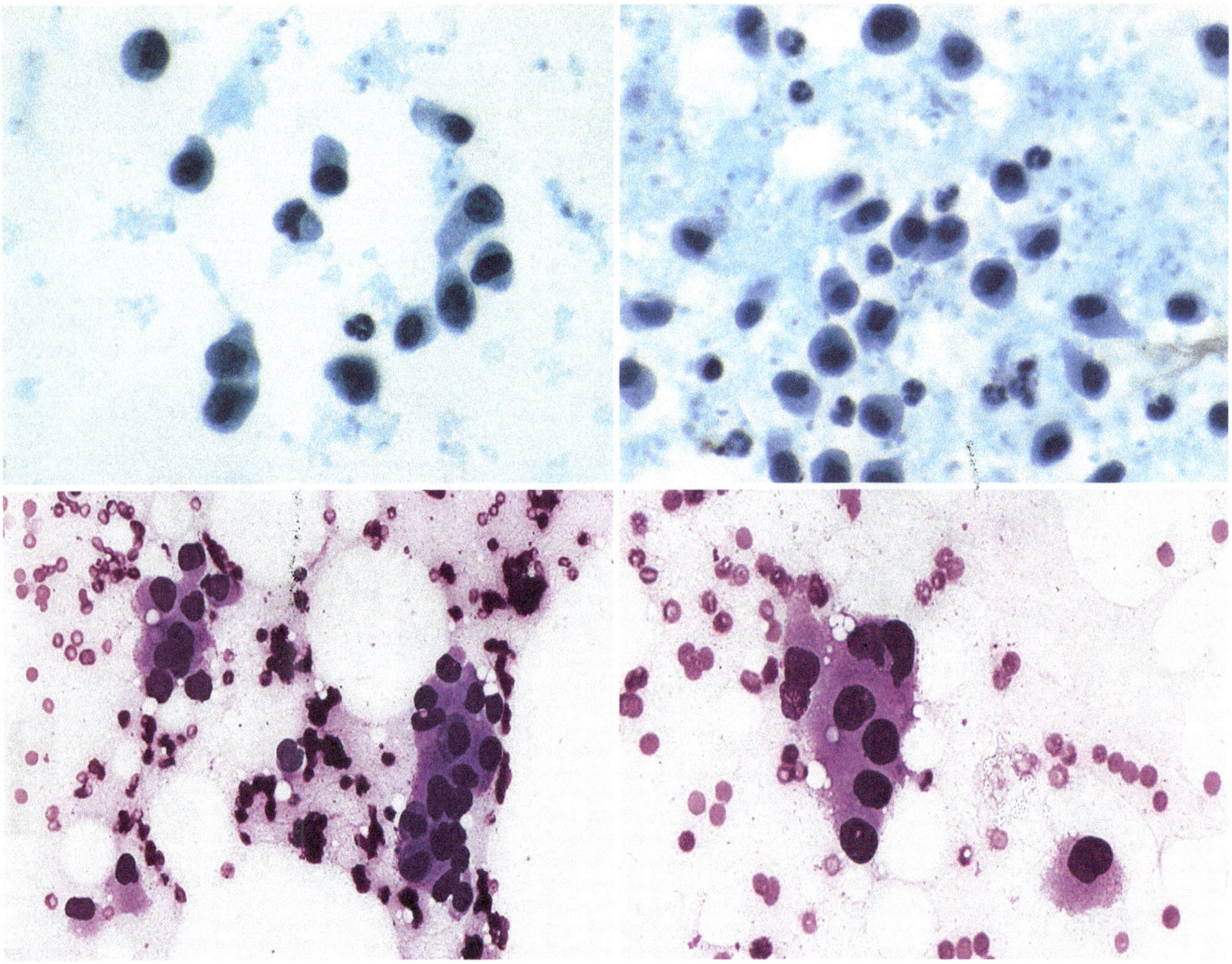

Fig. 10.64

Q-64. This nipple discharge smear is from a 64-year-old who has noticed a bloody discharge from the nipple of her right breast for the past week. On physical examination, the skin is normal, and a large mass located in the retro-areolar area is palpated. There is no axillary lymphadenopathy. The nipple discharge was smeared. Which of the following is the most likely diagnosis?

(a) Ductal carcinoma
(b) Fat necrosis
(c) Fibrocystic changes
(d) Fibroadenoma
(e) Intraductal papilloma

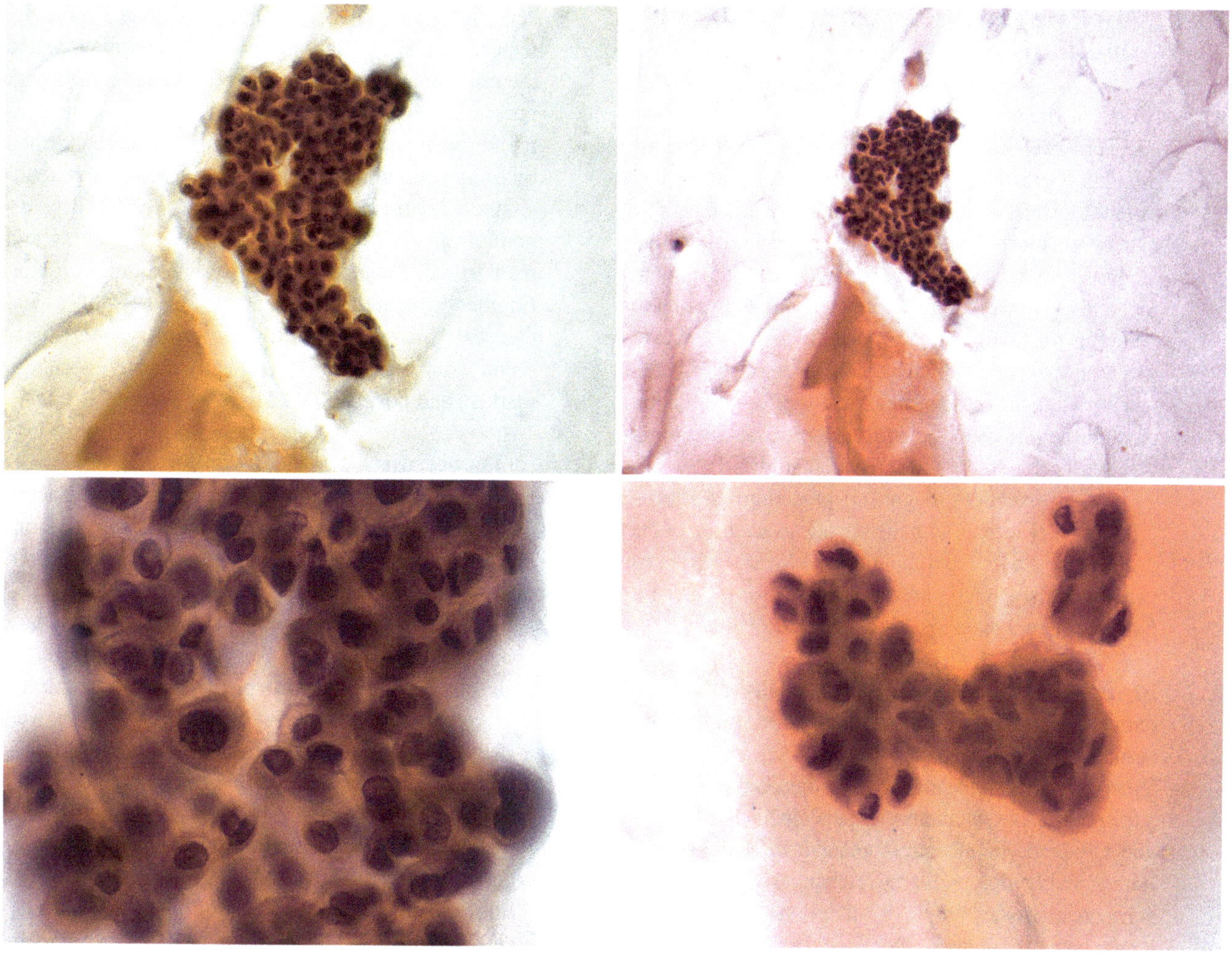

Fig. 10.65

Q-65. This ductal lavage smear is from a 44-year-old who has been on a screening program for her family history of breast cancer. Her physical examination is normal with no axillary lymphadenopathy. Which of the following is the most likely diagnosis?

(a) Unsatisfactory
(b) Ductal epithelium with mild cytological atypia
(c) Ductal epithelium with marked cytological atypia
(d) Ductal carcinoma
(e) Intraductal papilloma

10.4 Answers and Discussion of Text-Based Questions 1–5

A-1. **(e) All of the above**

Breast FBN is economical and cost-effective outpatient procedure. It is a minimally traumatic (physically and psychologically) with high acceptance rate and minimal or no morbidity. It provides rapid and accurate diagnosis offering stress relief of anxiety for the patient for benign diagnosis and more time for pretreatment planning for malignant diagnosis. It permits involvement of the patient in the decision-making process when malignancy is identified, and it offers evaluation of multiple nodules/lesions. It also provides sampling tumor for biomarkers and molecular studies.

It is an excellent diagnostic procedure of cystic/inflammatory lesions with therapeutic evacuation of the cyst. It also offers rapid diagnosis of locally advanced cancer, axillary lymph node metastases, or recurrence for better tumor staging and treatment decision.

A-2. **(d) It offers rapid diagnosis of locally advanced cancer or recurrence for better tumor staging and treatment decision**

Breast FNA lacks the ability to distinguish between in situ and invasive carcinoma, atypical ductal hyperplasia and low-grade in situ carcinoma and low-grade carcinomas and benign proliferative changes which require subsequent tissue biopsy of all lesions with atypical "gray zone" diagnoses. However, breast FNA is an excellent diagnostic procedure of cystic/inflammatory lesions with therapeutic evacuation of the cyst. It also offers rapid diagnosis of locally advanced cancer, axillary lymph node metastases, or recurrence for better tumor staging and treatment decision.

A-3. **(d) Needle tract seeding and epithelial displacement of tumor cells**

Complication of breast FNA includes bleeding, hematoma, infection, pneumothorax, vasovagal reaction, epithelial displacement, tumor seeding, and post-FNA changes that may interfere with image studies. Needle tract seeding and epithelial displacement are extremely rare in breast FNA.

A-4. **(e) Immunohistochemical staining for ER, PR, and GCDFP-15 is helpful**

Primary neuroendocrine carcinomas of the breast are a rare variant of breast carcinoma, constituting about 2–5 % of invasive breast carcinomas. Patients are usually older, in the 60–70-year-old age range. Most patients present with a palpable mass. On mammography, the tumor presents as a well-circumscribed nodule. The prognosis of these patients is grave. Smears are highly cellular and consist of a monotonous population of small round blue cells, arranged in a single cell discohesive pattern. There is nuclear molding, hyperchromasia, "salt-and-pepper" chromatin, and inconspicuous nucleoli. Karyorrhexis and mitoses with nuclear crush artifact are seen in cell clusters. The neuroendocrine nature of these tumors can be confirmed by using neuroendocrine markers. Differential diagnosis includes metastatic carcinoid or small cell carcinoma from the lung. A history of heavy smoking and mediastinal mass favor a metastatic tumor. Immunohistochemical staining for ER, PR, and GCDFP-15 is not helpful, since primary breast neuroendocrine carcinomas are usually negative for these markers and positive for TTF-1.

A-5. **(c) Fat necrosis**

Fat necrosis shows variable cellularity consisting of abundant lipid-laden macrophages (lipophages), hemosiderin-laden macrophages, amorphous (granular background) debris, and inflammatory cells including neutrophils, plasma cells, and lymphocytes. The lipophages have abundant vacuolated cytoplasm. Multinucleated foreign-body-type giant cells and spindle-shaped fibroblastic cells can also be present. Fragments of normal as well as degenerating adipose tissue with free lipid droplets are seen. Fat necrosis can mimic carcinoma both clinically and mammographically and is commonly seen in patients who have had a previous surgical biopsy or other trauma to the breast. Fat necrosis may present as a firm, irregular, fixed, and painful breast mass. It may create diagnostic problems if the history of injury is remote or is not recalled by the patient. Fat necrosis may also be encountered in male patients. Secretory carcinoma of the breast is a rare variant and it affects young female patients. It is characterized by large amounts of intracellular and extracellular secretions and cells with abundant, granular, eosinophilic cytoplasm arranged in papillary, tubular, or solid structures. Shinagawa and colleagues believe that the grapelike cluster of vacuolated cells may be a helpful cytological feature for the diagnosis of secretory carcinoma. Cytological findings of breast cystic hypersecretory duct carcinoma include the presence of mildly atypical epithelial cells arranged singly and in small groups and sheets of cells set in a background of abundant, intensely staining, pink-to-purple thyroid-like colloid material that has a bubbly, fractured, or cracking artifact appearance in the smears. The differential diagnosis includes lipid-rich carcinoma, characterized by the presence of abundant cytoplasmic fat in the majority of tumor cells. Smears consist of neoplastic cells with large, foamy, and vacuolated cytoplasm. Positive staining of fatty droplets with oil red O stain in lipid-rich carcinoma may be helpful in this differential. Basal-like carcinoma tends to occur in younger patients with an African ethnicity and is associated with a poorer prognosis. Basal-like breast carcinomas are characterized by highly pleomorphic cells.

10.5 Answers and Discussion of Image-Based Questions 6–65

A-6. **(a) Unsatisfactory for evaluation**

The images represent the cytological findings of an unsatisfactory (nondiagnostic) specimen. The unsatisfactory heading is used for various reasons: poor technique, obscuring blood or inflammation, paucicellular material, etc. We do not encourage the use of "negative for malignancy" term when a specimen is unsatisfactory for interpretation. A negative FNA result is more reliable when a specific diagnosis corroborates a clinical and radiological impression (e.g., fibroadenoma, lactating adenoma). The false-negative rate is greatly reduced in patients with a triple-negative test.

The M.D. Anderson Cancer Center Group proposes that four to six well-visualized cell groups consisting of at least six cells in each cluster and more than ten cells per flat sheet constitute an adequate specimen. On occasion, the diagnosis of breast carcinoma can be made on a scantly cellular specimen, while another case having abundant cellularity may not lend itself to a definitive diagnosis.

A-7. **(c) Lipoma**

The images represent the cytological findings of lipoma. Adipose tissue is commonly found in breast aspirates as a component of normal breast tissue. The presence of fat in the smears usually results from inadequate sampling of a palpable mass, representing inadvertent aspiration of the surrounding nondiagnostic breast adipose tissue. Although it is generally accepted that FNA specimens that lack epithelial cells are considered inadequate, there are certain exceptions. If a lesion regresses after aspiration or yields only fat when a lipoma diagnosis is suspected, smear may be deemed adequate even if it is paucicellular. However, the diagnosis of a breast lipoma can only be suggested if there is strong mammographic correlation.

A-8. **(c) Fat necrosis**

The images represent the cytological findings of fat necrosis. The smears show variable cellularity and consist of abundant lipid-laden macrophages (lipophages), hemosiderin-laden macrophages, amorphous (granular background) debris, and inflammatory cells including neutrophils, plasma cells, and lymphocytes. The lipophages have abundant vacuolated cytoplasm. Multinucleated foreign-body-type giant cells and spindle-shaped fibroblastic cells can also be present. Fragments of normal as well as degenerating adipose tissue with free lipid droplets are seen.

The rare hibernoma of the breast should be considered in the differential diagnosis when finely and coarsely vacuolated cells are encountered. Reactive epithelial atypia and epithelioid histiocytes associated with fat necrosis can be over-interpreted as breast cancer.

Fat necrosis can mimic carcinoma both clinically and mammographically and is commonly seen in patients who have had a previous surgical biopsy or other trauma to the breast. Fat necrosis may present as a firm, irregular, fixed, and painful breast mass. It may create diagnostic problems if the history of injury is remote or is not recalled by the patient. Fat necrosis may also be encountered in male patients.

A-9. **(d) Acute mastitis/breast abscess**

The images represent the cytological findings of acute mastitis. Smear cellularity depends on the clinical stage of the abscess: high cellularity in acute/active stage and low cellular in the subacute/chronic stage due to fibrosis. In acute phase, smears demonstrate abundant acute inflammatory cells: neutrophils and foamy macrophages with evidence of cytophagocytosis. Abundant cell debris is observed in the background. Isolated cells and clusters of epithelial cells with reactive (repair) atypia are also seen, which may lead to a suspicion of malignancy. In a repair reaction, however, the N:C ratios are usually within normal limits, with cells having a streaming pattern and no loss of polarity. Cytological features not supportive of a diagnosis of carcinoma also include limited epithelial cellularity and degenerating atypical cells in an inflammatory setting, as well as only a few intact single epithelial cells.

Breast abscess often presents as a palpable breast lesion with varying degrees of pain and tenderness. Most inflammatory lesions of the breast are secondary to bacterial infection. The breast can rarely be involved with tuberculosis, fungal, and/or viral infections. Aspiration can be a therapeutic procedure to evacuate the abscess. In addition, aspirated material provides enough material for microbiological studies.

A-10. **(d) Subareolar abscess**

The images represent the cytological findings of subareolar abscess. The smears are usually hypercellular and demonstrate a spectrum of cytomorphologic findings, including the presence of anucleated squamous cells associated with chronic inflammation, cholesterol crystals, keratinous debris, parakeratosis, and strips of squamous epithelium. A foreign-body reaction with sheets of histiocytes and multinucleated foreign-body-type giant cells can also be present. Ductal epithelium and granulation tissue with varying degree of reactive atypia can be appreciated. Subareolar abscess has also been reported in the FNA of the male breast with similar findings.

With the presence of nipple retraction and a mass, the lesion can be clinically confused with breast carcinoma. Subareolar abscess smears may demonstrate some of the potential diagnostic pitfalls for a false-positive diagnosis due to the presence of inflammatory or repair atypia and fragments of exuberant granulation tissue. The differential diagnosis includes a ruptured epidermal inclusion cyst arising in the skin overlying the breast. However, the peripheral location of the epidermal inclusion cyst should clearly distinguish this lesion from the central subareolar abscess.

Subareolar abscess is a specific clinicopathologic entity. It occurs in the subareolar region as a result of squamous metaplasia of lactiferous ducts, with subsequent keratin plugging, dilatation, and rupture of the ducts, associated with low-grade infection. Subareolar abscess has high recurrence, and surgery is the only line of curative treatment.

A-11. (**c**) **Plasma cell mastitis**

The images represent the cytological findings of plasma cell mastitis. The smears are characterized by amorphous debris with variable numbers of foamy macrophages and other inflammatory cells. Occasionally, ductal cells may be present, showing a variable degree of inflammatory atypia. The degree of atypia appears greater in the Romanowsky-stained air-dried smears (i.e., Diff-Quik stain) than in Papanicolaou-stained alcohol-fixed smears owing to greater cell size in the former type of smear. Appreciation of the inflammatory background in which the atypia is present serves as a check to avoid a false-positive diagnosis of malignancy.

Plasma cell mastitis is a common chronic inflammatory condition of the breast that may mimic carcinoma by showing nipple retraction with an underlying well-defined, centrally located lesion. Mammography may reveal calcifications. The aspirated material is characteristically thick, creamy, and homogenous.

A-12. (**d**) **Granulomatous mastitis**

The images represent the cytological findings of granulomatous mastitis. Smears are usually hypercellular and demonstrate granulomatous reaction in the form of single or loose clusters of epithelioid histiocytes, with or without associated multinucleated giant cells, lymphocytes, and plasma cells. Fragments of ductal epithelium with reactive atypia can be seen.

Granulomatous mastitis can be seen in different breast lesions including sarcoidosis, infectious granulomas (secondary to tuberculosis, fungi, leprosy, or brucellosis), fat necrosis, ruptured epidermal inclusion cyst, foreign-body reaction as in suture or silicone granulomas, and idiopathic granulomatous mastitis. Clues to the specific diagnosis include the presence of necrotic background in caseating granulomas, positive culture and special stains for organisms in infectious cases, foreign material in the foreign-body granulomatous inflammation, or tight non-caseating granulomas in sarcoidosis.

A-13. (**c**) **Silicone granuloma**

The images represent the cytological findings of silicone granulomas. Silicone granulomas are often associated with ruptured silicone tissue expanders. Exuberant proliferative tissue reaction may result in single or multiple nodules simulating malignancy. Smears are usually moderately cellular and contain amorphous, nonstaining material in Diff-Quik-stained smears (pools of liquid silicone), surrounded by epithelioid histiocytes and foamy macrophages containing numerous empty vacuoles with foreign-body-type giant cells "silicone granulomata." Degenerated vacuolated adipocytes mimicking fat necrosis can be seen.

A-14. (**d**) **Benign breast cyst**

The images represent the cytological findings of benign breast cysts. Single or multiple cysts are the most prevalent lesions of the female breast. Although aspiration of breast cysts is an ideal procedure for both diagnosis and treatment, some have questioned the utility of cytologically examining all cyst fluid. A lesion is considered to be a breast cyst when greater than 1 mL of fluid is aspirated. The aspirated cyst fluid may be clear, opaque, or turbid and may vary in color from green or brown to bloodstained. Fluid is almost always acellular or quite limited in cellularity, consisting of a few epithelial cells including apocrine cells and foam cells. Eosinophilic inclusions have been noted in breast cyst fluid and are believed to be giant lysosomes.

After complete aspiration of the cyst, it is especially important to reevaluate the area to determine if a residual breast mass is present. If a residual mass is found, a second aspiration should be performed. Intracystic carcinomas are suspected on the basis of physical examination, mammography, or when bloodstained fluid is aspirated.

A-15. (**d**) **Postsurgical seroma**

The images represent the cytological findings of seroma. In our experience, FNA of a seroma generally shows a clear yellow fluid that is paucicellular containing only a few degenerating foam cells. When squamous metaplasia of the cells lining the seroma cavity occurs, the smears may show epithelial atypia with cells having high nuclear-to-cytoplasmic (N:C) ratios and hyperchromatic nuclei. These atypical squamous metaplastic cells can be a potential pitfall for false-positive diagnoses of malignancy, particularly in the light of patient's history of breast cancer.

In one study, seroma occurred in 40 % of the patients with no closed suction drainage compared to 6 % of patients with closed suction drainage.

A-16. (e) **Fibrocystic changes** (FCC), **nonproliferative type**

The images represent the cytological findings of nonproliferative fibrocystic changes. Aspirations can have limited cellularity owing to the fibrotic nature of the lesions. Smears demonstrate usually cohesive fragments of uniform cells arranged in a honeycomb fashion associated with myoepithelial cells (bipolar stripped or naked nuclei). Benign apocrine cells are arranged as flat sheets; isolated cells are rare. Apocrine cells are large polygonal cells with abundant granular cytoplasm that stains pink or green with the Papanicolaou stain and gray with a Romanowsky stain. Nuclei are centrally located, round, and regular, with prominent eosinophilic nucleoli, and moderate nuclear atypia is present in some cases. Foam cells have abundant vacuolated cytoplasm. An important component of fibrocystic change and an excellent indicator of benignity is the presence of stripped (naked) bipolar nuclei of myoepithelial cells. They have a uniform hyperchromatic chromatin without nucleoli. A background of cystic debris and microcalcifications can occasionally be seen.

Fibrocystic change is the most common lump-producing lesion in women between 30 and 50 years old. The lesions are generally bilateral and multifocal. Presence of moderate and florid ductal hyperplasia is a marker for increased cancer risk, not seen in nonproliferative fibrocystic changes.

A-17. (c) **Fibrocystic changes, proliferative type**

The images represent the cytological findings of proliferative fibrocystic changes. Smears are usually moderately cellular and demonstrate tightly cohesive groups of ductal epithelial fragments and background of bipolar naked nuclei. There are crowded sheets with regular or irregular cell spacing and associated bipolar naked nuclei.

High cellularity, epithelial atypia, slight nuclear overlapping, and mild loss of polarity may lead to a potential false-positive diagnosis of malignancy. The benign nature of these lesions should be suspected when diverse cell types including apocrine, ductal, and histiocytic cells are present and bipolar naked nuclei are found in the smear background and within the epithelial clusters. Proliferative FCC includes a spectrum of breast lesions such as sclerosing adenosis, adenosis tumor, collagenous spherulosis, papillomatosis, and ductal hyperplasia. Proliferative changes are associated with an increased risk for breast cancer.

Adenosis tumor is an entity of proliferative FCC that can be clinically and histologically confused with breast carcinoma. Aspiration cytology reveals changes of proliferative fibrocystic disease without any features to suggest the specific diagnosis of adenosis. In sclerosing adenosis, acinar sheets, scattered individual epithelial cells, and small, dense, hyalinized stroma are usually found. Epithelial cells in sclerosing adenosis appear more frequently as acinar sheets and discohesive individual cells. Awareness of the presence of scattered individual epithelial cells in cytological smears of sclerosing adenosis can help prevent a misdiagnosis of malignancy.

It should be emphasized that differentiation between different entities of proliferative FCC on FNA specimens is challenging and in many times components of multiple lesions can be seen in the same specimen. The interobserver variability in the diagnosis of ductal proliferative lesions is extremely high with poor cytohistologic correlation.

A-18. (e) **Radial scar and sclerosing complex lesions**

Explanation: The images represent the cytological findings of radial scar/complex sclerosing lesion. These benign sclerosing lesions frequently have a small size and fibrosis which makes the aspiration of sufficient cells difficult. When a sample is obtained, it is generally scanty and shows a mixture of small groups and some dissociated epithelial cells and a few bipolar cells. Some cases of complex sclerosing lesions have increased cellularity with abundant three-dimensional atypical papillary clusters. Discohesive isolated single cells with intact cytoplasm, high N:C ratios, nuclear hyperchromasia, molding, and nuclear pleomorphism with atypia can be present which can lead to a false-positive diagnosis. Single cells can occasionally show vacuolated cytoplasm simulating a signet ring cell carcinoma. Although the presence of a dual cell population is the main differentiating criterion between benign and malignant papillary neoplasm, myoepithelial cells can also be seen in malignancy, since sampling can retrieve myoepithelial cells from nearby benign breast tissue. A recent study has recommended excision of all radial scar lesions since they may be associated with carcinoma in situ or invasive carcinoma.

A-19. (**a**) **Collagenous spherulosis**

The images represent the cytological findings of collagenous spherulosis. Smears are moderately cellular and consist of scattered, acellular eosinophilic metachromatically staining hyaline globules (best seen on Romanowsky stain), surrounded by monomorphic benign ductal epithelium, with focal branching papillary architecture.

Collagenous spherulosis is an unusual benign breast lesion, characterized by the presence of distinct globular material that can mimic adenoid cystic carcinoma. It is usually seen associated with intraductal papilloma, sclerosing adenosis, or radial scar. The major entity considered in the differential diagnosis is adenoid cystic carcinoma. Collagenous spherulosis is usually an incidental finding, whereas adenoid cystic carcinoma of the breast almost always presents as a palpable mass. The extracellular material of adenoid cystic carcinoma generally lacks the fibrillary appearance associated with collagenous spherulosis. In addition, there is an absence of significant cellular atypia and basaloid morphology of the cells, features usually seen in adenoid cystic carcinoma. A less likely diagnostic consideration is the rare intraductal signet ring carcinoma, distinguished by eccentrically placed atypical nuclei and "spherules" of intracellular mucin rather than the basement membrane material of collagenous spherulosis.

Mucinous spherulosis, a variant of collagenous spherulosis, is characterized by cribriform structures containing lightly basophilic material. Cytological features consist of intermediate to large round hyaline spherules, with or without surrounding myoepithelial cells. This entity can be potentially overdiagnosed as mucinous carcinoma in cytology and histology.

A-20. (**a**) **Adenomyoepithelioma**

The images represent the cytological findings of adenomyoepithelioma. FNA of adenomyoepithelioma usually yields specimens of moderate-to-high cellularity, consisting of a biphasic population of epithelial and myoepithelial cells in varying proportions. Myoepithelial cells can be seen as small, comma-shaped or ovoid, dark nuclei, located in a plane of focus either above or below that of the ductal epithelium or scattered in the background as bipolar, naked nuclei. They can also appear epithelioid, plasmacytoid (hyaline), or spindled, arranged singly or in small clusters. Intranuclear inclusions and intracytoplasmic vacuoles give the impression of a "soap-bubble" appearance and are characteristic for adenomyoepithelioma. A background of naked bipolar nuclei and metachromatic fibromyxoid stroma is seen.

In FNA cytology, the dispersed distribution of the epithelioid myoepithelial cells combined with the high cellularity may potentially lead to a misdiagnosis of carcinoma. Adenomyoepithelioma usually demonstrates more tridimensional and crowded groups and fewer sheets of ductal epithelium than those in fibroadenoma.

Adenomyoepithelioma of the breast is a rare benign neoplasm characterized by a biphasic proliferation of epithelial and myoepithelial cells. It usually presents as a solitary, unilateral lesion. Because of its histological heterogeneity, the diagnosis of adenomyoepithelioma can be challenging on both FNA and core biopsy.

A-21. (**c**) **Proliferative fibrocystic changes with atypia**

The images represent the cytological findings of proliferative fibrocystic changes with atypia (atypical ductal hyperplasia, ADH). Aspirates of ADH are generally highly cellular, with crowded groups consisting of atypical features such as variation in cell size and shape and loss of polarity. The nuclei of the epithelial cells show a greater degree of hyperchromasia, and nucleoli can be readily appreciated. There are small numbers of atypical single cells. Architectural atypia in the form of cribriform-like structures, three-dimensional epithelial fragments with lumens, and complex infolding of epithelial fragments is seen in ADH. However, in contrast to DCIS, myoepithelial cells (bipolar naked nuclei) are present. The epithelial cells have oval-to-round nuclei possessing a bland chromatin pattern.

There is a lack of well-defined criteria for the diagnosis of atypia, leading to high interobserver variability with poor cytohistologic correlation. The NCI has recognized this problem and has created a category of atypical/indeterminate. Some investigators subdivided this category into atypical, probably benign, suspicious, and probably malignant. They found that the majority of cases having suspicious findings proved to be malignant, while about 50 % of cases with atypical findings turned out to be carcinoma. Other investigators found no specific morphologic criteria to reliably differentiate benign from malignant lesions in cases diagnosed with atypia. In our study we implement the use of IHC such as CK5/6 and p63 on cell block as helpful markers. Cases show positive staining for CK5/6 in more than 25 % of the cells clusters proved to be benign epithelial proliferation.

It is generally agreed that FNA cytology cannot reliably distinguish ADH from a low grade of DCIS. Therefore, surgical biopsy confirmation is required. However, atypical hyperplasia can usually be distinguished from high-grade DCIS by markedly pleomorphic cells associated with a necrotic background. Cytological features favoring DCIS over ADH include more single discohesive atypical cells, loosely arranged epithelial fragments, prominent anisonucleosis, coarser nuclear chromatin, and a background of inflammatory cells.

In proliferative FCC without atypia, some of the epithelial clusters can be folded or angulated, and secondary irregular lumen formation can be present. Some cytological variation in cell size and shape is noted within the groups, but single intact epithelial cells are either not present or very scarce.

A-22. **(e) Pleomorphic adenoma**

The images represent the cytological findings of pleomorphic adenoma (chondroid syringoma, benign mixed tumor). Pleomorphic adenoma of the breast shows cytological features identical to its more common salivary gland counterpart. Smears are hypercellular and consist of cohesive epithelial fragments, stromal mesenchymal tissue, and myoepithelial cells. Prominent chondromyxoid stroma can be identified.

Pleomorphic adenoma of the breast is a rare benign tumor, with patients ranging age from 23 to 78 years. Clinically, pleomorphic adenoma presents as a firm, non-tender, and mobile mass. Mammogram can reveal a mass with poorly outlined borders that suggests a malignant process.

A-23. **(b) Lactating adenoma**

The images represent the cytological findings of lactating adenoma (LA). Smears are usually highly cellular and consist of clusters of large cells with prominent nucleoli and foamy cytoplasm. Cytoplasm is extremely fragile and wispy. There is a dirty background caused by disruption of the delicate, frayed pale cytoplasm and spillage of the secretory product into the background caused by the trauma of smearing the slides. There are numerous, round, naked, stripped nuclei in the background, with prominent nucleoli. Numerous inflammatory cells with few macrophages are seen. De novo lactating adenomas have few or no bipolar nuclei but contain scattered stripped epithelial nuclei.

Most breast lesions in pregnant and postpartum patients are benign and are secondary to hormonal stimulation of the breast tissue in pregnant patients. During pregnancy and lactation, the ductules of the terminal duct lobular unit become hyperplastic and manifest cytoplasmic vacuolization and luminal secretion. Although most breast masses in pregnancy are benign, breast carcinoma in a pregnant woman needs to be excluded. FNA in this setting may be especially useful because a diagnosis of pregnancy or lactational changes could at least postpone and even spare the woman an excisional biopsy.

Occasionally, a false-positive diagnosis of malignancy is possible due to nuclear atypicality and prominent nucleoli, mimicking breast carcinoma. It is especially important to appreciate the presence of cytoplasmic secretion characterized by cytoplasmic foaminess or vacuolation with fraying of cytoplasmic borders, in order to avoid a false-positive diagnosis. In addition, the prominent nucleoli of an LA are absent in invasive lobular cancers. In general, ductal cancers do not have the foamy background or the acinar structure seen in lactating adenoma. Also, the nuclei in ductal cancers are more hyperchromatic, the nucleoli are less prominent, and the cytoplasm is less wispy than in LA. Ductal carcinomas show a greater degree of nuclear atypia, necrosis, hyperchromasia, loss of polarity, and discohesion, with the presence of intact atypical single cells.

A-24. **(e) Fibroadenoma with lactational changes**

The images represent the cytological findings of fibroadenoma with lactational changes. Smears are usually highly cellular and show similar cytological features to fibroadenoma. Both lactating adenomas and fibroadenomas have similar cytological features. However, a history of preexisting breast nodule before pregnancy favors the diagnosis of fibroadenoma with lactational changes. Fibroadenoma generally produces a cell-rich smear pattern containing a biphasic pattern of epithelial clusters and numerous bipolar naked nuclei which are appreciated in addition to the lactational changes. In contrast, de novo lactating adenomas have few or no bipolar nuclei but contain scattered stripped epithelial nuclei.

A-25. **(d) Galactocele**

The images represent the cytological findings of galactocele. Galactocele arises shortly after pregnancy, during lactation. The diagnosis is confirmed by the aspiration of milk. The smears show abundant secretory material with scattered foamy macrophages and rare epithelial cells.

A-26. **(d) Gynecomastia**

The images represent the cytological findings of gynecomastia. Smears usually show moderate cellularity and consist of large cohesive ductal epithelial fragments, often papillary-like or as monolayered cells. The cytomorphologic spectrum ranges from benign ductal cells to florid gynecomastia changes including a fibroadenoma-like picture, with cohesive sheets of bland cells and columnar cells. Atypical discohesive single epithelial cells are rarely observed. A scattered background of bipolar naked myoepithelial nuclei and occasional fragments of metachromatic stroma/fibrous tissue are seen.

Breast carcinoma and carcinoid tumor have also been reported in male breast. The diagnosis of malignancy should be avoided unless the aspirate shows frankly malignant cytological features and totally lacks myoepithelial cells. It is important to remember that male breast carcinoma is extremely rare.

Gynecomastia is the male breast enlargement caused by both hypertrophy and hyperplasia of the ductal epithelial and stromal components as a result of hormonal activity. It occurs most frequently in adolescent and elderly male patients. Unlike HIV-infected women who present with different breast lesions, HIV-positive males will most likely present with gynecomastia associated with antiretroviral therapy. It is more often unilateral, although bilateral cases can occur (2:1 unilateral to bilateral).

A-27. (**b**) **Radiation effect**

The images represent the cytological findings of radiation effect. FNA cytology specimens in this setting are generally hypocellular and consist of small fragments and dissociated epithelial cells with significant cytological atypia. There is significant nuclear pleomorphism with large nuclei and occasional prominent eosinophilic nucleoli. However, the nuclei show degenerative changes, with nuclear and cytoplasmic vacuolization. In addition, the nuclear-to-cytoplasmic ratio is low. There are chronic inflammatory cells in the background.

Radiation change in normal breast epithelium is observed with increasing frequency because of the widespread use of lumpectomy and radiation to treat patients with breast cancer. The significant atypia induced by radiation can lead to an erroneous false-positive diagnosis of cancer on aspiration. Knowledge of prior irradiation therapy is crucial in order to avoid a potential false-positive diagnosis of malignancy. In addition, recurrent carcinomas usually demonstrate a moderately to highly cellular smear with many atypical cells with high nuclear-to-cytoplasmic ratio. The absence of isolated cells and necrotic cell debris is a useful finding to rule out cancer. Comparison with the morphology of the original tumor is recommended to confirm the diagnosis.

A-28. (**d**) **Amyloid tumor**

The images represent the cytological findings of amyloid tumor. The aspirate is sparsely cellular and shows aggregates of birefringent dense irregular amorphous material of varying sizes, some with embedded nuclei of lymphomononuclear cells. The waxy hyaline nature is highlighted on Pap stain. Congo red stain shows apple green birefringence. A background of numerous lymphocytes with occasional multinucleated giant cells is seen. The differential diagnosis includes adenoid cystic carcinoma and chondroid syringoma.

Primary amyloid breast tumor presents as an indeterminate mass clinically and radiologically. The breast can be involved in a localized amyloidosis or as part of systemic amyloidosis. Patients often do not have clinical or pathologic evidence of amyloidosis, such as monoclonal gammopathy or plasma cell dyscrasia.

A-29. (**d**) **Granular cell tumor of the breast**

The images represent the cytological findings of granular cell tumor. FNA cytological examination usually reveals a moderately cellular smear consisting of scattered groups of cells with low N:C ratio, abundant granular cytoplasm, and indistinct cell borders intersected by arborizing thin-wall blood vessels. The nuclei are round to oval, uniform in size, and have an evenly dispersed chromatin pattern, with inconspicuous nucleoli. Numerous naked "stripped-off" nuclei in a granular smear background are seen. The cytoplasm of granular cells stains red with Papanicolaou stain, and PAS stain accentuates the granules. Immunoperoxidase stains on cytological material demonstrate S-100 and carcinoembryonic antigen (CEA) positivity.

A discohesive nature of the cells with large amounts of granular cytoplasm may mimic histiocytes or apocrine carcinoma. Apocrine carcinoma should be suspected when there is hypercellularity, marked nuclear atypia, and pronounced cell dyshesion; however, occasional marked variation in nuclear size is also seen in some cases of granular cell tumor.

Granular cell tumor is an uncommon breast lesion, affecting mainly middle-aged black women. Clinically and radiologically, granular cell tumors of the breast can closely mimic breast carcinoma (often fixed to the overlying skin). FNA is crucial for the definitive diagnosis.

A-30. (**e**) **Intraductal papilloma**

The images represent the cytological findings of intraductal papilloma. Smears are usually moderately cellular and reveal large cohesive epithelial cells arranged in tight sheets or three-dimensional papillary clusters with fibrovascular cores. Clusters have often scalloped edges. Spindle-shaped stromal cells also are present occasionally. Smaller papillary fragments with intact tips or "anatomical edges" are often seen. Columnar epithelial cells with palisading arrangement and nuclear stratification can be seen. There is a background of blood, foam cells, and hemosiderin-laden macrophages.

Papillomas can also be confused with fibroadenomas, because both can have branching epithelial groups. The presence of columnar epithelial cells, stromal cores, or foam cells favors a papilloma, whereas increased numbers of bipolar naked nuclei favor fibroadenoma. Because differentiating a benign papilloma from a well-differentiated papillary carcinoma can be difficult, surgical excision is advised when a papillary lesion is encountered. Infarcted intraductal papilloma has the potential for a false-positive diagnosis of malignancy. The aspirates may yield a high number of degenerated atypical epithelial cells with necrotic debris, mimicking breast malignancy.

Papilloma is a benign tumor, often arising in one of the large subareolar lactiferous ducts. Solitary papillomas occur most frequently in women from 50 to 60 years of age. Patients often present with unilateral serous, bloody nipple secretion or discrete subareolar mass. Intraductal hyperplasia with papillary architecture, "papillomatosis," is a nonspecific entity and different from intraductal papillomas.

A-31. (**e**) **Papillary carcinoma**

The images represent the cytological findings of papillary carcinoma (PC). Characteristic cytological features include the presence of three-dimensional papillary groups, along with scattered columnar cells and a bloody diathesis with hemosiderin-laden macrophages. Papillary carcinoma generally demonstrates a monomorphous population of abundant isolated columnar cells with intact cytoplasm in a hemorrhagic background, raising the suspicion of malignancy.

The distinction between intraductal papilloma and PC is very difficult to establish by FNA. The National Cancer Institute (NCI) sponsored a conference for revising guidelines for FNA of the breast placed mammary papillary lesions into an indeterminate category, as the criteria for distinguishing benign from malignant papillary lesions by cytological examination are not well established. Cytological features that favor PC are high cellularity, monomorphic population, complex branching with numerous thin fronds, mostly thin fibrovascular cores, marked discohesion, crowded and disorderly columnar cells, and abundant single detached papillae with mild to moderate nuclear hyperchromasia. The presence and appearance of fibrovascular cores are significantly different in PC and papilloma: fibrovascular cores are thicker in papilloma and tend to be incompletely aspirated and appear either as a small thick fibrous portion of the periphery of the branching fragments or separately detached. In contrast, PC shows well-defined thin fibrovascular cores in the branching fragments. Atypical papillary lesions share with papillomas' thick fibrovascular cores, simple branching papillae, and polymorphous cell populations. It is best, therefore, to recommend an excisional biopsy when a breast mass has a papillary appearance on FNA.

The similarity of PC to an FA can be striking. FA often presents with folded branching clusters, with moderate-to-numerous bipolar nuclei in the background. Naked nuclei may also be present but considerably less than in fibroadenoma. In addition, the naked nuclei from papillary carcinoma are often larger, more elongated, and rounder than the benign bipolar nuclei of fibroadenomas.

PC represents 1–2 % of breast carcinomas and is associated with a favorable prognosis. About one-half of PCs arise in the central portion of the breast and cause a discharge from the nipple.

A-32. (**d**) **Fibroadenoma**

The images represent the cytological findings of fibroadenoma. The aspirate may appear sticky and tenacious, often clogging the needle lumen. Smears are usually highly cellular with a characteristic biphasic cell population (epithelial and mesenchymal/stromal components). Epithelial ductal cells demonstrate large sheets arranged in tightly cohesive honeycomb groupings. The branching antler-horn cluster pattern of the epithelial cells is fairly characteristic, but not absolutely specific for the diagnosis of fibroadenoma. Numerous naked bipolar nuclei are seen mainly scattered in the smear background with a "rice grain morphology"; some bipolar nuclei may be associated within sheets of epithelial cells. Smears show fragments of fibrous stroma with occasional chondromyxoid changes, having a bright metachromatic or magenta-colored appearance on Diff-Quik®-stained smears. Juvenile fibroadenoma tends to have a more monomorphic appearance with predominantly larger epithelial fragments of blander uniform columnar types of cells.

Fibroadenoma (FA) is the most common benign tumor of the female breast, more common in young women. FA usually presents as a solitary, firm, discrete, well-circumscribed nodule (usually 2–3 cm), freely mobile in the breast. It can be multiple and bilateral.

A-33. (**a**) **Fibroadenoma**

The images represent the cytological findings of fibroadenoma (FA). The aspirate may appear hypercellular with prominent cytological atypia and isolated cells with cytoplasm, a highly characteristic feature of ductal carcinoma, but seen in about 20 % of FA. Conversely, well-differentiated invasive ductal carcinoma and DCIS can show naked nuclei, mimicking the bipolar cells seen in FA. Most single epithelial cells on FNAs from carcinomas are round to oval with eccentric nuclei, and those from FAs are elongated or columnar with cytoplasm on both sides of the nucleus. Smears with equivocal findings should be reported as atypical. FCC is another differential diagnosis for FA. FAs are more cellular with more naked bipolar nuclei. Stromal fragments and papillary antler-like configurations, seen in many (but not all) FAs, are uncommon in FCC.

It has published that honeycomb sheets, antler-horn clusters, and stromal fragments are the most useful features in distinguishing fibroadenoma from ductal carcinoma. The presence of fingerlike projections (antler-like clusters) and bipolar naked nuclei in the background should suggest the correct diagnosis of fibroadenoma. In our and others' experience, there may be no significant cytological differences between phyllodes tumor and fibroadenoma in terms of stromal or epithelial appearance. The only reliable cytomorphologic feature discriminating between these lesions is the presence of long spindle cells comprising >30 % of the single cell background.

A-34. (**a**) **Phyllodes tumor**

The images represent the cytological findings of benign phyllodes tumor. Smears are usually highly cellular and consist of biphasic cell population. In benign phyllodes (the majority of cases), smears are epithelial predominant forming large folded bland-appearing cohesive epithelial fragments, associated with large stromal fragments. Stromal fragments are cellular with monomorphic cells. Dissociated spindle and stromal cells with plump fusiform nuclei, associated with myxoid or mucinous stromal tissue, are seen. Occasional multinucleated giant cells, apocrine cells, and foam cells are seen.

Cytological distinction of phyllodes tumor from fibroadenoma has been predominantly based on assessment of the cellularity of the stromal fragments. Highly cellular stromal fragments favor phyllodes tumor, in contrast to the relatively limited stromal cellularity of fibroadenoma in FNA specimens. Another helpful criterion favoring phyllodes tumor is the presence of spindle-shaped stromal cells enmeshed in a pink-staining matrix seen on metachromatic stains. In phyllodes tumor, the stromal cells are elongated and have long spindle nuclei with irregular nuclear membranes and occasional nucleoli, in contrast to the bipolar naked nuclei of stromal cells of fibroadenoma. Cytological differentiation of benign from malignant phyllodes tumor is based on the presence of atypical stromal cells and mitoses. In malignant phyllodes tumor, stromal fragments are more predominant and more cellular with significant atypia, mimicking fibrosarcoma.

Prominent epithelial component can be seen in both benign and malignant phyllodes tumor and could potentially lead to a false-positive diagnosis of breast carcinoma. Helpful cytological features suggestive of phyllodes tumor and unusual for breast carcinoma include increased numbers of naked nuclei and hypercellular stromal fragments.

Phyllodes tumors (PTs) are biphasic, composed of an epithelial and a stromal proliferation with prominent and cellular stroma. They are classified into benign, low grade (borderline), and malignant subtypes. They can mimic carcinoma by distorting the breast and even ulcerating the overlying skin. The average age of patients with phyllodes tumor is 45 years, about 20 years older than the average age of patients with fibroadenoma. Most of the patients present with a unilateral slowly enlarging breast mass, with an average size of 5 cm. Phyllodes tumors rarely metastasize, but recurrence has been reported in 15–20 % of cases.

A-35. (**a**) **Ductal carcinoma**

The images represent the cytological findings of an intraductal carcinoma (DCIS). The cytomorphology of DCIS varies according to whether comedo or non-comedo type of DCIS has been aspirated. Aspirates from non-comedo-type/low-grade DCIS show clusters of tumor cells arranged in three-dimensional structures with occasional acinar formation attempts and absence of myoepithelial cells. The background should lack hemorrhage and necrosis. The nuclei have finely granular chromatin with some condensation along the nuclear membrane and small nucleoli. FNA of comedo-type/high-grade DCIS reveals a cellular smear in which loosely cohesive groups of malignant cells show significant nuclear atypia with prominent nucleoli as well as necrosis and mitotic activity. Both comedo and non-comedo types of in situ carcinoma lack increased numbers of atypical single cells in contrast to invasive ductal carcinoma.

It is generally agreed that FNA cytology can differentiate ADH from comedo-type DCIS, although differentiation of ADH from the non-comedo/low-grade type of DCIS is not generally possible. Therefore, surgical biopsy confirmation is required. Similarly, it is not possible to separate comedo-type/

high-grade DCIS from invasive carcinoma, although invasive lesions are generally more cellular and show greater loss of cell cohesion. Extensive necrosis with markedly atypical cells is more often seen in a comedo type of DCIS than in invasive ductal carcinoma, although necrosis can be present in the latter, especially if the carcinoma is large. With the foregoing limitations and management implications, we sign our breast malignancies of ductal origin as ductal carcinoma rather than specify invasive carcinoma or DCIS, due to the inability of FNA to reliably differentiate invasive carcinoma from DCIS. DCIS accounts for 10–20 % of mammographically detected breast carcinoma.

A-36. **(b) Ductal carcinoma**

The images represent the cytological findings of invasive ductal carcinoma, NOS type. Smears usually demonstrate abundant cellularity with groups of loosely cohesive malignant cells and individually scattered tumor cells. The background can be bloody, with occasional necrotic debris, or rarely clean. The cellular pattern shows considerable variability, with tumor cells present in three-dimensional clusters, syncytial groupings, or occasionally in acinar (gland-like) arrangements. The malignant clusters show evidence of loss of polarity and nuclear molding. Individual tumor cells demonstrate malignant cytological features including anisonucleosis, irregular nuclear borders, high N:C ratios, and hyperchromatic, coarsely granular chromatin with small-to-prominent nucleoli. The nuclei can occasionally be eccentric, imparting a plasmacytoid appearance to the cells, most notably appreciated in the Diff-Quik preparation. This pattern is most often seen in aspirates of ductal carcinomas from older women.

Not surprisingly, invasive ductal carcinoma (IDC) and ductal carcinoma in-situ (DCIS) appear identical on cytological examination. The significance of malignant cells embedded in fat or stroma is controversial. Others have found this finding unreliable since benign ductal cells and DCIS are commonly seen in association with fatty tissue. Important clues to the presence of invasion are cell clusters with a tubular structure, cytoplasmic lumen formation in malignant cells, fibroblast proliferation, and fragments of elastoid stroma. Although these features may be specific, sensitivity is low. IDC is usually graded by a combination of nuclear and architectural features; thus, FNA is of limited use in grading breast carcinomas.

Invasive ductal carcinoma (IDC) is the most common malignant tumor of the breast, accounting for about 75 % of all breast cancers. IDC is almost invariably solid and can be detected by palpation or mammography. These tumors are rare in women below the age of 40. They usually present as a hard, painless, and fixed breast mass. Overlying skin may show puckering, peau d'orange changes, ulceration, or nipple retraction. Mammographically, breast carcinoma presents as a poorly defined spiculated mass with and without microcalcifications. Occasionally, IDC may present as a well-defined mass on mammography.

A-37. **(e) Tubular carcinoma**

The images represent the cytological findings of tubular carcinoma (TC). Smears show variable cellularity and consist of cohesive epithelial fragments with prominent tubular architecture. The tubules have rigid walls, often showing an open lumen with angulated tubular structures. This cytological feature is considered to be characteristic for TC. Cells show minimal atypia with nuclear monomorphism. A few fragments of densely collagenized fibrous tissue are seen.

TC usually tends to be smaller in size, with a more favorable prognosis than for those patients with IDC, NOS type. It constitutes 1–2 % of breast cancers with an average patient age of 50 years. TC can be multicentric and bilateral. The mammogram shows an ill-defined, spiculated mass, mimicking radial scar.

TC is an important cause of false-negative FNA results and can masquerade as fibroepithelial lesions. The diagnosis of tubular carcinoma is confounded by the presence of myoepithelial cells in some of the cases. However, the tumor cells tend to be arranged in smaller groups than those of fibroadenoma or ductal proliferative lesions. The presence of angular/rigid glands composed of atypical monomorphic cells, isolated epithelial cells, and nuclear atypia warrants consideration of the diagnosis of TC. Isolated cells with intact cytoplasm can also be seen in fibroadenoma. However, the presence of nuclear atypia and nuclear hyperchromasia is highly characteristic of malignancy. Nuclei with a single, small, uniform nucleolus, stromal fragments, and bipolar cells are characteristic of fibroadenoma.

A-38. **(b) Invasive lobular carcinoma**

The images represent the cytological findings of invasive lobular carcinoma (ILC). Aspirates are variable in cellularity but usually show low cellularity. Smears consist of a monomorphic population of mildly atypical cells arranged individually, in small aggregates, or thin linear cords, with an absence of myoepithelial cells, key features for the diagnosis of ILC. The presence of scant cytoplasm, vesicular nuclei with smooth/mildly irregular nuclear membranes, inconspicuous nucleoli, and low cellularity were found helpful in the correct diagnosis of lobular carcinoma. The cells are relatively small and have increased N:C ratios. The nuclei vary from hypochromatic to mildly hyperchromatic. Another helpful feature is the presence of eccentric nuclei with intracytoplasmic lumina containing mucin droplets, which can distort the nucleus. Because of the scant cellularity, most cases are diagnosed as "atypical" or "suspicious." The presence of signet-ring cells represents a poor prognostic factor.

ILC is one of the most difficult breast cancers to diagnose by FNA. Because of the limited cellularity and the presence of mild atypia of the cells, a false-negative diagnosis is quite possible. As with ductal carcinoma, it is not possible to distinguish ILC from its precursor lesion, lobular carcinoma in situ (LCIS), by FNA. Some authors believe that ILCs are more cellular and discohesive, with greater nuclear atypia and pleomorphism than LCIS.

Differentiating ductal from lobular carcinoma of the breast in FNA cytology specimens can be challenging. The presence of coarsely granular chromatin and large nuclei are helpful diagnostic cytological features of ductal carcinoma. On the other hand, intracytoplasmic vacuoles, nuclear grooves, and linear arrangement of the cells are features of lobular carcinoma.

ILC constitutes about 10–15 % of primary breast carcinomas. It usually presents as a vague breast lesion, which may be readily palpable or visible. Mammographically, it can present as an asymmetrical density with no clearly delineated margin and no or little architectural distortion, usually without microcalcifications. Multifocal infiltrating lobular carcinoma may present with minimal distortion with no significant mass or increased density. ILC has a different pattern of metastatic presentations and tends to involve skeletal, visceral, serosal, and meningeal areas with ovary and uterus as the most common sites of metastasis.

A-39. (**e**) **Invasive lobular carcinoma, pleomorphic type**

The images represent the cytological findings of pleomorphic type of invasive lobular carcinoma. In contrast to classic lobular carcinoma, the aspirate is highly cellular and demonstrates a pleomorphic population of atypical cells arranged individually, in small aggregates, or thin linear cords, with an absence of myoepithelial cells. The presence of scant cytoplasm, vesicular nuclei with smooth/mildly irregular nuclear membranes, and prominent nucleoli are helpful features for the correct diagnosis of lobular carcinoma.

Pleomorphic lobular carcinoma can be misdiagnosed as ductal carcinoma because of the presence of cells with large, hyperchromatic nuclei and irregular nuclear membrane. A helpful cytological feature to aid in recognition of pleomorphic lobular carcinoma is the linear arrangement of the malignant cells and the presence of cytoplasmic vacuoles. Immunostaining for E-cadherin can help to differentiate between the two entities, with loss of expression typically seen in lobular carcinomas.

Variants of lobular carcinoma such as those tumors having a solid, alveolar, or mixed pattern may be misclassified as ductal carcinomas owing to the larger size of the cells and increased cellularity. However, smears usually show similar features of lobular carcinoma.

A-40. (**a**) **Signet ring carcinoma**

The images represent the cytological findings of the signet ring variant of lobular carcinoma. Aspirates are usually highly cellular and consist of cells arranged as single cells, linear cords, or small loose clusters. The cells are small with crescent-shaped nuclei compressed to the cell periphery by mucin. The cells are mucicarmine and PAS positive. Other features of lobular carcinoma can also be seen.

The differential diagnosis includes metastatic carcinoma of gastrointestinal tract. The clinical history and the review of the original pathology with IHC will help in this setting. Colloid/mucinous carcinoma is another differential diagnosis. In signet ring breast carcinomas, the mucin is intracytoplasmic, while colloid carcinoma presents with clusters of tumor cells in large mucin pools.

Signet ring carcinoma is a rare tumor representing 2–4 % of all breast carcinomas and associated with an unfavorable prognosis. It usually affects older patients, from the mid- to late 50s. Signet ring carcinomas tend to be more aggressive with a higher incidence of lymph node metastases and a more advanced stage at presentation than NOS type. It can metastasize to involve the stomach, female genital tract, and urinary tract.

A-41. (**a**) **Inflammatory carcinoma**

The images represent the cytological findings of inflammatory carcinoma. Because this lesion usually does not form a discrete palpable mass, it is not as amenable to diagnosis by FNA as other breast lesions. Aspiration of the dermis, subcutaneous tissue, or underlying breast tissue with multiple passes may be required to obtain diagnostic material. Some investigators have suggested a tangential approach technique with a 23-gauge needle in all 4 breast quadrants including antigravity areas to produce adequate sample for diagnosis. Aspirates are usually paucicellular, and malignant cells are predominantly distributed in three-dimensional clusters and as loose single malignant cells with increased N:C ratio, pleomorphic nuclei, and macronucleoli. The underlying infiltrating carcinoma has no specific features and is similar to high-grade ductal carcinoma, NOS type.

The differential diagnosis includes acute mastitis/abscess and lactational/pregnancy changes. In acute mastitis, there is an inflammatory background (neutrophils) and lack of single malignant cells. For lactational changes, it is especially important to appreciate the presence of cytoplasmic secretions characterized by cytoplasmic foaminess or vacuolization with fraying of cytoplasmic borders, in order to avoid a false-positive diagnosis. Also, ductal carcinomas show a greater degree of nuclear atypia, necrosis, hyperchromasia, loss of polarity, and discohesion with the presence of intact atypical single cells.

Inflammatory carcinoma is an uncommon, aggressive form of breast carcinoma accounting for approximately 2–4 % of cases. Clinically, the breast shows diffuse erythema, induration, warmth, edema, and tenderness, with peau d'orange skin changes and histopathologic findings of malignant cells within the lymphatics of the overlying skin and breast parenchyma.

A-42. (e) **Glycogen-rich ductal carcinoma**

The images represent the cytological findings of glycogen-rich ductal carcinoma. Smears are usually highly cellular and consist of discohesive malignant cells with sharp cytoplasmic borders. The majority of neoplastic cells show abundant clear cytoplasm and are PAS positive, confirming the glycogen-rich cytoplasm. The nuclei are hyperchromatic with prominent nucleoli.

Differential diagnosis includes other "clear cell tumors" such as clear cell hidradenoma, adenomyoepithelioma, and metastatic renal cell carcinomas. Ancillary studies including immunohistochemistry will help to make the definitive diagnosis.

Glycogen-rich carcinoma is a rare variant of invasive breast carcinoma, comprising 1–3 % of all breast carcinomas. It usually affects middle-aged women between 41 and 78, with a median age of 57 years. Glycogen-rich carcinoma is more aggressive than NOS type, with a higher incidence of lymph node metastases on presentation.

A-43. (e) **Secretory carcinoma**

The images represent the cytological findings of secretory carcinoma. Secretory carcinoma of the breast, a rare variant, is characterized by large amounts of intracellular and extracellular secretions and cells with abundant, granular, eosinophilic cytoplasm arranged in papillary, tubular, or solid structures. Shinagawa and colleagues believe that the grapelike cluster of vacuolated cells may be a helpful cytological feature for the diagnosis of secretory carcinoma. Cytological findings of breast cystic hypersecretory duct carcinoma include the presence of mildly atypical epithelial cells arranged singly and in small groups and sheets of cells set in a background of abundant, intensely staining, pink-to-purple thyroid-like colloid material that has a bubbly, fractured, or cracking artifact appearance in the smears.

The differential diagnosis includes lipid-rich carcinoma, characterized by the presence of abundant cytoplasmic fat in the majority of tumor cells. Smears consist of neoplastic cells with large, foamy, and vacuolated cytoplasm. Positive staining of fatty droplets with oil red O stain in lipid-rich carcinoma may be helpful in this differential.

A-44. (e) **Paget's disease of the nipple**

The images represent the cytological findings of Paget's disease. Cytological diagnosis can be made by scraping the nipple or by FNA biopsy. Tumor cells are arranged individually and in clusters. Differentiation from malignant melanoma can be enhanced with the use of an immunocytochemical panel, which demonstrates positive staining of malignant cells in Paget's disease for ER, carcinoembryonic antigen, epithelial membrane antigen (EMA), Her2/neu, and cytokeratin versus positive cytoplasmic staining for S-100 protein or HMB-45 in malignant melanoma.

Paget's disease presents with an eczema-like change of the nipple and areola, occasionally associated with an underlying breast mass, and is most commonly associated with DCIS in the same breast.

A-45. (b) **Medullary carcinoma**

The images represent the cytological findings of medullary carcinoma (MC). Aspirates are usually highly cellular and consist of large pleomorphic malignant cells arranged in three-dimensional clusters and syncytial groupings along with individually scattered malignant cells. Tumor cells have large nuclei with macronucleoli and increased N:C ratios. Tumor cells are characteristically admixed with lymphocytes and some plasma cells. The surrounding basophilic to finely granular or vacuolated cytoplasm is scant to abundant. Large-tripped tumor nuclei with macronucleoli, better appreciated on Diff-Quik preparations, may be seen. A background of lymphocytes in close proximity to cellular syncytia is seen. In any aspirate of a breast mass demonstrating lymphoid cells, a diligent search for malignant epithelial cells should be made to avoid a false-negative diagnosis.

The relatively young age of many patients, the presence of a well-circumscribed mass, and the prominent inflammatory cell component may lead to a false-negative diagnosis. However, the diagnosis can be highly suspected when three cytomorphological features are present: pleomorphic atypical cells, naked highly atypical nuclei, and an infiltrate composed of lymphocytes and plasma cells.

Based on cytological features, the differential diagnosis includes poorly differentiated ductal carcinoma with lymphocytic infiltrate, metastatic carcinoma in an intramammary lymph node, lymphoepithelioma-like carcinoma and malignant lymphoma. In ductal carcinoma, the aspirates consist predominantly of pleomorphic cells arranged in three-dimensional clusters rather than syncytial groups. The distinction is sometimes based on the finding of circumscription of the tumor, suggesting the subclassification of a malignant tumor as MC. However, differentiating MC from poorly differentiated ductal carcinoma may be impossible based on cytology examination alone. Metastatic carcinoma in intramammary lymph node is another difficult differential diagnosis because the neoplastic cells are admixed with lymphocytes. Lymphoepithelioma-like carcinoma is another rare entity that is difficult to differentiate from MC. Smears contained cohesive clusters and isolated tumor cells in a hemorrhagic background with scattered lymphocytes. The cells have large, pleomorphic nuclei and scanty ill-defined cytoplasm. Finally, high-grade lymphoma presents as a discohesive population of malignant lymphoid cells, devoid of neoplastic epithelial cells. The tumor cells of MC are larger and more variable than those of large cell lymphoma, with cell clustering. In ambiguous cases, immunocytochemistry for leukocyte common antigen (LCA), keratin, and epithelial membrane antigen (EMA) is helpful.

Medullary carcinoma accounts for 1–7 % of breast tumors and has a better 5- and 10-year survival than the common infiltrating duct carcinoma (NOS type). It is more common in young patients. Clinically and mammographically, medullary carcinoma presents as a well-demarcated lesion that can be mistaken for a fibroadenoma, a colloid carcinoma, or a papillary carcinoma.

A-46. (c) **Mucinous carcinoma**

The images represent the cytological findings of mucinous (colloid) carcinoma (CC). Aspirates show abundant mucin with a gelatinous appearance.

Smears show variable cellularity and consist of loosely cohesive, minimally pleomorphic three-dimensional epithelial fragments, surrounded by abundant extracellular mucinous material that stains metachromatically with the Diff-Quik® stain. Occasional single malignant cells with intact cytoplasm are seen. Tumor cells may demonstrate only a slight degree of atypia with intracytoplasmic mucin vacuoles. Pools of mucin are seen in the background. The relatively bland appearance of the tumor cells coupled with decreased cellularity secondary to the abundant extracellular mucinous material can potentially lead to a false-negative diagnosis.

Differentiating benign from malignant mucinous lesions can be difficult in FNA. The presence of pools of mucicarcmine-positive material in FNA smears of the breast is not an exclusive feature of CC and can be seen in benign lesions such as mucocele. However, mucocele, a benign mucin-filled cyst, usually lacks the presence of neoplastic cells that are typical CC. Smears usually are scanty with muciphages and small epithelial fragments, lacking atypia. Although an FA can also have a myxoid background, it is more cellular, and the cells are arranged in large groups or in antler-like configurations rather than balls. In addition, FAs may have many single stromal or bipolar cells or stripped nuclei and myxoid stromal fragments. Recent analysis of data from CAP interlaboratory comparison program shows that fibroadenoma is the most common false negative diagnosis for CC. Because a definite distinction between a pure and a mixed mucinous and typical ductal tumor is not possible, terminology such as "carcinoma with prominent mucinous features" rather than an outright diagnosis of "mucinous carcinoma" is preferred.

CC accounts for about 5 % of all breast carcinomas and has a better 5–10-year survival than infiltrating duct carcinoma, NOS type. It usually presents as a slow-growing mass, soft and well circumscribed on palpation. It rarely metastasizes and has less nodal involvement than the usual type of ductal carcinoma.

A-47. (d) **Metaplastic carcinoma**

The images represent the cytological findings of metaplastic carcinoma, carcinosarcoma variant. The cytological diagnosis of metaplastic carcinoma is usually challenging, and cytological features depend on the specific tumor subtype. Smears are usually highly cellular and consist of a biphasic population of spindle mesenchymal cells with fusiform nuclei and epithelial malignant cells. Multinucleated malignant cells are occasionally seen. The mixed population of malignant ductal cells, spindle cells, and multinucleated giant cells is helpful to suggest the correct diagnosis. The sarcomatoid component can be undifferentiated spindle cells or in some cases show chondrosarcomatous or osteosarcomatous differentiation.

Metaplastic carcinoma should be considered when there are high-grade malignant features with mesenchymal or combined epithelial and mesenchymal elements, and especially with two or more elements. The differential diagnosis includes benign mixed tumor, malignant phyllodes, sarcomas, fibromatosis, and nodular fasciitis. A primary breast sarcoma can be cytologically indistinguishable from a sarcomatoid metaplastic carcinoma. Immunocytochemistry can be helpful, because tumor cells are immunoreactive for cytokeratin and EMA in metaplastic carcinoma.

Metaplastic carcinomas are uncommon breast tumors accounting for less than 1 % of all invasive breast carcinomas. They are a heterogeneous group of carcinomas with monophasic (spindle cell only) or biphasic (carcinosarcoma) differentiation. They usually have an aggressive behavior with a poor prognosis.

A-48. (**d**) **Metaplastic carcinoma**

The images represent the cytological findings of metaplastic carcinoma, squamous cell carcinoma subtype. Smears are highly cellular and consist of sheets of well-differentiated or poorly differentiated malignant squamous cells. Malignant cells demonstrate keratinization and intercellular bridges. Some of the tumor cells may show a tendency to spindle. There is a background of keratinous debris and extensive necrosis.

Although squamous cell carcinoma is considered a subtype of metaplastic carcinoma, it has a better prognosis than carcinosarcoma subtype. The prognosis is similar to conventional infiltrating ductal carcinoma. The differential diagnosis of malignant squamous cells in a breast aspirate includes squamous cell carcinoma metastatic to the breast.

Pure primary squamous cell carcinomas of the breast are quite rare, although squamous cell carcinoma mixed with ductal carcinoma is more common. Approximately 10–15 % of pure squamous cell carcinomas have axillary node metastasis.

A-49. (**c**) **Osteoclastic-type giant cell carcinoma**

The images represent the cytological findings of osteoclastic-type giant cell carcinoma. Smears are usually highly cellular and demonstrate cytological features similar to those of NOS type, with the exception of osteoclast-like giant cells that are admixed with carcinoma cells. The differential diagnosis includes osteosarcoma and other tumors with multinucleated giant cells.

Osteoclastic giant cell carcinoma is a rare variant of high-grade carcinoma, characterized by the presence of osteoclastic giant cells in the stroma. The majority of these cases present at a late stage with positive lymph nodes.

A-50. (**e**) **Apocrine carcinoma**

The images represent the cytological findings of apocrine carcinoma. The smears are highly cellular and consist of numerous cells both individually scattered and arranged in syncytial clusters with apocrine morphology. Tumor cells show abundant basophilic to eosinophilic granular cytoplasm and large nuclei with prominent nucleoli. Cells are often binucleated with distinct and well-defined cytoplasmic borders. There is nuclear overlapping, pleomorphism, and high nuclear-to-cytoplasmic ratios with occasional mitoses.

The differential diagnosis includes atypical squamous metaplasia, apocrine metaplasia, and granular cell tumors. Atypical squamous metaplasia is usually seen in patients with a history of lumpectomy followed by seroma formation. Aspiration usually results in an abundant amount of fluid with scantly cellular smears. In addition, the atypical nuclei are only focally present, in contrast to diffuse atypia seen in apocrine carcinoma. The presence of pleomorphic large nuclei, eccentrically located within the dense granular eosinophilic cytoplasm (comet shaped), is also useful because these are seen in carcinoma, whereas nuclei are centrally located in apocrine metaplasia. Granular cell tumor is characterized by bland nuclei with the absence of atypia. IHC for S100 and cytokeratin may be helpful in differentiating these entities, with the former showing positive staining in granular cell tumor and the latter showing positive staining in apocrine carcinoma.

Apocrine carcinoma is composed predominantly of apocrine cells and constitutes about 4 % of breast cancers. It is clinically indistinguishable from invasive ductal carcinoma, NOS type with a similar prognosis. Apocrine carcinoma occurs more commonly in the older age group between ages 60 and 70 years.

A-51. (**b**) **Adenoid cystic carcinoma**

The images represent the cytological findings of adenoid cystic carcinoma. The cytological features are similar to the FNA findings of the more common salivary gland neoplasm. Morphologically, the tumor consists of nests of small uniform basaloid cells surrounding globules and/or cylinders of pale blue hyaline material that is mucicarmine positive. Isolated cells stripped of cytoplasm can also be present. Tumor cells are small and hyperchromatic with very little cytoplasm and inconspicuous nucleoli.

Similar globules are seen in collagenous spherulosis associated with benign ductal hyperplasia. Adenomyoepithelioma is another rare tumor composed of myoepithelial cells that must be distinguished from adenoid cystic carcinoma. The cells of adenomyoepithelioma are arranged in tightly cohesive clusters with scant stromal material but lack the typical hyaline globules of adenoid cystic carcinoma. Another differential diagnosis is cribriform carcinoma. IHC may be helpful since cribriform carcinoma is usually ER/PR positive while adenoid cystic carcinoma is negative.

Adenoid cystic carcinoma represents about 0.1 % of breast cancers and is morphologically and cytologically identical to those arising in the salivary glands and other sites. It presents as a slowly enlarging breast mass. The mammogram demonstrates a lobulated and well-defined mass. Patients with adenoid cystic carcinoma of the breast, unlike those of its salivary gland counterpart, have an excellent prognosis.

A-52. (c) **Micropapillary carcinoma**

The images represent the cytological findings of micropapillary carcinoma. Smears are usually moderately cellular with multiple tightly cohesive three-dimensional tumor clusters "cell balls" or "morules." Papillary structures of hyperchromatic cells with crowded nuclei and scalloped borders are seen. However, well-developed papillary fronds with fibrovascular cores are not identified. Tumor cells show moderate cytological atypia or enlarged hyperchromatic nuclei, prominent nucleoli, and high nuclear-to-cytoplasmic ratios. Single discohesive atypical tumor cells are seen. There is a background of blood with hemosiderin-laden macrophages. These cytological features are also seen in the cell block sections.

In FNA cytology, micropapillary carcinoma may mimic metastatic adenocarcinoma (especially serous carcinoma). In metastatic serous carcinoma, psammoma bodies are more commonly encountered. Immunohistochemistry staining may be helpful: Serous carcinoma is positive for WT-1 and Ca-125 but negative for GCDFP-15.

Invasive micropapillary carcinoma is characterized by the formation of micropapillae within clear spaces separated by a fibrocollagenous stroma. Most frequently they are seen admixed with invasive ductal carcinoma, NOS type. Patients usually present with a solid mass, without microcalcifications. Micropapillary carcinoma has been associated with vascular invasion and a high incidence of lymph node metastases (75 % of the patients).

A-53. (e) **Neuroendocrine carcinoma**

The images represent the cytological findings of primary neuroendocrine carcinoma. Smears are highly cellular and consist of a monotonous population of small round blue cells, arranged in a single cell discohesive pattern. There are nuclear molding, hyperchromasia, "salt-and-pepper" chromatin, and inconspicuous nucleoli. Karyorrhexis and mitoses with nuclear crush artifact are seen in cell clusters. The neuroendocrine nature of these tumors can be confirmed by using neuroendocrine markers.

Differential diagnosis includes metastatic carcinoid or small cell carcinoma from the lung. A history of heavy smoking and mediastinal mass favors a metastatic tumor. Immunohistochemical staining for ER, PR, and GCDFP-15 is not helpful, since primary breast neuroendocrine carcinomas are usually negative for these markers and positive for TTF-1.

Primary neuroendocrine carcinomas of the breast are a rare variant of breast carcinoma, constituting about 2–5 % of invasive breast carcinomas. Patients are usually older, in the 60–70-year-old age range. Most patients present with a palpable mass. On mammography, the tumor presents as a well-circumscribed nodule. The prognosis of these patients is grave.

A-54. (e) **Ductal carcinoma, low grade**

The images represent the cytological findings of low-grade ductal carcinoma. Tumor grading performed on cytological material may be especially useful in those patients receiving chemotherapy before resection of their tumors. A number of studies have shown that grading of breast carcinoma can be performed on FNA smears. Nuclear grade I is defined as nuclei similar to those of normal duct epithelium, having minimal enlargement; round, smooth nuclear membranes; uniform, fine chromatin; and no nucleoli. Nuclear grade II reveals nuclei that can be twice the size of nuclear grade I nuclei, with smooth nuclear membranes and uniform chromatin, and that may show small nucleoli. A moderate degree of anisonucleosis may be present. Nuclear grade III demonstrates marked anisonucleosis in which the nuclei often show a threefold variation in nuclear diameter. Other features of nuclear grade III are marked hyperchromasia, irregular nuclear contours, coarse chromatin, and macronucleoli.

A-55. (a) **Positive for hormonal receptors**

Numerous studies have demonstrated that hormone receptors can be evaluated on FNA specimens and cytology imprints with excellent correlation with the surgical pathology status. Both formalin-fixed and Papanicolaou-stained (Carnoy-fixed) slides yield similar results, provided that antigen retrieval was applied. The NCI-sponsored consensus conference determined that "evaluation of prognostic and predictive factors in fine needle aspiration specimens of primary breast cancer should be largely confined to patients who will undergo neoadjuvant chemotherapy before surgery, and then only if core-needle biopsy samples are not available." In metastatic breast carcinoma, assessment of ER and PR is clinically useful because metastatic deposits can be negative for receptors when the primary tumor was positive or vice versa.

Amplification of Her2/neu gene is one of the most important genetic alterations associated with human breast cancer. Studies show that Her2/neu oncogene amplification can be detected in both cytological and surgical specimens with equal results. Some investigators recommend FISH studies as the first-line analysis because cytology material can be limited and membranous staining of HER2/neu in FNA preparation is difficult to interpret. In our experience, CISH testing on cell blocks and cytology specimens shows excellent correlation with Her2 testing on surgical specimens. Therefore, FISH/CISH testing is believed to be more reliable than IHC analysis in cytology specimens.

A-56. **(d) Spindle cell lesion**

The images represent the cytological findings of spindle cell lesions. The aspirate shows abundant, randomly arranged single and clustered benign spindle-shaped mesenchymal cells with scant cytoplasm and elongated or oval nuclei displaying a finely granular chromatin pattern and inconspicuous nucleoli. Nuclear grooves and occasional intranuclear inclusions are seen. There is no significant cytological atypia or mitotic figures. The cells are positive for desmin, actin, and vimentin.

The most important differential diagnosis of spindle cell breast lesions is metaplastic carcinoma, low-grade (fibromatosis-like metaplastic) carcinoma, or DCIS with spindle cell feature. Careful cytological examination should prevent overdiagnosis of the benign cases. Myofibroblastoma of the breast, a benign spindle cell neoplasm composed of myofibroblasts, should also be in the differential diagnosis. It occurs primarily in elderly men and women, with a mean age of 65 years. Classic myofibroblastoma is a circumscribed, nonencapsulated, slowly growing solitary tumor comprised of bipolar fusiform cells arranged randomly, or in fascicles alternating with broad collagenous bands. Mammography reveals a well-circumscribed solid mass, usually without microcalcifications.

Inflammatory myofibroblastic tumor (IMT) of the breast is another entity in the differential diagnosis. It is a rare lesion which can simulate a primary breast carcinoma, clinically and mammographically. The aspiration is usually hypocellular and demonstrates a polymorphous population of cellular connective tissue fragments of myofibroblasts, spindle cells, lymphocytes, and histiocyte-like cells. Sheets of benign uniform ductal epithelial cells with myoepithelial cells are seen. A small number of IMT may express ALK protein as a result of a chromosomal translocation involving 2p23 gene. Nodular fasciitis and fibromatosis can also occur in breast and show similar cytological features to lesions arising from other sites.

Reactive spindle cell nodules, uncommon benign nonneoplastic lesions, usually arise following an FNA procedure. It most commonly presents as unencapsulated nodules and results from needle trauma which incites myofibroblastic proliferation. Most of the cases are seen in association with papillary and complex sclerosing breast lesions. Smears demonstrate spindle cells with mild pleomorphism with fine arborizing capillary vessels. A background of inflammatory cells and macrophages is seen.

A-57. **(d) Non-Hodgkin lymphoma**

The images represent the cytological findings of non-Hodgkin lymphoma, large cell type. Non-Hodgkin lymphoma can involve the breast either as a primary neoplasm or secondary to systemic disease that involves lymph nodes. The majority has a B-cell phenotype, and the most common subtypes are diffuse large B-cell lymphomas (DLBL), follicular center cell lymphomas, and lymphomas of mucosa-associated lymphoid tissue (MALT). The cytological features are identical to those of lymphomas that arise in lymph nodes. The use of flow cytometry can improve subclassification significantly. Rarely, plasmacytoma or myeloma can also involve the breast with typical findings.

A-58. **(d) Angiosarcoma**

The images represent the cytological features of angiosarcoma of the breast. The cytological features of pure breast sarcoma are similar to sarcomas encountered in soft tissue. Smears are highly variable, depending on tumor differentiation. Since the majority of these cases are high-grade angiosarcoma, the smears are usually moderately cellular, composed of plump spindle and oval cells with a moderate amount of cytoplasm as well as isolated cells of the same type, set in a hemorrhagic background. Eccentric, large, pleomorphic, oval nuclei containing finely granular chromatin and centrally located, prominent nucleoli are seen. Vasoformative arrangements with cells containing intracytoplasmic erythrocytes are best appreciated in the cell block preparation. In general, the presence of a few single pleomorphic cells with intracytoplasmic hemosiderin deposits in a hemorrhagic background should raise the diagnostic possibility of angiosarcoma. Immunopositivity for endothelial markers are positive for CD31, CD34, factor VIII, and D2-40. The IHCs performed on cell blocks can be helpful in characterizing endothelial differentiation.

The differential diagnosis includes atypical hemangioma, radiotherapy-related changes, and resolving hematoma. Malignant fibrous histiocytoma (MFH) may also occur at the sites of irradiation and hence may be mistaken for tumor recurrence. FNA biopsy of MFH of the breast is hypercellular and consists of cells with extreme pleomorphism including numerous atypical mononucleated, binucleated, and multinucleated histiocyte-like and fibroblastic cells. Frequent atypical mitotic figures are readily identified. Touton-like and osteoclast-like giant cells are occasionally seen. The background is composed of blood and necrotic debris with numerous lymphocytes, plasma cells, and foamy macrophages. Leiomyosarcoma is a rare, slowly growing tumor. Smears show variable cellularity and consist of dissociated cells with sheets of spindle and round cells. Cells are positive for desmin.

Primary breast angiosarcoma is the most common primary breast sarcoma. The majority of these cases follow radiation therapy and breast-conserving surgery or are related to lymphedema due to mastectomy, with a latency period of 4–7 years after therapy. The lesion usually develops as a rapidly growing mass causing diffuse enlargement of the breast and associated with blue–red discoloration of the skin.

A-59. (c) **Metastatic malignant melanoma**

The images represent the cytological findings of metastatic malignant melanoma. The smears are highly cellular and consist of a discohesive cell pattern. The cells can be plasmacytoid, spindle, or epithelial like. The cells may contain pigment and/or intranuclear inclusions. Binucleated cells are seen. Typically, large prominent "cherry-red" nucleoli may also be present. Malignant melanoma is known as one of the great mimickers. IHC for S100, Melan-A, and HMB-45 can be helpful in confirming the diagnosis.

Malignancies metastatic to the breast have a clinically observed rate of only 0.4–2 % of all breast malignancies. In rare cases, cancers metastatic to the breast can be the initial presentation of malignancy and therefore simulate a primary breast carcinoma. The most common metastatic cancers to involve the breast in women are, in decreasing frequency, melanoma, lymphoma, lung cancer, ovarian carcinoma, and soft tissue sarcomas, followed by gastrointestinal, genitourinary, and CNS tumors. If the site of the primary tumor is known, comparison of the cytology with available prior morphology is often helpful for distinguishing a primary from a metastatic neoplasm. IHC of ER, PR, and GCFDP-15 may be helpful since primary breast carcinomas are usually positive for these markers.

Metastatic tumors are usually well circumscribed and freely mobile in the deep breast tissue. They are rarely predominantly cystic masses. Clinically, radiologically, and cytologically, metastatic tumors may mimic primary breast carcinomas.

A-60. (e) **Metastatic small cell carcinoma**

The images represent the cytological findings of small cell carcinoma. The smears are highly cellular and show similar cytological features of small cell carcinoma of lung. The differential diagnosis includes metastatic small cell carcinoma from the lung. IHC of ER, PR, and GCFDP-15 are not helpful, since both primary and metastatic small cell carcinoma can be negative. A past history of smoking and the presence of a hilar mass favor metastatic small cell carcinoma from the lung.

Tumors metastatic to the breast are especially difficult to diagnose, especially when breast metastasis is the first manifestation of an occult extramammary malignancy. Breast metastasis is the initial presentation of extramammary occult malignant neoplasms in approximately 25 % of patients. The most common sites of occult carcinomas presenting with breast metastases include lung (particularly small cell carcinoma), followed by kidney, stomach, intestine (carcinoid), ovaries, uterine cervix, and thyroid gland. Moreover, even in patients with a history of malignancy presenting with a single breast mass, a second primary breast lesion is always considered more probable than a metastasis. The majority of cases of extramammary malignancy metastatic to the breast have a history of primary malignancy.

A-61. (d) **Metastatic prostatic adenocarcinoma**

The images represent the cytological findings of metastatic prostatic adenocarcinoma. The smears are usually hypercellular. Cytomorphologic features usually depend on the primary tumor, representing various cell types including pleomorphic and spindle-shaped cells with varying sizes and cellular arrangement. In men, the prostate is the most common primary site of metastasis to the breast. The presence of a past history of prostatic carcinoma and positivity of the tumor cells for PSA are helpful to confirm the diagnosis.

Distinguishing primary from metastatic carcinoma can be challenging, if not impossible. Metastatic tumors have variable mammographic features ranging from features similar to those seen in proliferative fibrocystic changes, fibroadenoma, or medullary carcinoma. Microcalcifications are usually seen in primary carcinoma, with a few exceptions such as psammoma bodies in metastatic tumors of ovary or thyroid. In the presence of a past history of cancer, a careful review of clinical history and comparison of the primary to the breast tumor may help to differentiate between these entities. In difficult cases, a panel of IHC stains and ancillary studies may be helpful in confirming the diagnosis.

A-62. (**b**) **Physiologic nipple discharge**

The images represent the cytological findings of physiologic nipple discharge. Physiologic nipple discharge is generally paucicellular to acellular, consisting almost exclusively of proteinaceous background material. Sometimes, a predominant population of foam cells having coarsely vacuolated cytoplasm together with occasional benign ductal cells can be seen. The origin of these foamy cells has been controversial. The ductal cells are usually arranged in tightly cohesive, uniform groups, and the cells show minimal to no variation in size. Although the cells may have high N:C ratios, hyperchromasia with coarse chromatin is not present. Occasionally, apocrine cells can be present. Inflammatory and infectious conditions can also result in a nipple discharge with the expected inflammatory cell exudate. Tuberculosis can be suspected when the cytological examination reveals epithelioid histiocytes and giant cells; however, the definitive diagnosis needs to be confirmed by the presence of acid-fast bacilli. Galactorrhea is characterized by numerous foam cells set in a prominent lipoproteinaceous smear background.

A-63. (**e**) **Intraductal papilloma**

The images represent the cytological findings of intraductal papilloma (IP) in nipple discharge. Smears usually demonstrate three-dimensional clusters of cells in which considerable variation in cell size is evident. Although nuclear atypicality may be present within the clusters, single atypical cells, a useful feature of malignancy, are not seen with any significant frequency. A malignant cytological diagnosis should not be rendered in a nipple discharge specimen unless many individually scattered atypical cells are present. In addition, it is also recommended that if a malignant diagnosis is made, histologic confirmation should be obtained before definitive treatment. Evaluation for occult blood, mucin staining, carcinoembryonic antigen (CEA), and other biomarkers have been attempted to increase the sensitivity of nipple discharge sampling to detect nonpalpable breast cancer.

Benign ductal cells are arranged in tight clusters that are small and spherical or large and branching; isolated ductal cells are uncommon. Usually, the cells are small and have scant cytoplasm, but occasionally they are larger and have abundant cytoplasm.

A-64. (**a**) **Ductal carcinoma**

The images represent the cytological findings of ductal carcinoma in nipple discharge. The smears are hypocellular and show isolated malignant cells with intact cytoplasm, increased nuclear-to-cytoplasmic ratio, and occasional prominent nucleoli. Although nuclear atypia may be present within the clusters of intraductal papilloma, single atypical cells, a useful feature of malignancy, are not seen with any significant frequency. A malignant cytological diagnosis should not be rendered in a nipple discharge specimen unless many individually scattered atypical cells are present. In addition, it is also recommended that if a malignant diagnosis is made, histologic confirmation should be obtained before definitive treatment. Evaluation for occult blood, mucin staining, carcinoembryonic antigen (CEA), and other biomarkers have been attempted to increase the sensitivity of nipple discharge to detect breast cancer.

A-65. (**c**) **Ductal epithelium with marked cytological atypia**

The images represent the cytological findings of ductal epithelium with severe atypia in ductal lavage smears.

Ductal lavage is a relatively new and invasive method of sampling the ductal epithelium. It involves infusing 10–20 mL of saline into the duct through an inserted microcatheter. The saline "rinse," combined with breast compression, enables collection of breast ductal epithelial cells. The collection is deposited into preservative and commonly prepared as a ThinPrep slide.

The interpretation of ductal lavage fluid specimens is based on the morphology of ductal cells. The diagnosis is classified into one of the following categories: insufficient cellular material for diagnosis (fewer than 10 epithelial cells), benign epithelial cells, mild ductal cell atypia, marked ductal cell atypia, and malignant.

Ljung et al. evaluated 431 ductal lavage specimens for cell features including cell arrangements, cell size and variation, nuclear features, nucleoli, and background findings. Benign cases showed few or large epithelial clusters of ductal cells arranged in one layer and associated with myoepithelial cells in a slightly different plane of focus.

In mild cytological atypia, the ductal cells are moderately large, arranged in a monolayer and in small clusters. Nuclear membranes are regular and chromatin remains finely granular with small nucleoli. Mild atypia may represent histologic lesions of hyperplasia, ADH, or low-grade DCIS.

In marked cytological atypia, the ductal cells are arranged in large two-dimensional clusters. The cells demonstrate anisonucleosis with irregular nuclear membranes, coarse granular chromatin, and variable nucleoli. Increased N:C ratios with multinucleation and occasional mitotic figures are seen. These cells may be associated with ADH or low- to intermediate-grade DCIS.

Malignant cells demonstrate markedly large cells with high N:C ratios. Single cells are also found, along with two-dimensional cell clusters. Irregular arrangements and nuclear overlapping are present. Conspicuous anisonucleosis is present, with marked nuclear membrane irregularity and clumped, uneven chromatin granularity. Multinucleation and necrotic debris are noted. Ductal lavage lends itself not only to cytological evaluation but also to molecular studies.

Cellular atypia has been found to be predictive of an increased risk of developing breast carcinoma. Women who have atypical intraductal cellular proliferations have approximately a twofold greater risk of developing invasive breast cancer, independent of other risk factors, such as family history. When combined with other factors, they have a 12-fold greater risk than the general population. However, ductal lavage is not sensitive for breast cancer detection and should not be used as a substitute for screening or other diagnostic procedures and follow-up, including periodic physical examination and mammography.

Reading List

Amrikachi M, Green LK, Rone R, Ramzy I. Gynecomastia: cytologic features and diagnostic pitfalls in fine needle aspirates. Acta Cytol. 2001;45:948–52.

Bibbo M, Wilbur DC. Breast. In: Bibbo M, Wilbur DC, editors. Comprehensive cytopathology. 3rd ed. Philadelphia: Saunders/Elsevier; 2009.

ElAouni N, Athanasiou A, Mansouri D, et al. Medullary breast carcinoma: a case report with cytological features and histological confirmation. Diagn Cytopathol. 2006;34:701–3.

Fasih T, Jain M, Shrimankar J, et al. All radial scars/complex sclerosing lesions seen on breast screening mammograms should be excised. Eur J Surg Oncol. 2005;31:1125–8.

Frost AR, Terahata S, Yeh IT, et al. The significance of signet ring cells in infiltrating lobular carcinoma of the breast. Arch Pathol Lab Med. 1995;119:64–8.

Gupta RK, McHutchison AGR, Dowle GS, et al. Fine-needle aspiration cytodiagnosis of breast masses in pregnant and lactating women and its impact on management. Diagn Cytopathol. 1993;9:156–9.

Koss LG, Melamed MR. The breast. In: Koss LG, Melamed MR, editors. Koss' diagnostic cytology and its histopathologic bases. Philadelphia: Lippincott Williams & Wilkins; 2005.

Krishnamurthy S, Ashfaq R, Shin HJ, Sneige N. Distinction of phyllodes tumor from fibroadenoma: a reappraisal of an old problem. Cancer (Cancer Cytopathol). 2000;90:342–9.

Lynch LA, Moriarty AT. Localized primary amyloid tumor associated with osseous metaplasia presenting as bilateral breast masses: cytologic and radiologic features. Diagn Cytopathol. 1993;9:570–5.

McCluggage WG, McManus DI, Caughley LM. Fine needle aspiration (FNA) cytology of adenoid cystic carcinoma and adenomyoepithelioma of breast: two lesions rich in myoepithelial cells. Cytopathology. 1997;8:31–9.

Mooney EE, Kayani N, Tavassoli FA. Spherulosis of the breast. A spectrum of mucinous and collagenous lesions. Arch Pathol Lab Med. 1999;123:626–30.

Nogueira M, Andre S, Mendonca E. Metaplastic carcinomas of the breast: fine needle aspiration (FNA) cytology findings. Cytopathology. 1998;9:291–300.

Pieterse AS, Mahar A, Orell S. Granular cell tumor: a pitfall in FNA cytology of breast lesions. Pathology. 2004;36:58–62.

Saad RS, Silverman JF, Julian T, et al. Atypical squamous metaplasia of seromas in breast needle aspirates from irradiated lumpectomy sites: a potential pitfall for false positive diagnosis of carcinoma. Diagn Cytopathol. 2002;26:104–8.

Saad RS, Kanbour-Shakir A, Syed A, Kanbour A. Sclerosing papillary lesion of the breast: a diagnostic pitfall for malignancy in fine needle aspiration biopsy. Diagn Cytopathol. 2006;34:114–8.

Saad RS, Richmond L, Nofech-Mozes S, Ghorab Z. Fine needle aspiration biopsy of adenomyoepithelioma: a potential false positive pitfall and presence of intranuclear cytoplasmic inclusions. Diagn Cytopathol. 2012;40(11):1005–9. doi:10.1002/dc.21705. Epub 2011 May 4.

Shabb NS, Tawil A, Mufarri A, et al. Mammary carcinoma with osteoclast like giant cells cytologically mimicking benign breast disease: a case report. Acta Cytol. 1997;41:1284–8.

Silverman JF. Diagnostic accuracy, cost-effectiveness, and triage role of fine-needle aspiration biopsy in the diagnosis of palpable breast lesions. Breast J. 1995;1:3–8.

Silverman JF, Lannin DR, Unverferth M, Norris HT. Fine needle aspiration cytology of subareolar abscess of the breast: spectrum of cytomorphologic findings and potential diagnostic pitfalls. Acta Cytol. 1986;30:413–9.

Simsir A, Tsang P, Greenebaum E. Additional mimics of mucinous mammary carcinoma: fibroepithelial lesions. Am J Clin Pathol. 1998;109:169–72.

Sneige N, Staerkel GA. Fine-needle aspiration cytology of ductal hyperplasia with and without atypia and ductal carcinoma in situ. Hum Pathol. 1994;25:485–92.

Index

W.E. Khalbuss, M. Means (eds.), *Gynecological and Breast Cytopathology Board Review and Self-Assessment*, DOI 10.1007/978-1-4614-7270-4, © Springer Science+Business Media New York 2013

GPSR Compliance
The European Union's (EU) General Product Safety Regulation (GPSR) is a set of rules that requires consumer products to be safe and our obligations to ensure this.

If you have any concerns about our products, you can contact us on

ProductSafety@springernature.com

In case Publisher is established outside the EU, the EU authorized representative is:

Springer Nature Customer Service Center GmbH
Europaplatz 3
69115 Heidelberg, Germany

www.ingramcontent.com/pod-product-compliance
Lightning Source LLC
Chambersburg PA
CBHW081826250825
31638CB00027B/1047

9781461472698